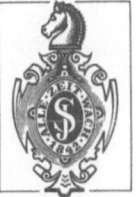

H.G. Beger M. Büchler
H. Ditschuneit P. Malfertheiner (Eds.)

Chronic Pancreatitis

Research and Clinical Management

With 246 Figures and 131 Tables

Springer-Verlag
Berlin Heidelberg New York
London Paris Tokyo Hong Kong

BEGER, H. G., M. D., Prof., FACS
BÜCHLER, M., M. D., Priv.-Doz.

Department of Surgery
University of Ulm
Steinhövelstrasse 9
D-7900 Ulm, W.-Germany

DITSCHUNEIT, H., M. D., Prof.
MALFERTHEINER, P., M. D., Priv.-Doz.

Department of Internal Medicine II
University of Ulm
Robert-Koch-Strasse 8
D-7900 Ulm, W.-Germany

ISBN-13: 978-3-642-75321-3   e-ISBN-13: 978-3-642-75319-0
DOI: 10.1007/978-3-642-75319-0

2119/3140/543210 – Printed on acid-free paper

Preface

There has been a continual increase in the incidence of pancreatic diseases in the Western industrialized countries. As a result, during the last 25 years a major effort has been made to achieve advances in research and clinical management of these diseases, concentrating on an analysis of the causes of inflammatory and neoplastic diseases and the implications for therapy.

The pathogenesis of chronic pancreatitis is unclear, although some most interesting but controversial concepts have been developed. Today we are, however, well aware of the clinical picture of chronic pancreatitis, including various complications that have been thoroughly described. Diagnostic measurements have been standardized, and in particular the developments in imaging procedures have contributed much to our understanding of chronic pancreatitis.

The therapeutic management of patients with chronic pancreatitis is a matter of debate, especially regarding the nature and duration of treatment. There seems to be no doubt about the fact that complications of chronic pancreatitis should preferably be treated by surgical measures, whereas an uncomplicated course of chronic pancreatitis is best managed by conservative protocols. Still we do not know if there is any chance to interrupt the natural course of the disease, which leads to irreversible functional damage.

This volume deals with all the aspects of chronic pancreatitis, including its etiology, morphology, pathophysiology, and conservative and operative treatment. It focuses on very recent data obtained from experimental and clinical research projects.

Special attention is paid to the topical subjects of feedback regulation, new aspects of conservative treatment in chronic pancreatitis, and the state of the art in interventional treatment protocols. Finally the role of surgery in chronic pancreatitis is elaborated, with special interest on organ-preserving procedures.

We have been most fortunate in having recruited a team of internationally recognized contributors, each of whom is an authority in his field. We hope that this volume will be of value to everyone interested in the fundamentals and clinical management of chronic pancreatitis.

There is no doubt that various items presented in this book are still a matter of controversy. We hope that this will stimulate further investigations and attempts to achieve a more concise understanding of chronic pancreatitis by the end of this century.

Ulm, May 1990   H. G. BEGER · M. BÜCHLER · H. DITSCHUNEIT · P. MALFERTHEINER

Contents

Pathophysiology

Feedback Regulation of Exocrine Function

Clinical Features

Complications

Interventional Treatment

Surgical Treatment: Indication

Surgical Treatment: Denervation and Drainage

Surgical Treatment: Resectional Procedures

Surgical Treatment: New Horizons

List of Contributors

Lüthen, R.   185
Lygidakis, N.   554

Maier, W.   309
Malfertheiner, P.   41, 77, 153, 221, 229, 358
Marks, I.N.   26, 218, 256
Meggiato, T.   283
Mössner, J.   198
Müller, S.   83

Naccarato, R.   283
Nauck, M.   235
Nelson, D.K.   229
Neoptolemos, J.   269
Niederau, C.   185
Niederau, M.   185

Otte, M.   350
Owyang, Ch.   171

Pap, A.   122
Permeth, J.   354
Pieramico, O.   221, 229
Pitchumoni, C.S.   15
Pour, P.M.   106
Prinz, R.A.   426

Reber, H.A.   253
Reinshagen, M.   178
Roscher, R.   439
Rossi, R.L.   551
Rösch, Th.   319
Rumpf, K.D.   454
Russel, R.C.G.   539

Sarner, M.   3
Sarr, M.   383
Scherbaum, W.   153
Schwall, G.   400
Schweiberer, L.   532
Senn, T.   41
Singer, M.V.   35, 115
Singh, M.   140
Steer, M.L.   245
Stöckmann, F.   235
Suzuki, M.   490

Toskes, Ph.   302
Traverso, L.W.   505
Trede, M.   400

van der Burg, M.P.M.   517
van der Heyde, M.N.   554
Vitas, G.J.   383

Warshaw, A.L.   395
Weihe, E.   83
Wilker, D.   532
Winslet, M.C.   269
Wolff, H.   496
Worning, H.   8
Wresky, H.P.   198

Yanaihara, N.   83

Zentel, H.J.   83
Zirngibl, H.   481

Definition · Epidemiology · Etiology

Update in the Classification of Chronic Pancreatitis

M. Sarner[1]

Classification of any disease has two functions. The first is to answer the three questions "What is wrong?" "What is going to happen?" and "What can be done?" The second is to provide a lingua franca among those caring for the patients. No classification system is perfect, and any one simply reflects the state of the art at the time that it is promulgated.

It is non-controversial that the term chronic pancreatitis means an irreversibly damaged gland. This carries the implication that the damage, be it morphological or functional, is either static or getting worse, and that repair back to normality does not occur. However, this may not be true since the extent of disease as documented at the time of study may reflect merely the balance between repair and regeneration, on the one hand, and destruction and fibrosis, on the other. In other words, pancreatic inflammation may be a continuing or dynamic process. In addition, the concept of a scarred, but normally functioning gland must be borne in mind, just as a post-myocardial infarction heart may function entirely normally.

What advances have occurred in our understanding of chronic pancreatitis since the reviews of 1984 and 1986 [1–3], and how do these advances shed light on any classification system? In this chapter five areas are identified in which possibly useful change has occurred that may help us to define our understanding in the categorisation of the disease; with increasing sophistication of investigation, better grading of severity of the disease is also available.

Natural History

Studies of Ammann et al. [4] in following the natural history of their patients, many of whom suffered from alcohol-induced disease, have been most valuable. This is the bonus of long-term follow-up of a defined group of patients by one physician. In studying the natural history of nearly 300 patients, of whom two-thirds had alcohol induced disease, more than 60% became painfree if followed long enough, and this was irrespective of cause. It has also become apparent that as many as one-third of the alcohol-induced cases have non-progressive disease, with preservation of endocrine function. Finding the reason why this occurs and the early identification of these patients are important.

Is an alcohol-induced aetiology a reliable guide to progress of the disease? The longer the period of observation, the more pain seems to be relieved [5, 6]. In a more

[1] Dept. Gastroenterology, University College Hospital, London W.C.I., UK

Chronic Pancreatitis
Ed. by Beger, Büchler, Ditschuneit, and Malfertheiner
© Springer-Verlag Berlin Heidelberg 1990

recent paper [7] 107 patients with chronic calcified pancreatitis, in 84 of whom alcohol induced, all showed decreasing calcification as the disease wore on. Stone dissolution was related to the duration of the disease but was also facilitated by drainage procedures. Unfortunately, factors such as secretory pressures or ductal stasis are not documented, but it is certain that calcification may regress and does so as part of the progression of the disease in its late phase.

These studies of the natural history of the disease also reveal that the non-alcoholic patient can be clinically differentiated. In these patients the disease seems to progress more slowly, it is more likely to be painless, and malabsorption and diabetes are less marked. The need for surgery is less, and so it seems that the disease which is not due to alcohol is less severe than its alcohol-induced counterpart.

From these data I believe that it is crucial to include the term "alcohol induced" in any statement of diagnosis. This aetiology carries important prognostic implications in respect of pain, preservation of function and calcification. If the alcohol is given up, the disease may slow, but death from other alcohol-related disease is much more common in this group of patients. Of 210 cases followed by Levy et al. [8], 57 died, the bulk of deaths being due to alcohol-related disease that was not pancreatic. Thus it is crucial to separate alcohol as a cause; alcohol-induced chronic pancreatitis is a discrete entity.

Imaging

Two imaging modalities – endoscopic retrograde pancreatography (ERP) and ultrasound, – have had a major impact in refining our approach to chronic pancreatitis. Perhaps ERP is beginning to lose its value as a diagnostic tool, whilst the non-invasive ultrasound procedure is becoming increasingly sophisticated and accurate. At present, using high-resolution linear array scanners in experienced hands, it is possible to acquire all or more information than is available from ERP, since the ultrasonic study gives some idea as to the state of the acinar cells and also allows access for percutaneous biopsy, pressure measurements and, via an endoscope, endoscopic ultrasound.

Correlation studies between ultrasonic appearances and histopathology are not well worked out, and at present both parameters are needed for accurate diagnosis.

Ductal obstruction, which is an important guide for the surgeon, remains crucial, and the very best grading of severity still rests in the area of imaging, given the current levels of sensitivity of function testing. The grading system proposed 5 years ago by Axon [9] (normal, equivocal, mild, moderate and marked), has been modified in practice by Jones et al. [10] who in their review of 58 patients produced excellent correlation between ERP and ultrasound findings. Large cavities (larger than 1 cm) or calculi are indicative of chronic pancreatitis, and since intraduct filling defects may be transient, they can now be removed from classification. Jones et al. dropped the phrase "as above with one or more of" and simply require two or more abnormal features to establish a diagnosis. Ultrasound can provide us with a non-invasive technique correlating well with ERP, which grades pancreatitis accurately by adding the terms "mild, moderate or marked" to the classification.

At present, of the various systems advocated for classifying ERP findings, that promulgated at Cambridge seems most widely accepted. In respect of the correlation between imaging and function, this has been reviewed in detail, and a high correlation occurs in the later but not in the earlier stages of the disease [11], as one would expect for a gland that may carry severe morphological change without necessarily showing important impairment of function. The status of the "evocative" test for ductal obstruction remains uncertain, and we are now obtaining information from the ultrasound examination in respect of changes found in old age. The correlation between morphology and function is high only in the late stages of the disease, and in early or moderate change ERP and intubation tests remain the best combination. At present the conclusion must be that grading may carry an implication for function, but high correlation is not present at the moment unless the disease is very far advanced.

Histopathology

Major advances are now heralded by the use of the ultrasound-guided bioptic gun, and the situation is comparable to that found in liver disease a generation ago, although today's histopathologists have the sophistication of immunohistochemistry, electron microscopy, etc. Histology has provided us with information in respect of pancreatic "ageing" – an involutionary change due to vascular or metabolic alterations; in addition we now may be able to acquire information in respect of the pathogenesis of pain, which is possibly related to changes in the nerves seen in the gland [12]. Histological staining for most pain mediators has not been available, but the presence of giant nerves and increase in nerve tissue found in the chronically inflamed gland must have something to do with pain, and this should be correlated. Mean nerve diameter is increased by one-third and the area served by any individual nerves increased by two-thirds. These estimations are not quantitated, and how or why the gland eventually becomes painless is not understood, but bioptic techniques are likely to be helpful here. Using immunohistochemistry, the presence of sensory mediators such as calcitonin gene-related protein have been shown but, again, have not been quantitated.

These sampling and staining techniques may enable us to derive a histopathological basis for our classification and certainly help to explain pain.

The use of the bioptic needle is of value in determining the distribution of lesions, and it has been shown that severe chronic pancreatitis may be found in one part of the gland, which is normal elsewhere. Thus an anatomical classification may also be possible, for example, chronic dorsal pancreatitis.

One variety of pancreatitis that may be differentiated because of histopathology is chronic obstructed pancreatitis (obstructive pancreatopathy) with its characteristic histological pattern of diffuse fibrosis surrounding the lobule – a peri-lobular scarring.

This entity is associated with duct dilatation but shows little inflammatory infiltrate in the parenchyma; protein plugs and calculi are not common. Function may be related to flow rate, and the relief of the obstruction may cure the disease (but is this chronic pancreatitis?).

Pancreatic Duct Pressure – Hypertensive/Obstructive Pancreatopathy

A further group of patients with chronic pancreatitis may be differentiated [13]: those with pancreatic duct obstruction in the region of the sphincter of Oddi. The mechanism by which ductal hypertension actually causes pancreatitis is unknown, but its relief will cure. Ductal obstruction may be congenital or acquired; if there is failure of fusion of the dorsal and ventral outpouchings, disease may develop. For example, if the dorsal anlage fails to develop, the pancreatic body, tail, minor papilla and Santorini duct will all fail to drain adequately, and this may be partial or total. Stenosis of the main pancreatic duct may be congenital and may be associated with concretions in the juice which are non-opaque. How ductal hypertension is associated with this change is not understood [14]. As stated, histology is typical, and there is very rarely damage to the ductular epithelium.

Acquired causes may include small ampullary tumours such as carcinoids, islet cell tumours, ectopic pancreatic tissue at the ampulla, or cancer [15, 16]. In respect of pressures the main pancreatic duct pressure may be higher in patients with chronic pancreatitis, but this needs to be correlated with the other parameters for identifying the disease, and this is as yet not a classifier. Pancreatic juice viscosity may also be increased, but this is not yet capable of being accurately and repeatably measured. There are a small number of cases in which gall stones are associated with chronic pancreatitis; here the linking factor seems to be recurrent odditis caused by a stenosis of the sphincter of Oddi consequent on the passage of small stones. Basal pressure is raised above 40 mmHg, and it is important to measure pressures if possible [17]. It is now possible to measure pancreatic duct pressures via the minor papilla, and, again, raised pressures have been demonstrated in the dorsal duct. Thus manometry of the sphincter of Oddi is useful, and the concept of ductal hypertension (which may also be graded) can be very helpful for the surgeon.

The Stone Protein

The status of the stone (fibrillary or thread) protein remains uncertain. Its absence may be congenital and therefore the cause of chronic calcific pancreatitis (CCP) in the hereditary cases. Molecular pathology of CCP is being established at this stage, and if the stone protein is confirmed, diminution in cases of CCP may be primary or secondary. At present, the presence, diminution or absence of stone protein has not reached a level of confidence to influence a classification system.

Many questions remain to be answered in respect of a classification system which will help in management. These include the relationships between pain and function, which patients will become pain-free, and when and which patients will require surgery for a disease which is not really surgical. We have yet to understand the dynamics of chronic pancreatitis and the place of cholecystokinin as a injection therapy to stimulate regeneration. The comings and goings of calcification in CCP are observed but not understood, and the question as to whether non-calcific chronic pancreatitis is in fact post-calcific must be raised. We have yet to achieve a histological grading similar to that found in chronic inflammatory liver disease, and we want confidence in our interpretation of change in respect of its reversibility or otherwise.

The impact of magnetic resonance imaging has yet to be felt, and the role of bacteria in the pathogenesis of stone is not yet assessed. In respect of alcohol the genetic predisposition is very difficult to know.

At present I propose the following classification system. Chronic pancreatitis should be defined as a permanent morphological or functional change of the gland, and whenever this diagnosis is made, a statement should be added as to aetiology (e. g. alcohol, obstructive or other), and whether pain is present or absent. The degree of severity (mild, moderate or severe) should be stated, and complications such as cysts, portal hypertension, diabetes mellitus should be noted.

For the future we require agreed criteria for mild, moderate and marked disease. Only in this way will we be able to compare series from around the world.

References

1. Gyr KE, Singer MV, Sarles H (1984) Pancreatitis concepts and classification. Excerpta Medica, Amsterdam
2. Sarner M, Cotton PB (1984) Classification of pancreatitis. Gut 25:756–759
3. Sarles H (1986) Aetiopathogenesis and definition of chronic pancreatitis. Dig Dis Sci 31:91S–107S
4. Ammann RW, Buehler H, Meunch R, Freiburghaus AU, Siegenthaler W (1987) Differences in the natural history of idiopathic (non-alcoholic) and alcoholic chronic pancreatitis. Pancreas 2:368–377
5. Hayakawa T, Takaharu K, Tokimune S, Yoshiyuki S, Motoji K (1989) Chronic alcoholism and evolution of pain and prognosis in chronic pancreatitis. Dig Dis Sci 34:33–38
6. Gullo L, Barbara L, Labo G (1988) Effect of cessation of alcohol use on the cause of pancreatic dysfunction in alcohol in pancreatitis. Gastroenterology 95:1063–1068
7. Ammann RW, Meunch R, Otto R, Buehler H, Freiburg Haus AU, Siegenthaler W (1988) Evolution and regression of pancreatitic calcification in chronic pancreatitis. Gastroenterology 95:1018–1028
8. Levy T, Chantal M, Pignon JP, Baitz A, Bernadez P (1989) Mortality factors associated with chronic pancreatitis. Gastroenterology 96:1165–1172
9. Axon ATR (1989) Endoscopic retrograde cholangiopancreatography in chronic pancreatitis. Radiol Clin North Am 27:39–49
10. Jones SN, Lees WR, Frost RA (1988) Diagnosis and grading of chronic pancreatitis by morphological criteria derived by ultrasound and pancreatography. Clin Radiol 39:43–48
11. Malfertheimer P, Buchler M (1989) Correlation of imaging and function in chronic pancreatitis. Radiol Clin North Am 27:51–64
12. Bockman DE, Buchler M, Malfertheimer P, Beger HG (1988) Analysis of nerves in chronic pancreatitis. Gastroenterology 94:1459–1469
13. Venu RP, Geenen JE, Hogan W, Stone J, Johnson GK, Soergel K (1989) Idiopathic recurrent pancreatitis. Dig Dis Sci 34:56–60
14. Staritz M, Meyer zum Buschenfelde KH (1988) Elevated pressure in the dorsal part of pancreas divisum: the cause of chronic pancreatitis? Pancreas 3:108–110
15. Sarles H, Cambon P, Choux R, Payan MJ, Odaira S, Laugier R, Sahal J (1988) Chronic obstructive pancreatitis due to tiny benign tumours obstructing the pancreatic ducts: report of 3 cases. Pancreas 3:232–237
16. Lowes JR, Rode J, Lees WR, Russell RCG, Cotton PB (1988) Obstructive pancreatitis unusual causes of chronic pancreatitis. Br J Surg 75:1129–1133
17. Okazaki K, Yamamoto Y, Kagiyama S, Tamura S, Salamoto Y, Nakazawa Y, Morita M, Yamamoto Y (1988) Pressure of papillary sphincter zone and pancreatic main duct in patients with chronic pancreatitis in the early stage. Scand J Gastroenterol 23:501–507

Incidence and Prevalence of Chronic Pancreatitis

H. Worning[1]

Introduction

Chronic pancreatitis has been known as a pathoanatomical abnormality for many years. The prevalence in autopsy materials has differed between 0.04% [1] and 5% [2]. The clinical picture was only sporadically mentioned in the medical literature up to 1946, when Comfort et al. [3] presented the first detailed clinical material of chronic pancreatitis, comprising 29 cases. Since that time, studies on etiology, clinical picture, medical and surgical treatment, prognosis, and complications of chronic pancreatitis have resulted in a huge number of publications. However, epidemiological studies, especially studies of the frequency (incidence and prevalence) of the disease, are very few. Only one prospective study concerning incidence and prevalence of chronic pancreatitis exists, collected in the city of Copenhagen in 1978–1979 and presented in 1981 [4]. On the other hand, epidemiological data are available either from retrospective studies [5–7] or by calculation from data given in clinical material [8–10; Ammann, personal communication].

Incidence

The figures from the prospective study in Copenhagen [4] are given in Table 1. The incidence was equivalent to 8.2 new cases/100000 inhabitants per year. The prevalence was found to be 27.4 cases/100000 inhabitants. Combination of these two figures indicates an expected mean life time for patients with chronic pancreatitis of around 3.3 years. However, even the disease seems to shorten life expectancy, the published data for mean survival time being much longer (vide infra). The conclusion must be that, if the figure for incidence is correct, the figure for prevalence must be higher than given in Table 1 or vice versa. However, the incidence rate was very near to figures

Table 1. Incidence and prevalence of chronic pancreatitis (CP) in Copenhagen City 1978–1979 [4]

	Incidence $100000^{-1}year^{-1}$	Prevalence 100000^{-1}
Possible CP	4.2	14.4
Verified CP	4.0	13.0
Total CP	8.2	27.4

---

[1] University of Copenhagen, Medical Department F, Glostrup Hospital, 2600 Glostrup, Denmark

---

Chronic Pancreatitis
Ed. by Beger, Büchler, Ditschuneit, and Malfertheiner
© Springer-Verlag Berlin Heidelberg 1990

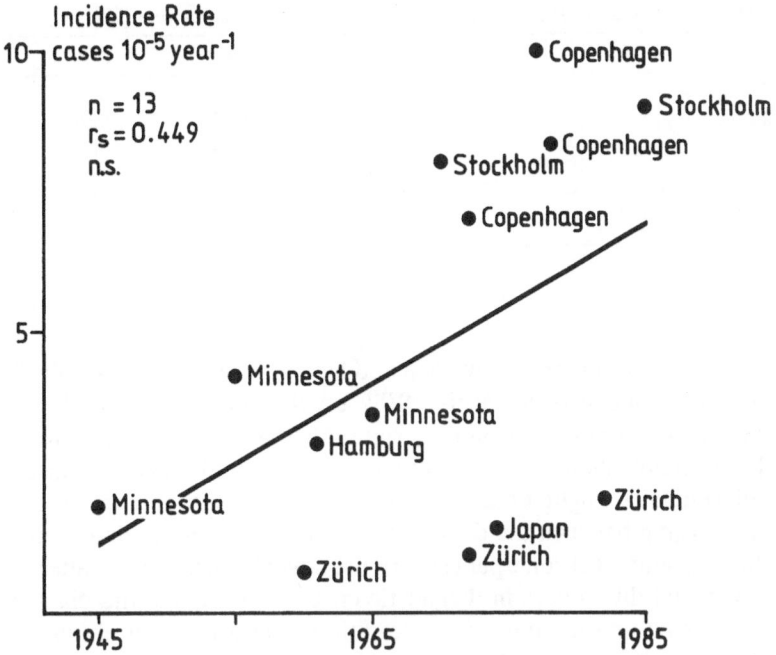

Fig. 1. Incidence rate of chronic pancreatitis through the years 1945–1985. [4, 5–7, 8–10; Ammann, personal communication]

observed in Copenhagen County collected in the same period (Fig. 1). It is worth mentioning that the proportion between incidence and prevalence is the same in the two groups: possible pancreatitis (3.3) and verified pancreatitis (3.4) in Table 1. This phenomenon indicates the population to be homogeneous in composition and, if so, the technique used for the estimation of the prevalence was insufficient. Not all cases of chronic pancreatitis were registered.

Incidence data collected in the literature from the period 1946–1985 are shown in Fig. 1. The slope of the regression curve is not significantly different from zero. An overall increase in incidence rate during the period studied is consequently not substantiated. However, in four areas, where repeated data have been published (Minnesota, Zürich, Stockholm, and Copenhagen), the incidence rate within all these four areas increased during the time of investigation (Fig. 1). Figure 1 demonstrates clearly the enormous differences in incidence rate between different areas collected in nearly the same period (Zürich 1983: 2.0%, Copenhagen 1976: 10%).

Alcohol consumption has known to be an essential factor for the development of chronic pancreatitis. Around 70% of cases are characterized as alcohol-induced disease [11]. The registered alcohol consumption in a number of countries in the period 1950–1976 is shown in Table 2. Japan has traditionally a very low alcohol intake fitting with the low incidence rate of chronic pancreatitis (Fig. 1). However, for the years studied Switzerland has a substantially higher alcohol consumption than observed in Denmark and Sweden (Table 2). Even so, the disease is rather rare in

Table 2. Alcohol consumption, liters 100% ethanol/capita per year [12]

	1950	1960	1970	1976
Denmark	3.6	4.2	6.8	9.2
France	17.2	17.3	15.6	16.5
Japan	0.2	2.4	4.7	5.1
Sweden	3.6	3.7	5.7	5.9
Switzerland	7.9	9.8	10.5	10.3
United States	5.0	4.8	6.3	8.1

Switzerland compared to Sweden and Denmark. What protects the Swiss population against alcoholic pancreatitis? Why do the Swedish population develop chronic pancreatitis at a lower alcohol consumption than the Danes? No answers can be given. The question about the different epidemiology of the alcohol consumption in different countries might be of relevance for the question, but studies to clarify the relationship between the distribution of alcohol consumption in the population and the frequency of chronic pancreatitis has never been made. An alternative mechanism is regional differences in diagnostic criteria for making the diagnosis chronic pancreatitis or, put another way, the different awareness of chronic pancreatitis as a reason for the complaints presented by the patients (vide infra).

Prevalence

The prevalence was, as mentioned above (Table 1), found to be 27.4 cases/100000 inhabitants in the city of Copenhagen in 1978–1979. Survival rates of chronic pancreatitis from four different materials are shown in Fig. 2. The differences in the cumulative survival in Denmark and Switzerland are obvious and no explanation for this difference can be given. If the difference in incidence rates mentioned above were dependent on diagnostic criteria, one would expect the Swiss material to be composed of more advanced cases than the Danish material. If so the prognosis should be expected to be even worse in Switzerland than in Denmark. However, the survival rate of chronic pancreatitis is identical in Illinois and Copenhagen (Fig. 2).

Based on the above-mentioned figures for incidence rates (Fig. 1) and the figures for median survival time (Fig. 2) the prevalence of chronic pancreatitis in Copenhagen and Switzerland can be calculated (Table 3). Equivalent figures from other places are not available as corresponding figures for incidence rate and mean survival are only present from Zürich and Copenhagen.

Table 3. Chronic pancreatitis: calculated prevalences/100000 inhabitants

	Incidence	Mean survival (years)	Prevalence
Zürich	2.0	20	40
Copenhagen	10	7	70

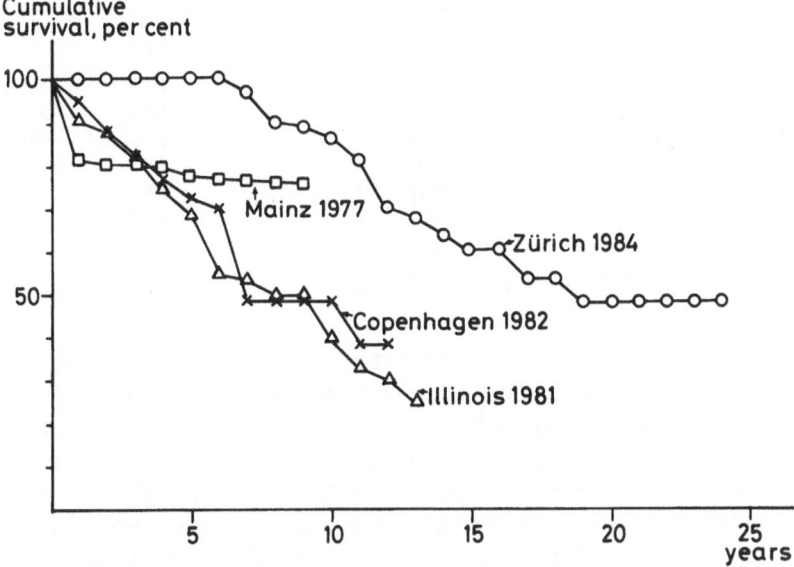

Fig. 2. Cummulative survival in chronic pancreatitis in four series. [13–16]

The prevalence of chronic pancreatitis in Copenhagen center (Table 1), Copenhagen County (Table 3), and Zürich (Table 3) ranges from 27 and 70. Is it reasonable to believe these differences to be real or is it an indication of differing diagnostic practice and the difference due to focusing on chronic pancreatitis in gastrointestinal patients? (vide infra).

Specific Prevalence

As the epidemiological studies of incidence and prevalence of chronic pancreatitis are few in number and far from optimal in methodology, one has to look for the prevalence in selected groups of patients. Figures are available in the literature from two groups:

1. patients characterized by abdominal symptoms indicating gastrointestinal diseases and
2. the total number of patients admitted to inpatient departments specifically and scientifically engaged in the field of chronic pancreatitis.

1. In 8 series of patients collected through the years 1975–1988 (Table 4) patients sent to investigations for different reasons were characterized by the final diagnosis, and the prevalence of chronic pancreatitis in these series is given in Table 4. The series are not fully comparable. The series by Møllmann et al. [17] and Horrock and DeDombal [18] comprised patients with upper dyspepsia (whatever that means). Harvey et al. [20] gave final diagnoses in 2000 consecutive patients referred to an outpatient gastroenterology clinic. The series by Andersen et al.

Table 4. Prevalence of chronic pancreatitis (%) among patients with "dyspepsia" (n)

Authors		Year	n	%
Møllmann et al.	[17]	1975	197	0
Horrock and DeDombal	[18]	1978	360	0
Andersen et al.	[19]	1982	460	35
Harvey et al.	[20]	1983	2000	0
Enslev et al.	[21]	1984	80	31
Lankish et al.	[22]	1986	218	38
Skude et al.	[23]	1987	36	14
Møller-Petersen et al.	[24]	1988	105	34

[19], Enslev et al. [21], Lankish et al. [22], and Møller-Petersen et al. [24] comprised patients with unexplained abdominal pain in combination with diarrhea and/or weight loss, whereas Skude et al. [23] studied patients with dyspepsia consulting their general practitioner. Even with these differences in the composition of the material, the variability in the prevalence is unexplained. A specific prevalence of 38% [22] among 218 patients compared to a prevalence of zero among 2000 patients [20] indicates big differences in the diagnostic approach to patients with gastrointestinal complaints. In the three series with prevalences of zero [17, 18, 20] diagnostic tests for pancreatic diseases were probably not included in the routine diagnostic armamentarium. In contradistinction, a prevalence in patients with abdominal pain, diarrhea, and weight loss of 38% [22] indicate chronic pancreatitis to be a common disease, a standpoint certainly not generally accepted.

2. The specific prevalence of chronic pancreatitis calculated as the percentage of patients totally admitted to different departments finally diagnosed as suffering from chronic pancreatitis is illustrated in Table 5. The specific prevalence calculated in this way ranges between 0.008% [8] and 0.476% [6]. These figures are certainly more difficult to compare than those given above, but even so a factor of 60 between the department with the highest prevalence and that with the lowest prevalence is difficult to explain. The departments presented in Table 5 are selected by their documented interest, scientifically and clinically, in chronic pancreatitis.

The lowest figure in Table 5 (0.008%) is equivalent to a prevalence of 8/100000 inhabitants. The figure is much lower than even the lowest figure given above in

Table 5. Chronic pancreatitis. Prevalence of chronic pancreatitis (%) among patients admitted to different medical and surgical departments

Authors		Period	Total admissions (n_1)	Chronic pancreatitis (n_2)	Prevalence %
White et al.	[25]	1956–65	403539	179	0.044
Haemmerli et al.	[8]	1958–62	194980	15	0.008
Creutzfeldt et al.	[26]	1955–69	86000	60	0.070
Freiburg		1955–63	55000	20	0.036
Göttingen		1964–69	15000	29	0.194
Anrau		1965–68	16000	11	0.069
Nyboe Andersen et al.	[6]	1970–79	26452	127	0.476

the total population and of course the specific prevalence of patients admitted to inpatient clinics specializing in chronic pancreatitis must be much higher than that in the general population. The figures in Table 5 point even more to the above-mentioned problem about differences in clinical practice in different centers. However, the probable heterogeneity of the populations admitted to the different hospitals mentioned in Table 5 may be taken into consideration.

Conclusion

The figures for frequency of chronic pancreatitis (incidence and prevalence) are collected with different techniques. The figures differ markedly from one center to another with no systematic tendency toward an increased incidence. The enormous differences are probably not based only on a real difference in frequency, but point strongly to considerable regional differences in selection of patients, clinical practice, diagnostic approach, and awareness of the disease chronic pancreatitis.

Valid and comparable figures for the incidence and prevalence of chronic pancreatitis must wait for careful prospective epidemiological studies based on systematized diagnostic criteria.

References

1. Sarles H (1973) An international survey on nutrition and pancreatitis. Digestion 9:389–407
2. Skyhøj Olsen T (1978) The incidence and clinical relevance of chronic inflammation in the pancreas in autopsy material. Acta Pathol Microbiol Scand [A] 86:361–365
3. Comfort MW, Gambile EE, Baggenstoss AH (1946) Chronic relapsing pancreatitis. Gastroenterology 6:239–285, 376–408
4. Copenhagen Pancreatitis Study (1981) An interim report from a prospective epidemiological multicenter study. Scand J Gastroenterol 16:305–312
5. O'Sullivan JN, Nobrega FT, Morlock CG, Brown AL jr, Bertholomew LG (1972) Acute and chronic pancreatitis in Rochester Minnesota 1940 to 1969. Gastroenterology 62:373–379
6. Nyboe Andersen N, Thorsgaard Pedersen N, Scheel J, Worning H (1982) Incidence of alcoholic chronic pancreatitis in Copenhagen. Scand J Gastroenterol 17:247–252
7. Schmidt DN (1989) Apparent risk factors for acute and chronic pancreatitis in Stockholm country: spiritus but not wine and beer. In: Ebbehøj N, Thorsgaard N (eds) Pancreas in focus. Meda, Copenhagen, pp 197–204
8. Haemmerli UP, Hefti ML, Schmid M (1962) Chronic pancreatitis in Zürich 1958 through 1962. Bibl Gastroenterol 7:58–74
9. Müller-Wieland K (1965) Analyse der Klinik der chronischen Pankreatitis. Z Klin Med 158:371–378
10. Sato T (1957) The annual report of Ministry of Health and Welfare, Chronic Pancreatitis Committee, Japan 1951. The Ministry of Health and Welfare, Tokyo (in Japanese)
11. Worning H (1984) Chronic pancreatitis: pathogenesis, natural history and conservative treatment. Clin Gastroenterol 13:871–894
12. Moser J (1980) Prevention of alcohol related problems. World Health Organization, Toronto
13. Ammann RW, Buehler H, Muench R, Freiburghaus AW, Siegenthaler W (1987) Differences in the natural history of idiopathic (nonalcoholic) and alcoholic chronic pancreatitis. A comparative long-term study of 287 patients. Pancreas 2:368–377
14. Mangold G, Neher M, Oswald B, Wagner G (1977) Ergebnisse der Resektionsbehandlung der chronischen Pankreatitis. Dtsch Med Wochenschr 102:229–234

15. Prinz RA, Greenlee HB (1981) Pancreatic duct drainage in 100 patients with chronic pancreatitis. Ann Surg 194:313–318
16. Thorsgaard Pedersen N, Nyboe Andersen B, Pedersen G, Worning H (1982) Chronic pancreatitis in Copenhagen. A retrospective study of 64 consecutive patients. Scand J Gastroenterol 17:925–931
17. Møllmann K-M, Bonnevie O, Gudmand-Höyer E, Wulff HR (1975) A diagnostic study of patients with upper abdominal pain. Scand J Gastroenterol 10:805–809
18. Horrock JC, DeDombal FT (1978) Clinical presentation of patients with "dyspepsia". Gut 19:19–26
19. Andersen BN, Scheel J, Rune SR, Woring H (1982) Exocrine pancreatic function in patients with dyspepsia. Hepatogastroenterology 29:35–37
20. Harvey RF, Salih SY, Read AE (1983) Organic and functional disorders in 2000 gastroenterology outpatients. Lancet 1:632–634
21. Enslev L, Andersen BN, Fahrenkrug J, Magid E, Thorsgaard Pedersen N (1984) Serum immunoreactive trypsin, pancreatic polypeptide and pancreatic isoamylase as diagnostic tests for chronic pancreatitis. Scand J Gastroenterol 19:204–208
22. Lankish PG, Koop H, Otto J (1986) Estimation of serum pancreatic isoamylase: its role in the diagnosis of exocrine pancreatic insufficiency. Am J Gastroenterol 81:365–368
23. Skude G, Andrén P, Hallert C, Kalin S, Lorentzson S, Pettersson B-G, Sassner P (1987) Pancreatic disease in dyspepsia. Digestion Suppl 1 37:14–17
24. Møller-Petersen J, Pedersen JO, Thorsgaard Pedersen N, Andersen BN (1988) Serum cathodic trypsin-like immunoreactivity, pancreatic lipase, and pancreatic isoamylase as diagnostic tests of chronic pancreatitis or pancreatic steatorrhea. Scand J Gastroenterol 23:287–296
25. White TT, Mural J, Morgan A (1968) Pancreatitis. Review of 733 cases of pancreatitis from three Seattle hospitals. Northwest Med 67:731–734
26. Creutzfeldt W, Fehr H, Schmidt H (1970) Verlaufsbeobachtungen und diagnostische Verfahren bei der chronisch-rezidivierenden und chronischen Pankreatitis. Schweiz Med Wochenschr 100:1180–1189

Role of Nutrition in Chronic Pancreatitis

C. S. Pitchumoni[1]

Throughout the evolution of multicellular organisms, the pancreas has acquired the capability to adapt to a wide variety of physiological and pathological stimuli, the most prominent of which are nutritional in origin. Normal pancreatic function and structure are altered by a number of nutritional factors which include changes in intake of major dietary components (proteins, carbohydrates, and fats) as well as vitamins and other micronutrients and trace elements [1].

It is not surprising that pancreatic injury occurs in protein deprivation since the pancreas has a very high turnover of proteins compared with other organs in the body. Experimental and clinical studies have documented that functional and structural abnormalities of the pancreas occur in advanced states of malnutrition in children [2]. Steatorrhea and creatorrhea have been observed in kwashiorkor. In clinical malnutrition deterioration of pancreatic secretory status progresses steadily. Lipase is the first enzyme to be affected followed by amylase and, in far advanced cases, enzyme secretion ceases almost completely. On light microscopy of the pancreas in children dying of kwashiorkor, a generalized reduction in the size of the pancreas associated with extreme acinar cell atrophy and fibrosis could be seen [2]. The pancreatic acinar pattern was disrupted and the cells appeared in small, irregular ring-like clusters with accumulation of fat. The basal apical polarity seen in healthy acinar cells was lost, associated with a marked decrease in both endoplasmic reticulum and zymogen granules. The mitochondria were decreased and were abnormal.

The earlier clinical and experimental studies, however, attributed all the alterations seen in the pancreas solely to protein deficiency and ignored the role of micronutrients. Micronutrients are nutrients essential for humans which are needed only in microgram to milligram amounts per day. In the field of nutrition, the term "essential" is given to those nutrients which must be consumed on a regular basis because the body cannot synthesize the compounds. It has only recently become clear that all the changes noted in organs in clinical malnutrition are not solely attributable to protein deficiency. Data suggest that deficiencies of certain vitamins, provitamins, and trace elements also induce acinar and islet changes. Trace elements play a major role in human physiology. Many of these micronutrients have at least three major biological roles:

1. as inorganic constituents in a number of metalloenzymes,
2. as donors or acceptors of electrons in oxidation-reduction reactions, and
3. in the transport and release of oxygen.

[1] Division of Gastroenterology and Clinical Nutrition, Our Lady of Mercy Medical Center, Bronx, New York 10466, USA

Chronic Pancreatitis
Ed. by Beger, Büchler, Ditschuneit, and Malfertheiner
© Springer-Verlag Berlin Heidelberg 1990

Some of the above functions are closely related to protection of tissue injury by "free radicals," a topic of intensive study today in various branches of medicine. A discussion on "free-radical" injury to the pancreas is beyond the scope of this presentation, but the reader is referred to an excellent review by Southorn and Powis [3]. Briefly, when a reactive molecule contains one or more unpaired electrons the molecule is termed a "free radical." These potentially harmful free radicals are scavenged by antioxidants. Many of these antioxidants are either essential nutrients or essential nutrients that are part of enzymes (Table 1) [4] which maintain the critical balance between free radical generation and destruction.

Table 1. Antioxidant micronutrients. (Modified from [4])

Nutrient	Property
Vitamin A	Cannot quench singlet oxygen, a poor scavenger of free radicals
β-Carotene	Most efficient quencher of singlet oxygen, can function as an antioxidant
Vitamin E (∞-tocopherol)	Lipid-soluble antioxidant protects against lipid peroxidation, reacts with superoxide, singlet oxygen
Zinc	Required for the activity of superoxide dismutases
Selenium	Constituent of glutathione peroxidase
Copper	Constituent of superoxide dismutase
Manganese	Constituent of superoxide dismutase

Although malnutrition was known to injure the pancreas and cause acinar atrophy and fibrosis, the importance of nutritional deficiency as a cause of chronic pancreatitis became obvious only since 1959 with a series of reports on a type of nonalcoholic chronic pancreatitis from various developing countries [5]. Although the etiopathogenesis of this entity, known variously as tropical, Afro-Asian, or nutritional pancreatitis, juvenile tropical pancreatitis syndrome, or fibrocalcific pancreatic diabetes is not clear, some form of malnutrition appears to be intimately related to the pathogenesis [6].

A totally different situation exists in affluent Western nations, where alcoholic pancreatitis is prevalent. The pathogenesis of chronic alcoholic pancreatitis, despite extensive studies, remains controversial. The fact that only some alcoholics develop chronic pancreatitis has baffled clinicians. This question has led to a number of studies looking for concomitant factors of synergistic importance, such as genetic predisposition, nutritional factors, and the effects of cigarette smoking.

I have attempted here to summarize the data on
1. tropical pancreatitis and
2. nutritional factors in alcoholic pancreatitis and subsequently identify common nutritional deficiencies of pathogenetic importance in these conditions.

Tropical Pancreatitis

Definition

Tropical pancreatitis is a term used in the past 30 years to describe a calcific pancreatic disease that has been observed in children and young adults, predominantly of the low income groups in many Afro-Asian countries [5]. The clinicopathological descriptions of this disease entity closely resemble the alcoholic type of chronic pancreatitis of the Western nations. The prevalence of the disease almost exclusively in the impoverished sectors of developing nations, the presence of clinical signs of malnutrition in the large majority of affected individuals, and the total absence of the other known causes of calcific pancreatitis strongly implicated malnutrition as a major etiologic factor.

Epidemiology

The disease was originally described by Zuidema [7] in Jakarta, Indonesia, where he studied 18 patients who were poor and had nonketotic diabetes mellitus and disseminated pancreatic calcification. Marked emaciation, bilateral parotid gland enlargement, and hair and skin changes resembling kwashiorkor were the associated findings. Shaper [8] reported a similar syndrome from Kampala, Uganda. Most of the patients were poor peasants of Uganda who consumed a low-protein, low-fat, high-carbohydrate diet. Shaper considered protein malnutrition as the etiologic factor although he exercised caution in suggesting that it was important to identify additional factors [8]. A similar syndrome of chronic pancreatitis associated with pancreatic calculi and diabetes mellitus was subsequently reported from different Afro-Asian countries, which included Malawi, Zaire, Uganda, Sri Lanka, Nigeria, Brazil, Tunisia, and a number of other countries.

The single largest series of cases to date is from the southwestern state of Kerala in India. GeeVarghese and Pitchumoni [9] observed this disease in endemic proportions in two major medical college hospitals of the state. To date more than 1000 cases have been carefully studied by GeeVarghese [10]. The natural history of nutritional pancreatitis is succinctly summarized by GeeVarghese [10] as "recurrent abdominal pain in childhood, diabetes around puberty and death at the prime of life".

Although a large number of cases of the calcific type of chronic pancreatitis have been reported from the state of Kerala, the disease is not uncommon elsewhere in the country. Cases studied by others in the state and in other parts of India were the subject of a recent symposium in 1987 [6].

In addition to the classical calcific pancreatitis, a type of diabetes occuring in the young associated with malnutrition is frequently recognized in many parts of India and Africa. At this time this entity is discussed in the diabetes literature as malnutrition-related diabetes mellitus (MRDM) with its subtype, namely, protein-deficient pancreatic diabetes (PDPD) [11]. The diabetologists in India consider this type of diabetes of the young malnourished to be a variant of chronic pancreatitis of fibrocalculous pancreatic disease (FCPD). A number of questions are unanswered with regard to the entity of MRDM and PDPD. In view of lack of definitive studies evaluating pancreatic structure and function in the above group of patients it is difficult to say whether MRDM is a noncalculous variant of chronic pancreatitis of the tropics. The controversies are discussed in the proceedings of "tropical diabetes workshop" held in London in June 1988 [12].

Abdominal pain characterizes the onset of tropical pancreatitis. Recurrent pain, lasting for hours to days radiating to the back, aggravated by food was noted in 95% of the patients. Most of the patients had diabetes at the time of admission to the hospital and abdominal flat plate abdomen then invariably showed diffuse pancreatic calculi. Although no genetic pattern of transmission of the disease was noted, we observed several families with multiple cases of pancreatitis [5]. The onset of diabetes was a few years after the onset of pancreatalgia. A pain-free period of 1 or 2 years and an apparent transient improvement in the clinical picture prior to the onset of diabetes was not unusual. The age of onset of diabetes was below 30 years in 72% of the 325 cases studied initially [9]. The fasting blood sugar ranged between 200 and 400 mg/dl. Severe forms of diabetes with higher blood sugar levels were not uncommon. Pancreatic diabetes is characteristically brittle with marked fluctuations of blood glucose. Hypoglycemic episodes may complicate the picture. Insulin resistance was seen in a number of patients.

Pathology

Macroscopically the pancreas in tropical pancreatitis appears small and firm to touch. The consistency varies in different regions of the pancreas. Homogeneous areas, early fibrosis, advanced fibrosis, cystic dilatation of the glands, and advanced stages of calculi formation can be seen in the same pancreas. Pancreatic calculi of different sizes and shapes are distributed throughout the major duct and ductules.

Microscopically, dilatation of the ducts, pancreatic lithiasis, chronic inflammatory cell infiltration, and atrophy of the parenchyma are seen. The main ducts and ductules show marked dilatation. Denudation of the ductal epithelium and squamous metaplasia are seen.

Pancreatic calculi of varying size, some as small as sand particles. and others as big as 3 cm in diameter and weighing up to 20 g are seen. These calculi are composed of calcium carbonate. Using X-ray diffraction studies we demonstrated that the nidus of the stones contains an amorphous material and the periphery is rich in calcite [13]. These findings were confirmed by scanning electron microscopic studies [14]. The elemental analysis of the calculus using energy-dispersive X-ray fluorescence (EDXRF) showed that the nidus is rich in iron, chromium, and nickel, but deficient in calcium or phosphorus. This observation is contradictory to the earlier data on pancreatic stone protein claimed to be a phosphoprotein [15]. The outer areas contain poorly formed crystals of calcium carbonate and at least 17 other elements including iron, chromium, potassium, chloride, silica, aluminum, magnesium, and sodium. The structure and composition of these calculi are identical with those from patients with alcoholic pancreatitis.

Etiopathogenesis

The etiology of tropical pancreatitis is not yet clearly determined although there is agreement that malnutrition is a common denominator in most of the cases [1, 5–13]. There are, however, exceptions as the disease has been reported in professionals and business men in India [16], casting doubts on malnutrition theories. In the field of epidemiology such exceptions are not uncommon in studies of etiopathogenesis of any disease, and certainly they do not form the basis to exclude general observations.

Protein Malnutrition

Early observers categorically stated that the disease was secondary to protein malnutrition or childhood kwashiorkor. Some of the signs of tropical pancreatitis such as the hair and skin changes and bilateral parotid gland enlargement observed in Indonesian patients were seen in classic kwashiorkor [7]. Pancreatic fibrosis was noted in kwashiorkor [8]. However, recent observations have indicated that tropical pancreatitis is not a consequence of kwashiorkor. The prevalence of the two diseases does not always overlap in many Afro-Asian countries. The high prevalence of tropical pancreatitis in the state of Kerala, which has the lowest infant mortality rate in India (40/1000 in Kerala vs. 90/1000 in the rest of India), is contradictory to the idea that infant malnutrition is a major etiologic factor. Patients with tropical pancreatitis do not have a history of childhood kwashiorkor. The features of advanced malnutrition noted in patients with tropical pancreatitis may be, mostly, the result of the disease.

The conflicting data have raised doubts as to whether protein malnutrition is an initiating factor in the pathogenesis of tropical pancreatitis [17]. The weight of evidence is in favor of a nutritional deficiency not elucidated currently or a nutritional toxin as the major etiologic factor [5, 6, 10, 12].

Dietary Toxin

A potential toxic effect of cassava *(Manihot esculenta)* through its content of cyanogenetic glycosides, linamarin, and linamarase is cited as a possible etiologic factor based on epidemiologic data [5, 6, 10, 12, 16]. Cassava root contains 65 mg toxic glycosides/100 g. The concentration varies depending on the method of preparation of the meal, and preservation. Hydrocyanic acid is liberated when the glycosides react with hydrochloric acid in the stomach. The enzyme rhodanase acts on hydrocyanic acid leading to thiocyanate production in the presence of adequate amounts of methionine and cystine. Cassava is consumed in large quantities by the majority of poor people in southern Nigeria, Kerala, Indonesia, Uganda, Malawi, and Thailand, areas where tropical pancreatitis is prevalent. In epidemiological studies there are conflicting observations which suggest that not all populations which consume cassava develop pancreatitis and the disease also occurs in individuals with no history of cassava consumption. However, the strength of association between malnutrition and cassava diet is not weakened by these exceptions. In any chronic disease the suggested etiologic factor cannot be demonstrated in 100% of cases. The possible role of the cassava diet in injuring the pancreas and leading to fibrocalcific pancreatic diabetes was discussed at length in a recent meeting [12].

Cyanogens impair a number of enzymes including superoxide dismutase, an important scavenger of free radicals which are proposed to cause cell injury [18–20]. The interactions between malnutrition and cyanogen toxicity are conducive to unopposed free radical injury. Associated nutritional deficiency, such as deficiencies of methionine, zinc, copper, and selenium common in malnutrition, interferes with the detoxification of cyanogens. Methionine deficiency in experimental animals causes pancreatitis. Cassava diet is not only deficient in protein, but also in methionine, cyanogens in the presence of malnutrition thus creating an ideal setting for free radical injury by promoting the generation of free radicals, and by decreasing the ability to scavenge them.

Miscellaneous Factors

Genetic predisposition, ductal anomalies, and pancreatic ductal stasis as a result of recurrent bacterial, viral, and parasitic infections are other postulated causes with weak scientific evidence at this time [6, 10, 21].

Diet and Alcoholic Pancreatitis

Experimental and epidemiological studies have indicated that the risk for alcoholic pancreatitis is higher on high-fat high-protein diet. Sarles et al. described focal lesions of chronic pancreatitis in more than half of Wistar rats that ingested ethanol for 20–30 months [22]. Pancreatic juice in these animals contained significantly higher protein concentrations than controls. These conditions appeared to be similar to the pathological changes observed in clinical pancreatitis. Recently Tsukamoto et al. [23] have developed a rat model of chronic ethanol intoxication which achieved sustained blood ethanol levels. When intragastric infusion of 5% (low fat), 25% (high fat), and 35% (extra high fat) of total calories as fat (corn oil rich in polyunsaturated fatty acids) was given to rats for 30–160 days while maintaining a blood alcohol level of 210 mg/dl, differing grades of pancreatic injury were noted. With the low dietary intake of corn oil fat, chronic ethanol intoxication produced only mild pancreatic injury. However, focal lesions of chronic pancreatitis were observed in animals fed higher amounts of fat. The fivefold or sevenfold increases of dietary fat resulted in striking potentiation of ethanol-induced pancreatic injury. These studies demonstrated potentiation by dietary fat, in particular unsaturated fat in ethanol-induced pancreatic injury.

It has been observed in many European countries (Table 2) that alcoholics consuming a high-fat and -protein diet are predisposed to chronic pancreatitis [24]. Noncalcific chronic pancreatitis and acute pancreatitis predominate in northern Europe in patients with a high protein and fat intake. The amount of total protein intake is related to the logarithm of the relative risk of developing chronic pancreatitis. But fat intake was related quadratically to the risk of developing pancreatitis. Sarles [24] noted that the risk was less with average consumption of fat, but was increased by both high (> 100 g) and low (< 85 g) fat intake [25]. It is highly debatable whether this

Table 2. Alcohol and dietary intake in chronic pancreatitis

Country	Reference		Protein	Fat
France	Sarles	[24]	113 ± 38	111 ± 35
Marseilles	Gastard	1973 [39]	137.00	156.00
Rennes	Goebell/Hotz	1975 [40]	112 ± 66	156 ± 94
Federal Republic				
of Germany	Sarles	[24]	89 ± 33	87 ± 31
Cape Town	Sarles	[24]	43 ± 26	22 ± 17
New York City	Pitchumoni	1980 [26]	67 ± 22	59 ± 33
Baltimore	Mezey et al.	[28]	57.1 ± 4.8	53.8 ± 4.2

range between 85 and 100 g would make a difference in the risk for pancreatitis and whether 85 g fat can be considered a low-fat diet.

The observations in European studies could not be supported by data from centers in the United States and Australia [26–28]. Although a high-fat and/or -protein diet may predispose to pancreatitis, such a diet is not a prerequisite for development of pancreatitis in chronic alcoholics (Table 2 summarizes the data from various countries).

Some of these conflicting data may be observed because of differences in genetic predisposition, quantity of alcohol, and the type of fat (saturated versus polyunsaturated) consumed by various population groups in different countries.

Trace Elements, Vitamins, and Provitamin Deficiencies in Pancreatic Injury

The importance of micronutrients in the structural integrity of the pancreas is currently being studied in experimental animals. Very little information is available with regard to their role in clinical medicine.

Zinc is a component of many metalloenzymes including procarboxypeptidases A and B produced in pancreatic acinar cells and carbonic anhydrase produced in both gastric epithelium and pancreatic duct cells. Zinc is required for the optimal activity of other enzymes such as DNA polymerase, RNA polymerase, and reverse transcriptase required for nucleic acid synthesis. Long-term feeding of a zinc-deficient diet in rats resulted in acinar cell degeneration [29].

Copper deficiency in experimental rats induced a selective and progressive atrophy of pancreatic acinar tissue [30], sparing ductules and islets. At the ultrastructural level copper deficiency in the rat led to enlargement and degeneration of mitochondria, extensive degeneration of the rough endoplasmic reticulum, and a failure of zymogen granule formation in the acinar pancreas [31]. A marked decrease in the cytochrome oxidase (high copper content) activity was observed. It has been postulated that decreases in ATP production could affect protein synthesis and secretion and phospholipid biosynthesis.

Magnesium deficiency similarly induces mitochondrial changes in the acinar cell [1].

Selenium-deficient diets in chicken resulted in atrophy of the pancreas in addition to diminished growth and feathering [32]. The role of selenium deficiency in pancreatic injury is being studied extensively.

There is some evidence that chronic alcoholics suffer from deficiency of a number of trace elements, particularly of zinc and selenium [33]. Several of the essential minerals listed above are incorporated into protective antioxidant enzymes. Zinc, copper, and manganese are required for the activity of both types of superoxide dismutase. Selenium is an essential component of glutathione peroxidase which plays a major role in controlling endogenous formation of peroxides from unsaturated fatty acids in cell membranes.

Antioxidant enzymes are mostly intracellular and hence extracellular free radicals, either endogenously produced or from the environment, must be inactivated by the circulating antioxidants which include vitamins and provitamins [4]. (Ceruloplasmin, a copper-containing protein, is also a circulating antioxidant). Recent studies have emphasized the role of these circulating antioxidants (see Table 1). Vitamin C interacts with the tocopherol radical and promotes regeneration of reduced tocopherol, an important antioxidant function of the vitamin. Vitamin E protects the conjugated double bonds of betacarotene from oxidation. Further vitamin E can protect against many of the symptoms of selenium deficiency and vice versa. Betacarotene, a pigment found in all plants, is a major carotenoid precursor. It is the most efficient quencher of singlet oxygen. The reactivity of molecular oxygen is enhanced during the course of certain reactions involving molecular oxygen that invert the spin of one of the electrons of the two outer orbitals producing singlet oxygen which is highly reactive [3]. Betacarotene deactivates reactive chemical species such as triplet photochemical sensitizers, free radicals, and singlet oxygen which cause tissue damage.

Cigarette Smoking and Chronic Pancreatitis

Chronic pancreatitis is predominantly a disease of men. Smoking and drinking are common coexisting social habits. One has to admit that it would be difficult to study the separate effects of these two toxins in most populations. A strong association with ethanol and cigarette smoking with chronic pancreatitis was noted in men and not in women [34]. Lowenfels et al. [35] recently studied a unique population group, the southwestern American Indians, who had history of chronic alcoholism but very little or no associated cigarette smoking. The risk for pancreatitis in cigarette-smoking alcoholics was noted to be much higher than in non-cigarette-smoking alcoholics. The study, when repeated in another population group, yielded the same results [36]. The epidemiological observations can be partly explained based on our current knowledge of cigarette smoke. One of the most powerful exogenous sources of free radicals includes tobacco smoke. Cigarette smoke not only increases free radical production, it also effectively interferes with the scavenging free radicals by decreasing antioxidant levels. Studies have shown that levels of vitamin C and B carotene are markedly diminished in smokers [37].

Our preliminary data on provitamins in chronic alcoholics and those with pancreatitis (Table 3) indicate that there is a trend for low levels of these substances [38]. Further studies are needed to evaluate the role of provitamin deficiencies on pancreatic injury.

Table 3. Plasma vitamin and provitamin antioxidant levels in chronic pancreatitis

Alcoholic pancreatitis	Ascorbic acid (0.4 mg/dl)	Tocopherol Alpha (0.7–2.0 mg/dl	Tocopherol Gamma (?)	Retinol (20–180 mg/dl)	Betacarotene (10 mg/dl)
Cigarette smokers					
1	0.74	0.72	0.10	19.1[a]	14.0
2	0.36[a]	0.78	0.45	11.5[a]	< 0.4[a]
3	0.84	0.72	0.14	13.2[a]	5.9
3		0.21[a]	0.94	37.9	12.6
5		0.58[a]	0.11	45.3	< 0.4[a]
No cigarettes					
6	0.64	0.47[a]	0.15	28.5	4.6[a]
7	0.63	0.35[a]	0.28	31.3	6.2[a]
8	0.42	0.84	0.10	62.6	< 0.4[a]
Miscellaneous: anorexia nervosa					
9	1.28	0.34[a]	0.06	48.1	5.1[a]
Idiopathic					
10	0.79	0.74	0.12	79.9	11.2

[a] Indicates low levels

Summary and Conclusion

It is clear that the pancreas is sensitive to malnutrition, which includes not only deficiency of macronutrients but also many micronutrients, which include trace elements, vitamins, and provitamins. The pathogenesis of Afro-Asian pancreatitis is not established, but may be partly explained by micronutrient-antioxidant deficiencies and unopposed free radical injury by dietary cyanogens. Epidemiologic data of Afro-Asian pancreatitis do not suggest kwashiorkor or severe protein malnutrition as a major cause of this disease. The pathogenesis of alcoholic pancreatitis is also not firmly established. In some countries increased intake of fat enhances the predisposition to the disease. This observation is not confirmed in studies from the United States, South Africa, and Australia. The observation that the risk of pancreatitis in the cigarette-smoking alcoholic is increased fits in well with the hypothesis of unopposed free radical injury to the pancreas. Cigarette smoking, in addition to promoting free radical generation, inhibits a number of normal defense mechanisms, by depleting many antioxidants. The possible depletion of antioxidant enzymes in the malnourished populations of developing nations exposed to dietary cyanogens and in the cigarette-smoking alcoholics of the affluent Western nations creates the same environment for unopposed free radical injury. The common pathway although highly hypothetical at this time offers new opportunities for future studies.

References

1. Pitchumoni CS, Scheele G, Lee PC, Lebenthal E (1986) Effects of nutrition on the exocrine pancreas. In: Go VLW, et al. (eds) The exocrine pancreas: biology, pathobiology and diseases. Raven, New York, pp 387–406
2. Blackburn WR, Vinijchaikul K (1969) The pancreas in kwashiorkor: an electron microscopic study. Lab Invest 20:305–331
3. Southorn PA, Powis G (1988) Free radicals in medicine. I. Chemical nature and biologic interactions. II. Involvement in human disease. Mayo Clin Proc 63:381–408
4. Machlin LW, Bendich A (1987) Free radical tissue damage: protective role of antioxidant nutrients. FASEB J 1:441–445
5. Pitchumoni CS (1984) Special problems of tropical pancreatitis. Clin Gastroenterol 13: 941–959
6. Balakrishnan V (1987) Tropical pancreatitis – epidemiology, pathogenesis and etiology. In: Balakrishnan (ed) Chronic pancreatitis in India. Indian Society of Pancreatology, pp 81–85
7. Zuidema PJ (1959) Cirrhosis and disseminated calcification of the pancreas in patients with malnutrition. Trop Geogr Med 11:70–74
8. Shaper AG (1960) Chronic pancreatic disease and protein malnutrition. Lancet 1:1223–1224
9. GeeVarghese PJ, Pitchumoni CS (1966) Pancreatic diabetes in Kerala. Based on a clinico-pathological study of 325 diabetic patients with pancreatic calculi. In: Patel JC, Talvalcar NG (eds) Proceedings of the world congress on diabetes in the tropics. Bombay, pp 223–229
10. GeeVarghese PJ (1986) Calcific pancreatitis. Causes and mechanisms in the tropics compared with those in the subtropics. St Joseph's Trivandrum
11. Mohan V (1988) Clinical manifestations of MRDM in southern India. Tropical diabetes workshop June 30–July 2, Wellcome Tropical Institute, London
12. Tropical Diabetes Workshop (1988) Proceedings of the meeting held in June 30–July 2. Wellcome Tropical Institute, London
13. Schultz AC, Moore PB, GeeVarghese PJ, Pitchumoni CS (1986) X-ray diffraction studies of pancreatic calculi associated with nutritional pancreatitis. Dig Dis Sci 31:476–480
14. Pitchumoni CS, Viswanathan KV, GeeVarghese PJ, Banks PA (1987) Ultrastructure and elemental composition of human pancreatic calculi. Pancreas 2:152–158
15. DeCaro A, Multiligner L, Lafont H, Lomardo D, Sarles H (1984) The molecular characteristics of a human pancreatic acid phosphoprotein that inhibits calcium carbonate crystal growth. Biochem J 222:669–677
16. Narendranathan M (1981) Chronic calcific pancreatitis of the tropics. Trop Gastroenterol 2:40–45
17. GeeVarghese PJ, Pitchumoni CS, Nair SR (1969) Is protein malnutrition an initiating cause of pancreatic calcification. J Assoc Physicians India 17:417–419
18. Braganza JM (1983) Pancreatic disease: a causality of hepatic "detoxification"? Lancet 2:1000–1002
19. Braganza JM (1986) The pancreas. In: Pounder RE (ed) Recent advances in gastroenterology. Livingston, Edinburgh, 251–280
20. Pitchumoni CS, Jain NK, Lowenfels AF, DiMagno EP (1988) Chronic cyanide poisoning. Unifying concept for alcoholic and tropical pancreatitis. Pancreas 3:220–222
21. Nwokolo C, Oli JM (1980) Pathogenesis of juvenile tropical pancreatitis syndrome. Lancet 1:456–459
22. Sarles H, Figarella C, Clemente F (1971) The interaction of ethanol, dietary lipids and proteins on the rat pancreas. Pancreatic enzymes. Digestion 4:13–22
23. Tsukamoto H, Towner SJ, Yu GSM, French SW (1988) Potentiation of ethanol-induced pancreatic injury by dietary fat. Induction of chronic pancreatitis by alcohol in rats. Am J Pathol 131:246–257
24. Sarles H (1973) An international survey on nutrition and pancreatitis. Digestion 9:389–403
25. Durbec JP, Sarles H (1978) Multicenter survey of the etiology of pancreatic diseases. Relationship between the relative risk of developing chronic pancreatitis and alcohol, protein, and lipid consumption. Digestion 18:337–350
26. Pitchumoni CS, Sonnenshein M, Candido FM, Panchacharam P, Cooperman JM (1980) Nutrition in the pathogenesis of alcoholic pancreatitis. Am J Clin Nutr 33:631–636

27. Wilson JS, Bernstein L, McDonald C, Tsait A, McNeil D, Pirola RC (1985) Diet and drinking habits in relation to the development of alcoholic pancreatitis. Gut 26:882–887
28. Mezey E, Kolman C, Mae Diehl A, Mitchell MC, Herlong FL (1988) Alcohol and dietary intake in the development of chronic pancreatitis and liver disease in alcoholism. Am J Clin Nutr 48:148–151
29. Koo SI, Turk DE (1977) Effect of zinc deficiency on the ultrastructure of the pancreatic acinar cells and intestinal epithelium in the rat. J Nutr 107: 896–908
30. Muller HB (1979) Der Einfluß kupferarmer Kost auf das Pankreas. Lichtmikroskopische Untersuchungen am exokrinen Teil der Bauchspeicheldrüsen weißer Ratten. Birchows Arch [Pathol Anat] 350:353–367
31. Fell BF, King TP, Davies NT (1982) Pancreatic atrophy in copper deficient rats. Histochemical and ultrastructural evidence of a selective effect on acinar cells. Histochem J 14:665–680
32. Thompson JN, Scott ML (1969) Role of selenium in the nutrition of the chick. J Nutr 97:335–342
33. Dutta SK, Miller PA, Greenberg LB, Lavander OA (1983) Selenium and acute alcoholism. Am J Clin Nutr 38:713–718
34. Yen S, Hsieh C, MacMahon B (1982) Consumption of alcohol and tobacco and other risk factors for pancreatitis. Am J Epidemiol 116:407–411
35. Lowenfels AB, Zwemer FL, Jhangiani S, Pitchumoni CS (1987) Pancreatitis in a native American Indian population. Pancreas 2:694–697
36. Lowenfels AB, Abdelsayed GG, Pitchumoni CS, Welty TK, Cash J (1989) Smoking and the risk of pancreatitis in a native American Indian population (Abstr). American Pancreatic Association, 2–3 Nov 1989
37. Chow CK, Thacker RR, Chamgchint C, Bridges RB, Rehm SR, Humble J, Turbek J (1986) Lower levels of vitamin C and carotenes in plasma of cigarette smokers. J Am Coll Nutr 5:305–312
38. Norkus EP, Vazquez W, Pitchumoni CS (1989) Plasma vitamin and provitamin antioxidant levels in patients with alcoholic pancreatitis (Abstr). Federation for Clinical Research, Eastern Section Meeting
39. Gastard J, Joubaud F, Farbos T, Loussouarn J, Marion J, Pannier M, Ranaudet F, Faldazo R, Gosselin M (1973) Etiology and course of primary chronic pancreatitis in Western France. Digestion 9:416–428
40. Goebell H, Hotz H (1975) Nutritional Aspects of Chronic Pancreatitis in Germany. Biol Gastroenterol (Paris) 8:365–370

Alcohol, the Alimentary Tract and Pancreas: Facts and Controversies*

I. N. MARKS[1]

Historical Aspects

Alcohol has been used, and abused, since biblical times. Noah, of Ararat fame, was perhaps the first drunkard – "and he drank of the wine, and was drunken; and he was uncovered within his tent" (Genesis 9:21). Lot's daughters plied their father with drink to suit their own nefarious ends – "come, let us make our father drink wine, ... that we may preserve seed of our father" (Genesis 19:32), while Samson's mother was told to avoid alcohol to ensure a successful pregnancy – "now therefore beware, I pray thee, and drink no wine, nor strong drink" (Judges 13:4). The prophets of old, it seems, were fully aware of the fetal alcohol syndrome.

The method of making pure alcohol was discovered by the alchemist Lully (1235–1315), who enthused: "The taste of it exceedeth all other tastes, and the smell of it all other smells." He considered alcohol "of marveylous use and commoditie a little before joyning of battle to styre and encourage the soldiers' minds" [9]. It does more. In South Africa, alcohol abuse accounts for 60% of adult drownings, 70% of pedestrian deaths, and 80% of driving fatalities within the first 2 h of an accident.

Alcohol Abuse: General Aspects

Ethyl alcohol (alcohol) is widely available in a number of different beverages with an alcohol content of 4–35 g/100 ml. One tot of spirits, one glass of wine, or half a reputed pint of beer (i. e., about 200 ml) contain approximately 10 ml or 8.0 g absolute alcohol. The effects of alcohol on the CNS are directly proportional to the blood alcohol concentrations. Levels below 0.05 g% tend to produce a subjective feeling of well-being, but incoordination and impaired reflexes manifest themselves at levels between 0.05 and 0.10 g%, and frank intoxication with blurred vision, loss of sensory perception, ataxia, and slurred speech occurs at higher levels. The risk of an auto accident rises almost exponentially in drivers with blood alcohol levels in excess of 0.08 g%, the legal limit for drivers of vehicles in most countries.

The Widmark formula $(A = p \times c \times r)$ may be used to calculate the amount of alcohol required to produce a given blood alcohol level in a particular individual. The

* Support from the South African Medical Research Council is acknowledged
[1] Gastrointestinal Clinic, Groote Schuur Hospital and Department of Medicine, University of Cape Town, Observatory 7925, South Africa

Chronic Pancreatitis
Ed. by Beger, Büchler, Ditschuneit, and Malfertheiner
© Springer-Verlag Berlin Heidelberg 1990

amount of alcohol absorbed in g *(A)* = body weight in kg *(p)* × blood alcohol concentration in g/1000 ml *(c)* × diffusion rate *(r)*. The diffusion rate varies according to the build of the individual and is about 0.5 in the obese, 0.75 in the muscular and 0.67 in a person of average build [9]. A 70 kg man of average build thus attains a blood alcohol level of 0.08 g% after absorbing 38 g alcohol. This is roughly equivalent to four or five tots of spirits, three reputed pints of beer, or 500 ml dry wine. This generalization does not allow for absorption variables such as delayed gastric emptying or a possible dilution factor, or for variability in the rate of elimination. The fall in blood levels is of the order of 0.01–0.02 g%/h, equivalent to about one tot per hour.

Alcohol generates 7.1 kcal/g when combusted and may be overlooked as a source of calories. However, alcohol does not provide a caloric food value equivalent to that of carbohydrates. Isocaloric replacement of carbohydrate calories by alcohol (50% of total calories) in a balanced diet results in a decline in body weight [30].

Chronic alcohol abuse may be associated with a wide spectrum of diseases. These comprise a variety of neurological, muscular, hematological, and gastrointestinal disorders and a number of vitamin deficiencies. This presentation will consider some of the alimentary disorders and focus, in particular, on a few of the current controversies in alcohol-induced pancreatitis (AIP).

Alimentary Tract

Nonspecific abdominal symptoms are common in heavy drinkers. These include early morning nausea and retching, anorexia, heartburn, right upper quadrant discomfort, and diarrhea.

Esophagus

Excessive drinking is commonly associated with heartburn and linked, characteristically, with varices and emetogenic injuries of the esophagus.
1. Heartburn may be related simply to relaxation of the lower esophageal sphincter but is due more frequently to exacerbation of reflux esophagitis in patients with a preexistent hiatus hernia. Severe retching in this setting may produce blood-stained vomitus. Painful dysphagia due to superficial ulceration is a rare complication of acute alcohol insult.
2. Frank hematemesis in an alcoholic always raises the possibility of bleeding from esophageal varices.
3. Severe bleeding may also be due to mucosal tears of the lower esophagus or gastroesophageal region following retching (Mallory-Weiss syndrome).

Spontaneous rupture of the esophagus (Boerhaave's syndrome) is a rare, but catastrophic, complication of retching; it manifests itself, almost invariably, as an overwhelming retrosternal pain.

Stomach and Duodenum

The association between alcohol abuse and transient erosive gastritis is wellrecognized. Beaumont [4] observed gastric erythema and gastritis in Alexis St. Martin following the "free use of ardent spirits for a few days," but found the mucosa to be normal after 4–5 days. Wolf and Wolff [40] noted the development of gastric hyperemia and turgidity in their gastrostomy subject, Tom, following the intake of 30 ml of 90% proof whisky (i. e., 45% by volume). Changes were maximal after 45 min and the mucosa appeared normal some 90 min later. These early observations were extended by Palmer [28] in a gastroscopic study in a group of 24 young soldiers. An alcoholic binge in these volunteers was followed, within 6 h, by the development of hyperemia, petechiae, and erosions associated with histological evidence of necrobiosis of the mucosal neck region. This was followed by exfoliation and development of erosions. The changes reverted to normal within 7–20 days. Palmer [28] also dispelled the notion that chronic alcoholism predisposes to chronic gastritis. A group of 141 chronic alcoholics showed normal gastric biopsies without evidence of chronic gastritis.

The widely held view that excessive alcohol intake causes peptic ulcer has not been confirmed epidemiologically, and there is no evidence that moderate drinking adversely affects ulcer healing. However, alcohol has a potentiating effect on gastric and duodenal mucosal injuries due to aspirin or nonsteroidal antiinflammatory drugs (NSAIDS) [19].

Small Bowel

Diarrhea in the alcoholic may be due to effects on motility, active transport mechanisms, and bile salt metabolism. Other contributory factors include portal hypertension, pancreatic insufficiency, alterations in bowel flora, and possible nutritional deficiencies. Impaired absorption of folate, thiamine, vitamin B_{12}, fat, and xylose may occur, with recovery after alcohol withdrawal [36]. Depressed levels of intestinal lactase and sucrase with recovery following alcohol withdrawal have also been described [29].

Liver Disease

Alcohol abuse is frequently associated with a wide spectrum of liver disorders. This includes fatty change alone, acute alcoholic hepatitis with or without fatty change, and cirrhosis. Other variants of alcohol-induced liver disease include acute or chronic hyaline necrosis, cholestatic liver disease, hepatic iron overload, and hepatic porphyria; and alcoholic cirrhosis may be complicated by hepatocellular carcinoma.

The clinical presentation depends on the nature and severity of the particular liver disorder. These are wellrecognized and beyond the scope of this presentation. It should be stressed, however, that early forms of the disease may manifest themselves with little more than early morning nausea, anorexia, and right upper quadrant discomfort. The finding of a raised AST/ALT ratio, a raised GGT, or macrocytosis is a useful pointer to alcohol abuse in such patients [26].

Pancreatitis

Early reports linked alcoholism with not only chronic pancreatitis [13], but also with the more acute, and indeed fatal, hemorrhagic varieties of the disease [12, 37]. Alcohol is now recognized as being the major etiologic factor in chronic pancreatitis, and one of the more important causes of clinically acute pancreatitis. Many workers are of the opinion that chronic pathologic changes in the pancreas are invariably present even at this clinically acute stage of the disease, but this is probably an over-statement [23]. This, and other controversial issues relating to alcohol-induced pancreatitis (AIP), will be considered.

Does Alcohol Cause Acute Pancreatitis?

Alcohol is an important cause of clinically acute pancreatitis, the incidence varying according to the frequency of gallstones and the drinking habits of a particular community or country. The incidence of alcohol-induced disease in different countries is in the order of 9% in the United Kingdom, 31% in Europe, 50% in the United States and 61% in South Africa [21]. The latter figure derives mainly from a 1-year prospective study of 150 patients seen at Groote Schuur Hospital – alcohol accounted for 61%, gallstones 11%, miscellaneous causes 16%, and idiopathic causes 11% [20].

The vast majority of patients with clinically acute AIP have evidence of chronic pancreatitis, and this applies even to patients at the time of their first attack. The finding of normal pancreatic function in a small number of patients some months or years after a clinically acute attack of AIP, however, suggests that the latter is not incompatible with acute pancreatitis in the Marseilles context.

Although the Bologna group were unable to find a single patient with normal pancreatic function in a series of 21 patients tested 1–19 years after their first attack [17], the Cape Town group reported normal function in 6 of 21 patients when tested 6 months and 11 years after their first attack [25]. The Zurich group reported normal exocrine function in no fewer than 49 of 144 patients with AIP followed up for 2–10 years and, on the basis of these findings, coined the term "acute nonprogressive, alcoholic pancreatitis" [3]. The use of serial stool chymotrypsins rather than the more discriminatory pancreatic function test in their study almost certainly resulted in an overestimate of the true incidence of acute pancreatitis in AIP. Despite this, histologic evidence of chronic pancreatitis was found in only two of seven patients with "acute, nonprogressive AIP" in whom histology became available. These results contrast with those of an earlier follow-up study carried out by the same group [1].

It may be argued that a normal ERCP or pancreatic function test does not necessarily exclude early chronic pancreatitis, and that histology is mandatory to exclude such early lesions. Autopsy evidence is indeed available.
1. Weiner and Tennant [39] in their Yale study, found histologic changes of acute pancreatitis unassociated with chronic change in 25 of 27 patients who died during

the course of acute alcohol intoxication. One of these, a 16-year-old girl, died within 6 h of the onset of severe pain and vomiting which followed the drinking of "two large glasses of Italian wine."

2. Clark [8] reported on the autopsy findings in 36 cases of pancreatic disease in chronic alcoholics who died at the Bellevue Hospital, New York, over a 5-year period. Death was attributed to acute AIP in 15 of the 36 patients, and varying degrees of associated pancreatic fibrosis were found in 10 of the 15 cases.

3. A 29-year retrospective autopsy study from Los Angeles provides the most convincing evidence of the existence of acute AIP in the Marseilles context [32]. Four hundred and five of more than 50000 patients in the study were judged to have died from clinically acute pancreatitis. The pancreatitis was due to alcohol abuse in 247 and, of these, no fewer than 64% died during their first attack. Histologic evidence of chronic pancreatitis was present in addition to the acute changes in 116 (47%) cases, but no chronic changes were noted in the remaining 131 (53%). These three studies point very strongly to the existence of acute AIP in the Marseilles context in patients dying of clinically acute AIP. However, the high incidence of acute AIP in these autopsy studies does not necessarily reflect the overall incidence in AIP. The vast majority of the latter survive the clinically acute attack and, in them, the incidence is clearly lower.

Does the Magnitude of Alcohol Intake Influence Rate of Development of AIP?

While the etiologic role of alcohol in AIP is not in question, the precise mechanism of action of alcohol in the causation of this disease remains unclear. The pathogenesis of calcific AIP championed by Sarles et al. [34] is universally accepted and the sequence of protein plugs in the ducts, duct obstruction and dilatation, acinar cell atrophy, fibrosis, and eventual calcification of the plugs is beyond dispute. But there is less unanimity as to the primary alcohol-induced derangement at the molecular level in both acute and chronic AIP.

Other controversial aspects relate to the threshold of alcohol intake in AIP, the time interval between the onset of drinking and the first attack, and the influence of the magnitude of alcohol intake on the latter.

1. The threshold of alcohol intake in AIP was believed to be of the order of 50 g/day, but there is evidence to suggest that the threshold may be even lower [10, 33]. Most investigators, however, regard a minimum daily intake of 100 g [7] or even 120 g [17] as necessary to warrant inclusion in an AIP study group.

2. Although the occasional patient may develop AIP within a year of the commencement of heavy drinking, the vast majority suffer their first attack after about 3–20 years of alcohol overindulgence. More controversial is the observation that attacks tend to start on "the afternoon after the night before" [22]. This may be attributable to variations in the drinking pattern in different countries.

3. Sarles et al. [35] drew attention to the correlation between the magnitude of alcohol intake and the duration of alcoholism prior to the onset of calcification. This was supported by their observation that Japanese patients, with a mean intake of only 100 g/day, develop calcific AIP at the age of 45 years, whereas Brazilian patients, with a mean daily intake of about 400 g, develop their disease some 10

years earlier. Durbec and Sarles [10], surprisingly, were unable to confirm this correlation between mean daily intake and the duration of drinking in patients with AIP. The latter study raises the question of an individual susceptibility to alcohol.

These studies highlight problems in the assessment of alcohol intake, the reliability of such data in dedicated drinkers, and possible differences in the entry point of patients into a study (i. e, onset of first attack versus onset of calcification).

Disproportionate Steatorrhea

The natural history of chronic pancreatitis is that of progressive pancreatic dysfunction with the development of diabetes and steatorrhea. In the majority of patients diabetes precedes the onset of steatorrhea which, in our experience, is usually a late sequel of the disease. However, a small proportion of patients with chronic pancreatitis present with steatorrhea associated with only a mild or no abnormality, in glucose tolerance. We have designated this group, in which the magnitude of exocrine insufficiency is out of proportion to the endocrine dysfunction, as having "disproportionate steatorrhea." Girdwood et al. [15] were able to reconcile this clinical observation with the ERCP finding of an increased incidence of complete or incomplete obstruction of the proximal portion of the main pancreatic duct in patients with disproportionate steatorrhea. They concluded that proximal obstruction of the pancreatic duct, either complete or incomplete, contributes largely to the dominant clinical presentation of steatorrhea in some patients with chronic pancreatitis. The concept of disproportionate steatorrhea is shared by workers in Italy, Portugal, and Brazil, but is not accepted by others in the United Kingdom and the United States. It is not clear why pancreatic steatorrhea should be a late sequel of chronic pancreatitis in some countries, but not in others.

Incidence of Cirrhosis in AIP

Alcoholic cirrhosis, suprisingly, is an uncommon finding in patients with calcific pancreatitis. This certainly applies to France, Italy, and South Africa, where the prevalence of overt cirrhosis is of the order of only 2%–3%. Routine liver biopsies in 56 of our South African patients with calcific AIP revealed a frequency of the early changes of cirrhosis of only 9%. It should be noted, however, that rates as high as 40% have been reported from the United States in patients with less advanced forms of chronic pancreatitis.

On the other hand, about 50% of patients with alcoholic cirrhosis unassociated with abdominal pain show abnormal pancreatic function on testing [27]. This finding is supported by autopsy data in patients with portal cirrhosis [31, 39]. The study of Renner et al. [31] is of interest in that pancreatic disease was present in 49% of 783 autopsies in cases of lethal alcoholic liver disease. Of these, 8% were identified as acute AIP and the remaining 41% as chronic (20%), calcific (4%), and dominant fibrosis (17%). The frequency of classic ERCP changes of chronic pancreatitis in alcoholic cirrhosis remains uncertain [11], but the 4% incidence of calcific disease in the study by Renner et al. [31] supports the view that the association of cirrhosis with calcific AIP is an uncommon one.

Again, the available data do not answer the question as to whether involvement of the liver or pancreas reflects an individual susceptibility of one or other of these organs to alcohol.

Does the Pancreas Burn Itself Out?

The natural history of chronic AIP is characterized by recurrent attacks of pain which tend to diminish in frequency and severity with the passage of time. This is associated with progressive parenchymal fibrosis and eventual calcification, changes reflected by the progressive impairment of endocrine and exocrine function on the one hand, and increasingly abnormal ERCP changes on the other.

This generalization would appear to apply to the majority of patients and, in them, a good correlation has been found between diminution in the severity of attacks and progressive pancreatic dysfunction [2, 14]. The role of alcohol and/or pancreatic duct stricture or dilatation in the causation of pain, so important in the early stages of the disease, appears less relevant in patients with calcific AIP and this, too, has been linked with progressive pancreatic insufficiency [5, 6, 24].

These findings have given rise to the perception that, with time, the painful pancreas will "burn itself out." Dr Ammann & Dr Girdwood will probably address this burning issue during the course of this meeting, but I would like to end with a note of caution. The concept may be flawed by a statistical bias since the higher early mortality in patients with severe disease may reduce the incidence of pain in late follow-up groups [18]. And there is the real possibility that the concept may have little relevance in the subgroup of surgical candidates with intractable pain. The reluctance of surgeons to temporize with medical measures while waiting for the pancreas "to burn itself out" [38] appears to have been vindicated by the results of a 10-year prospective study in patients with intractable pain unassociated with cyst formation [16]. Despite alcohol withdrawal, the intractable pain continued to haunt the patients and their doctors.

References

1. Ammann RW, Hammer B, Fumagalli I (1973) Chronic pancreatitis inZurich 1963–1972. Digestion 9:404–415
2. Ammann RW, Largiader F, Akovbiantz A (1979) Pain relief by surgery in chronic pancreatitis? Relationship between pain relief, pancreatic dysfunction, and alcohol withdrawal. Scand J Gastroenterol 14:209–215
3. Ammann RW, Buehler H, Bruehlmann W, Kehl D, Muench R, Stamm B (1986) Acute (non-progressive) alcoholic pancreatitis: prospective longitudinal study of 144 patients with recurrent alcoholic pancreatitis. Pancreas 1:195–203
4. Beaumont W (1959) Experiments and observations on the gastric juice, and the physiology of digestion. Dover, New York (Original 1833)
5. Bornman PC, Marks IN, Girdwood AH, et al. (1980) Is pancreatic duct obstruction or stricture a major cause of pain in calcific pancreatitis? Br J Surg 67:425–428

6. Bornman PC, Girdwood AH, Marks IN, Hatfield ARW, Kottler RE (1982) The influence of continued alcohol intake, pancreatic duct hold-up, and pancreatic insufficiency on the pain pattern in chronic noncalcific and calcific pancreatitis: a comparative study. Surg Gastroenterol 1:5–9

7. Cavallini G, Angelini G, Vantini I, Scuro LA (1984) Relationship between morphological (ERP) and functional (secretin-caerulin infusion test) findings in chronic relapsing pancreatitis and following acute pancreatitis. In: Gyr KE, Singer MV, Sarles H (eds) Pancreatitis: concepts and classification. Excerpta Medica, Amsterdam, pp 307–315

8. Clark E (1942) Pancreatitis in acute and chronic alcoholism. Am J Dig Dis 9:428–431

9. Cooper WE, Schwär TG, Smith LS (1979) Alcohol, drugs and road traffic. Juta, Cape Town

10. Durbec JP, Sarles H (1984) Epidemiology of chronic pancreatitis. Alcohol and dietary habits. In: Gyr KE, Singer MV, Sarles H (eds) Pancreatitis: concepts and classification. Excerpta Medica, Amsterdam, pp 352–353

11. Elsborg L, Bruusgaard A, Strandgaard L, Reinicke V (1981) Endoscopic retrograde pancreatography and the exocrine pancreatic function in chronic alcoholism. Scand J Gastroenterol 15:395–399

12. Fitz RH (1889) Acute pancreatitis: a consideration of pancreatic hemorrhage, hemorrhage, suppurative, and gangrenous pancreatitis and of disseminated fat necrosis. Med Rec NY 35:197

13. Friedreich N (1878) Diseases of the pancreas. In: Cyclopedia of the practice of medicine, vol 8. Wood, New York

14. Girdwood AH, Marks IN, Bornman PC, Kottler RE, Cohen M (1981) Does progressive pancreatic insufficiency limit pain in calcific pancreatitis with duct stricture or continued alcohol insult? J Clin Gastroenterol 3:241–245

15. Girdwood AH, Marks IN, Hatfield ARW, Bornman PC, Kottler RE (1985) Disproportionate steatorrhoea in alcohol-induced pancreatitis. S Afr Med J 68:876–877

16. Girdwood AH, Bornman PC, Marks IN (1987) Intractable pain in alcohol-induced chronic pancreatitis – can one wait for the pancreas to burn itself out? S Afr Med J 72:64

17. Gullo L, Durbec JP (1984) Epidemiology and etiology of pancreatitis. In: Gyr KE, Singer MV, Sarles H (eds) Pancreatitis: concepts and classification. Excerpta Medica, Amsterdam, pp 371–376

18. Hayakawa T, Kondo T, Shibata T, Sugimoto Y, Kitagawa M (1989) Chronic alcoholism and evolution of pain and prognosis in chronic pancreatitis. Dig Dis Sci 34:33–38

19. Lanza FL, Royer GL, Nielson RS, Rack MF (1982) A single blind randomized study of the potentiating effect of alcohol on the gastric and duodenal mucosa injury seen with aspirin and ibuprofen. Am J Gastroenterol 77:699

20. Madden MV, Goodman H, Bornman PC, Lipschitz EM, Marks IN (1986) Causes of acute pancreatitis and incidence and course of peripancreatic fluid collections. S Afr Med J 70:53

21. Marks IN (1986) Epidemiology of pancreatitis. Dig Dis Sci 31:526S

22. Marks IN, Bank S (1963) The etiology, clinical features and diagnosis of pancreatitis in the South Western Cape: a review of 243 cases. S Afr Med J 37:1039–1053

23. Marks IN, Bank S (1985) Chronic pancreatitis: etiology, clinical aspects, and medical management. In: Berk JE (ed) Bockus gastroenterology, vol 6, 4th edn. Saunders, Philadelphia, pp 4020–4040

24. Marks IN, Girdwood AH, Banks S, Louw JH (1980) The prognosis of alcohol-induced calcific pancreatitis. S Afr Med J 57:640–643

25. Marks IN, Girdwood AH, Bornman PC, Feretis C (1984) The prevalence and etiology of pancreatitis in Cape Town. In: Gyr KE, Singer MV, Sarles H (eds) Pancreatitis: concepts and classification. Excerpta Medica, Amsterdam, pp 345–346

26. Marotta F, Lipschitz EM, Marks IN, Bornman PC, Madden M, Kirsch RE (1987) AST/ALT ratio, MCV and GGT in acute pancreatitis – an aid in differentiating the etiology. S Afr Med J 72:63

27. Mezey E, Jow E, Slavin RE, Tobon F (1970) Pancreatic function and intestinal absorption in chronic alcoholism. Gastroenterology 59:657–664

28. Palmer ED (1954) Gastritis. A re-evaluation. Medicine (Baltimore) 33:199–290

29. Perlow W, Baraona E, Lieber CS (1977) Symptomatic intestinal disaccharidase deficiency in alcoholics. Gastroenterology 72:680–685

30. Pirola RC, Lieber CS (1972) The energy cost of the metabolism of drugs including alcohol. Pharmacology 7:185–196
31. Renner IG, Savage WT, Stace NH, Pantoja JL, Schultheis WM, Peters RL (1984) Pancreatitis associated with alcoholic liver disease: a review of 1022 autopsy cases. Dig Dis Sci 29:593–599
32. Renner IG, Savage WT, Pantoja JL, Renner VJ (1985) Death due to acute pancreatitis: a retrospective analysis of 405 autopsy cases. Dig Dis Sci 30:1005–1018
33. Sarles H (1985) Review: chronic calcifying pancreatitis. Scand J Gastroenterol 20:651–659
34. Sarles H, Payan H, Tasso F, Sahel J (1976) Chronic pancreatitis, relapsing pancreatitis, calcifications of the pancreas: pathology. In: Bockus HL (ed) Gastroenterology, vol 6, 3rd edn. Saunders, Philadelphia, pp 1040–1051
35. Sarles H, Sahel J, Staub JL, Bourry J, Laugier R (1979) Chronic pancreatitis. In: Howat HT, Sarles H (eds) The exocrine pancreas. Saunders, London, pp 402–439
36. Shaw S, Lieber CS (1988) Nutrition and diet in alcoholism. In: Shils ME, Young VR (eds) Modern nutrition in health and disease, 7th edn. Lea and Febiger, Philadelphia, pp 1423–1449
37. Symners WSTC (1917) Acute alcoholic pancreatitis. Dublin J Med Sci 143:244
38. Warshaw AL (1984) Pain in chronic pancreatitis: patients, patience and the impatient surgeon. Gastroenterology 86:987–989
39. Weiner HA, Tennant R (1938) A statistical study of acute hemorrhagic pancreatitis (hemorrhagic necrosis of pancreas). Am J Med Sci 196:167–176
40. Wolf S, Wolff HG (1943) Human gastric function. An experimental study of a man and his stomach. Oxford University Press, Oxford

Non-Alcohol-Related Etiologies in Chronic Pancreatitis

P. LAYER and M. V. SINGER[1]

In addition to alcohol, which is the most important cause of chronic pancreatitis, several other, nonalcoholic conditions have been associated with chronic pancreatitis; thus, nutritional, metabolic, and mechanical disturbances, as well as a hereditary disposition, have been implicated:

1. Tropical	6. Trauma
2. Hyperlipidemia (?)	7. Pancreas divisum (?)
3. Hyperparathyroidism	8. Hereditary
4. Biliary disease (?)	9. Idiopathic
5. Obstruction	

However, not all of these etiologies are proven, and some are unlikely or controversial.

Tropical chronic pancreatitis

Tropical chronic pancreatitis, which is one of the major nutritional forms of chronic pancreatitis, is an important disease among juveniles and young adults in several countries in tropical Africa, Indonesia, and southern India. Its etiology and pathogenesis are not known. Traditionally, it had been associated with protein malnutrition, but more recent evidence suggests that other factors such as toxic products in certain nutritional components (cassava) or deficiency of trace elements (selenium, zinc, copper) may be more important [21]. A more detailed description of tropical chronic pancreatitis will be given in another chapter.

Hyperlipemia

Hyperlipemia, an important cause of acute pancreatitis, has also been considered a cause of chronic pancreatitis but so far there is no convincing evidence.

---

[1] Abteilung für Gastroenterologie, Zentrum für Innere Medizin, Universitätsklinikum, Hufelandstr. 55, 4300 Essen 1, FRG

Chronic Pancreatitis
Ed. by Beger, Büchler, Ditschuneit, and Malfertheiner
© Springer-Verlag Berlin Heidelberg 1990

Hyperparathyroidism

Hyperparathyroidism can be complicated by both acute and chronic pancreatitis; calcifications are found frequently. The pathomechanism is hypothetical.

Effects of Hypercalcemia on Pancreatic Enzyme and Volume Secretion

Acute hypercalcemia is a potent stimulus of human pancreatic enzyme secretion [9, 16]. Experimental evidence suggests that both direct action of high extracellular calcium concentrations on the acinar cellular level [18] and indirect mechanisms such as release of cholecystokinin and other peptide hormones [16] are involved in its mediation. Therefore it had been assumed that hyperparathyroidism may cause continuous and excessive, pathological stimulation of the acinar cell which then could lead to pancreatitis. However, chronic disturbance of acinar cell function in vivo due to elevated serum calcium levels is unlikely, because experimental chronic hypercalcemia for up to 3 months did not lead to continuous stimulation of enzyme secretion [13]. Rather, hypercalcemia caused significant reduction in volume and bicarbonate secretion.

Effect of Hypercalcemia on Pancreatic Calcium Secretion

Chronic hypercalcemia causes a strong increase in pancreatic calcium secretion. This has been observed both in patients with hyperparathyroidism [8] and in experimental animals [13]. In the latter studies, a major proportion of intraductal calcium precipitated in native pancreatic juice. This was partly due to elevated interstitial calcium concentrations in hypercalcemia, because the enzyme-independent calcium fraction in pancreatic juice is secreted proportional to serum calcium levels [14]. Moreover, chronic hypercalcemia caused a significant decrease in the pancreatic diffusion barrier between the interstitial compartment and the ductular system (Fig. 1). Therefore, the intrapancreatic permeability for calcium increased, with the consequence that excessive amounts of calcium diffused from the interstitial fluid into the juice: Per millimole calcium in the serum, significantly more calcium appeared in the pancreatic juice [13, 14].

Hypothetical Pathomechanism

In combination, increased serum calcium levels and increased intrapancreatic permeability for calcium (Fig. 1), as well as inhibition of fluid secretion, may be responsible for the pancreatic changes induced by chronic hypercalcemia: Excessive quantities of calcium in reduced pancreatic juice may promote intraductal calcium precipitation in alkaline secretion, leading to a pathogenic pathway that is discussed for alcoholic chronic pancreatitis. Conversely, diffusion of protein-independent calcium into pancreatic juice increases in the course of chronic pancreatitis [7, 17], which may lead to further damage of the organ.

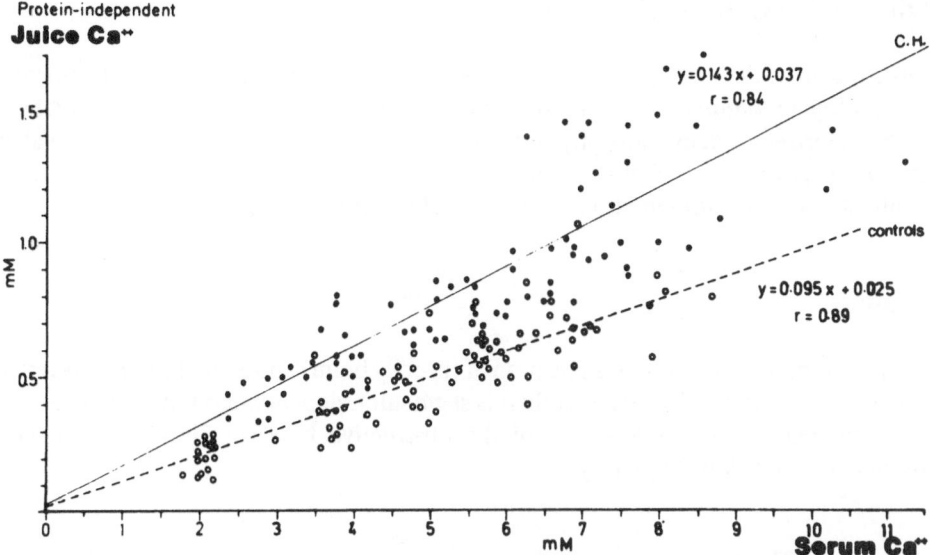

Fig. 1. Pathogenesis of hypercalcemia-induced pancreatitis: Correlation between protein-independent juice calcium and serum calcium concentrations in chronic hypercalcemia *(CH)* and controls. The significantly steeper slope in *CH* indicates increased permeation of calcium into the juice at a given serum calcium level, suggesting increased permeability due to decreased diffusion threshold (From ref. [13] with permission)

Incidence

The incidence of pancreatitis in hyperparathyroidism was estimated to be 5%–10% in earlier studies [20], but more recent surveys suggest that it may be no more than 1%–2% [4]; moreover, the majority of cases are now acute pancreatitis, often precipitated by acute hypercalcemic crises [12]. These data suggest that the incidence of chronic pancreatitis in hyperparathyroidism may be decreasing. A likely explanation is that serum calcium concentration is now measured routinely in virtually all patients that undergo a medical checkup. As a consequence, hyperparathyroidism does not remain undiscovered and untreated for many years; by contrast, before routine measurement of serum calcium levels, hyperparathyroidism used to be a very insidious disease, usually diagnosed only by its late complications [5, 20]. Due to its early detection, hyperparathyroidism is now a rare cause for chronic pancreatitis.

Gallstones

Biliary disorders are important causes for acute pancreatitis; they may induce relapses if not removed intermittently. However, it is unlikely that gallstones can also cause chronic pancreatitis.

Obstructive Chronic Pancreatitis

Obstruction of the main pancreatic duct by tumor, benign Vaterian stenosis, fibrotic scars (often in *traumatic pancreatitis*), and pseudocysts leads to a distinct entity which is characterized by acinar atrophy and fibrosis that may be reversible upon removal of the obstructive cause. Similarly, resulting exocrine insufficiency is reversible. In contrast to other, inflammatory forms, ductal structures are preserved.

Trauma

Traumatic pancreatitis is a complication of (usually blunt) abdominal trauma, often in the median portion. Most frequently it is segmental, dependent on the site of lesion. Its pathogenesis may follow that of the obstructive type, but inflammation and pseudocysts develop frequently.

Pancreas Divisum

Whether pancreas divisum disposes to chronic pancreatitis [6] is disputed controversially; the topic is covered in a separate article.

Hereditary Chronic Pancreatitis

Hereditary chronic pancreatitis often appears in childhood, at a mean age of 10–12 years, but a later onset of symptoms is possible. The disease is inherited through an autosomal-dominant gene of incomplete penetrance. This pattern explains the even sex distribution of the disease [10]. There is no evidence that specific HLA haplotypes are coupled to pancreatitis [15]. The diagnosis should be suspected if several members develop pancreatitis in the absence of alcohol consumption or other causes of chronic pancreatitis. An example of the distribution of the disease in the offspring from both marriages of a man married twice is shown in Fig. 2.

Idiopathic Chronic Pancreatitis

Epidemiology

In the Western World nonalcoholic chronic pancreatitis of defined etiology is rare; together this group comprises < 5% of all cases. Most investigators agree that the major form of nonalcoholic chronic pancreatitis in Europe and North America is of the idiopathic type (10%–40%). A subgroup of older patients within idiopathic pancreatitis was first described by Ammann, who suggested that this senile form of nonalcoholic chronic pancreatitis might be caused by arteriosclerosis ("vascular chronic pancreatitis" [1–3].

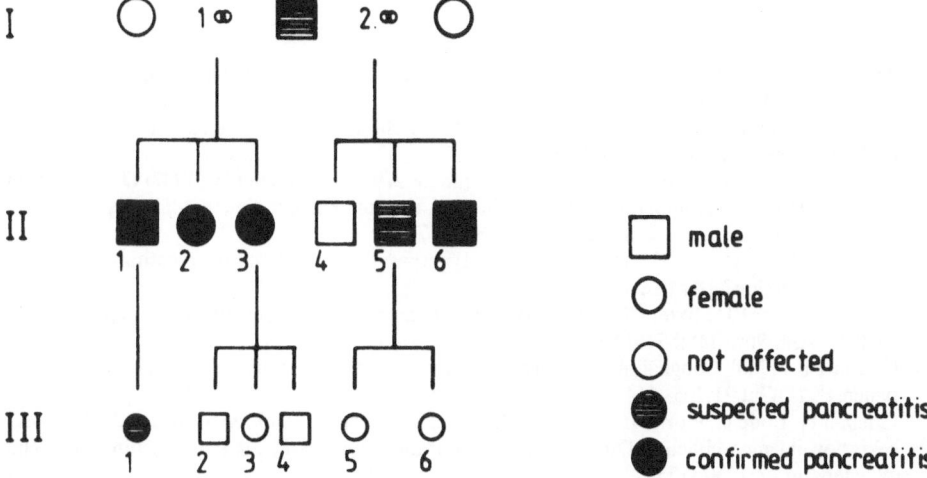

Fig. 2. Hereditary pancreatitis: family tree with three generations of a family with hereditary pancreatitis. (From ref. [15]; with permission)

Own data obtained in patients with definite idiopathic chronic pancreatitis suggest that this group may be composed of two distinct groups: a juvenile type of idiopathic chronic pancreatitis with a median age of 18 years at onset of symptomatic disease, and a senile type with an incidence peak at approximately 60 years. By contrast, age distribution at onset of symptomatic disease in the alcoholic group follows a typical bell-shaped pattern with an incidence peak between 35 and 45 years. In both idiopathic groups, both sexes were equally distributed [11, 19], while the male sex is more prevalent in alcoholic pancreatitis. Epidemiology and natural course of both types of idiopathic chronic pancreatitis differ from each other and from definite alcoholic disease.

Natural History

In juvenile chronic pancreatitis, severe pain dominates the clinical picture at initial presentation, whereas, in senile chronic pancreatitis, primary painless disease is frequent. The further course appears to differ among both groups: Compared with alcoholic patients, juvenile idiopathic chronic pancreatitis tended to develop calcification, exocrine insufficiency, diabetes, and complications of chronic pancreatitis less often and later. On the other hand, in senile idiopathic chronic pancreatitis, initially a large proportion of patients present with exocrine insufficiency, diabetes and/or calcification. This reflects the manifestation of symptomatic disease in primary painless chronic pancreatitis [19].

References

1. Ammann RW (1976) Zur vaskulären Genese der chronischen Pankreatitis. Dtsch Med Wochenschr 101:867–868
2. Ammann RW, Sulser H (1976) Die „senile" chronische Pankreatitis – eine neue nosologische Einheit? Schweiz Med Wochenschr 106:429–437
3. Ammann RW, Buehler H, Muench R, Freiburghaus AW, Siegenthaler W (1987) Differences in the natural history of idiopathic (nonalcoholic) and alcoholic chronic pancreatitis. A comparative long-term study of 287 patients. Pancreas 2:368–377
4. Bess MA, Edis AJ, van Heerden JA (1980) Hyperparathyroidism and pancreatitis – chance or causal association? JAMA 243:246–247
5. Cope O, Culver PJ, Mixter CG, Nardi GL (1957) Pancreatitis, a diagnostic clue to hyperparathyroidism. Ann Surg 145:857–863
6. Cotton PB (1980) Congenital anomaly of pancreas divisum as cause of obstructive pain and pancreatitis. Gut 21:105–114
7. Goebell H, Bode C, Horn HD (1970) Einfluß von Sekretin und Pankreozymin auf die Calciumsekretion im menschlichen Duodenalsaft bei normaler und gestörter Pankreasfunktion. Klin Wochenschr 48:1330–1339
8. Goebell H, Horn HD, Bode C, Gossmann HH (1970) Primärer Hyperparathyreoidismus und exokrine Pankreasfunktion: Störungen der Enzym- und Elektrolytsekretion im Duodenalsaft. Klin Wochenschr 48:810–819
9. Goebell H, Steffen C, Baltzer G, Bode C (1973) Stimulation of pancreatic secretion of enzymes by acute hypercalcemia in man. Eur J Clin Invest 3:98–104
10. Gross JB (1986) Hereditary pancreatitis. In: Go VLW, et al. (eds) The exocrine pancreas. Raven, New York
11. Kalthoff L, Layer P, Clain JE, DiMagno EP (1984) The course of alcoholic and nonalcoholic chronic pancreatitis. Dig Dis Sci 29:953
12. Kelly RT, Falor WH (1968) Hyperparathyroid crises associated with pancreatitis. Ann Surg 168:917–926
13. Layer P, Hotz J, Schmitz-Moormann HP, Goebell H (1982) Effects of experimental chronic hypercalcemia on feline exocrine pancreatic secretion. Gastroenterology 82:309–316
14. Layer P, Hotz J, Goebell H (1983) Calcium secretion from the feline pancreas: influence of hormonal and cholinergic secretagogues and of serum calcium. Digestion 26:89–98
15. Layer P, Balzer K, Goebell H (1985) Hereditary pancreatitis: presentation of another family. Hepatogastroenterology 32:31–33
16. Layer P, Hotz J, Eysselein VE, Jansen JBMJ, Lamers CBHW, Schmitz-Moormann HP, Goebell H (1985) The effects of acute hypercalcemia on exocrine pancreatic secretion in the cat. Gastroenterology 88:1168–1174
17. Layer P, Hotz J, Noske A, Goebell H (1986) Duodenal calcium in chronic pancreatitis: is it of diagnostic value? Digestion 34:22–27
18. Layer P, Hotz J, Cherian L, Goebell H (1987) In vitro stimulation of pancreatic enzyme discharge by elevated extracellular calcium concentrations. Gut 28:1215–1220
19. Layer P, Kalthoff L, Clain JE, DiMagno EP (1985) Nonalcoholic chronic pancreatitis – two diseases? Dig Dis Sci 30:980
20. Mixter CG, Keynes WM, Cope O (1962) Further experience with pancreatitis as diagnostic clue to hyperparathyroidism. N Engl J Med 266:265–272
21. Pitchumoni CS (1984) "Tropical" or "nutritional pancreatitis" – an update. In: Gyr KE, Singer MV, Sarles H (eds) Pancreatitis – concepts and classification. Elsevier, Amsterdam

Chronic Pancreatitis with Inflammatory Mass in the Head of the Pancreas: A Special Entity?

M. Büchler, P. Malfertheiner, H. Friess, T. Senn, and H. G. Beger[1]

From a histopathological point of view, chronic alcoholic pancreatitis generally involves the whole pancreas [1–3]. However there is a small subgroup of patients (5%–10%), obviously in an early phase of the development of the disease, who suffer from focal lesions of chronic pancreatitis. Mainly data from surgical literature have shown that patients with chronic pancreatitis undergoing surgery for pain or complications often exhibit a preponderant lesion either in the right (head) or in the left part (body and tail) of the gland. For this reason, surgical techniques in chronic pancreatitis have been developed and applied either to resect the pancreatic head and preserve the body and tail or vice versa [4, 5].

It is surprising how few data exist regarding the prevalence of preponderant pathological lesions involving the head, body, or tail of the pancreas which lead to specific complications of the disease. This phenomenon must have something to do with the improved technique of imaging procedures which have only recently begun to be applied routinely in patients with chronic pancreatitis.

There are several reasons why we have been specifically interested in patients showing an inflammatory mass in the head of the pancreas as part of a focal lesion:

1. From a pathophysiological and pathogenetic point of view, it seems likely that an inflammatory process located in the head of the pancreas influences the natural course of the disease like a "pacemaker" of chronic pancreatitis [6]. This is due to the complications resulting from this inflammatory tumor in the head of the pancreas such as obstruction of the main pancreatic duct system, obstruction of the extrahepatic bile duct, obstruction of the duodenum, and sometimes involvement of major intestinal vessels such as the superior mesenteric vein and artery.

2. Resection of the head of the pancreas in these patients, either by a modification of the Whipple procedure or by a pancreatic head resection which preserves the duodenum, leads to excellent results in pain relief [7–9], and the excision of the inflammatory pancreatic head region alone provides favorable long-term results in chronic pancreatitis, which might be due to an interruption of the so-called natural course of chronic pancreatitis [10, 11].

3. We recently demonstrated that the inflammatory changes in patients suffering from pancreatic head enlargement are specific lesions with regard to nerve histopathology and ultrastructure [12], neurotransmitter changes [13, 14], and the type of inflammatory cellular elements inducing these alterations [15].

---

[1] Departments of Surgery and Gastroenterology, University of Ulm, Steinhövelstrasse 9, D-7900 Ulm, FRG

Chronic Pancreatitis
Ed. by Beger, Büchler, Ditschuneit, and Malfertheiner
© Springer-Verlag Berlin Heidelberg 1990

The aim of this investigation was to analyze the prevalence and clinical role of an inflammatory mass in the head of the pancreas in patients with chronic pancreatitis.

Definition

An inflammatory pancreatic head enlargement was defined as a vertical pancreatic head diameter of 4 cm or more, as shown by ultrasonography, contrast enhanced computed tomography (CT) scan and/or intraoperative findings. Patients with solid, cystic, or mixed solid and cystic inflammatory masses in the head of the pancreas were included.

The size of 4 cm or more was chosen to characterize an inflammatory enlargement after a previous ultrasonographic investigation in healthy volunteers had shown a mean vertical pancreatic head diameter of 20.8 ± 0.6 mm (x $\pm$ SEM) [16]. Moreover several investigations have demonstrated that the human pancreatic head diameter is considered to be normal up to 25–30 mm [17] using ultrasonographic criteria.

Patient Population

Since 1982, 279 patients suffering from chronic pancreatitis (216 male, 63 female) have been recruited and treated in the Departments of General Surgery and Gastroenterology at the University of Ulm. The mean age of these patients was 42 years (range 19–76 years). The diagnosis of chronic pancreatitis was based upon at least one imaging procedure [endoscopic retrograde cholangiopancreatography (ERCP) and/or ultrasonography and/or contrast-enhanced CT scan] and one exocrine pancreatic function test (urine and/or serum pancreolauryl test and/or secretin-ceruletide test). In addition, histological confirmation of chronic pancreatitis was provided in 195 (70%) out of 279 study patients undergoing surgery.

Prevalence of Pancreatic Head Enlargement in Patients with Chronic pancreatitis

Out of 279 patients with chronic pancreatitis, 138 (49%) had an inflammatory pancreatic head enlargement shown by imaging procedures or intraoperative findings. The age and sex distributions were comparable in patients with and without pancreatic head enlargement (Table 1).

Table 1. Age and sex distribution of patients with and without pancreatic head enlargement

	Patients with pancreatic head enlargement	Patients without pancreatic head enlargement
mean age (range)	44.5 (22–76)	42.2 (19–76)
no. of men (%)	110 (79%)	108 (77%)
no. of women (%)	28 (21%)	33 (23%)

History and Clinical Signs

Of all patients included, 82% showed a clear-cut clinical history of long-term over-indulgence in alcohol; there were no differences between those patients with inflammatory pancreatic head enlargement and those without. The duration of symptoms (pain) up to the diagnosis of chronic pancreatitis was comparable in both groups (Table 2), whereas the median duration of symptoms until surgery was 70% longer (54 months) in the patients without inflammatory pancreatic head enlargement (Table 2).

Table 2. Duration of symptoms until diagnosis in patients with and without pancretic head enlargement

Duration until diagnosis	Patients with head enlargement ($n = 138$)	Patients without head enlargement ($n = 141$)
< 24 months	58%	63%
24–48 months	15%	13%
> 48 months	27%	24%

The quality and intensity of pain was scored as follows:

Stage I   slight or no pain
Stage II   frequent pain attacks
Stage III   daily pain attacks
Stage IV   daily severe pain

Two thirds of patients with pancreatic head enlargement suffered from daily (Stage III) or daily severe (Stage IV) pain, whereas 60% of those without pancreatic head enlargement had pain scores in Stages I and II (Table 3).

Table 3. Pain scores in patients with and without pancreatic head enlargement

Stage	Patients with head enlargement ($n = 138$)	Patients without head enlargement ($n = 141$)
I	6%	17% ⎫
		⎬ 60%
II	27%	43% ⎭
III	33% ⎫	32%
	⎬ 67%	
IV	34% ⎭	8%

Of all patients, 121 (88%) with and 72 (51%) without inflammatory head enlargement underwent surgery during the observation period. The surgical procedures performed were duodenum-preserving pancreatic head resection in 129 patients, cystojejunostomy in 35 patients, left resection of the pancreas in 11 patients, a Puestow procedure in 9 patients, and other procedures in 11 patients.

Complications of Chronic Pancreatitis

Patients with pancreatic head enlargement suffered significantly more frequently from complications of chronic pancreatitis (Table 4). There was a cholestasis syndrome in 46% and 11% of patients with and without head enlargement, respectively. Similarly, more patients with pancreatic head enlargement suffered from duodenal obstruction (30% versus 7%) and pancreatic duct stenosis (53% versus 32%). There was no difference regarding the prevalence of pancreatic pseudocysts (61% versus 51%) and vascular involvement (15% versus 8%) in our patients with chronic pancreatitis.

Table 4. Complications of chronic pancreatitis in patients with and without pancreatic head enlargement

Type of complication	Patients with head enlargement	Patients without head enlargement
Common bile duct obstruction	64/138 (46%)	16/141 (11%)
Pancreatic duct stenosis	72/135 (53%)	45/141 (32%)
Duodenal obstruction	37/122 (30%)	9/121 (7%)
Cysts	77/127 (60%)	43/ 85 (51%)
Vascular involvement	18/122 (15%)	6/ 73 (8%)

Pancreatic Function

To check pancreatic exocrine function, we performed a urine pancreolauryl test [18] in 43 patients and a serum pancreolauryl test [19] in 60 patients. The median T/K ratio of urine pancreolauryl test was 27% (4%–76%) in patients with head enlargement (11 patients tested) and 16% (0.2%–75%) in patients without head enlargement (32 patients tested). A comparable relationship showing impaired but better preserved exocrine pancreatic function in patients with pancreatic head enlargement was demonstrated by the test results of the serum pancreolauryl investigation (Fig. 1). Patients without pancreatic head enlargement had a significantly worse serum fluorescein concentration curve (area under the curve) than those with head enlargement.

Endocrine pancreatic function was analyzed by administrating an oral glucose load. Insulin-dependent diabetes mellitus was shown to be present in 18% (25/138) of patients with head enlargement and in 30% (42/141) ($p < 0.05$) of patients without.

Final Considerations

Our hypothesis seems to be valid that an inflammatory pancreatic head enlargement is a frequent and, with regard to clinical implication, important specific entity in chronic pancreatitis. Patients with an inflammatory mass in the head of the pancreas (diameter 4 cm or more) show a higher pain score, more typical complications of chronic pancreatitis, and, at the time of clinical presentation, better preserved pancreatic

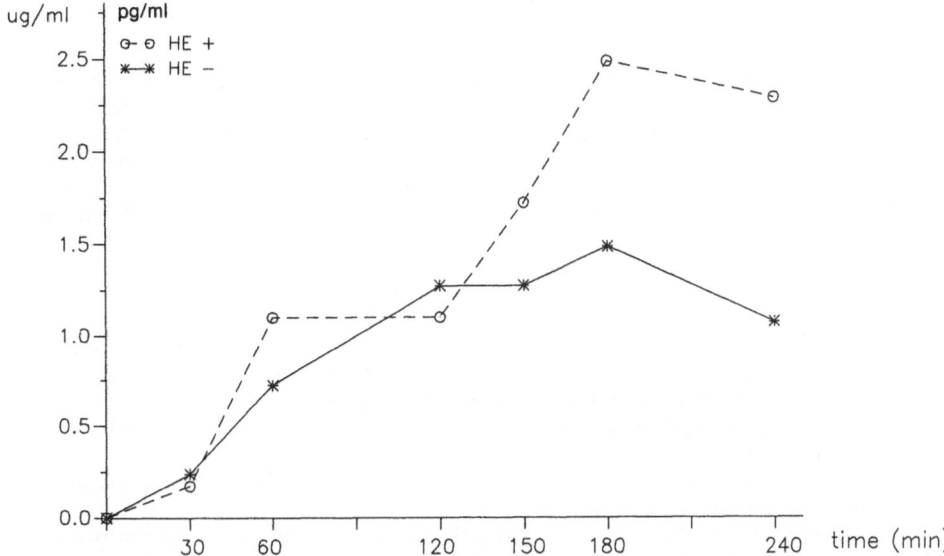

Fig. 1. Serum course of fluorescein following oral ingestion (test meal) of 0.5 mmol fluorescein dilaurate and simultaneous i.v. administration of metoclopramide and secretin. The normal range (healthy volunteers) of peak serum fluorescein is above 4.5 µg/ml. Both serum curves of the patients ($n = 60$) analyzed are in a pathological range. However, the area under the serum curve of patients suffering from pancreatic head enlargement *(HE +)* is significantly greater than that of patients with chronic pancreatitis but without head enlargement *(HE −)*. Values are medians

exocrine and endocrine function than patients without pancreatic head enlargement. The prevalence of almost 50% of patients with pancreatic head enlargement in our patient population is certainly caused in part by a selection bias in the Ulm population. Many patients with head enlargement are referred to us for a duodenum-preserving pancreatic head resection. On the other hand, it would be worthwhile to compare the Ulm population with other large patient populations to clarify the real prevalence of this entity.

It seems completely uncertain why some patients with chronic pancreatitis develop an inflammatory tumor in the head of the pancreas while others, probably the majority, do not from an embryological point of view. It seems likely that underlying anatomical features may play an important role such as ductal morphology.

It might well be that the development of pancreatic head enlargement during the natural course of chronic pancreatitis leads to an earlier diagnosis of chronic pancreatitis because pain and complications induce the patient to seek the advice of a doctor. On the other hand, patients who do not develop an inflammatory mass in the head of the pancreas come to the clinic later. Therefore, one might speculate that the whole problem of pancreatic head enlargement is a phenomenon occurring early during the natural course of disease.

However, in nerves and immune cells the specific inflammatory changes in the pancreatic head region and the favorable long-term results obtained after pancreatic head resection in these patients support the hypothesis of a specific disease entity.

References

1. Becker V (1984) Chronische Pankreatitis, Klinische Morphologie, In: Bartelheimer H, Kühn HA, Becker V, Stelzner F (eds) Gastroenterologie und Stoffwechsel, vol 21. Thieme, Stuttgart
2. Reber HA (1987) Chronic pancreatitis, etiology, pathology, and diagnosis. In: Howard JM, Jordan GL Jr, Reber HA (eds) Surgical diseases of the pancreas. Lea and Febiger, Philadelphia, pp 475–495
3. Münch R, Ammann RW (1989) Entwicklungsstadien der chronischen Pankreatitis. Internist 30:738–746
4. Howard JM (1987) Surgical treatment of chronic pancreatitis, principles, applications, results. In: Howard JM, Jordan GL Jr, Reber HA (eds) Surgical diseases of the pancreas, Lea and Febiger, Philadelphia, pp 496–521
5. Adson MA, McIlrath DC (1986) Surgical treatment of chronic pancreatitis. In: Go VLW, Gardner JD, Brooks FP, Lebenthal E, DiMagno EP, Scheele GA (eds) The exocrine pancreas: biology, pathobiology, and diseases. Raven, New York, pp 587–599
6. Traverso LW (1990) Preservation of the pylorus during pancreaticoduodenectomy for chronic pancreatitis. (This volume)
7. Greenlee HB, Prinz RA, Aranha GV (1990) Long-term results of side-to-side pancreatico-jejunostomy. World J Surg 14:70–76
8. Zirngibl H, Gall FP (1990) Results of the Whipple procedure in combination with pancreatic duct occlusion. (this volume)
9. Beger HG, Krautzberger W, Bittner R, Büchler M, Limmer J (1985) Duodenum-preserving resection of the head of the pancreas in patients with severe chronic pancreatitis. Surgery 97:467–473
10. Beger HG, Büchler M, Bittner R, Oettinger W, Roscher R (1989) Duodenum-preserving resection of the head of the pancreas in severe chronic pancreatitis – early and late results. Ann Surg 209:273–278
11. Beger HG, Büchler M (1990) Duodenum-preserving resection of the head of the pancreas in chronic pancreatitis with inflammatory mass in the head. World J Surg 14:83–87
12. Bockman DE, Büchler M, Malfertheiner P, Beger HG (1988) Analysis of nerves in chronic pancreatitis. Gastroenterology 94:1459–1469
13. Büchler M, Malfertheiner P, Weihe E, Frieß H, Beger HG (1988) Neurotransmitters in nerves in chronic pancreatitis. Pancreas 3:592
14. Weihe E, Büchler M, Müller S, Frieß H, Zentel HF, Yanaihara N (1990) Peptidergic innervation in chronic pancreatitis. (This volume)
15. Büchler M, Weihe E, Malfertheiner P, Frieß H, Bockman DA, Beger HG (1989) Changes in peptiderigic innervation and neuroimmune cross-talk in chronic pancreatitis. Digestion 43[3]:134
16. Büchler M, Malfertheiner P, Frieß H, Seitz J, Rolle K, Nustede R, Schafmayer A, Beger HG (1989) Pancreatic and GI-hormone adaptation following long-term camostate treatment in man. Pancreas 5:612
17. Weill FS (1978) Ultrasonography of digestive diseases. Masby, St. Louis
18. Lankisch PG, Schreiber A, Otto J (1983) Pancreolauryl test. Dig Dis Sci 28:490–493
19. Malfertheiner P, Büchler M, Müller A, Ditschuneit H (1987) Fluorescein dilaurate serum test: a rapid tubeless pancreatic function test. Pancreas 2:53–60

Natural History of Chronic (Progressive) Pancreatitis: A Life Experience

R. W. Ammann[1]

Problems of Diagnosis and Classification

The controversies on diagnosis and therapy of chronic pancreatitis (CP) are as marked today as 30 years ago despite many international meetings of classification [1], a marked improvement of diagnostic technics, and, the large and increasing amount of literature.

There are many reasons for these controversies, but probably most important is the fact that "pancreatitis still means many things to many people" [1]. According to the definition of Marseille, two forms of pancreatitis are distinguished, namely acute and chronic pancreatitis. In 1989 we have to accept that the definitions of 1963/1984 have not solved the problem of classification of pancreatitis for clinical practice mainly for two reasons:

1. There is a broad overlap between acute and chronic pancreatitis in regard of clinical, functional, and morphological changes in early phases of the disease. A clear differentiation between acute (reversible) and chronic (progressive) pancreatitis is only possible based upon the long-term profile (Fig. 1).
2. Paradoxically in the definition of Marseille the diagnosis of CP is essentially based upon histopathology despite the fact that histopathology is rarely available and postacute (nonprogressive) pancreatitis may be indistinguishable histopathologically from CP in early phases of the disease [1].

Ductal changes visualized by endoscopic retrograde pancreatography (ERP) have been advocated as the "gold standard" of CP [2]. However, the classification based upon ERP changes has never been validated in regard of CP, and it has not been accepted by the expert group of Marseille 1984. ERP like histopathology tends to overestimate the incidence of CP because postacute (nonprogressive) changes will be interpreted as CP (Fig. 2). Thus, the prevalence of CP in autopsy studies is about 100–1000 times higher than clinical studies on epidemiology [1]. It is therefore questionable if morphologically diagnosed "early" CP ("mini"-CP) has anything in common with clinical progressive CP except some morphological abnormalities [1].

---

[1] Gastroenterology Service, Dept. of Medicine, University Hospital, 8091 Zurich, Switzerland

Chronic Pancreatitis
Ed. by Beger, Büchler, Ditschuneit, and Malfertheiner
© Springer-Verlag Berlin Heidelberg 1990

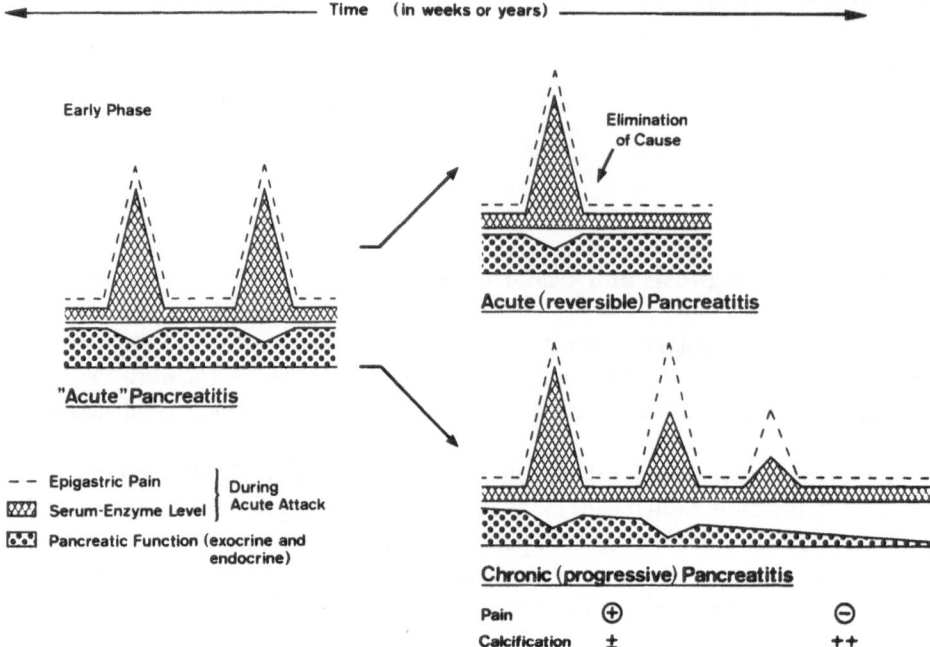

Fig. 1. Clinical classification of pancreatitis. Note: Identical episodes of "acute" pancreatitis are typical for acute (reversible) and chronic (progressive) pancreatitis in early phases of disease. In late phases the characteristic long-term profiles clearly separate the two entities. (From Ammann [1])

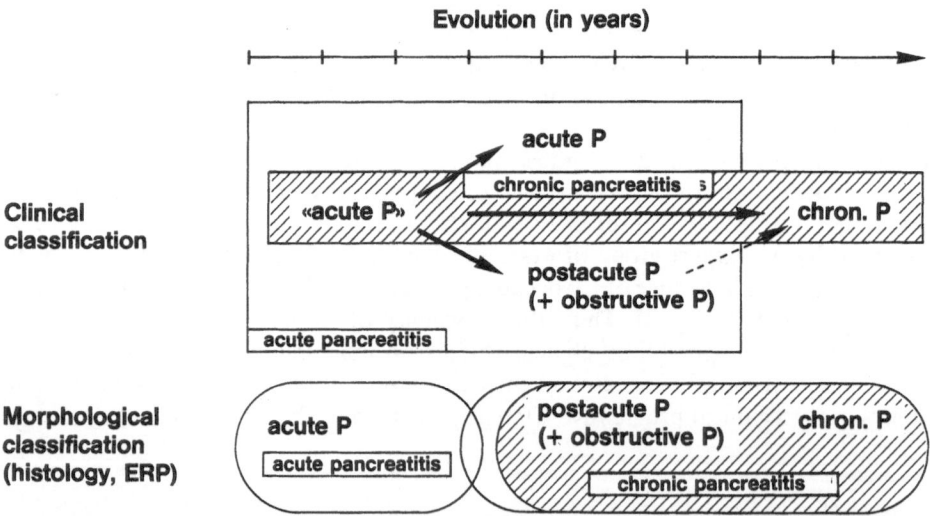

Fig. 2. Differences of clinical and morphological classifications of chronic (progressive) pancreatitis. Note: Morphology (ERP, histopathology) overestimates the incidence of "chronic" pancreatitis, particularly because postacute and obstructive pancreatitis are indistinguishable morphologically from CP in early disease [1]. Clinical classification will primarily overestimate the incidence of "acute" pancreatitis. Based upon long-term studies, however, chronic progressive pancreatitis is accurately differentiated from acute reversible pancreatitis, as well as from nonprogressive "chronic" pancreatitis, e. g., postacute and obstructive forms

Main Variables of CP

In the last 25 years a large number of patients with suspected or proved CP have been studied prospectively according to a protocol as outlined before [3]. In particular all cooperative patients had control studies at yearly intervals in regard to clinical symptoms, etiology, morphology (mainly plain films of the abdomen in three projections centered on the pancreas), and studies of exocrine and endocrine function. Data of 287 patients with proved CP worked up until December 1986 have been published [4]. At the present time our study comprises 323 patients with CP and with a median observation time of 7 years (from time of diagnosis) and over 2200 fecal chymotrypsin data (estimated at yearly intervals) (e. g., function studies for over 2200 patients/ years).

A close correlation between the CCK secreton and the fecal chymotrypsin test in CP has been demonstrated [5]. In Fig. 3 the correlation of fecal chymotrypsin and

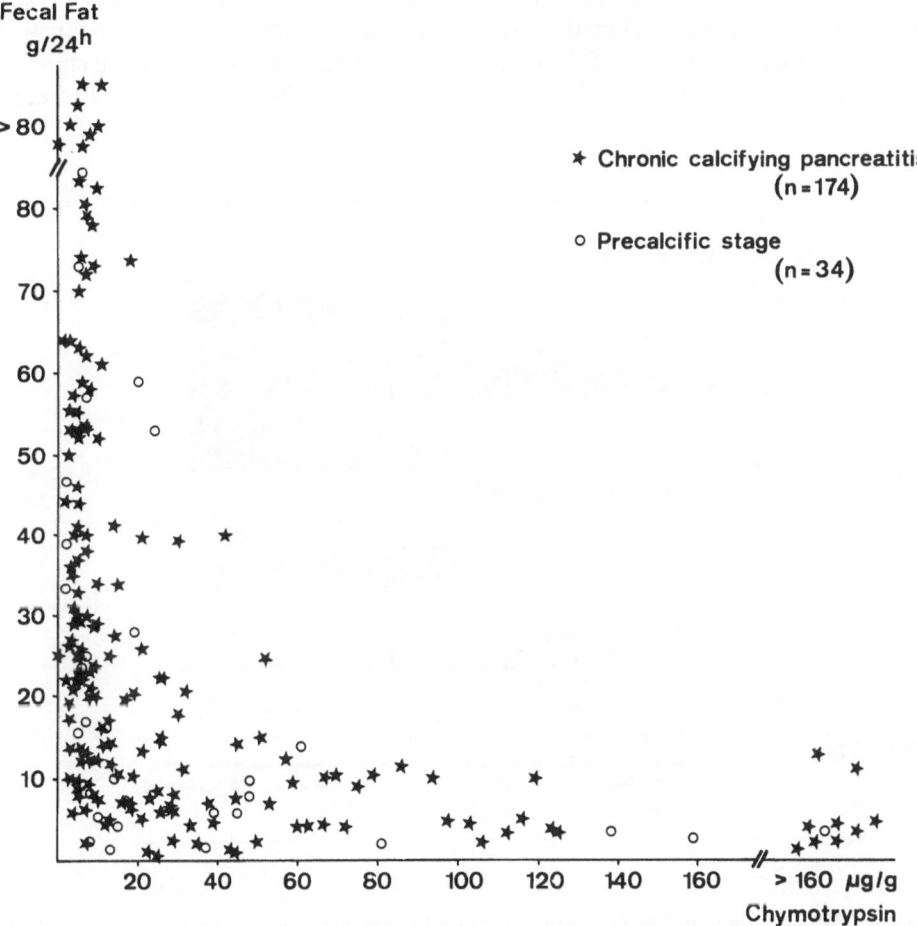

Fig. 3. Correlation of fecal chymotrypsin and fecal fat excretion in CP. Note: Steatorrhea (> 10 g/24 h) becomes manifest only in patients with marked reduction of fecal chymotrypsin (< 60 μg/g). (Normal fecal chymotrypsin: > 120 μg/g). (From Ammann et al. [5])

fecal fat excretion is shown indicating that steatorrhea becomes manifest only in patients with marked reduction of fecal chymotrypsin (the lower limit of normal being 120 µg/g).

The natural history of CP is defined by five factors, namely:
1. etiology,
2. clinical features,
3. morphology,
4. function, and
5. evolution.

Factors 1 to 4 are of equal importance, but a time lag in manifestation of clinical features and of morphological and functional abnormalities exists (Fig. 4). There is a close relationship between clinical symptoms, morphology, and function in relation to duration of CP. Most experts agree that CP is a dynamic progressive process characterized by continuous destruction of glandular tissue leading to "cirrhosis" of the pancreas. There is an interval (on the average of 5.5 years) between onset of CP and the manifestation of typical markers of CP, e. g., progressive pancreatic dysfunction and/or calcification (Fig. 1). This interval is the "black box" period for the clinician during which a definite diagnosis of CP is virtually impossible. Particularly pancreatic

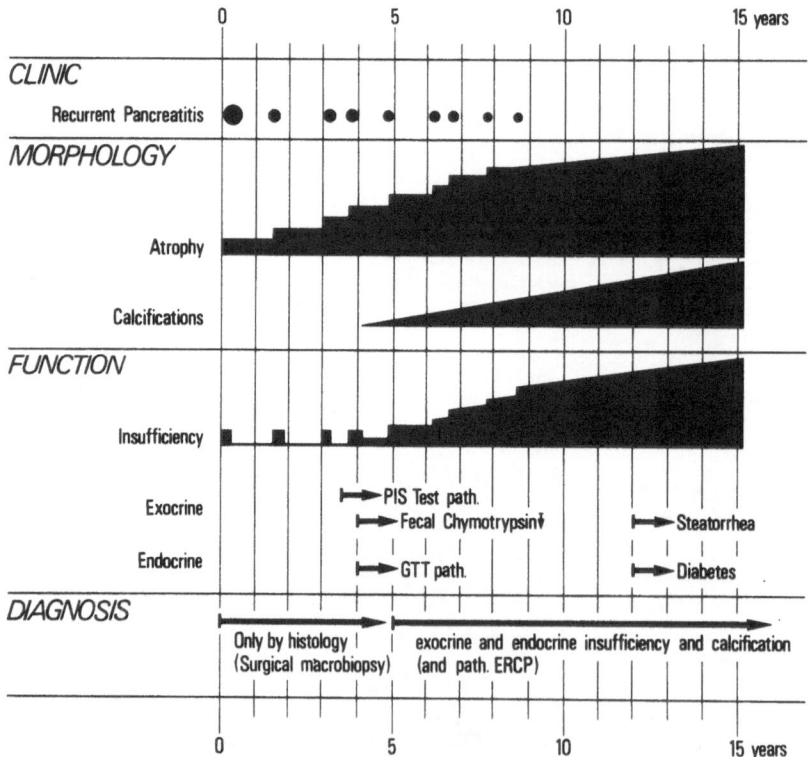

Fig. 4. Natural history of CP. Time course in onset (or manifestation) of the main variables of CP, e. g., clinical, morphology, pancreatic calcification, and dysfunction. Progressive dysfunction (secondary to glandular atrophy) becomes apparent only in advanced CP (on the average 5.5 years from clinical onset), usually in association with pancreatic calcifications (see Fig. 5)

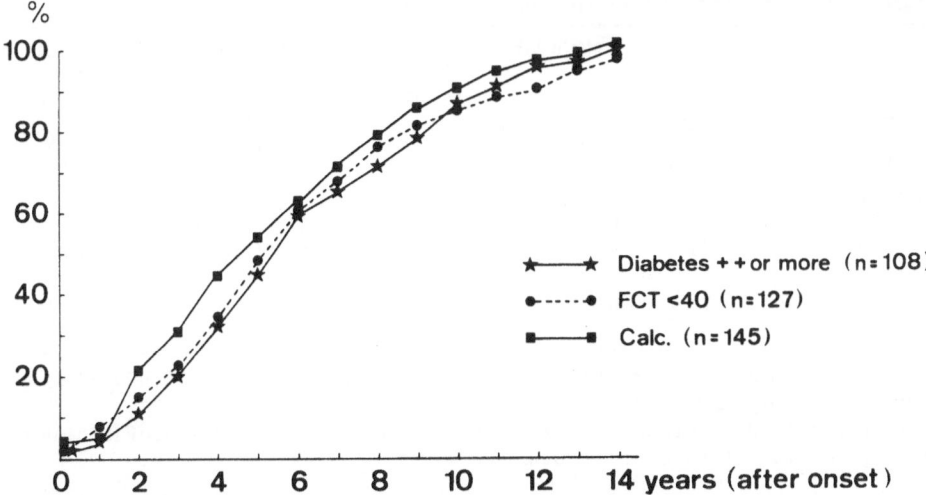

Fig. 5. Rate of manifestation of exocrine insufficiency, diabetes, and pancreatic calcification in relation to duration of alcoholic CP from onset ($n = 145$). (FCT; fecal chymotrypsin, normal $> 120 \mu g/$ g). (From Ammann et al. [3])

dysfunction (usually reversible) may occur in acute and postacute pancreatitis in the early course and in severe chronic alcoholism. Thus pancreatic function tests like the CCK-secretin test may yield pathological results in these conditions and may wrongly be interpreted as evidence of CP [1]. Serial function tests are necessary to differentiate acute (reversible) and chronic (progressive) pancreatitis [1]. Thus CP can be diagnosed precisely by the clinician only in the late phases, e.g., a posteriori. Most patients of our series with alcoholic CP have been classified initially as having "acute" recurrent pancreatitis.

The close covariation of calcification and exocrine and endocrine insufficiency in relation to duration [3] is documented for alcoholic CP in Fig. 5. It is evident that the cumulative incidence of the three markers amounts to about 40% at 4 years, to about 60% at 6 years, and reaches over 90% at 12 years from onset. It should be noted that the gold standard of CP in all patients was pancreatic calcification. In addition it is evident that in some patients it may take 10 years or longer until calcification and irreversible pancreatic dysfunction become apparent [3]. Progression of pancreatic dysfunction has not been confirmed in some series of the literature [4]. That may be due in part to a rather short follow-up of the patients and perhaps also to the fact that the progression of exocrine insufficiency occurs at a slower rate in nonalcoholic CP (see below).

Etiology and Long-Term Course

Etiology plays an important role in evolution of pancreatitis. Most experts will agree that biliary pancreatitis virtually never progresses to CP [1]. On the contrary alcoholic pancreatitis will progress to CP in a high percentage of patients, but exceptions to this

Table 1. Pertinent clinical data of AICP and NAICP. [4]

	N	Calcific CP %	Sex % M F	Age (at diagnosis) Median (range)	ppCP %
AICP	205	85	91 9	42.5 (26–72)	4.9
NAICP	82	77	80 20		53.7
Subgroups					
1. IJCP	15	93	87 13	32.0 (9–50)	0
2. ISCP	49	69	88 12	65.8 (44–75)	69.4
3. Rare					
Causes	18	83	56 44	46.0 (16–78)	55.6

AICP, alcoholic CP; NAICP, nonalcoholic CP; IJCP, idiopathic juvenile CP; ISCP; idiopathic senile CP; ppCP, primary painless CP
Note: Primary painless CP is very rare in AICP ($< 5\%$), but occurs in $> 50\%$ of NAICP (in particular in idiopathic senile CP and in CP due to rare causes)

rule are probably not as rare as often stated in the literature [6]. In a personal prospective long-term study over 10 years on 144 patients with recurrent alcoholic pancreatitis we found that over 30% of patients showed no evidence of progression to CP at the end of the study [6]. Accordingly, alcoholic etiology appears not to be a reliable marker to predict the course of pancreatitis.

There are also marked differences of the natural history of alcoholic versus nonalcoholic CP as reported by others (Layer et al., see above) and by our group [4]. As shown in Table 1, clinically primary painless CP (ppCP) is very rare in alcoholic CP ($<$ 5%) but very common in nonalcoholic CP (over 50%). A markedly higher progression rate of exocrine and endocrine insufficiency in relation to duration of disease has been noted in alcoholic than in nonalcoholic CP [4]. For instance the incidence of diabetes in severe steatorrhea (over 16 g/day) was 58% in alcoholic compared to only 23% in nonalcoholic CP (Table 2) [4].

Table 2. Relationship between steatorrhea and diabetes. [4]

		Diabetes			
		Present		Absent	
	n	n	%	n	%
Group A (no. of cases 137)					
Steatorrhea					
Absent (0–7 g)	64	14	21.9	50	78.1
Mild (8–15 g)	50	23	46.0	27	54.0
Severe (> 16 g)	91	53	58.2	38	41.8
Total no. of estimations	205	90		115	
Group B (no. of cases 58)					
Steatorrhea					
Absent (0–7 g)	12	3	25	9	75
Mild (8–15 g)	6	2	33	4	67
Severe (> 16 g)	43	10	23.3	33	76.7
Total no. of estimations	61	15		46	

Group A, AICP; Group B, NAICP

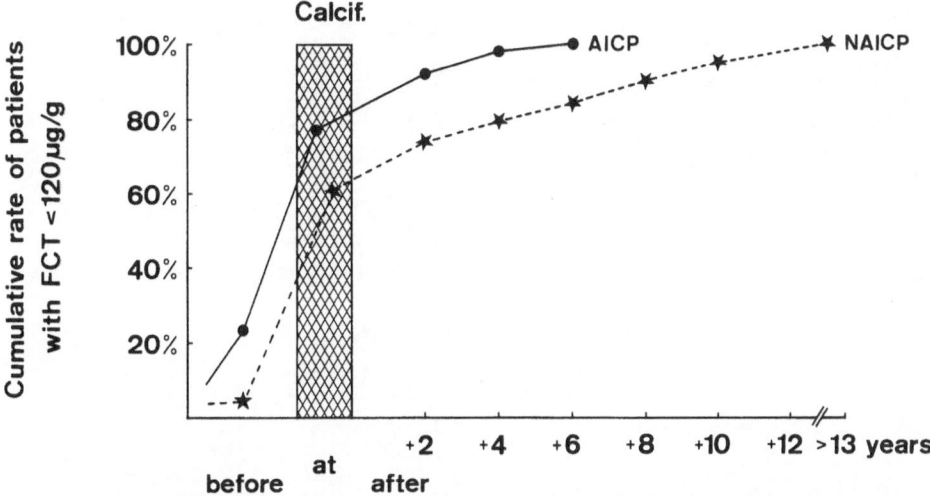

Fig. 6. Onset of calcification in relation to exocrine insufficiency (*FCT*, fecal chymotrypsin test, normal > 120 µg/g). In alcoholic CP *(AICP)* about 90% of patients have exocrine insufficiency at or within 2 years from onset of calcification. In nonalcoholic CP (NAICP) pancreatic calcifications precede exocrine insufficiency in about 40% of patients up to 13 years or longer. (From Ammann et al. [4])

Evolution and Regression of Calcification in CP

According to the current concept pancreatic calcifications (intraductal stones) increase in density in relation to duration of CP and up to 95% of cases develop calcification in series with a long follow-up [7]. The onset of calcification is closely related to the onset of exocrine insufficiency in alcoholic CP (Fig. 6) [7]. In nonalcoholic CP, calcifications precede exocrine insufficiency in about 40% of patients up to 13 years. This fact explains in part the lack of correlation between pancreatic calcification and exocrine insufficiency as pointed out previously [4]. Recent studies have shown that, at variance with the current concept, pancreatic calcifications tend to decrease spontaneously late in the course of CP [7].

A typical example is shown in Fig. 7. The evolution of pancreatic calcification (Fig. 8) suggests that lithogenesis and regression of pancreatic calcification represent a biological phenomenon with two antagonizing mechanisms, namely factors which promote and other factors which inhibit stone formation. The true nature of the mechanisms involved remains to be elucidated.

The "Burning out" Thesis and the Role of Pancreatic Surgery

Pain ist the major therapeutic problem early in the course of CP. To wait ("burning out") or to operate in CP is a major item of debate between internists and surgeons. The often-cited editorial: "patients, patience, and the impatient surgeon" characterizes the issue [8]. The statement in the surgical literature „some internists advocate

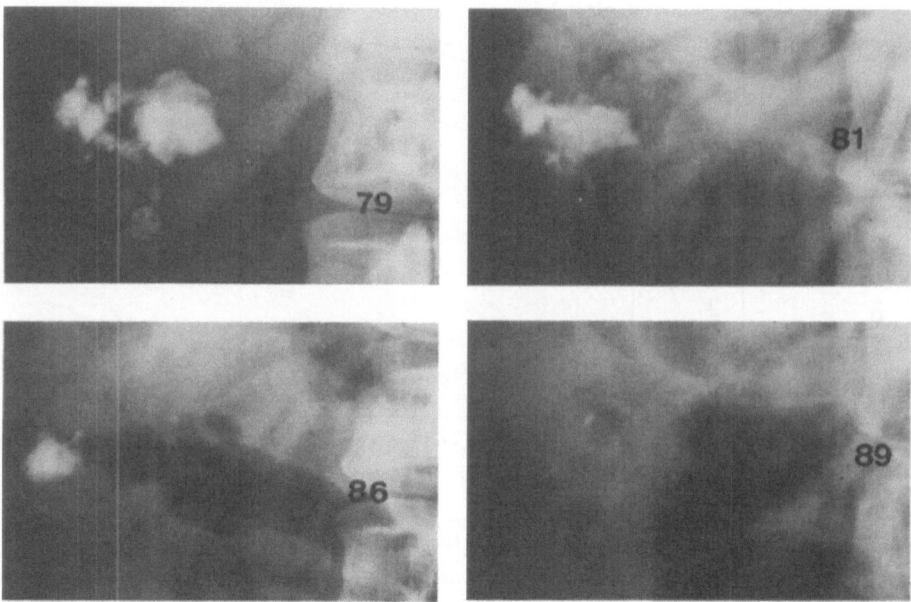

Fig. 7. Typical example of spontaneous regression of pancreatic calcification within 10 years (1979–1989) in patient with nonalcoholic CP. (From Ammann et al. [7])

that no surgery is necessary for pain relief in CP" and that "pain relief will come spontaneously if you wait long enough" [9] is the result of misinterpretation of results published by our group [3], mainly for two reasons. First, our results are based on the common experience of internists and surgeons in Zurich in the often cited paper [3] (R. A. is the only internist, F. L. and A. A. are expert pancreatic surgeons in Zurich and G. S. is an epidemiologist). Second, it has been clearly emphasized in the paper that 50% of the patients needed pancreatic surgery for pain relief [3].

It is a fact that about 50% of patients with alcoholic CP receive lasting pain relief spontaneously without pancreatic surgery in relation to three factors [1, 3, 9]: a) duration of CP, b) in association with pancreatic dysfunction, and/or c) with alcohol abstinence (early phases of CP).

These patients have uncomplicated CP and none of them ever experienced severe persistent pain. In uncomplicated CP an inverse relationship exists between recurrent pancreatitis and pancreatic function (Fig. 9), e.g., lasting pain relief occurs in advanced CP in association with marked pancreatic dysfunction [1, 3, 9].

Three types of pain pattern should be distinguished in recurrent pancreatitis (acute or chronic) (Fig. 10). (1) Uncomplicated recurrent pancreatitis is characterized by short episodes of pancreatitis and rather long pain-free intervals *(type A pain)*. (2) CP may run a primary painless course or may become painless in the course of advanced, uncomplicated CP as discussed *(type C)*. (3) Persistent severe pain (or repeated episodes of type A pain without pain-free intervals) are typical for *type B pain*. Type B pain is usually due to local complications which are easily visualized by imaging

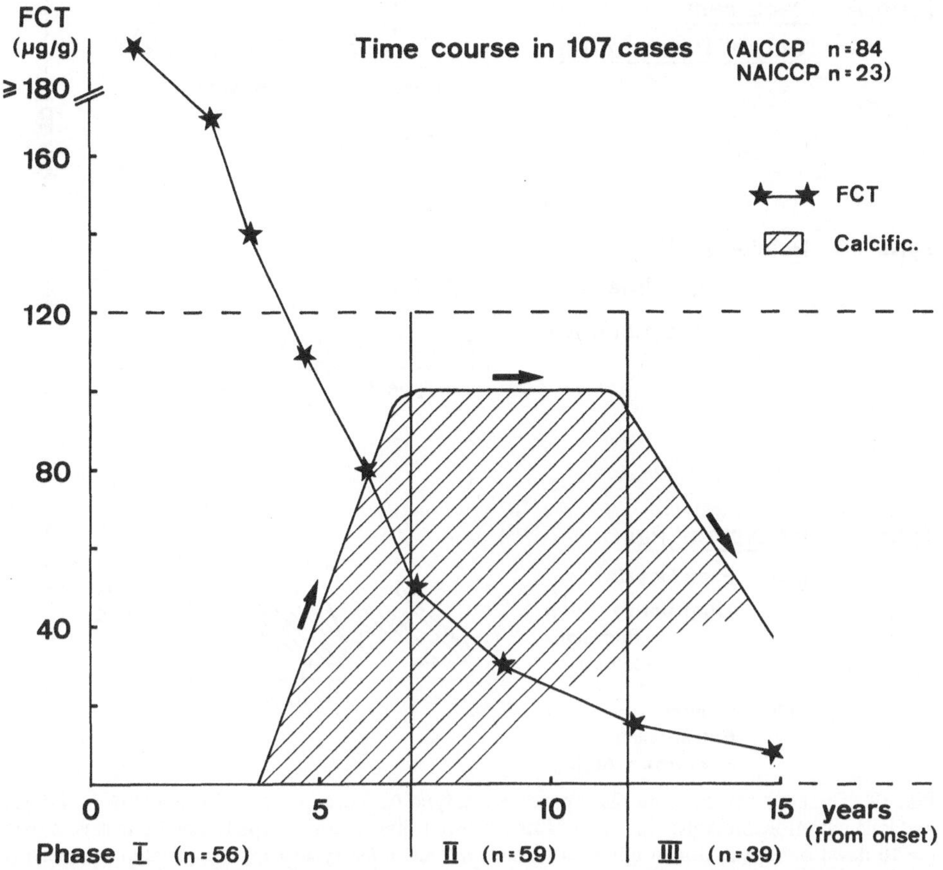

FCT
(μg/g)

Time course in 107 cases (AICCP n = 84
                                      NAICCP n = 23)

★——★ FCT

▨ Calcific.

Phase Ⅰ (n = 56)   Ⅱ (n = 59)   Ⅲ (n = 39)

Fig. 8. Evolution of pancreatic calcification in relation to duration of CP from onset. After an initial increase (phase I) about 50% of patients showed stationary calcification (phase II). In the late phase (III), regression of calcification occurred in about 35% of patients. (Ammann et al. [7])

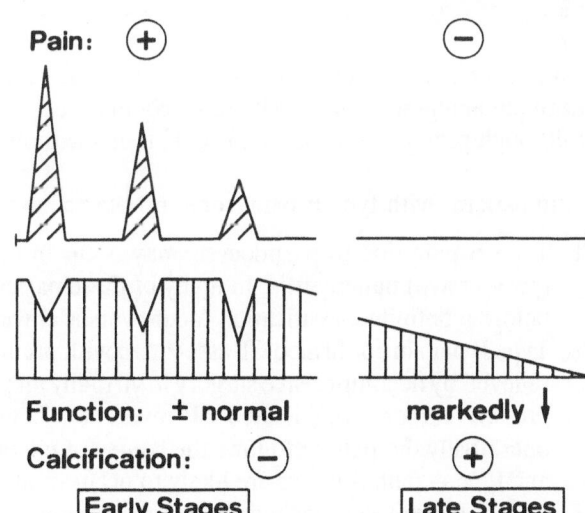

Fig. 9. Typical inverse relationship of pain and pancreatic function in uncomplicated CP. In advanced CP, spontaneous lasting pain relief is regularly found in association with marked pancreatic dysfunction (e.g., "burning out"). (From Ammann [1, 9])

Pain: ⊕   ⊖

Function: ± normal   markedly ↓

Calcification: ⊖   ⊕

Early Stages   Late Stages

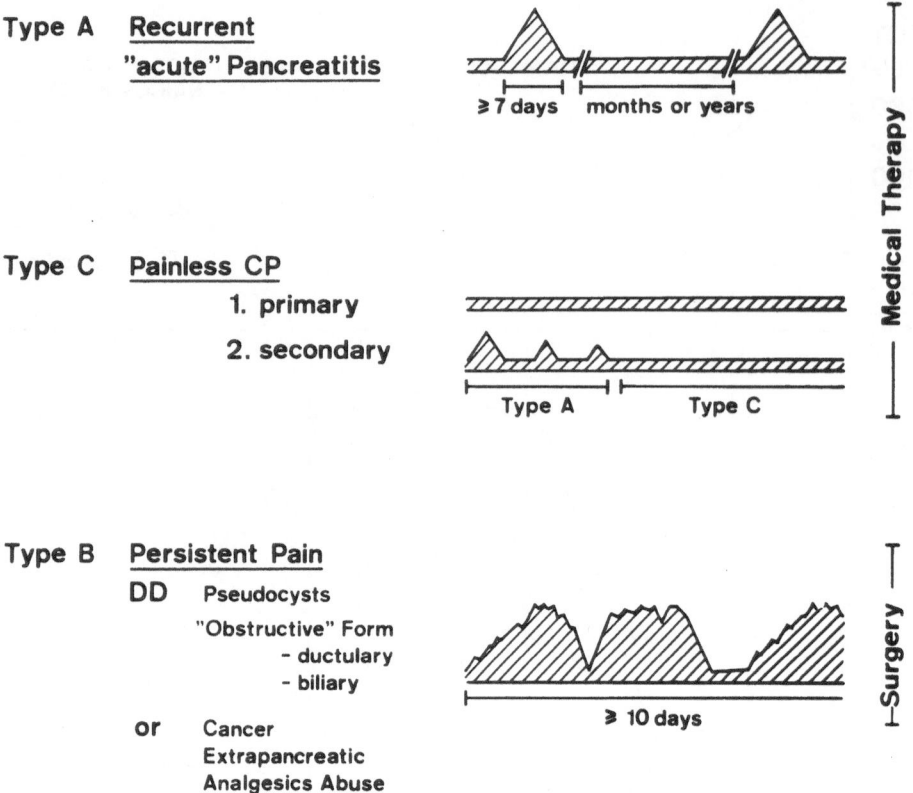

Fig. 10. Three typical pain patterns of pancreatitis: type A; short episodes of pancreatitis ($<$ 7 days) and long pain-free intervals; typical for acute or chronic pancreatitis. Type B; persistent severe pain ($>$ 10 days) or repeated pain episodes without intemissions; typical for complicated pancreatitis particularly pseudocysts in acute or CP, ductal "hypertension" in CP, or other causes like cancer and biliary obstruction. Type C: primary painless CP or secondary painless advanced CP

studies and may occur in acute and in CP (or may be due to extrapancreatic causes, for example analgesic abuse). The most common cause of type B pain are pseudocysts (although pseudocysts may occur in patients without pain).

In patients with type B pain, three problems have to be kept in mind:

1. Type B pain due to pseudocysts may occur in acute (reversible) and in chronic (progressive) pancreatitis. In many of these patients surgery has to be performed before a definite classification (acute versus chronic) is possible.
2. Type B pain in confirmed CP associated with pseudocysts or ductal hypertension is relieved by decompressive surgery in virtually all patients. Please note: By decompressive surgery complicated CP reverts back into uncomplicated CP [9]. Postoperatively the patient follows the course of uncomplicated CP as outlined above and type A pain relapses are likely to occur if: alcohol abuse is continued and the patient has not yet reached the advanced phase of painless CP.

It should be noted that in the surgical literature postoperative type A pain relapses are often classified as surgical failures. In our opinion type A relapses are primarily the patient's failure which should be treated by alcohol abstinence rather than by surgery (inclusive large resections) [9]. In patients with continued alcohol abuse postoperatively waiting for "burning out" appears appropriate in patients with uncomplicated CP.

3. Type B pain is primarily a problem of diagnosis, particularly in patients without proved CP in CP without local complications, or in advanced CP associated with marked pancreatic dysfunction. In such instances other causes of pain are likely to be found.

Nonprogressive "Chronic" Pancreatitis

In clinical practice there is a large number of patients with suspected CP and some of the clinical conditions mimic CP very closely in regard to etiology, clinical symptoms, morphology, or pancreatic function. Despite the progress in diagnosis, particularly with the imaging studies, pancreatic cancer still may be missed and even at surgery a considerable percentage of patients operated for CP prove to have pancreatic cancer at later time.

Here is a typical case history: A male patient, born in 1912 (F. Moritz), suffered from repeated episodes of typical "acute" pancreatitis since 1975 over a period of about 4 years (Fig. 11). Normal exocrine and endocrine function was demonstrated

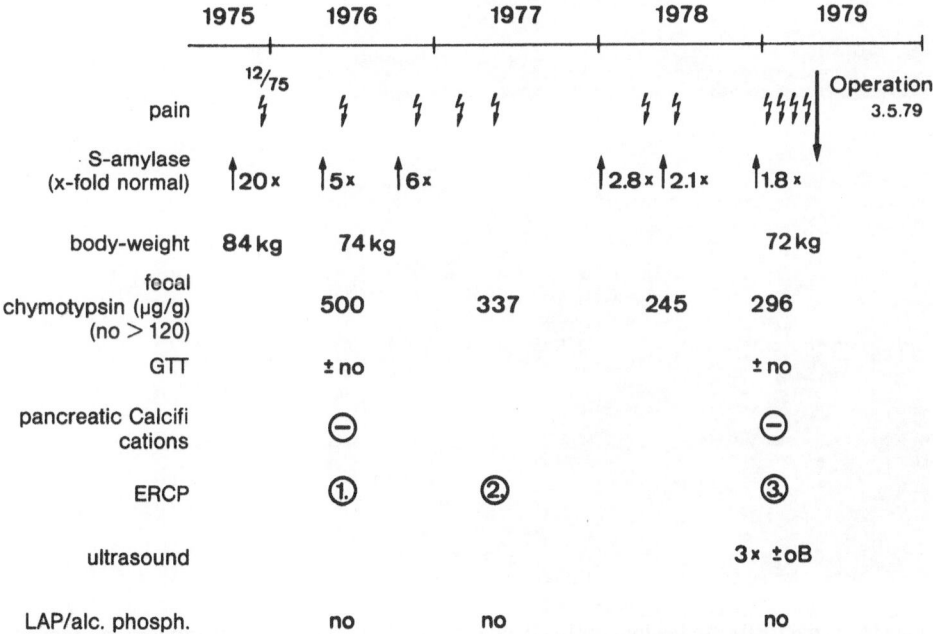

Fig. 11. Case report F, Moritz, 1912: long-term course with apparently typical recurrent "acute" pancreatitis (see Fig. 12.1–12.3)

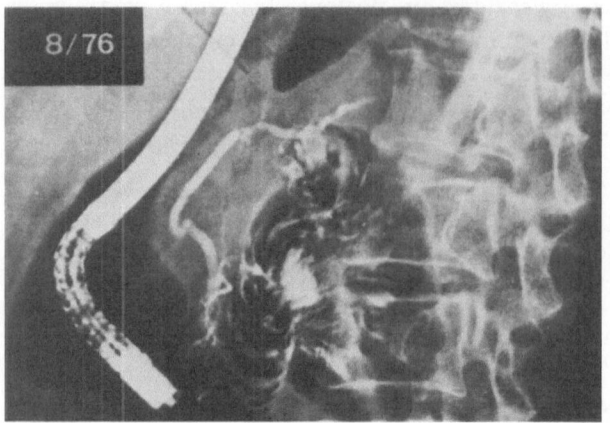

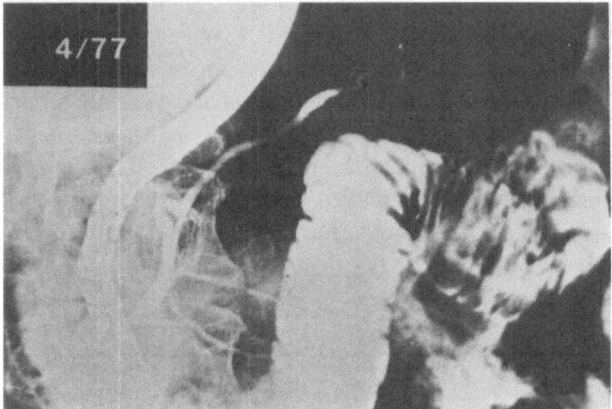

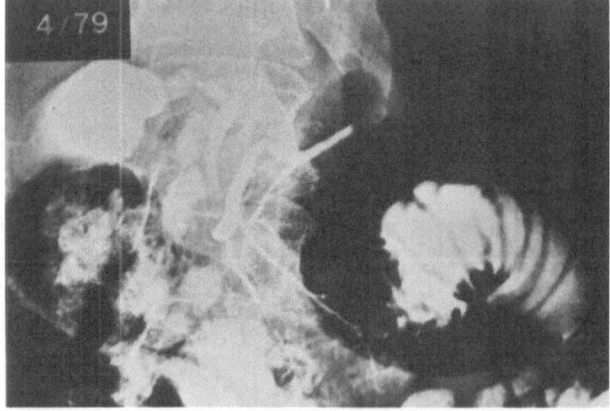

Fig. 12. Serial ERP examinations (1976–1979) of F, Moritz (see Fig. 11) with progressive segmental ductal changes in the pancreatic tail; complete stop in the last ERP 1979. At laparotomy 1979 (4 years from onset): inoperable pancreatic cancer with liver metastases

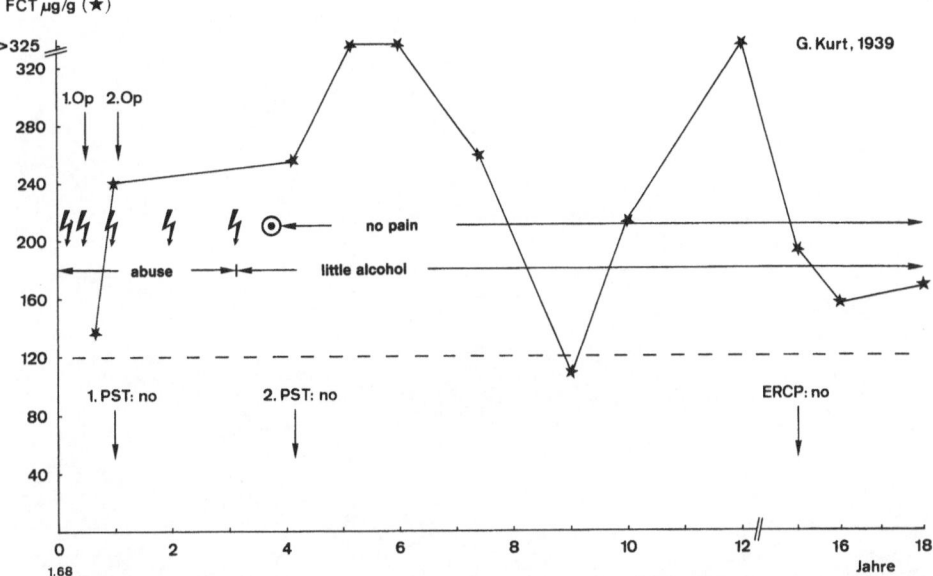

Fig. 13. Case report G, Kurt, 1939: long-term course (18 years) of recurrent alcoholic pancreatitis. Acute pancreatitis was confirmed twice by laparotomy 1968 and at a second laparotomy performed for a severe attack and suspected ulcer perforation (no pancreatic intervention). No evidence of exocrine insufficiency based upon two PSTs (CCK-secretin test) within the first 4 years and repeated fecal chymotrypsin examinations, over 18 years (FCT; normal > 120 μg/g). ERP was performed (for scientific reasons) 15 years from onset for diagnostic purpose (acute versus chronic pancreatitis) (see Fig. 14)

repeatedly and no evidence of calcification was found. Sonography (three times) showed no pancreatic pathology. ERP was performed three times within 3 years (Fig. 12) and showed marked irregularities of the duct of the tail of the pancreas and in the last examination a complete stop. A laparotomy (May 1979; e. g., 4 years after onset) an inoperable pancreatic cancer was found.

Often the classification remains in doubt until CP can be proved (or excluded) unequivocally based on a long observation time.

Figure 13 shows another typical case history: This male patient, born in 1939 (G., Kurt), with chronic alcohol abuse started with recurrent episodes of "acute" pancreatitis in 1972 over a period of about 4 years. Lasting pain relief occurred in association with alcohol abstinence. Exocrine and endocrine function has remained normal now for 16 years and no pancreatic calcifications have developed. Recently an ERP was performed for scientific reasons (Fig. 14). Mild irregularities of the ductal system in the tail are seen. Interpretation: "Small duct CP? segmental CP? or postacute (nonprogressive) pancreatitis? In some series such a case may be classified as CP. According to our experience such a case should be put into a separate category because it does not fulfill the strict criteria of chronic (progressive) pancreatitis.

The next case is particularly well documented (Fig. 5): This medical doctor, born 1919 (P. Hermann), suffered from a very severe episode of "acute pancreatitis" in

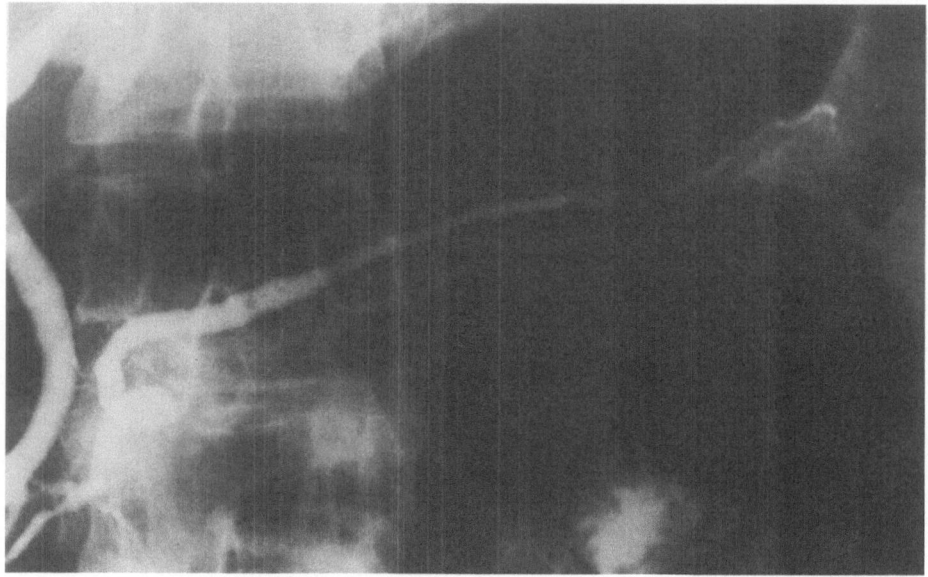

Fig. 14. Endoscopic retrograde pancreatography of G, Kurt, 1949 (see Fig. 13) shows discrete ductal abnormalities in the tail of the pancreas. Interpretation: "postacute" changes? or "small duct chronic pancreatitis"? or segmental "chronic" pancreatitis? (see text)

1968. The cause of pancreatitis remained undetermined. A cholecystectomy 1968 revealed no biliary stones. Over the next 12 years the patient experienced repeated mild episodes of pancreatitis. Four serial ERPs were performed in the period 1973–1983 (Fig. 16) which revealed marked, nonprogressive changes of the distal duct system. The patient consulted two to three expert surgeons and all agreed with our suggestion that because of the mild symptoms no surgery was indicated. In the last 7 years the patient has remained asymptomatic. The patient, who had intensively studied our publications, lately visited me again to thank me for not having sent him to operation. He concluded that we were right to wait since his pancreatitis had "burned out" as we anticipated. The statement of this medical doctor emphasizes the difficulty of communicating the message of "burning out." This patient always preserved a normal exocrine and endocrine function and developed no calcifications (Fig. 15). According to our strict criteria this patient never had true progressive CP. Cases like that should therefore be classified separately as "segmental, nonprogressive pancreatitis."

In conclusion our observations suggest that more data on the natural history inclusive long-term function studies are needed mainly for three reasons:

1. To give a more precise classification of individual patients having a true clinical progressive CP
2. As a basis of comparison of different series of CP (medical and surgical)
3. For developing a common strategy of treatment for CP.

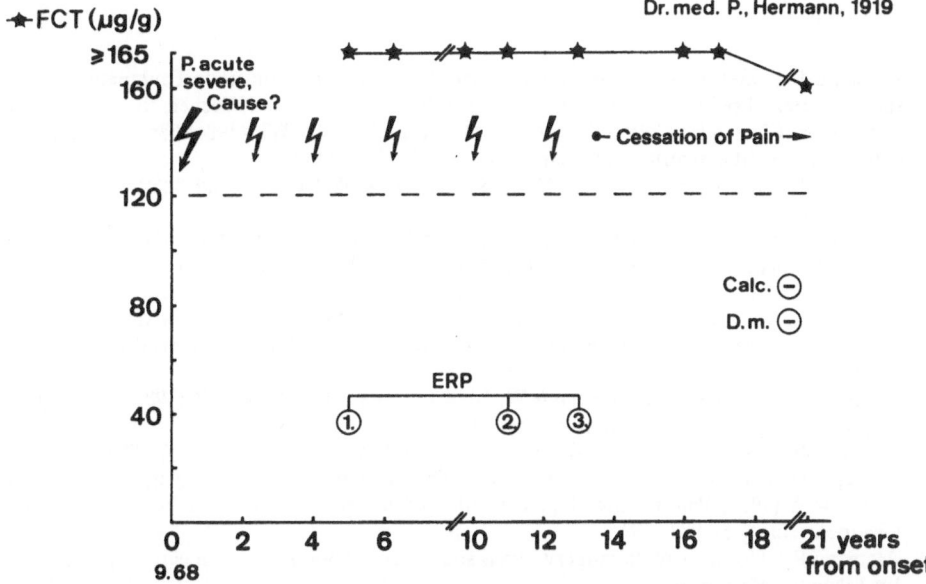

Fig. 15. Case report P, Hermann, 1919: long-term course (21 years) of recurrent, nonalcoholic pancreatitis after an initial severe episode 1968 of unknown origin (no biliary stones at cholecystectomy 1969). No diabetes, no calcification, and no exocrine insufficiency over 21 years (*FCT,* fecal chymotrypsin test, normal > 120 μg/g). For ERCP see Fig. 16

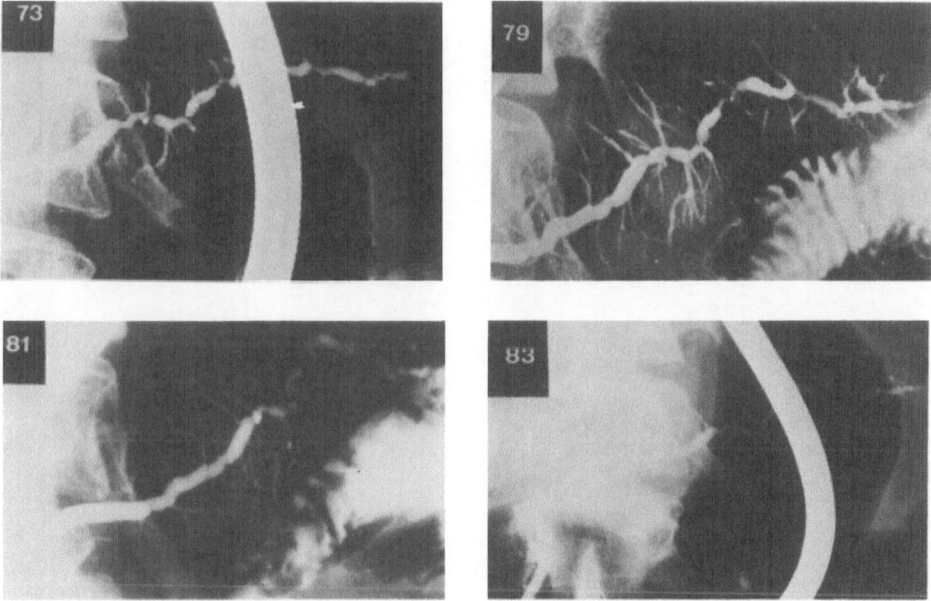

Fig. 16. The four ERP examinations of P, Hermann (1973–1983) (Fig. 15) show marked segmental (but nonprogressive) ductal changes in the distal pancreas. Interpretation "postacute" changes? or segmental "chronic," nonprogressive pancreatitis?

References

1. Ammann R (1989) Klinik, Spontanverlauf und Therapie der chronischen Pankreatitis. Unter spezieller Berücksichtigung der Nomenklaturprobleme. Schweiz Med Wochenschr 119:696–706
2. Axon ATR, Classen M, Cotton PB, Cremer M, Freeny PS, Lees WR (1984) Pancreatography in chronic pancreatitis: international definitions. Gut 25:1107–1112
3. Ammann R, Akovbiantz A, Largiadèr F, Schueler G (1984) Course and outcome of chronic pancreatitis. Gastroenterology 86:820–828
4. Ammann R, Buehler H, Muench R, Freiburghaus A, Siegenthaler W (1987) Differences in the natural history of idiopathic (non-alcoholic) and alcoholic chronic pancreatitis. Pancreas 2:368–377
5. Ammann R, Akovbiantz A, Haecki W, Largiadèr F, Schmid M (1981) Diagnostic value of the fecal chymotrypsin test in pancreatic insufficiency, particularly chronic pancreatitis. Digestion 21:281–289
6. Ammann R, Buehler H, Bruehlmann W, Kehl O, Muench R, Stamm B (1986) Acute (non-progressive) alcoholic pancreatitis. Pancreas 1:195–203
7. Ammann R, Muench R, Otto R, Buehler H, Freiburghaus A, Siegenthaler W (1988) Evolution and regression of pancreatic calcification in chronic pancreatitis. Gastroenterology 95:1018–1028
8. Warshaw A (1984) Pain in chronic pancreatitis: patient, patience, and the impatient surgeon. Gastroenterology 86:987–989
9. Ammann R (1989) Pancreatic surgery versus spontaneous "burning out" in chronic pancreatitis. Int J Pancreatol (in press)

Morphology

Exocrine and Endocrine Morphologic Changes in Chronic Pancreatitis

V. Becker[1]

Chronic pancreatitis is a mild inflammation of the pancreas which is determined by the substances secreted by the pancreas. It is characterized by chronicity, by relapsing attacks of pain and pathologically anatomically by severe loss of parenchyma and massive scarring. The decisive ethiologic factor is the chronic abuse of alcohol – this was discovered by our chairman Prof. Henri Sarles more than 30 years ago [4].

There are numerous characteristics of the pathological anatomy, and the whole gland is frequently affected (Fig. 1). The pancreatic duct is large, the parenchyma being nearly completely replaced by the surrounding cicatricial tissue. The whole gland has changed into a "cord of iron." More or less extensive calcifications are found in the lumen of the duct or in the cicatricial tissue in about the half of all cases [10].

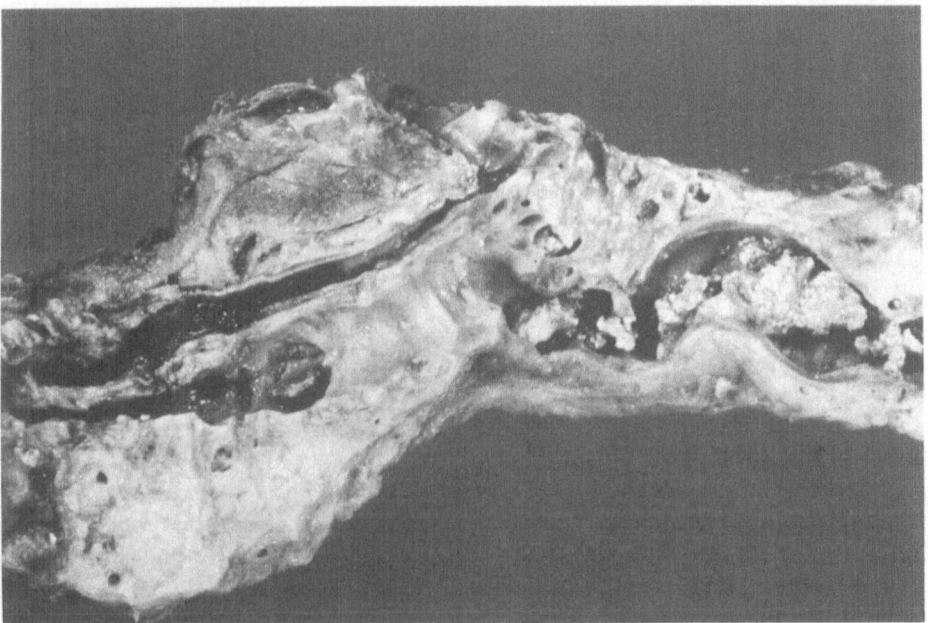

Fig. 1. Large, curved duct in a case of chronic pancreatitis. Calculi of different size in the duct. Survey, flat section

---

[1] Pathologisches Institut, Universität Erlangen/Nürnberg, Krankenhausstrasse 8–10, D-8520 Erlangen, FRG

Chronic Pancreatitis
Ed. by Beger, Büchler, Ditschuneit, and Malfertheiner
© Springer-Verlag Berlin Heidelberg 1990

Frequently, a real quarry is situated in the area next to the papilla of Vater. Pseudo-cysts indicating a preceding tryptic necrosis were found in 63% of the cases in our material. Sometimes, there are lots of small pseudocysts.

In 36% of the cases of our material, only a segment of the gland was affected, often only the head of pancreas. In this case, the affected segments are sharply demarcated from the remaining tissue; no explanation of this fact can be found in the ductal system or in the blood supply.

Two principally different histological forms can be distinguished: common chronic pancreatitis, which is caused by the effect of the saliva in the form of tryptic necrosis or inflows into the cicatricial tissue – and secondly obstructive pancreatitis. An occlusion of the excretion ducts slowly leads to the destruction of the organ, as can also be observed in other glands. In the case of the pancreas, fibrosis develops, the paren-chyma dies off in an almost regular manner, and the islet system remains. As is generally known the discovery of insulin by Banting and Best is based on this principle, but also the modern therapy of occlusion by the installation of Ethibloc. In this case, the main ducts are not influenced, the ductuli are of intermediate diameter, and the epithelium is flattened. The gland is slowly strangled by the surrounding connective tissue.

Obstructive pancreatitis develops by total occlusion of the duct of Wirsung by calculus or tumor – so one can find it in all stages of carcinoma of the papilla or of the head of the pancreas. It is a result of tumorous occlusion. Obstructive pancreatitis, which is acknowledged by the Marseille nomenclature of 1984, must be distinguished from chronic pancreatitis. In it, the duct is large and the epithelium of the duct is burst, being occasionally proliferated and forming single reactive nodes. The pancreatic parenchyma is spread out irregularly. The inslets of Langerhans are, step by step, first isolated and then also affected. There are epithelial reactions around the calculi, which are reminiscent of papillary dysplasia and which can be regarded as one. Cicatricial tissue develops around calcifications of the ductuli, and sometimes real granulomata are formed [9].

There are other indications of the slow, steady loss of parenchyma. As an adaption, the supplying vessels sustain a fibrosis of the intima, so that the lumen comes up to the diameter of a capillary [3]. This process only takes place in the case of a slow reduction, never in the case of the loss of the organ caused by pancreatic cancer. For this reason the adaption of the intima indicates chronic pancreatitis. Similarly, hyper-plasia of Brunner's glands is found in the case of chronic pancreatitis – this may be an endoscopic indication of the pancreatopathy [7].

The difference between obstructive and chronic pancreatitis cannot only be recog-nized by the different histological pattern of destruction, but also by the fact that in the case of a chronic tryptic pancreatitis the saliva can still pass the main pancreatic duct. With all so-called special kinds of pancreatitis, it is common that the excretion is made more difficult. The chronic pancreatitis is maintained by the reduced ability to excrete.

Such a reduction may be:
– The quarry near the papilla
– The cysts of the duodenal wall, which are seen in 33% of cases of chronic pan-creatitis (Fig. 2).
– The diverticulum near the papilla of Vater and many others.

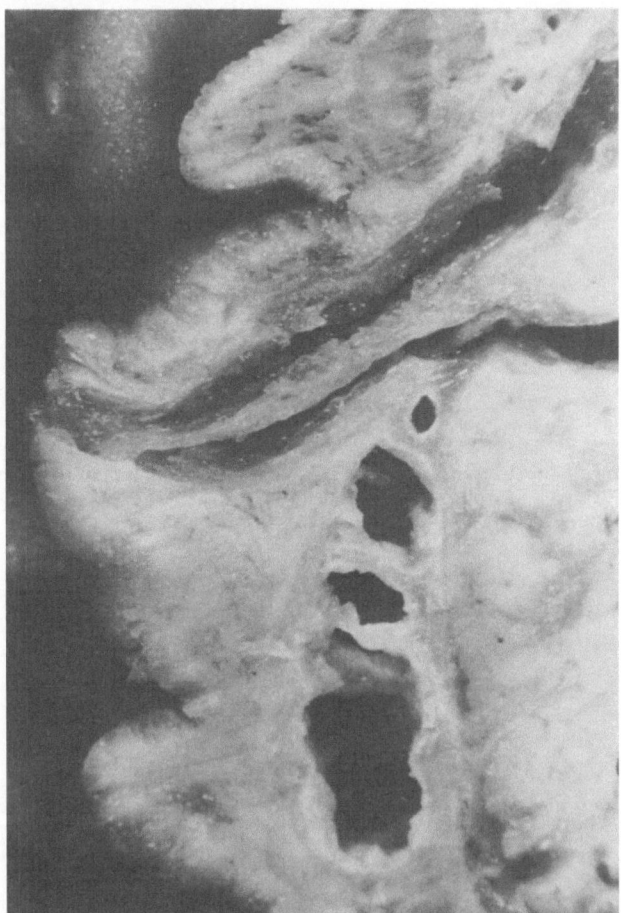

Fig. 2. Chronic pancreatitis in a case of cysts of the duodenal wall. Flat section through the papilla of Vater. Duodenum *on the left,* bile duct *above,* duct of Wirsung *below,* narrowed by a system of cysts, situated in the wall of the duodenum; therefore not pseudocysts of the pancreas!

With all these kinds it is common that the excretion duct is narrowed, but not totally occlused. It should be emphasized that the method of anatomical preparation of the specimen is very important for knowledge of the special kinds of pancreatitis and for knowledge of their characteristics [6]. We have, in the same way, histologically prepared about 1500 surgical specimens (with different surgical techniques) provided by many German hospitals. We have shown the connection to ERCP by means of anatomic pancreatography (Fig. 3). We tried to imitate the tonus of the living state by tightly filling the duodenum (Fig. 4). This helped us to discover the numerous cysts of the duodenal wall which may hinder the clinician if they are of sufficiant diameter. One particular type of pancreatitis, groove pancreatitis (Fig. 5), was also discovered by means of tight filling on the one hand, and by roentgenological ductography on the other hand [5, 8].

Groove pancreatitis belongs to the segmental forms of pancreatitis, which break out of the head of the pancreas filling up the groove between the duodenum and the

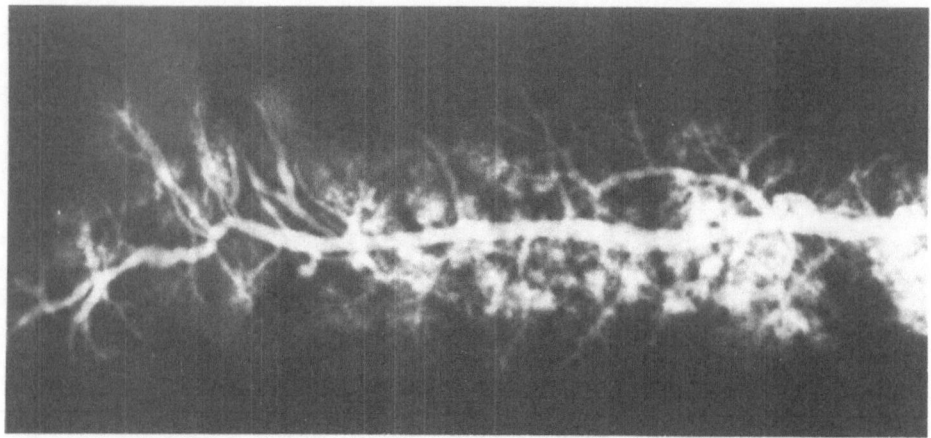

Fig. 3. Anatomic pancreatography analogous to ERCP. Iconography of the duct and its branches by instillation of contrast media. Histological examination of the areas shown up by pancreatography

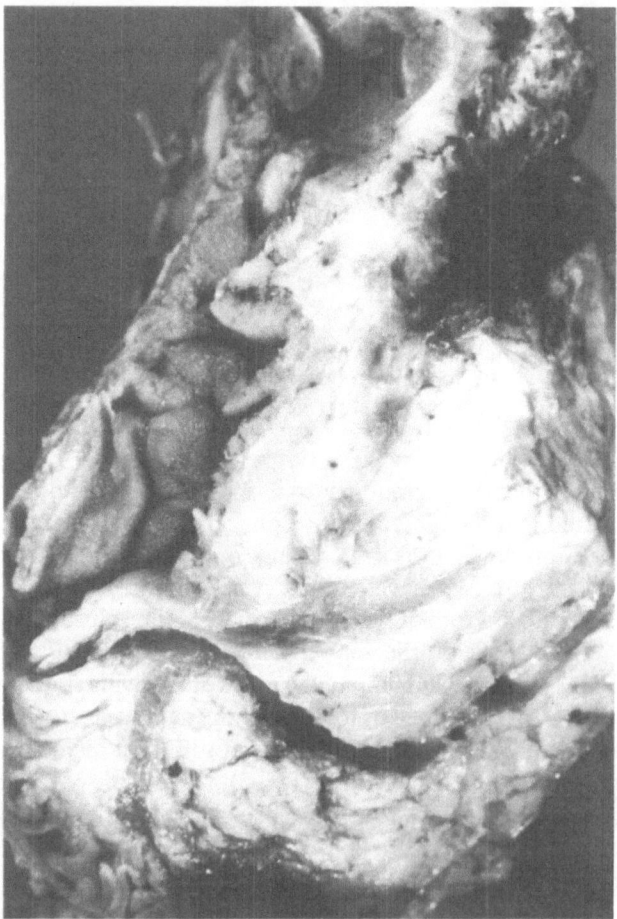

Fig. 4. Groove pancreatitis. *On the left,* duodenum cut open, below the duct of Wirsung; *in the middle,* narrowed bile duct, which is moved to the caudal part. Between the wall of the duodenum and the bile duct there is strong cicatricial tissue: scarring of the "groove"

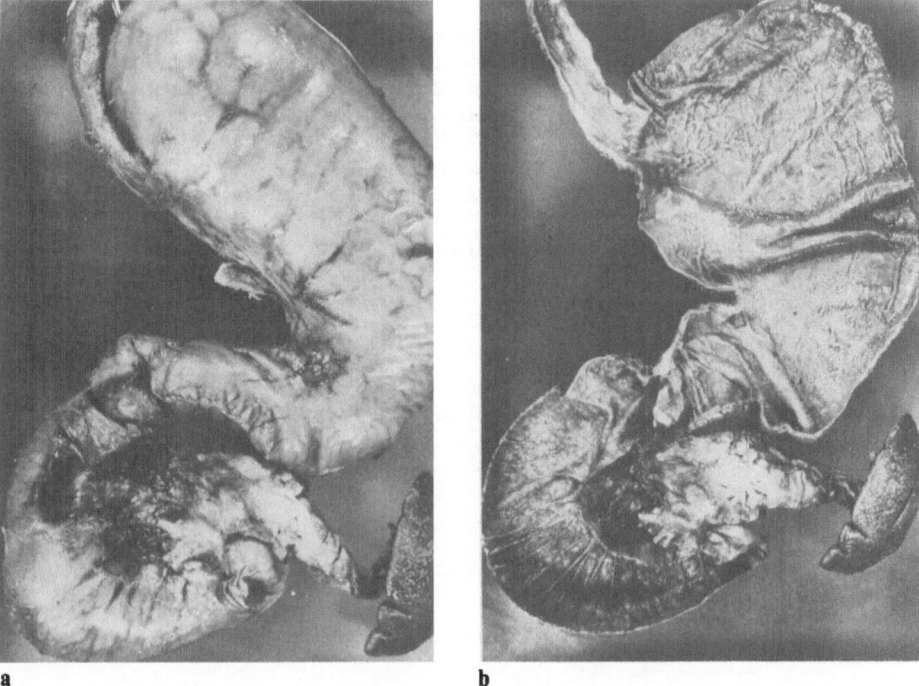

a   b

Fig. 5a, b. Tight filling of stomach and duodenum with formalin. **a** Filled specimen of stomach and duodenum; **b** flat section of the same specimen with a stretched duodenum

head of pancreas with cicatricial tissue. In this way, the duodenum and occasionally the bile duct is narrowed, similar to a carcinoma of the head of the pancreas. The clinical differential diagnosis between groove pancreatitis and carcinoma of the head of the pancreas is difficult [1, 2]. But since groove pancreatitis has been familiar to our clinicians, it has also been included in clinical differential diagnosis and has been diagnosed more frequently. The ERCP of the duct of Wirsung is totally inconspicuous, groove pancreatitis being based on the axis of the duct of Santorini.

Chronic pancreatitis is a comparatively recent disease. It has been known since the end of the 1950s, and was first described by Sarles. The pathologic anatomy of chronic pancreatitis gives us the chance to study the morphologic reactions of the pancreas, and, above all, to study the influence of the functional apparatus on the disease.

References

1. Becker V (1984) Chronische Pankreatitis. Klinische Morphologie. Thieme, Stuttgart
2. Becker V (1990) Rinnenpankreatitis. Z Gastroenterol (in press)
3. Kaiser G, Hommel G (1975) Morphometrisch-statistische Analyse der Pankreasarterien bei chronischer Pankreatitis. Virchow Arch Pathol Anat 365:103–118
4. Sarles H, Muratore R, Sarles J-C, Guien C (1959) Pancréatites chroniques de l'adulte à propos de 64 cas. Tijolschr Gastroenterol 2:617

5. Stolte M (1984) Chronische Pankreatitis. Morphologie – Pankreatographie – Differentialdiagnose. perimed, Erlangen
6. Stolte M, Schaffner O (1978) Entfaltungsfixation und röntgenologische Pankreas-Gang-Darstel-
   lung als Pfadfinder für die pathologisch-anatomische Diagnostik. Verh Dtsch Ges Pathol 62:400
7. Stolte M, Schwabe H (1977) Chronische Pankreatitis und Hyperplasie der Brunnerschen Drüsen.
   In: Creutzfeldt W, Classen M (eds) Ergebnisse der Gastroenterologie. Demeter, Gräfelfing
8. Stolte M, Weiß W, Volkholz H, Rösch W (1982) A special form of segmental pancreatitis:
   "groove pancreatitis". Hepatogastroenterology 29:198–200
9. Stürmer J, Becker V (1987) Granulomatous pancreatitis – granulomas in chronic pancreatitis.
   Virchow Arch [A] 410:327–338
10. Toskes PP (1988) Pancreatic calcification: new lessons from an old observation. Gastroenter-
    ology 95:1144

Focal Necrosis: Primary Event in the Pathogenesis of Chronic Pancreatitis?

G. Klöppel[1]

Pancreatic pseudocyst, the residual of focal fat necrosis in acute pancreatitis [11, 12], is also a common finding in chronic pancreatitis [1, 2, 17, 20]. Yet its significance for the pathogenesis of chronic pancreatitis has been neglected for many years, owing to the widely accepted view that acute and chronic pancreatitis differ in etiology and pathogenesis [18]. Here we will briefly review the pathology of focal necrosis and pseudocysts in chronic pancreatitis and discuss their possible role in the pathogenesis of the disease.

Pathology

The reported incidence of pseudocyst in chronic pancreatitis ranges from 11% to 50% [2–4, 6, 7, 17, 19, 20]. In our own study reviewing the pathology of 57 pancreas resection specimens and 9 autopsy pancreata of patients with chronic pancreatitis we found pseudocysts in 41% of the cases [10]. The majority of these lesions were found outside the parenchyma of the gland in the peripancreatic fatty tissue. Their wall was formed by granulation tissue and dense collagen, and there was no epithelium lining of the inner surface of the cystic cavities (Fig. 1). The latter observations contradict findings reported by Sarles et al. [15, 16], who demonstrated duct epithelium in some areas of cystic cavities associated with chronic pancreatitis [5]. Therefore they regarded these lesions as retention cysts and separated them from pseudocysts caused by acute pancreatitis. We cannot confirm these findings. Instead, we believe that the pseudocysts encountered in chronic pancreatitis are essentially the same as those found in acute pancreatitis. Although pseudocysts in chronic pancreatitis usually have a thicker wall (due to an increased amount of dense collagen) than those of acute pancreatitis, their principal structure is identical and in both diseases composed of an inner layer of granulation tissue followed by connective tissue rich in collagen. In some cases of chronic pancreatitis marked cystic dilatations of the main pancreatic duct may mimic intrapancreatic pseudocysts, because the lining epithelium of the dilated duct may be destroyed by calculi (Fig. 2). However, by careful histological analysis using step sections, these ulcerated ducts were easily separated from pseudocysts [10].

---

[1] Department of Pathology, Academic Hospital, Free University of Brussels, Laarbeeklaan 101, B-1090 Brussels, Belgium

Chronic Pancreatitis
Ed. by Beger, Büchler, Ditschuneit, and Malfertheiner
© Springer-Verlag Berlin Heidelberg 1990

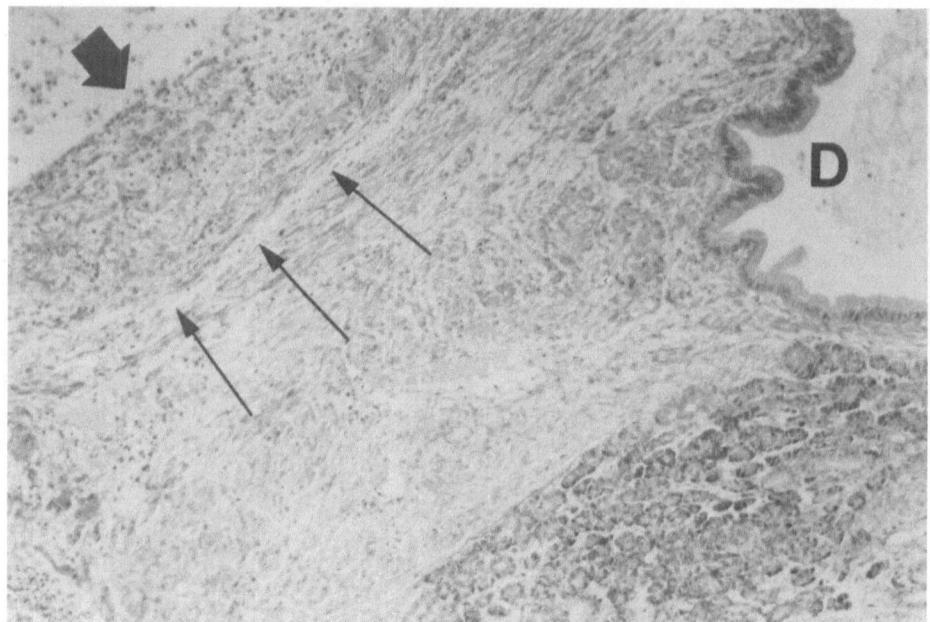

Fig. 1. Chronic pancreatitis: wall of an intrapancreatic pseudocyst composed of granulation tissue and loosely arranged collagen *(small arrows)*. There is no epithelium lining the inner surface of the cyst *(large arrow)*. D, Duct. H&E, × 125

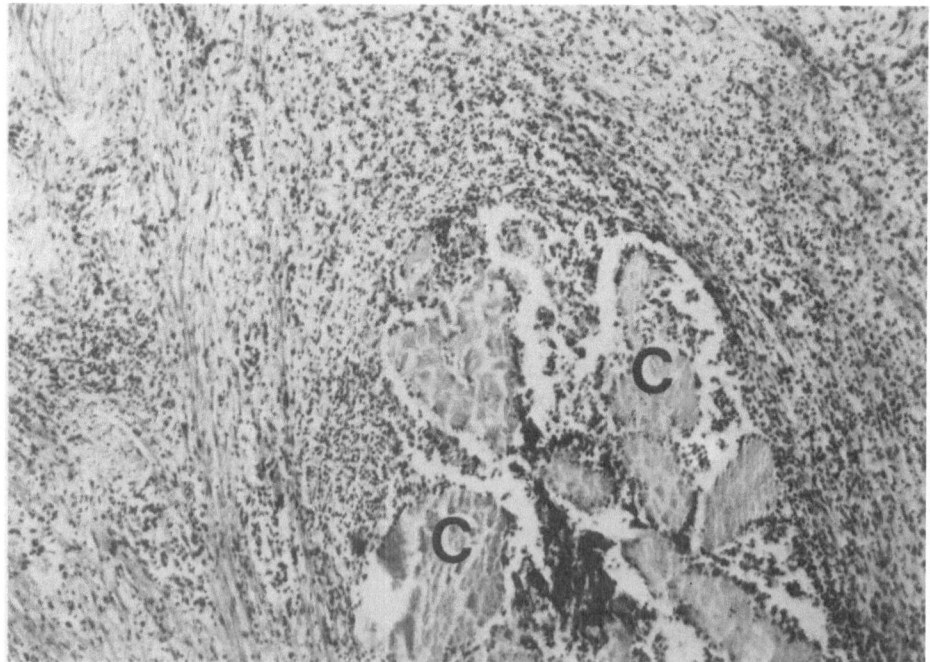

Fig. 2. Chronic pancreatitis: duct filled with calculi *(C)* and surrounded by chronically inflamed tissue. Due to destruction duct cells are absent. H&E, × 125

Pathogenesis

Pseudocysts in acute pancreatitis are residues of focal fat necrosis due to autodigestion by activated pancreatic proenzymes [8, 11, 12]. If, as we assume, pseudocysts in chronic pancreatitis have the same cause, focal necrosis and transitions of focal necrosis to pseudocyst should also be present in chronic pancreatitis, at least in some cases. Moreover, focal necrosis and pseudocysts should be more frequent in pancreatic specimens with little fibrosis and still numerous acinar cells (that can produce enzymes) than in pancreata showing advanced fibrosis and only few remaining acinar cells. In our series of pancreatic specimens with chronic pancreatitis we found 19 cases with recent focal necrosis and transitions of focal necrosis to pseudocyst (Fig. 3). Furthermore, pseudocysts as well as focal necroses were more common in pancreatic specimens with limited fibrosis (56%) than in those with extensive fibrosis (32%) [10]. Taken together, these findings lend support to our assumption that the pathogenetic process underlying pseudocyst development in chronic pancreatitis is identical to that in acute pancreatitis. With respect to the pathogenesis of chronic pancreatitis this implies that chronic pancreatitis may be the late stage of relapsing acute pancreatitis.

If chronic pancreatitis is related to acute pancreatitis the question remains how the sequelae of the acute process can produce the chronic lesions. The working hypothesis we have proposed [9] centers arround the late sequelae of extensive fat necrosis in severe acute pancreatitis. Depending on its localization and extent, fat necrosis may give rise to two different lesions. The large fat necrosis that occurs outside the pancreas usually leads to pseudocyst formation. In contrast, resolution of the smaller intrapancreatic foci of fat necrosis (located within the interlobular spaces) only rarely

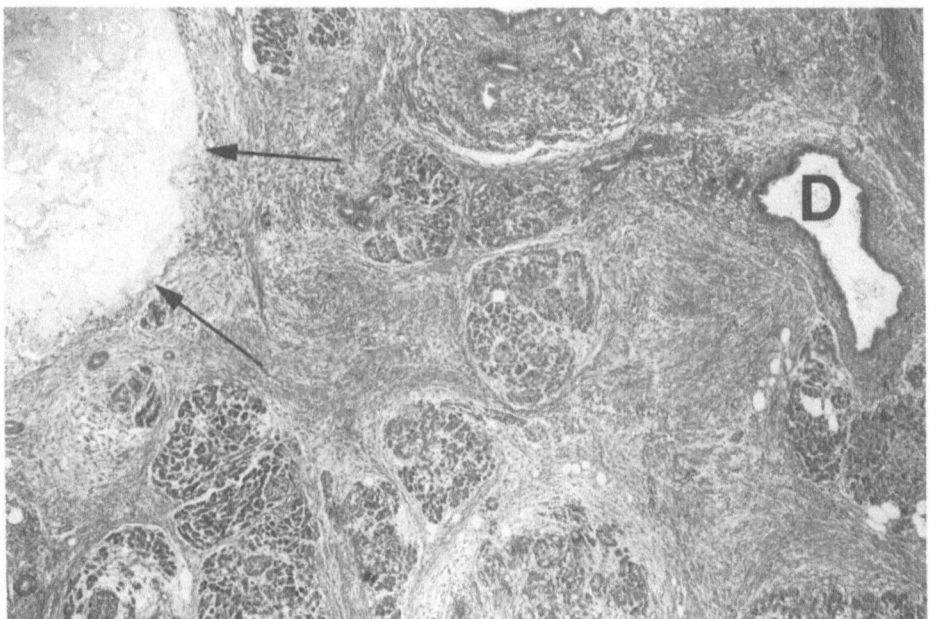

Fig. 3. Chronic pancreatitis with recent fat necrosis *(arrows)* and extensive perilobular fibrosis involving a duct *(D)*. H&E, × 40

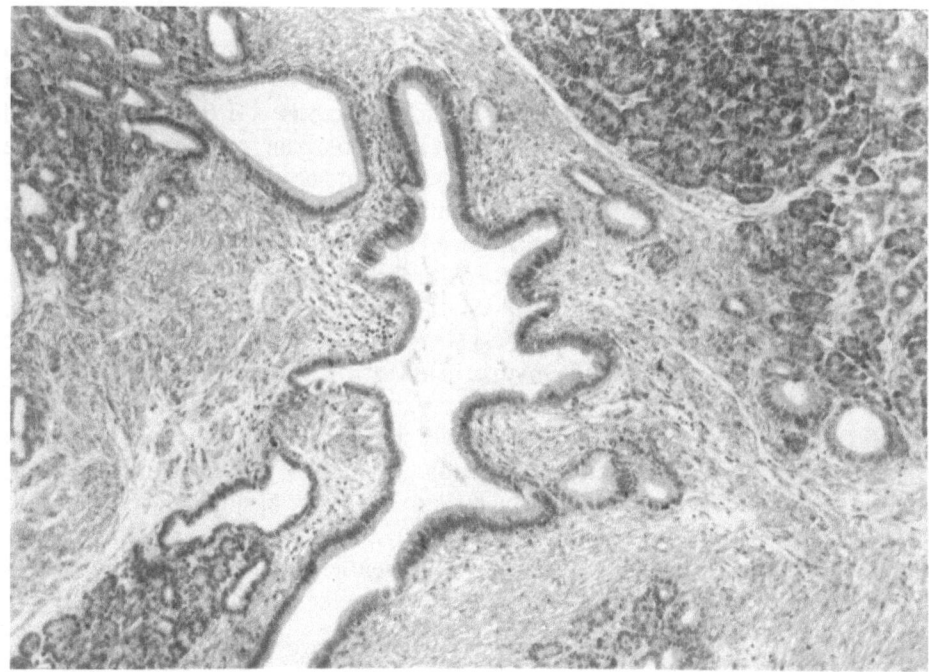

Fig. 4. Chronic pancreatitis: distorted interlobular duct surrounded by fibrosis. H&E, × 125

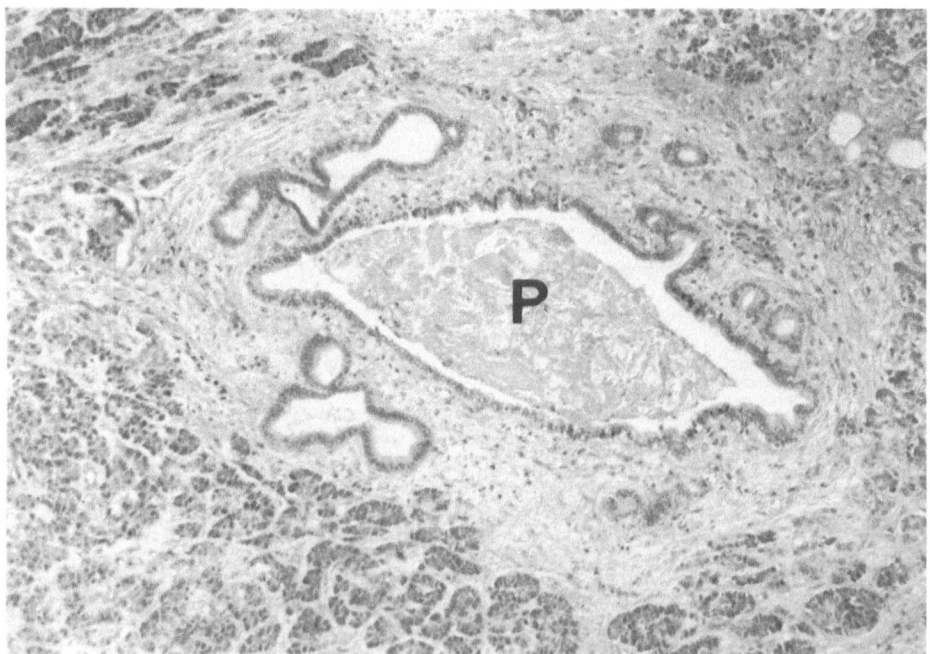

Fig. 5. Chronic pancreatitis: protein precipitate *(P)* in an interlobular duct entrapped in fibrotic tissue

results in pseudocysts, but rather induces perilobular fibrosis. The development of fibrosis in the interlobular spaces then most likely affects the wall of the interlobular ducts (Fig. 4). This may cause duct sacculations and strictures. Irregularities in duct caliber in turn may hamper the flow of pancreatic secretion and promote precipitation of proteins (Fig. 5) with subsequent calcification, as was experimentally demonstrated in dogs by partial pancreatic duct ligation for 4 months and longer [13]. In time the acinar cells of lobules drained by obstructed ducts disappear and are replaced by fibrotic tissue. In this way perilobular fibrosis extends into the lobule and eventually leads to diffuse lobular fibrosis. If the fibrotic process does not affect the main pancreatic duct, the disease most likely does not progress, unless acute pancreatitis relapses there and increasingly involves the remainder of the pancreas.

Conclusions

Focal necrosis and pseudocysts, the hallmarks of acute pancreatitis, are also present in chronic pancreatitis. This suggests a pathogenetic relationship between acute and chronic pancreatitis. The working hypothesis connecting the pathogenesis of acute pancreatitis with that of chronic pancreatitis focuses on the induction of perilobular fibrosis by the resolution of intrapancreatic fat necrosis, and the subsequent duct distortions by periductal fibrosis, with the consequences to pancreatic secretion and the drainage of acinar tissue.

References

1. Ammann RW, Akovbiantz A, Largiader F, Schueler G (1984) Course and outcome of chronic pancreatitis. Longitudinal study of a mixed medical-surgical series of 245 patients. Gastroenterology 86:820–828
2. Ammann RW, Buehler H, Bruehlmann W, Kehl O, Muench R, Stamm B (1986) Acute (non-progressive) alcoholic pancreatitis: prospective longitudinal study of 144 patients with recurrent alcoholic pancreatitis. Pancreas 1:195–203
3. Becker V (1984) Chronische Pankreatitis. Klinische Morphologie. In: Bartelheimer H, Kühn HA, Becker V, Stelzner F (eds) Gastroenterologie und Stoffwechsel, vol 21. Thieme, Stuttgart
4. Berens JJ, Baggenstoss AH, Gray HK (1954) Ductal changes in chronic pancreatitis. AMA Arch Surgery 68:723–733
5. Bourliere M, Sarles H (1989) Pancreatic cysts and pseudocysts associated with acute and chronic pancreatitis. Dig Dis Sci 34:343–348
6. Edmondson HA, Bullock WK, Mehl JW (1950) Chronic pancreatitis and lithiasis. II. Pathology and pathogenesis of pancreatic lithiasis. Am J Pathol 26:37–49
7. Gambill EE, Comfort MW, Baggenstoss AH (1948) Chronic relapsing pancreatitis. An analysis of 27 cases associated with disease of the biliary tract. Gastroenterology 11:1–33
8. Gyr K, Heitz PU, Beglinger C (1984) Pancreatitis. In: Klöppel G, Heitz PU (eds) Pancreatic pathology. Livingstone, Edinburgh, pp 44–72
9. Klöppel G (1986) Pathomorphology of chronic pancreatitis. In: Malfertheiner, Ditschuneit H (eds) Diagnostic procedures in pancreatic disease. Springer, Berlin Heidelberg New York, pp 135–139
10. Klöppel G, Maillet B (1990) Pseudocysts in chronic pancreatitis: a morphological analysis of 57 resection specimens and 9 autopsy pancreata. Pancreas (in press)

11. Klöppel G, von Gerkan R, Dreyer T (1984) Pathomorphology of acute pancreatitis. Analysis of 367 autopsy cases and 3 surgical specimens. In: Gyr KE, Singer MV, Sarles H (eds) Pancreatitis – concepts and classification. Excerpta Medica, Amsterdam, pp 29–35
12. Klöppel G, Dreyer T, Willemer S, Kern HF, Adler G (1986) Human acute pancreatitis: its pathogenesis in the light of immunocytochemical and ultrastructural findings in acinar cells. Virchows Arch [Pathol Anat] 409:791–803
13. Konishi K, Izumi R, Kato O, Yamaguchi A, Miyazaki I (1981) Experimental pancreatolithiasis in the dog. Surgery 89:687–691
14. Sarles H (1965) Pancreatitis. Symposium Marseille 1963. Karger, Basel
15. Sarles H, Muratore R, Sarles JC (1961) Etude anatomique des pancréatites chronique de l'adulte. Sem Hop Paris 25:1507–1522
16. Sarles H, Martin M, Camatte R, Sarles JC (1963) Le démembrement des pancréatites: les pseudokystes des pancréatites aigues et des pancréatites chroniques. Presse Med 5:237–240
17. Sarles H, Sarles JC, Camatte R, Muratore R, Gaini M, Guien C, Pastor J, Le Roy F (1965) Observations on 205 confirmed cases of acute pancreatitis, recurring pancreatitis, and chronic pancreatitis. Gut 6:545–559
18. Sarles H, Sahel J, Staub JL, Bourry J, Lauguer R (1979) Chronic pancreatitis. In: Howat HT, Sarles H (eds) The exocrine pancreas. Saunders, Philadelphia, pp 402–439
19. Stolte M (1984) Chronische Pankreatitis: Morphologie, Pankreatographie, Differentialdiagnose. perimed, Erlangen
20. Uys CJ, Bank S, Marks IN (1973) The pathology of chronic pancreatitis in Cape Town. Digestion 9:454–468

Morphology of Nerves in Chronic Pancreatitis and the Interrelationship with Inflammatory Tissue

D. E. BOCKMAN, M. BÜCHLER, P. MALFERTHEINER, and H. G. BEGER[1]

Changes Which Occur with Chronic Pancreatitis

Chronic pancreatitis causes profound changes to occur in the makeup of the pancreas. There is functional and morphological regression of the exocrine parenchyma. Acinar cells in affected areas contain fewer or no zymogen granules; the cells decrease in height. The result of this reversion is tubular complexes, which are derived from a combination of acini and small ducts, but which have the appearance of a collection of ducts [5]. These areas are sometimes interpreted as resulting from ductular proliferation, but there is a notable paucity of mitoses. The acinar tissue disappears with time. Some of the loss comes about by a process which has been termed apoptosis because the apical part of the acinar cell is sloughed off. Some of the cells simply disintegrate and become part of the amorphous material which may be drained away by patent ducts or retained in the connective tissue space.

There is a concomitant increase in the proportion of connective tissue in the pancreas, because of the fibrosis which is characteristic of chronic pancreatitis (Fig. 1). The fibrosis separates, and penetrates, lobules. It is common to find, upon histological examination, areas which are predominantly collagenous connective tissue, with islands of pancreatic parenchyma. The parenchyma may be relatively

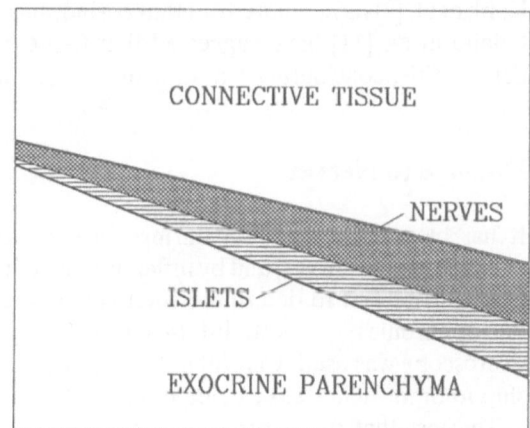

Fig. 1. Diagrammatic representation of the changing proportions of pancreatic elements with the progression of chronic pancreatitis. As one progresses from left to right, there is a decrease in exocrine parenchyma, but an increase in connective tissue, islets, and nerves

[1] Department of Anatomy, Medical College of Georgia, Augusta, Georgia, U.S.A., and Departments of Surgery and Internal Medicine, University of Ulm, FRG

Chronic Pancreatitis
Ed. by Beger, Büchler, Ditschuneit, and Malfertheiner
© Springer-Verlag Berlin Heidelberg 1990

normal in appearance, or may be reduced to strands of cells dispersed among the collagenous fibers. If acinar regression has progressed to the proper stage, the isolated parenchyma presents as tubular complexes.

It is also common to find islets of Langerhans either isolated in fibrous stroma, or prominent in lobules which have been reduced in size. Thus the proportion of islet tissue, relative to exocrine parenchyma, is elevated.

Pancreatic nerves are more prominent in the pancreas from patients with chronic pancreatitis [6]. The mean diameter of nerves is significantly greater than controls. Furthermore, the mean area of tissue which is served per nerve is significantly decreased. In short, the nerves seem to be larger and more numerous. They are dispersed mainly, but not exclusively, in the connective tissue.

Inflammatory Foci

Foci of inflammatory cells frequently are found within the substance of the pancreas from patients with chronic pancreatitis. These foci, furthermore, often are closely associated with pancreatic nerves, and with intrapancreatic ganglia. Inflammatory foci may surround, be in the vicinity of, or be unrelated to nerves.

The predominant cells in the inflammatory foci of chronic pancreatitis are lymphocytes. A smaller number are macrophages. Neutrophils in varying quantities may be present. Eosinophils [9] and tissue mast cells [11] are sometimes found. All of these cells are present in greater quantities in chronic pancreatitis than in healthy pancreas.

All of the cells which comprise these foci are capable of liberating powerful, biologically active products. Lymphocytes may liberate cytokines which attract other cells, and cause them to release bioactive materials. Macrophages and neutrophils liberate a plethora of biologically active materials, including hydrolytic enzymes [3]. Keith et al. [9] have pointed out that eosinophils are a source of a neurotoxin [7], while Odaira et al. [11] have suggested that tissue mast cells may play a role in chronic pancreatitis, considering that they produce a large variety of chemical mediators.

Damage to Nerves

It has been suggested that during chronic pancreatitis pain is caused by fibrosis constricting the nerves, and by inflammation of the nerves [8, 14]. Recent studies have been carried out to determine what changes might be present in pancreatic nerves during chronic pancreatitis [6]. In addition to light microscopic investigation, electron microscopy was used. Careful morphometric determination of the nerves in relationship to other tissue was carried out as well.

The fact that the nerves are larger argues against pain being caused by fibrosis constricting the nerves.

The nerves are altered, however. The organization of organelles, such as microtubules, which are evident in individual nerve fibers, is disrupted. There may be some breakdown of intrafiber organelles.

Perhaps most significantly, the perineurium is damaged (Fig. 2). The perineurium is a multilayered covering which surrounds each nerve bundle. It is composed of layers

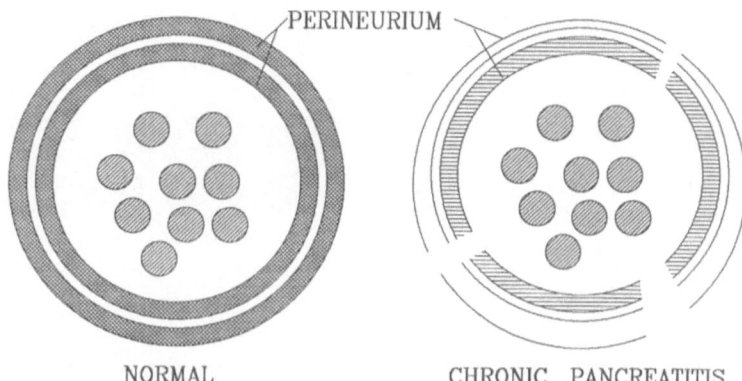

NORMAL CHRONIC PANCREATITIS

Fig. 2. Representation of the damage to the perineurium which occurs in chronic pancreatitis. The intact perineurium in the normal condition provides a barrier which insures a specialized environment for the nerves inside, whereas the damaged perineurium allows penetration of biologically active materials from the surrounding extracellular matrix

of epithelioid cells, each layer of which has a basement membrane on both sides. The perineurium serves as a barrier between the internal parts of the nerve bundle and the connective tissue space through which it is traveling.

Connections of Nerves

The autonomic nervous system provides sympathetic and parasympathetic motor fibers to the pancreas. In addition, sensory fibers run alongside motor fibers [1, 12] (Fig. 3). The nerves of the pancreas are distributed along blood vessels which supply the pancreas and adjacent structures. The nerves lie very close to the blood vessels.

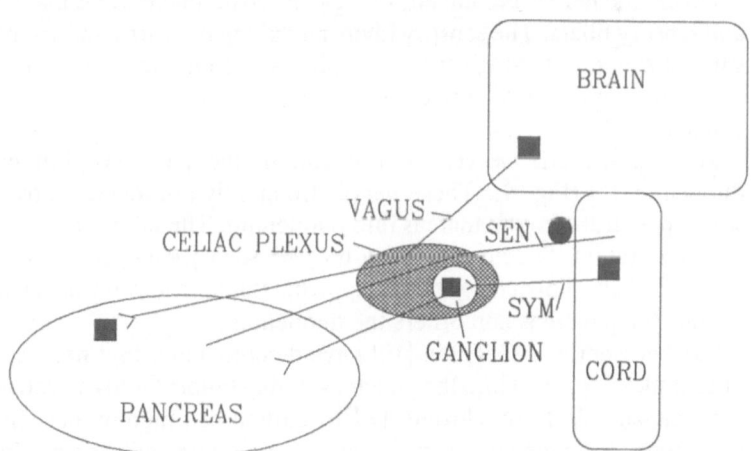

Fig. 3. Diagram showing the autonomic and sensory (SEN) innervation of the pancreas, as connected with the CNS. Although all fibers pass through the celiac plexus, only those of the sympathetic system (SYM) synapse in the celiac ganglion

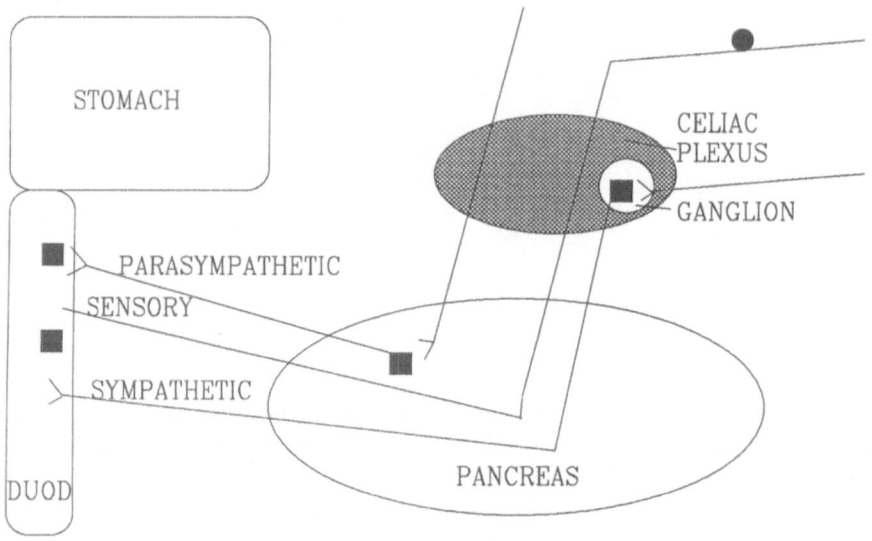

Fig. 4. Diagram showing the continuation of innervation through the pancreas into the duodenum. Autonomic and sensory fibers are shown, and all are presumed to be present in the nerves which run between pancreas and duodenum

Parasympathetic fibers are carried in the vagus nerve. They pass through the celiac plexus without synapse to end upon ganglia located within the pancreas.

Sympathetic fibers arise in the thoracic spinal cord and are conducted through the splanchnic nerves to the celiac plexus, where they synapse in the celiac ganglia. The postganglionic sympathetic fibers are then conducted, in company with vagal fibers, from the celiac plexus to the pancreas, where they associate with blood vessels.

Pancreatic nerves are mixed; a single nerve bundle may be made up of both motor and sensory fibers. The sensory fibers mediating pain are conducted toward the CNS, without synapse, through the celiac plexus, through the splanchnic nerves, to enter the thoracic spinal cord. The cell bodies of these neurons are located in the dorsal root ganglia.

Some pancreatic nerves do not end in the pancreas, but continue into the duodenum [4] (Fig. 4). These nerves frequently are located close to blood vessels which penetrate from pancreas into duodenum. The nerves connect with the enteric nervous system. Specifically, they may be seen joining the myenteric plexus. Tiscornia [13] has shown that nerves supplying this area may branch, with some branches serving the pancreas and others the duodenum.

Kirchgessner and Gershon [10] have demonstrated that nerves originating in the enteric plexus project into the pancreas. Using FluoroGold as a retrograde tracer, and the lipid-soluble fluorochrome DiI to outline cell membranes, they demonstrated projections from the myenteric ganglia of duodenum and stomach into pancreas (Fig. 5). Labeled neurons in the stomach were clustered, suggesting a subset of specialized gastric ganglia that innervate the pancreas. The number of labeled neurons was greater in the upper part of the duodenum, but continued caudally as far as 2 cm

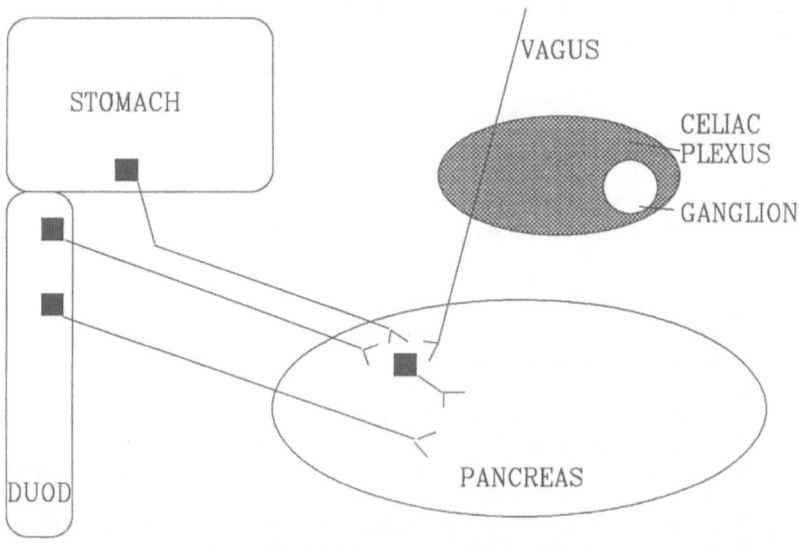

Fig. 5. Diagram showing the projection of enteric nerves into the pancreas. These nerves originate in stomach and duodenum, and are distributed to multiple sites in the pancreas

beyond the ampulla of Vater. Axons terminated in the pancreas in association with ganglia, acini, ducts, blood vessels, and islets. The enteropancreatic neural axis may thus affect exocrine and endocrine function.

Functional Consequences

The nerves of the pancreas, in patients with chronic pancreatitis, are retained, perhaps increased, in an environment of acinar regression, fibrosis, and inflammation. The barrier which normally separates the nerve fibers from the extracellular matrix is damaged. Specifically, the perineurium no longer provides a protective covering which maintains a specialized milieu within the nerve. The nerve is therefore maintained in a condition that is conductive to the initiation of nerve impulses. Several possible consequences result from this condition.

Pain would result from the continual stimulation of the sensory fibers which run in these nerves.

Parasympathetic and sympathetic fibers run in the same nerves. Continual stimulation of the parasympathetic fibers would cause stimulation of secretion, perhaps leading to the same consequences as overstimulation of secretion by cerulein. Continual stimulation of sympathetic fibers would cause alterations in the vasculature of the pancreas, the main target of these fibers.

Furthermore, because of the continuation of nerves through the pancreas into the duodenum, secondary effects in the duodenum might be expected, mediated through the enteric nervous system. These effects are consistent with the observation that a variably inflamed, rigid duodenum may be found at the time of surgery for pancreatic disease [2].

References

1. Alvarado F (1955) Distribution of nerves within the pancreas. J Int Coll Surg 23:675–699
2. Beger HG, Krautzberger W, Bittner R, Büchler M, Limmer J (1985) Duodenum-preserving resection of the head of the pancreas in patients with severe chronic pancreatitis. Surgery 97:467–473
3. Bockman DE (1987) Gut-associated macrophages. In: Brostoff J, Challacombe SJ (eds) Food allergy and intolerance. Baillière Tindall, London, pp 67–87
4. Bockman DE (1988) Systems underlying involvement of the duodenum in pancreatic disease. Pancreas 3:592
5. Bockman DE, Boydston WR, Anderson MC (1982) Origin of tubular complexes in human chronic pancreatitis. Am J Surg 144:243–249
6. Bockman DE, Büchler M, Malfertheiner P, Beger HG (1988) Analysis of nerves in chronic pancreatitis. Gastroenterology 94:1459–1469
7. Durack DT, Ackerman SJ, Loegering DA, Gleich GJ (1981) Purification of human eosinophil-derived neurotoxin. Proc Natl Acad Sci USA 78:5165–5169
8. Frey CF (1973) Ninety-five percent pancreatectomy. In: Carey LC (ed) The pancreas. Mosby, St Louis, pp 202–229
9. Keith RG, Keshavjee SH, Kerenyi NR (1982) Neuropathology of chronic pancreatitis in humans. Can J Surg 28:207–211
10. Kirchgessner AL, Gershon MD (1989) Innervation of the rat's pancreas: analysis of direct projections from neurons in myenteric ganglia of the duodenum and stomach and intrapancreatic ganglia. Gastroenterology 96:A258
11. Odaira C, Koizumi M, Sawai T (1987) Quantitative study on tissue mast cells in pancreatic disease. Digestion 38:50
12. Richins CA (1945) The innervation of the pancreas. J Comp Neurol 83:223–236
13. Tiscornia OM (1977) The neural control of exocrine and endocrine pancreas. Am J Gastroenterol 67:541–560
14. White TT (1982) Pain. In: Bradley EL III (ed) Complications of pancreatitis. Saunders, Philadelphia, pp 203–222

Peptidergic Innervation in Chronic Pancreatitis*

E. Weihe[1], M. Büchler[2], S. Müller[1], H. Friess[2], H. J. Zentel[1], and N. Yanaihara[3]

Introduction

The reason for the generation and continuation of chronic pain in chronic pancreatitis is unclear [6, 10, 11, 13, 61, 117]. Current concepts of the neurobiology of pain point to the possible role of various neuropeptides in pain processing and inflammation [8, 29, 32, 33, 44, 60, 64, 65, 68, 79, 104, 112]. A key function has been ascribed to the proinflammatory and pronociceptive peptides of the tachykininin (TK) family (8, 44, 104, 109]. That the tachykinin substance P (SP) may be involved in chronic inflammatory and painful disease of the gastrointestinal system is evidenced by a selective increase in the density of tachykinin receptors in the bowels of patients suffering from Crohn's disease and ulcerative colitis [62, 63, 64].

A recent study of pancreatic nerves from patients suffering from chronic pancreatitis revealed an increase in their number and diameter and striking ultrastructural changes consisting mainly of damage to the perineurial sheath [10]. This was taken as evidence to suggest that alterations of pancreatic nerves themselves might sustain pancreatic pain.

In the present study we aimed to clarify whether the neuronal changes in chronic pancreatitis concerned peptidergic pancreatic nerves. In the light of their presumed pronociceptive and proinflammatory function, we concentrated on TKs and calcitonin gene-related peptide (CGRP). Since vasoactive intestinal polypeptide (VIP) was recently shown also to play a role in primary afferent nociceptive processing, we included in our analysis this peptide and its gene coproduct, peptide histidine isoleucine (PHI) as well as the human form of PHI, peptide histidine methionine (PHM) [41, 112]. In the light of accumulating evidence for a crucial role of sympathetic fibers in chronic inflammatory pain we further investigated the response of neuropeptide Y (NPY), known to be present in postganglionic sympathetic fibers [45, 47, 71, 78, 80]. The view of a potential antinociceptive and anti-inflammatory role of endogenous opioids and opioid receptors in the periphery prompted us to look also for pancreatitis-induced changes of pancreatic opioid innervation [22, 49, 66, 67, 81, 85, 88, 89, 102, 105, 106, 107, 112].

---

* Supported by the German Research Foundation

[1] Department of Anatomy, University of Mainz, Saarstrasse 19–21, D-6500 Mainz, FRG
[2] Department of General Surgery, University of Ulm, Steinhövelstrasse 9, D-7900 Ulm, FRG
[3] College of Pharmacy, University of Shizuoka, 395 Yada, Shizuoka-shi, Shizuoka-ken, 422, Japan

Chronic Pancreatitis
Ed. by Beger, Büchler, Ditschuneit, and Malfertheiner
© Springer-Verlag Berlin Heidelberg 1990

Materials and Methods

Patients

Tissue from 20 patients with chronic alcohol-induced pancreatitis was prepared for analysis after duodenum-preserving resection of the pancreatic head [6]. Samples were removed from the resected portion of the gland. All 20 patients had advanced chronic pancreatitis. The proportion of fibrotic tissue exceeded that of parenchyma. This was verified by independent analysis of sections routinely stained with H&E. Specimens from the pancreatic head removed from 12 organ donors were prepared in parallel to serve as controls. Approval by the institution's human research review committee was obtained, and appropriate written informed consent was secured before taking tissue from organ donors [13].

Tissue Processing and Immunocytochemical Procedure

Specimens were processed for light-microscopic enzyme and double-immunofluorescence immunohistochemistry on deparaffinized serial sections after fixation in acid-free Bouin's solution as described in more detail elsewhere [102, 103, 104, 106, 114].

Primary antisera

TK immunoreactivity was visualized with a variety of anti-TKs. SP was localized with a monoclonal antibody (rat ascites) directed against its C-terminus (Serotec, UK, or Seralab, UK and used at a dilution of 1:40 and 1:400, respectively) [112].

Rabbit polyclonal anti-neurokinin A (NKA) and anti-neurokinin B (NKB) were obtained from Peninsula (UK) and used in a dilution ranging from 1:5000 to 1:20000.

CGRP was stained by a rabbit polyclonal anti-CGRP (Amersham, UK; dilution of 1.6000) which recognized the two human forms of CGRP [69].

A polyclonal antiserum, raised in rabbit, to NPY was purchased from Amersham (UK) and used at a dilution of 1:8000.

The polyclonal antiserum used to localize VIP was directed against its C-terminal (Cambridge Research Biochemicals, UK; dilution of 1:30000). Polyclonal rabbit antisera against PHI (code 8403; dilution 1:20000) and against PHM (code R8501; dilution 1:20000) were both raised by one of the authors (N. Yanaihara) [41].

Specificity of antisera

The specificity of the immunostaining was established by preabsorption of the diluted antisera with synthetic homologous antigens. Peptides for preabsorption studies were purchased from Peninsula (UK) and Bachem (Switzerland).

Anti-NPY exhibited minor cross-reactivity with peptide YY. Anti-rat CGRP cross-reacted with human CGRP but did not differentiate between CGRP I and II [69, 112].

Anti-VIP and anti-PHI did not mutually cross-react. Anti-PHI but not anti-VIP recognized PHM. Anti-PHM recognized PHI. Anti-PHI and anti-PHM were found to be equally potent to visualize PHI as well as PHM [41, 112].

Anti-SP cross-reacted with other mammalian TKs, namely with NKA and NKB [112]. Anti-NKA did not cross-react with SP but with NKB. Anti-NKB recognized not only NKB but also SP. Thus, none of the anti-TKs was very specific for a particular TK. Nevertheless, they were all found to be useful for tracing TK-immunoreactive (ir) fibers without claiming molecular identification [106, 112, 113].

Proenkephalin opioids were visualized with a polyclonal rabbit antiserum (E. Weber, Oregon, USA) directed against the octapeptide Met-enkephalin-Arg-Gly-Leu (ME-RGL). This antiserum specifically recognized the octapeptide and did not cross-react with other proenkephalin derivatives or with prodynorphin or proopiomelanocortin opioids [102, 106, 111, 114]. There was no evidence for mutual cross-reactions of the antisera used. They did not cross-react with unrelated peptides. Immunoreactivities are designated according to the antigen against which the antisera/antibodies are directed without claiming molecular specificity [112].

Results

Organ Donor Pancreas

NPY. NPY-ir nerve fibers supplied predominantly arterial blood vessels regardless of caliber. They formed dense periarterial plexus (Fig. 1a, c). Some NPY-ir fibers were also present in paravascular nerves. NPY-ir innervation of veins and venules was less dense than that of arteries and arterioles (Fig. 1c). In addition, a substantial number of NPY-ir varicose fibers were seen in the exocrine parenchyma and around ducts (Fig. 1a, d). Close contact with acinar cells and with ducts was frequent. Some peri- and intrainsular NPY-ir fibers were also seen. In intrinsic ganglia, a very minor population of neuronal cell bodies and a moderate number of fibers stained for NPY (Fig. 3a). Nonvascular inter- and intralobular nerves of varied caliber contained some NPY-ir fibers. A subpopulation of islet cells and of duct cells was weakly stained by anti-NPY, indicating that there was some cross-reaction with peptide YY, known to be present in such cells [94].

VIP/PHI/PHM. Antisera against VIP-, PHI, or PHM produced virtually identical results. The best staining against low background was obtained with the anti-PHI whereas anti-VIP immunocytochemistry was hampered by relatively high-background staining in spite of the use of highly diluted VIP antisera (up to 1:50000). Nevertheless, it was possible to reveal that the distribution of VIP, PHI-, and PHM-immunoreactivities completely overlapped, suggesting coexistence. Since PHI and PHM antisera mutually cross-reacted, it was impossible to specify exactly the molecular nature of PHI and PHM immunoreactivities. On the other hand, the noncross-reactivity of anti-VIP with PHI/PHM and of anti-PHI/PHM with VIP indicated that VIP as well as its coproduct PHI/PHM was present. VIP/PHI/PHM-ir varicose nerve fibers supplied the larger blood vessels less densely than NPY-ir fibers. The perivascu-

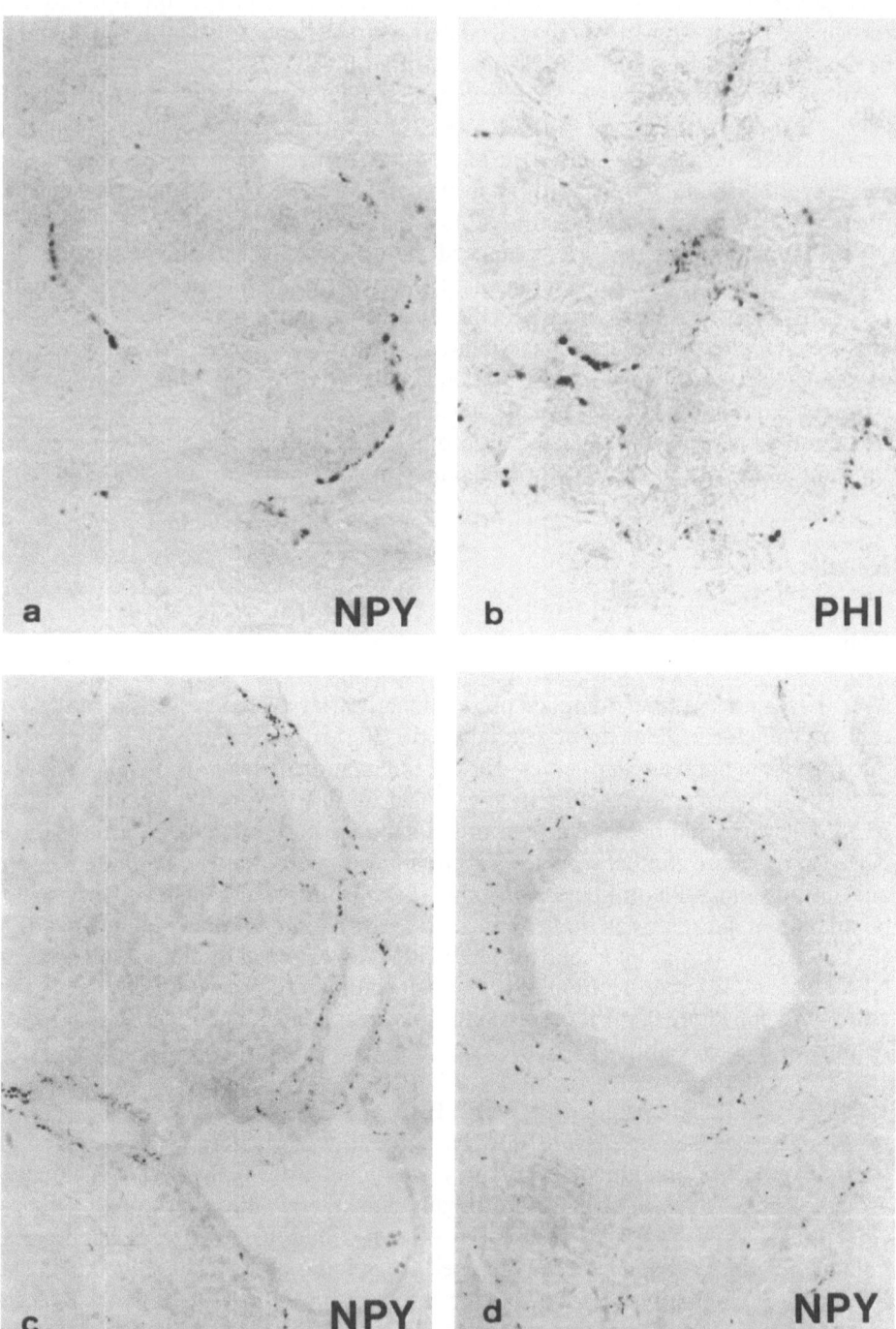

Fig. 1a–d. Organ donor pancreas. The distribution and density of NPY- and PHI-ir varicose nerve fibers in the exocrine parenchyma is similar (**a, b**); NPY-ir varicose nerve fibers form dense periarterial plexus but are less dense around veins (**c**). NPY-ir nerve supply to periductal tissue is relatively dense (**d**). (**a, b,** × 540; **c, d** × 80)

lar VIP//PHI/PHM-ir plexus in small-caliber blood vessels was almost as dense as the perivascular NPY-ir plexus. VIP/PHI-ir varicose fibers were frequently seen in the exocrine parenchyma (Fig. 1b), where they showed a distribution pattern similar to that of NPY. Occasionally they occurred within and around insulae. Numerous ganglionic cell bodies of intrinsic ganglia regularly stained for coexisting VIP and PHI/PHM, as revealed on adjacent sections. The intensity of cell body staining varied from weak to very strong. Numerous VIP/PHI/PHM-ir varicose fibers were present between VIP/PHI/PHM-ir and non-ir ganglionic cell bodies. Small groups of ganglionic cell bodies in the exocrine parenchyma or neuronal cell bodies located singularly in the parenchyma also stained for coexisting VIP/PHI/PHM. A subpopulation of islet cells and duct cells stained for VIP and PHI/PHM.

SP/NKA/NKB and CGRP. SP and NKB immunoreactivities were identical. This was not surprising because anti-SP and anti-NKB mutually cross-reacted. The number of NKA-ir fibers was lower than that of SP- or NKB-ir fibers. This indicated that the anti-NKA was relatively specific in staining only a subpopulation of the pan-TK immunoreactivity. The SP immunoreactivity referred to in the following must be interpreted as representing pan-TK immunoreactivity and not SP as molecular identity.

With the exception of parenchmal innervation, most of the SP- and CGRP-immunoreactive fibers coincided (Fig. 2). Double-immunofluorescence revealed almost complete coexistence of SP and CGRP immunoreactivities. However, there was a clear-cut difference between SP- and CGRP-ir fiber populations with regard to parenchymal innervation. While CGRP-ir fibers were almost completely absent from the exocrine parenchyma (Fig. 2d), some parenchymal SP-ir fibers were regularly seen (Fig. 2a, b, c). In contrast, the vascular innervation with SP and CGRP fibers completely coincided. Periarterial fibers staining for SP/CGRP were less frequent than those staining for NPY. In paravascular nerves, SP/CGRP-ir fibers outnumbered NPY-ir fibers. Only very rarely were intrinsic nerve cell bodies immunoreactive for SP, and in only a very few instances some very weakly ir-CGRP were seen in neuronal perikarya. Non-SP/CGRP-ir neuronal cell bodies of intrinsic ganglia (and of small groups of ganglionic cells or of individual neuronal cell bodies in the exocrine parenchyma) were surrounded by a dense plexus of SP/CGRP-ir fibers (Fig. 3b, c). Double-immunofluorescence revealed that VIP/PHI-ir ganglionic cell bodies were targetted by SP-ir varicose fibers. In inter- and intralobular nerve bundles, SP/CGRP-ir fibers were also much more frequent than those staining for NPY. Some SP/CGRP-ir peri- and intrainsular fibers were present. Ir-CGRP but not ir-SP were regulary present in a minor population of insular cells.

Opioid (ME-RGL). ME-RGL-ir fibers were sparse. They were present in a few nerve fibers running with paravascular, interlobular, and some intralobular nerves. Further, ME-RGL-ir fibers were seen in intrinsic ganglia where they surrounded non-ir ganglionic cell bodies. There was no evidence for opioid innervation delivered to the exocrine parenchyma.

Coexistence Patterns of Unrelated Peptides. Most if not all ir-CGRP coexisted with ir-SP as revealed by double-immunofluorescence (see also above). Double-immuno-

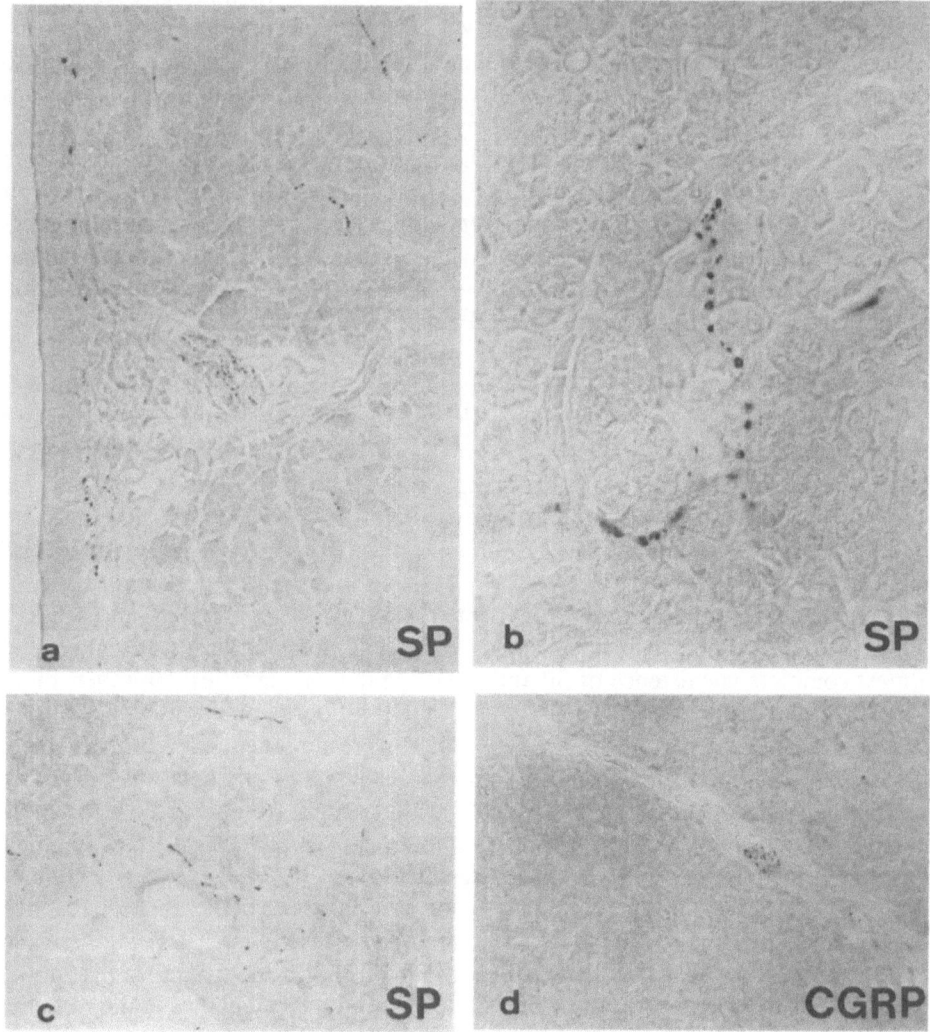

Fig. 2a–d. Organ donor pancreas: SP-ir nerve fibers are present in a small interlobular nerve (**a**). A moderate number of SP-ir fibers are seen in the exocrine parenchyma as shown at low magnification (**a, c**) and at high magnification (**b**). CGRP-ir fibers are present in a small interlobular nerve but absent from the exocrine parenchyma (**d**). (**a, c, d** × 40; **b** × 580)

fluorescence provided no evidence that significant proportions of SP and NPY immunoreactivities coexisted. In contrast, coexistence of ir-SP and ir-PHI was seen in a considerable proportion of fibers. There was no evidence for coexistence of ME-RGL with the nonopioid peptides investigated. It could not yet be determined whether CGRP and VIP/PHI/PHM were cocontained. Neither was it possible to answer the question as to whether NPY and VIP/PHI/PHM coexisted.

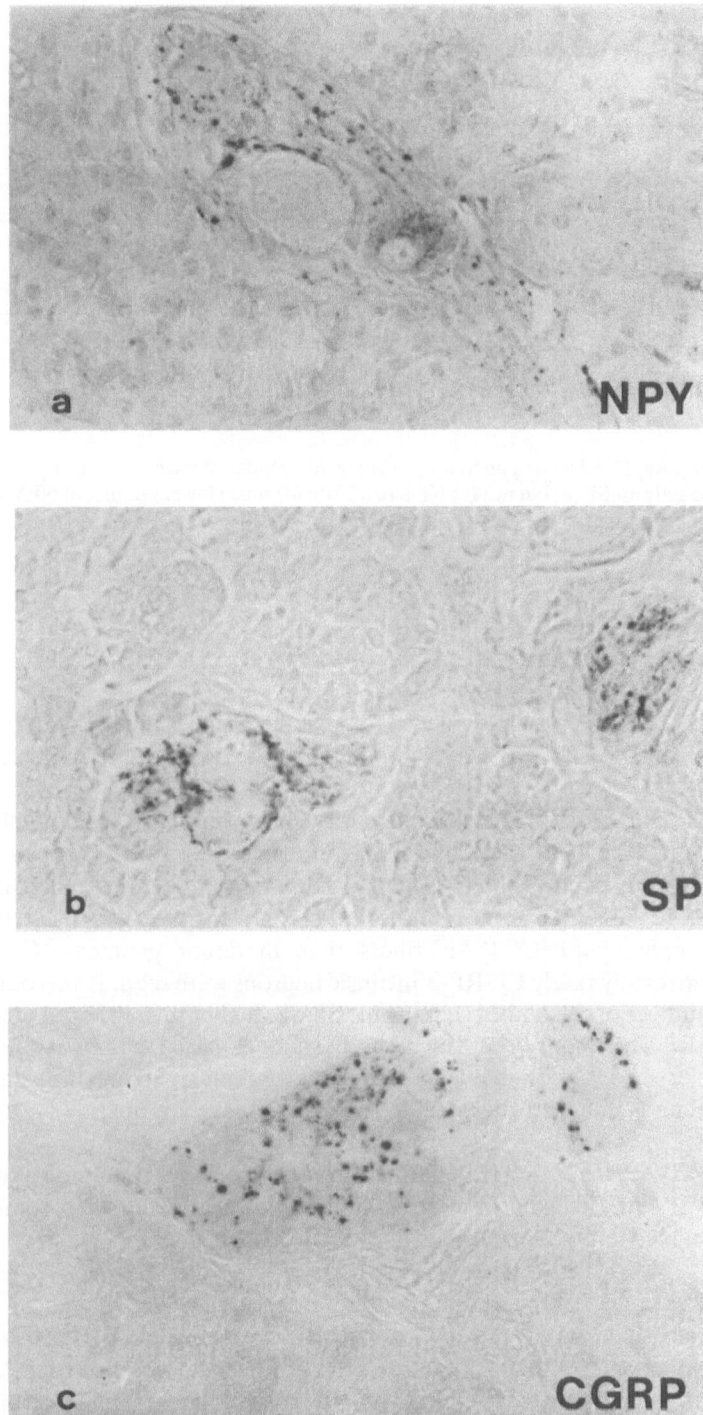

Fig. 3a–c. Organ donor pancreas. NPY (**a**) but not SP (**b**) or CGRP (**c**) immunoreactivity is present in a neuronal cell body of a small intrinsic ganglion. Note that the number of SP- and CGRP-ir intraganglionic and juxtaganglionic varicose fibers excedes that staining for NPY. (**a–c** × 350)

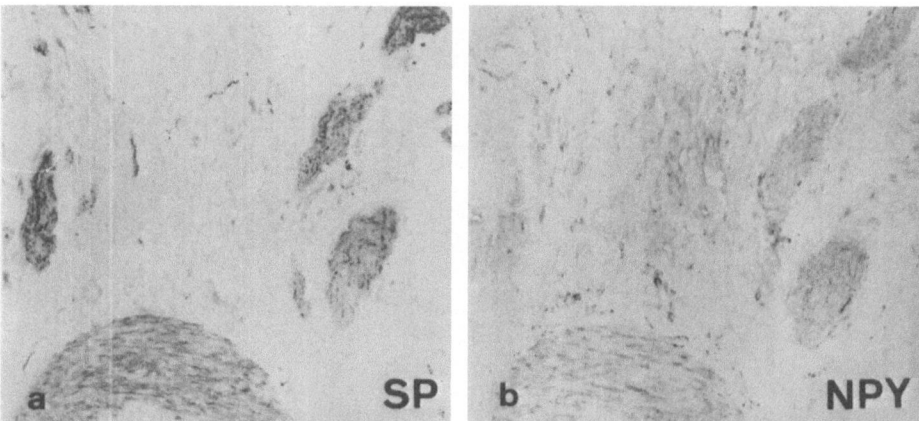

Fig. 4a, b. Chronic pancreatitis. Adjacent sections showing enlarged paravascular nerves staining heavily for SP (**a**) but not for NPY (**b**). Note the much lower number of NPY fibers as compared to SP fibers present in the enlarged nerves. (**a, b** × 80)

Changes in Pancreatitis

NPY. There was no evidence for striking changes in NPY innervation. In contrast to SP and CGRP, NPY fibers in enlarged nerves were little affected (Fig. 4).

SP and CGRP. The most striking change in peptidergic innervation pattern concerned the previously described altered nerves. It consisted of an intensification of the immunostaining for CGRP and SP in numerous fibers contained in these enlarged and more numerous nerves (Figs. 4a, 5b, c, d). Intrinsic ganglia received an even denser supply by SP/CGRP-ir fibers than in donor pancreas. Occasionally, SP- and extremely rarely CGRP-ir intrinsic neurons were seen. It was our impression that the number of cell bodies staining for SP was higher than in organ donors though still very low. The intensity of SP cell body staining varied from weak to moderately strong. Nerve bundles in the vicinity of or in continuity with intrinsic ganglia also contained abundant and strongly stained SP/CGRP-ir nerve fibers.

VIP/PHI/PHM. The enlarged nerve bundles also contained a substantial number of VIP- and PHI/PHM-ir nerve fibers. However, they were somewhat less intensely stained and less numerous than SP/CGRP-ir fibers.

Coexistence. Double-immunofluorescence revealed that most ir-SP and ir-CGRP coexisted in fibers present in enlarged nerves (Fig. 6a, b). However, some SP-ir fibers were not CGRP-ir, and some CGRP-ir fibers did not stain for SP. A subpopulation of fibers contained SP and PHI (Fig. 6c, d) immunoreactivities while ir-NPY, as a rule, was not coexisting with ir-SP. Thus, coexistence patterns were principally similar to that in donor pancreas but more easily visualized because SP/CGRP- and VIP/PHI-ir fibers were more frequent than in donor pancreas.

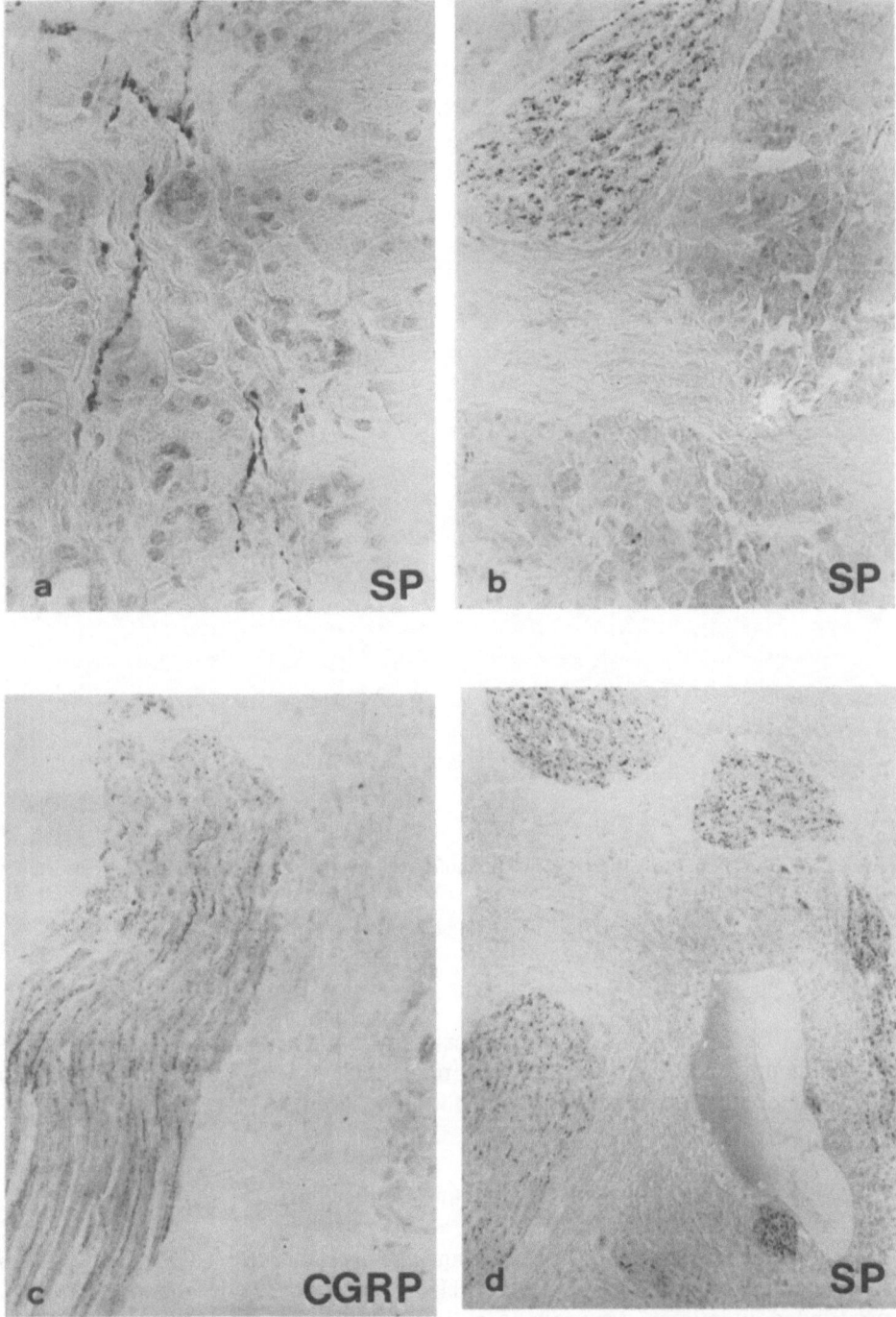

Fig. 5a–d. Chronic pancreatitis. Enlarged nerves in areas with little exocrine parenchyma (**b**) or devoid of exocrine parenchyma (**c, d**) contain abundant SP (**b, d**) and CGRP (**c**) immunoreactive nerve fibers. A region of remaining exocrine parenchyma contains SP-ir varicose fibers running between exocrine cells (**a**). (**a** × 335; **b** × 160; **c, d** × 80)

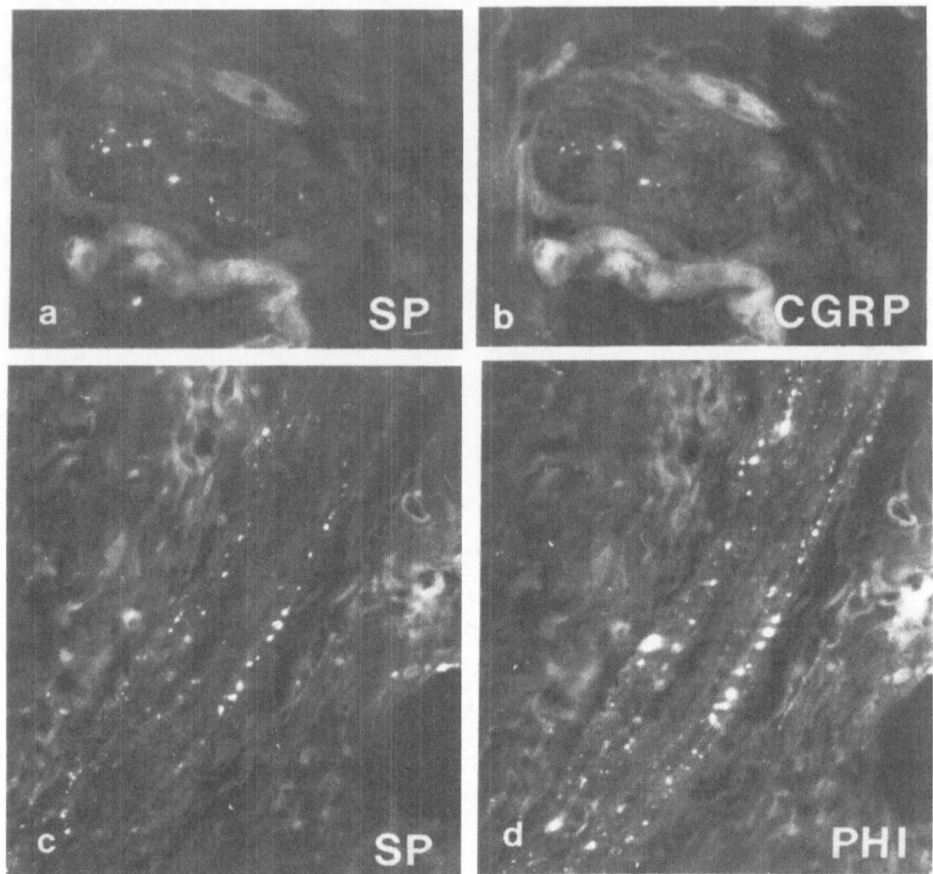

Fig. 6a–d. Chronic pancreatitis. Double immunofluorescence showing almost complete coexistence of SP (**a**) and CGRP (**b**) in an interlobular nerve. Note partial coexistence of ir-SP (**c**) and ir-PHI (**d**). (**a–d** × 450)

ME-RGL. No striking changes of pancreatic opioid innervation determined as ME-RGL immunoreactivity (proenkephalin related) have been detectable so far. No coexistence with other peptides was found to be "lit up" in pancreatitis.

"Lighting up" of Peptidergic Neuroimmune Connections

The nerve bundles containing numerous and heavily stained SP/CGRP-ir fibers (and somewhat less intensely stained VIP/PHI-ir and rare NPY-ir fibers) were often surrounded by inflammatory cells (Fig. 7a, b). In some areas, SP-ir and CGRP-ir fibers (and less frequently VIP/PHI-ir but extremely rarely NPY-ir fibers) branched off into the fields of inflammatory cells and formed close contacts with immunocytes (Fig. 7c, d). Inflammatory cells also accumulated around some ganglia. In some

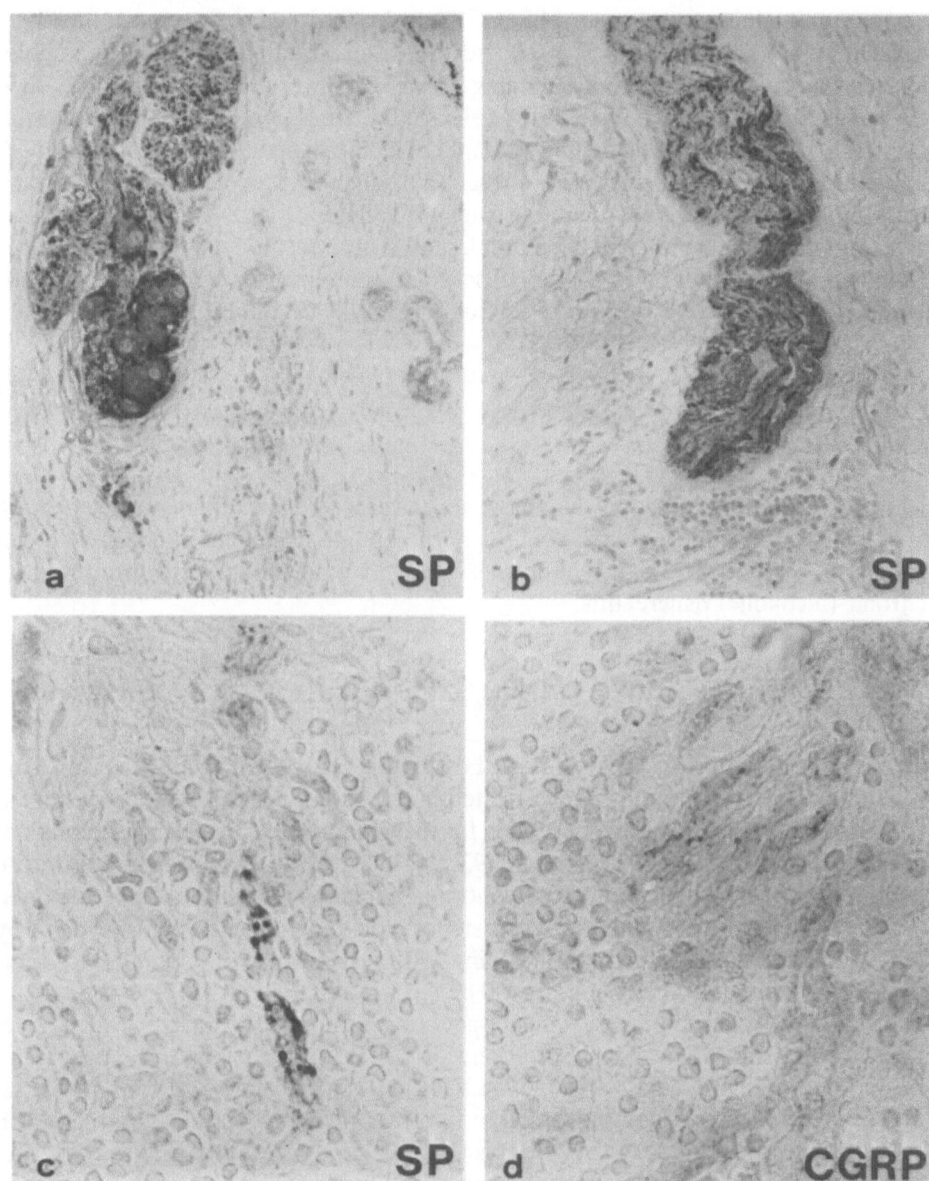

Fig. 7a–d. Chronic pancreatitis. An intrinsic ganglion with a iuxtaganglionic nerve (**a**) and an enlarged nerve abutting in a tissue area filled with inflammatory cells (**b**); note abundant nerve fibers heavily staining for SP in **a** and **b**; areas infiltrated by immune cells (mostly T- and B-lymphocytes) are targeted by SP- (**c**) and less strongly by CGRP-immunoreactive fibers (**d**); note close contacts of peptidergic varicose fibers with immune cells. (**a, b** × 165; **c, d** × 345)

regions, inflammatory cells infiltrated these nerve bundles and ganglia that contain nerve fibers staining for coexisting SP/CGRP or for PHI/PHM. In some of the fibers forming neuroimmune contacts ir-SP and ir-PHI coexisted, as revealed by double-immunofluorescence. Cell bodies staining for VIP/PHI were also seen to be located in the vicinity of infiltrated inflammatory cells. In the areas of neuroimmune interrelations, NKB immunoreactivities completely overlapped with ir-SP. NKA immunoreactivity represented only a fraction of but coexisted with ir-SP. The spectrum of inflammatory cells comprised mainly T-lymphocytes and B-lymphocytes whereas macrophages were not preponderant. These results obtained with double staining of nerve fibers by peptide antisera and immunocytes by monoclonal antibodies directed against subsets of immunocytes will be published in more detail elsewhere.

Discussion

The present light-microscopic immunohistochemical study has characterized peptide staining patterns in nerves supplying the normal human pancreas and has evaluated changes in peptidergic pancreatic innervation in patients suffering from painful chronic (alcoholic) pancreatitis.

Heterogeneity and Coexistence Patterns of Peptidergic Innervation

The normal peptidergic (NPY-, VIP-, PHI-, PHM, CGRP-, SP-, NKA-, NKB-, and opioid-ir) innervation pattern, investigated in organ donors, was found to be essentially similar to that previously described for the mammalian pancreas in general (if at all reported) [2, 13, 43, 59, 70, 84, 90, 92, 94, 99]. Newly recognized details of the peptidergic innervation specific for the normal human pancreas and a more detailed presentation of until now unknown coexistence/non-coexistence patterns revealed by our double-immunofluorescence including a wider spectrum of peptides, and their interrelation to classical transmitters will be reported elsewhere. However, we would like especially to point out a few new aspects at this point. We have provided novel evidence for a partial coexistence of SP and VIP/PHI in a subpopulation of pancreatic nerve fibers (Fig. 6c, d). Coexistence of VIP/PHI and SP has been also reported in other tissues. By demonstrating that SP-ir fibers supplying blood vessels or running in inter- and intralobular nerve bundles, as a rule, did not contain ir-NPY or tyrosine-hydroxylase (the marker enzyme of sympathetic nerves) we provide clear evidence against their being sympathetic [13, 40, 70].

Further, we have shown that the opioid (octapeptide) innervation of the human pancreas is more restricted than in other mammals, for example, in rodents where we have reported the presence of an extensive proenkephalin-related innervation of the exocrine parenchyma [106].

However the origin of the opioid innervation (preganglionic, postganglionic sympathetic/parasympathetic, or even sensory) remained unclarified [102, 103, 105, 106, 107, 108].

The extensive overlap of VIP//PHI/PHM and NPY immunoreactive varicose fibers and the fact that ir-VIP/PHI/PHM and ir-NPY (less frequently) occurred in intrinsic pancreatic neurons is suggestive of at least partial coexistence of NPY and VIP-related peptides. This constellation would be not unusual because there is accumulating evidence that NPY and VIP-related peptides coexist in neurons of various systems, particularly in the respiratory tract and in cranial ganglia, giving rise to the innervation of exocrine glands [107, 108, 112]. Although SP was found to occur in nerve fibers mainly independent of NPY, the possibility of coexistence of SP and NPY, in a minor subpopulation of pancreatic innervation, is conceivable [112].

Mixed Origins of Peptidergic Innervation

Contrary to the more simplistic view in the past that SP and CGRP are of sensory, VIP/PHI/PHM of postganglionic parasympathetic, and NPY of postganglionic sympathetic origin [17, 45, 100, 107, 112], our present results in conjunction with accumulating data in the literature indicate a far more mixed pattern of peptide phenotypes in the main divisions of the pancreatic innervation than previously believed. Nevertheless, SP and particularly CGRP may be still regarded as being mainly sensory although there may exist a so far neglected component of intrinsic SP innervation [112]. However, with regard to the nonspecificity of the SP antibodies available we must be aware that the SP innervation revealed in this study may represent not only SP but also other TKs. It would be intriguing if some of the apparently present intrinsic SP innervation would turn out to be NKB which is not expressed in sensory but possibly in intrinsic (parasympathetic?) neurons [112]. The partial coexistence of SP and PHI may reflect that there is a primary sensory or an intrinsic SP/VIP/PHI/PHM system, or oven both. The origin of pancreatic NPY innervation is probably dual, intrinsic (postganglionic parasympathetic) and extrinsic (postganglionic sympathetic) [45, 55, 107, 112]. However, a third (sensory) origin of pancreatic NPY innervation is not absolutely unlikely because our recent studies of sensory ganglia revealed some NPY-ir neuronal cell bodies in spinal ganglia of rodents (Weihe, unpublished). Similar observations were made in a nerve injury model in the rat by G. Bennett (Dahlem Conferenzen, Berlin, personal communication).

Clearly, the plasticity, coexistence patterns, and most likely mixed origins of peptidergic nerves in the human pancreas need further clarification (also discussed below) and should not be simplified [9, 55, 112].

Changes in Pancreatitis

The changes in peptidergic innervation in patients suffering from painful chronic pancreatitis appeared to be rather selective. They concerned predominantly interlobular and intralobular nerve bundles and the transmitter candidates SP and CGRP and, to a lesser extent, VIP/PHI/PHM [13, 70].

Thus, exactly those nerves which were found to be increased in number and diameter as shown in a preceeding analysis of nerves in chronic pancreatitis [10] contained a very large number of fibers staining intensely for mostly coexisting SP and

CGRP. A somewhat lower but still substantial number of fibers stained for VIP/PHI/ PHM. In contrast, such nerves contained comparatively low numbers of NPY fibers.

The absence of major changes in NPY, a cotransmitter candidate in postganglionic sympathetic neurons and, as suggested more recently, also in some intrinsic neurons underlines the selectivity of the neuronal response to chronic pancreatitis [45, 55, 112].

Although the opioid system did not seem to be strikingly affected, the involvement of opioids derived from other precursors than proenkephalin as investigated here, e.g., from prodynorphin or proopiomelanocortin is conceivable and still an open question [106, 107, 112].

It is not surprising that most of the staining for SP and CGRP in nerve fibers was equally intensified because these peptides are known to coexist in spinal and vagal primary sensory afferents of a variety of mammals, including humans [17, 45, 112].

That a substantial part of the altered nerves are of sensory nature is deducible from animal studies. Combined tracing and immunohistochemical studies revealed that the SP innervation of the rat pancreas is sensory. Its major part stems from spinal ganglia and can be expected to run with splanchnic nerves. Only a minor portion appears to originate from vagal sensory ganglia [84]. The staining of only rare cell bodies of intrinsic neurons for SP and CGRP is compatible with the view that the majority of altered nerve fibers does not originate from postganglionic parasympathetic neurons.

However, the possibility that a substantial intrinsic SP component is recruited in pancreatitis is not unlikely. In fact, the more obvious coexistence of SP and VIP/PHI/ PHM in pancreatitis as compared to donor pancreas may be indicative of such a nonsensory SP component being "lit up" and intensified in pancreatitis. On the other hand, the coexistence of SP and PHI in pancreatic nerves may reflect that some of the intensified VIP/PHI/PHM innervation is sensory. In fact, VIP and PHI can be regarded as primary sensory transmitter candidates, where they may coexist with SP and possibly CGRP [17, 45, 111]. Although there are still many uncertainties, all these observations taken together lead us to conclude that the innervation which appears to be predominantly affected in patients suffering painful chronic pancreatitis is mainly sensory.

The Neuroimmune Connection: Possible Pathophysiological Significance in Sustaining pain and Inflammation

The most striking and probably pathophysiologically important change was the "lighting up" of close interrelation between peptidergic neuronal elements and inflammatory cells in chronic pancreatitis. Interestingly, mainly the SP/CGRP and the VIP/PHI components formed frequent and close contacts with immune cells while the NPY fibers were much more rarely seen to branch off from blood vessels to intermingle with infiltrated immune cells. Thus, those peptidergic nerve fibers predominating in the enlarged and altered nerves also predominated in forming neuroimmune connections in inflamed areas. The neuroimmune link was, notably, most striking in the case of SP.

The function of the presumed sensory nerves which contain SP and/or CGRP or VIP/PHI as well as other TKs, (NKA and NPY) is probably heterogeneous. There appears to be consensus that SP can be regarded as a pain transmitter candidate in spinal primary afferents [8, 44, 60, 65, 112]. Immunization of rats against TKs results in hypoalgesia [25]. SP and CGRP interact in a complex manner, with CGRP inhibiting the degradation of SP [74], enhancing its pronociceptive (and immune-signaling?) action in the spinal dorsal horn and its proinflammatory (and pronociceptive?) action in the periphery [112]. Whether CGRP is transmitting pain on its own is unclear although anti-CGRP antisera given intrathecally produce antinociception in animals [50]. Interestingly, also VIP is involved in some qualities of nociceptive transmission [112]. In the light of their analgesic action, it will be particularly important to elucidate further the possible involvement and change of the various opioid peptides and receptors, though proenkephalin – derived ME-RGL appeared to be unaffected. Pain could be caused not only by increase in tonic activity of proalgesic substances but also by an insufficiency of endogenous antinociceptive system. Therefore, it will also be of interest to determine the possible involvement of neurotensin and galanin, which have antinociceptive actions [17, 45, 112]. Neurotensin receptors are present on visceral sensory fibers [51]. The possible involvement of somatostatin, having some actions related to pain also needs to be investigated [45].

Since pain over decades is the major symptom of chronic pancreatitis, we are tempted to postulate that the increase in SP/CGRP innervation in painful chronic pancreatitis is related to the pancreatic pain syndrome. Pancreatic nerves have been shown in a previous study to exhibit morphological signs of severe barrier loss at the interface of the perineurial sheath [10].

Therefore, activators and sensitizers of nociceptors, e. g., bradykinin, 5-HT, protons, ATP, prostaglandins, leukotrienes, lipoxygenase products, various cytokines, and growth factors, may have freer access to the small-diameter SP/CGRP and VIP/PHI sensory fibers enriched in these barrier-loss nerves [3, 5, 7, 23, 24, 37, 38, 40, 93, 95, 98]. It is particularly noteworthy that bradykinin receptors are present on small-diameter sensory fibers, and that peripherally applied bradykinin antagonists act antinociceptively [91]. Similar mechanisms apply to 5-HT$_3$ agonists and antagonists [26, 39], respectively. The specific properties of SP may perhaps be of crucial significance in the peripheral mechanism sustaining pain and inflammation or both. Experimental evidence supporting our view is derived from the recent observation that in the rat low doses of SP cause inflammatory hyperalgesia by sensitizing nociceptors to its own action and to the action of other mediators [72]. The increase of SP in pancreatic nerves in pancreatitis may indicate that there is an increase in peripheral SP signaling resulting in pain and chronic inflammation [52, 58, 120]. Release of SP-sensitizing nociceptors may occur not only at terminals but also along the fibers in nerves with barrier loss [73].

Thus, the involvement of SP and CGRP in chronic pancreatitis is not necessarily limited to pain transmission. Barrier damage would allow for freer access of inflammatory mediators to nerve fibers and of neuronal peptides to the surrounding tissue and thus provide the basis for local bidirectional communication between the nervous and the immune systems [21]. The chemoanatomical substrate for a neuroimmune dialogue at the peripheral level is seen not only in inflamed tissue but also in normal lymphoid tissue such as thymus, lymph nodes, and spleen where sensory and autonomic peptidergic nerves have been detected [30, 112, 113, 115]. Further, immune cells are present within nerves [27]. Peptides, particularly SP and VIP but also CGRP, are potent immunomodulators [18, 35, 36, 113]. The fact that SP is mitogenic for fibroblasts could indicate that it is involved in the fibrotic process [18]. Further, there is the intriguing possibility of reciprocal functional interrelation between neuropeptides, immune cells, cytokines, and nerve growth factor [1, 42, 56, 75, 76, 93, 97, 98, 116]. The possible importance of such a constellation in sustaining pain and inflammation has recently been suggested [57, 112]. A "soup" of mediators derived from nerves, various immune cells, endothelial cells, fibroblasts, etc. is most likely involved [58, 112]. Oncogenes may also participate in the neuroimmune cross-talk [86]. Complicatingly, immune cells, particularly when stimulated, express mRNA for neuropeptides and produce (and possibly release) a wide spectrum of neuropeptides [14, 85, 109]. Thus, neuropeptides are recently regarded to be not only neuromessengers but also cytokines [14]. Of perhaps crucial importance is the fact that opioids are contained in T-lymphocytes and other immune cells [14, 85]. They may have autocrine, paracrine, and cytokine actions, and they may even interfere with the primary sensory nerve fibers nearby because primary sensory (and sympathetic) neurons contain opioid receptors which may be important in peripheral nociception/antinociception and inflammatory/anti-inflammatory mechanisms [81, 88, 89, 109, 119]. Specific subclasses of opioid receptors present on immunocytes may be involved [87]. The fact that interleukin 1 has recently been shown to be contained in peripheral and central neurons and in the adrenal medulla possibly adds to the complexity of the interactive "soup" of neuroimmune mediators in chronic pancreatitis [83].

Experimental evidence for the functional involvement of SP innervation playing a major role in chronic pain comes from recent experiments employing the model of chronic inflammatory pain in the arthritic rat [4, 31, 112]. In this animal model it has been revealed that the message for the pronociceptive peptides SP and CGRP is upregulated in those primary nociceptive afferents which supply the inflamed limb [4, 22]. Thus, the levels of the messenger RNAs encoding SP and CGRP and the respective gene products are increased in the target-specific sensory neurons [22]. SP and CGRP fibers target spinal opioid neurons "lit up" in arthritic inflammatory pain [109, 110, 114]. There is evidence for peripheral sprouting of SP and CGRP nerve fibers into areas infiltrated by inflammatory cells, and the immunostaining for SP and CGRP coexisting in these fibers is intensified [53, 96, 109]. Further, the spinal release of SP in arthritic rats is increased [4]. Although we have no direct evidence for striking alterations in sympathetic or parasympathetic innervation in the course of pancreatitis, their possible involvement in the pain mechanisms of chronic pancreatitis should not be dismissed. The crucial importance of the sympathetic system in sustaining nociceptive behavior in the arthritic rat has been elegantly documented [4]. That sympathetic nerves play a role in human pain is well known. However, the possible contribution of peptide cotransmitters in sympathetically maintained pain is unelucidated. Therefore, the involvement of NPY and galanin, comessenger peptides in the sympathetic system [45], needs further investigation. On the other hand, changes in classical transmitters and their receptors and receptor subtypes may be worthwhile to be studied with respect to changes and influences in chronic pancreatitis. In this line, the possibility of cholinergic mechanisms in pancreatic pain should be also further elucidated [78]. Sensory autonomic interactions in the periphery are not inconceivable. Interestingly, NPY (a sympathetic messenger candidate) influences sensory nerves [34].

Certainly, multiple classical (amines, amino acids) and peptide neuromessengers and receptors are playing a complex interactive role in pain mechanisms, both in the periphery and centrally [4, 7, 19, 29, 33, 34, 37, 60, 68, 71, 112]. As regards the sensory peptidergic innervation (presumed capsaicin-sensitive) it will be interesting to see which second messenger systems are preferentially involved in mechanisms of chronic inflammatory pain [118].

For both human and animal inflammatory pain it has been argued that neuropep-tides are important not only in pain mechanisms but possibly also in the pathogenesis of chronic inflammation [20, 62, 64, 112, 121]. These considerations apply not only to arthritis but also to ulcerative colitis and Crohn's disease. In these chronic inflammat-ory and mostly painful diseases, a rather selective increase in SP receptor binding sites has recently been demonstrated [62, 64]. Interestingly, SP binding sites have been found to coincide with areas rich in immune cells. No major change in peptidergic innervation was seen. However, we have preliminary evidence that SP innervation is augmented in Crohn's disease, particularly in areas with neuroimmune overlap. We may predict that SP receptors are also increased in pancreatitis and possibly particu-larly augmented in areas where immune cells accumulate. We are even tempted to speculate on a hypothesis that the peptidergic (in particular SP-ergic) innervation may be not only a sustaining but even an initiating factor of the chronic inflammatory and painful process in chronic pancreatitis. We suggest that there is a vicious circle of disturbance in neuroimmune functioning sustaining pain and inflammation in chronic pancreatitis. Supportive of such a view is the fact that peripherally applied SP sensitizes nociceptors resulting in a hyperalgesia and intensification of inflammatory signs [72].

Textbook knowledge says that chronic alcohol abuse damages neuronal and influ-ences immune functions [48]. We feel provoked to speculate that neuroimmune disorder may be an underlying mechanism in the persistence of chronic alcoholic pancreatitis is in part a neuroimmune disorder. The diabetic syndrome associated with chronic pancreatitis may be related to such presumed mechanisms. An autoim-mune link triggered during the course of alcoholic pancreatitis is conceivable. It may be worthwhile to develop therapeutic strategies that pay attention to the intriguing possibility of a neuroimmune link in chronic alcoholic pancreatitis. Perhaps, immune therapy (as successfully performed in corticosteroid-resistant Crohn's disease) [12, 82] together with analgesics, including peripherally acting opioids, 5-HT$_3$ antagonists, and others or newly developed SP antagonists will prove to be a promising combinat-ory strategy to treat pain and inflammation in chronic pancreatitis [15, 16, 26, 28, 46, 49, 54, 71, 78, 89, 101, 112, 119].

References

1. Abramchik GV, Yermakova SS, Kaliunov VN, Tanina RM, Tumilovich MK (1988) The immunomodulatory effect of nerve growth factor. J. Neurosci Res 19:349–356
2. Ahren B, Martensson H, Ekman R (1989) Pancreatic nerve stimulation releases neuropeptide Y- but not galanin- or calcitonin gene-related peptide like-immunoreactivity from pig pancreas. J Autonom Nerv Syst 27:11–16
3. Balkwill FR, Burke F (1989) The cytokine network. Immunol Today 10:299–304

 4. Basbaum AI, Menetrey D, Presley R, Levine JD (1988) The contribution of the nervous system to experimental arthritis in the rat. In: Besson JM, Guilbaud G (eds) The arthritic rat as a model of clinical pain? Elsevier, Amsterdam New York Oxford, pp 41–53
 5. Beck PW, Handwerker HO (1974) Bradykinin and serotonin effects on various types of cutaneous nerve fibres. Pflügers Arch 347:209–222
 6. Beger HG, Büchler M, Bittner R, Oettinger W, Roscher R (1989) Duodenum-preserving resection of the head of the pancreas in severe chronic pancreatitis: early and late results. Ann Surg 209:13–18
 7. Benton HP, Jackson TR, Hanley MR (1989) Identification of a novel inflammatory stimulant of chondrocytes. Biochem J 258: 861–867
 8. Besson JM, Chaouch A (1987) Peripheral and spinal mechanisms of nociception. Physiol Rev 67:67–186
 9. Black IB, Adler JE, LaGamma EF (1988) Neurotransmitter plasticity in the peripheral nervous system. In: Björklund A, Hökfelt T, Owman C (eds) Handbook of chemical neuroanatomy, vol 6. The peripheral nervous system. Elsevier, Amsterdam New York Oxford, pp 51–64
10. Bockman DE, Büchler M, Malfertheiner P, Beger HG (1988) Analysis of nerves in chronic pancreatitis. Gastroenterology 94:1459–1469
11. Bradley EL (1982) Pancreatic duct pressure in chronic pancreatitis. Am J Surg 114:313–316
12. Brynskov J, Freund L, Rasmussen SN, Lauritsen K, Schaffaltzky-DeMuckadell O, Williams N, MacDonald AS, Tanton R, Molina F, Campanini MC, Bianchi P, Ranzi T, QuartoDiPalo F, Malchow-Moller A, Thomsen OO, Tage-Jensen U, Binder V, Rus, P (1989) A placebo-controlled, double-blind, randomized trial of cyclosporine therapy in active chronic Crohn's disease. New Engl J Med 321:845–850
13. Büchler M, Weihe E, Müller S, Bockmann DE, Malfertheiner P, Friess H, Beger HD (in press) Changes in peptidergic innervation in chronic pancreatitis. Pancreas
14. Carr DJJ, Blalock JE (1989) Cells of the immune system produce opioid peptides and express their receptors. In: Alan R (ed) Neuroimmune networks: physiology and diseases. Liss, New York, pp 99–104
15. Case JP, Lorberboum-Galski H, Lafyatis R, FitzGerald D, Wilder RL, Pastan I (1989) Chimeric cytotoxin IL2-PE40 delays and mitigates adjuvant-induced arthritis in rats. Proc Natl Acad Sci USA 86:287–291
16. Connolly KM, Stecher VJ, Danis E, Pruden DJ, LaBrie T (1988) Alteration of interleukin-1 production and the acute phase response following medication of adjuvant arthritic rats with cyclosporin-A or methotrexate. Int J Immunopharmac 10:717–728
17. Dalsgaard CJ (1988) The sensory system. In: Björklund A, Hökfelt T, Owman C (eds) Handbook of chemical neuroanatomy, Vol 6: The peripheral nervous system. Elsevier, Amsterdam New York·Oxford, pp 599–636
18. Dalsgaard CJ, Hultgardh-Nilsson A, Haegerstrand A, Nilsson J (1989) Neuropeptides as growth factors. Possible roles in human diseases. Regul Peptides 25:1–9
19. DeBiasi S, Rustioni A (1988) Glutamate and substance P coexist in primary afferent terminals in the superficial laminae of spinal cord. Proc Natl Acad Sci USA 85:7820–7824
20. Devillier P, Weill B, Renoux M, Menkes C, Pradelles P (1986) Elevated levels of tachykinin-like immunoreactivity in joint fluids from patients with inflammatory rheumatic diseases. N Engl J Med 314:1323–1325
21. DiMarzio V, Tippins JR, Morris HR (1989) Neuropeptides and inflammatory mediators: bidirectional regulatory mechanisms. TIPS 10:91–92
22. Draisci G, Iadarola MJ (1989) Temporal analysis of increases in c-*fos*, preprodynorphin and proenkephalin mRNAs in rat spinal cord. Mol Brain Res 6:31–37
23. Dray A, Bettaney J, Forster P, Perkins MN (1988) Bradykinin-induced stimulation of afferent fibres is mediated through protein kinase C. Neurosci Lett 91:301–307
24. Dray A, Bettaney J, Forster P (1989) Capsaicin desensitization of peripheral nociceptive fibres does not impair sensitivity to other noxious stimuli. Neurosci Lett 99:50–54
25. Elliot PJ, Krause JE, Cuello AC (1989) Diminished nociceptive response in mice following immunization with neurokinins. Peptides 10:69–71
26. Eschalier A, Kayser V, Gilbaud G (1989) Influence of specific 5-HT$_3$ antagonists on carageenan-induced hyperalgesia in the rat. Pain 36: 249–255

27. Esiri MM, Reading MC (1989) Macrophages, lymphocytes and major histocompatibility complex (HLA) class II antigens in adult human sensory and sympathetic ganglia. J Neuroimmunol 23:187–193
28. Ferreira SH, Lorenzetti BB, Bristow AF, Poole S (1988) Interleukin-1β as a potent hyperalgesic agent antagonized by a tripeptide analogue. Nature 334:698–700
29. Ferreira SH, Romitteli M, DeNucci G (1989) Endothelin-1 participation in overt and inflammatory pain. J Cardiovasc Pharmacol 13 (Suppl 5):S220–S222
30. Fink T, Weihe E (1988) Multiple neuropeptides in nerves supplying mammalian lymph nodes: messenger candidates for sensory and autonomic neuroimmunomodulation? Neurosci Lett 90:39–44
31. Fitzgerald M (1989) Arthritis and the nervous system. TINS 12:86–87
32. Gates TS, Zimmerman RP, Mantyh CR, Vigna SR, Mantyh PW (1989) Calcitonin gene-related peptide-α receptor binding sites in the gastrointestinal tract. Neuroscience 31:757–770
33. Giad A, Gibson SJ, Ibrahim NBN, Legon S, Bloom SR, Yanigisawa M, Masaki T, Varndell IM, Polak JM (1989) Endothelin 1, an endothelium-derived peptide, is expressed in neurons of the human spinal cord and dorsal root ganglia. Proc Natl Acad Sci USA 86:7634–7638
34. Guiliani S, Maggi CA, Meli A (1989) Prejunctional modulatory action of neuropeptide Y on peripheral terminals of capsaicin-sensitive sensory nerves. Br J Pharmacol 98:407–412
35. Goetzl K, Kodama KT, Turck CW, Schiogoley SA, Sreedharan SP (1989) Unique pattern of cleavage of vasoactive intestinal peptide by human lymphocytes. Immunol 66:554–558
36. Gourlet P, Robberecht P, DeNeef P, Tastenoy M, Damien C, Christophe J (1989) Presence of a new subclass of VIP receptors in human SUP-T1 lymphoblasts: the helodermin receptor. In: Aubry A, Marraud M, Vitoux B (eds) Second forum on peptides. Colloque INSERM. Libbey, pp 151–154
37. Guellner HG (1983) The interactions of prostaglandins with the sympathetic nervous system – a review. J Autonom Nerv Sys 8:1–12
38. Haley JE, Dickenson AH, Schachter M (1989) Electrophysiological evidence for a role of bradykinin in chemical nociception in the rat. Neurosci Lett 97:198–202
39. Hamon M, Gallissot MC, Ménard F, Gozlan S, Bourgoin S, Vergé D (1989) 5-HT$_3$ receptor binding sites are on capsaicin-sensitive fibres in the rat spinal cord. Eur J Pharmacol 164:315–322
40. Harrison LC, Campbell IL (1988) Cytokines: an expanding network of immuno-inflammatory hormones. Mol Endo 2:1151–1156
41. Hartschuh E, Weihe E, Yanaihara N (1989) Immunohistochemical analysis of chromogranin A and multiple peptides in the mammalian Merkel cell: further evidence for its paraneural function? Arch Histol Cytol 52: Suppl, pp 423–431
42. Heumann R, Lindholm D, Bandtlow C, Meyer M, Radeke MJ, Misko TP, Shooter E, Thoenen H (1987) Differential regulation of mRNA encoding nerve growth factor and its receptors in rat sciatic nerve during development, degeneration and regeneration: role of macrophages. Proc Natl Acad Sci USA 84:8735–8739
43. Holst JJ, Fahrenkrug J, Knuhtsen S, Jensen SL, Nielsen OV, Lundberg JM, Hökfelt T (1987) VIP and PHI in the pig pancreas: coexistence, corelease, and cooperative effects. Am J Physiol 252:182–189
44. Holzer P (1988) Local effector functions of capsaicin-sensitive sensory nerve endings: involvement of tachykinins, calcitonin gene-related peptide and other neuropeptides. Neuroscience 24:739–768
45. Hökfelt T, Millhorn D, Seroosy K, Tsuruo Y, Ceccatelli S, Lindh B, Meister B, Melander T, Schalling M, Bartfai T, Terenius L (1987) Coexistence of peptides with classical neurotransmitters. Experientia 43:768–774
46. Jacobs C, Young D, Tyler S, Callis T et al. (1988) In vivo treatment with IL-1 reduces the severity and duration of antigen-induced arthritis in rats. J Immunol 141:2967–2974
47. Jänig W (1989) The sympathetic nervous system in pain: physiology and pathophysiology. In: Stanton-Hicks M (ed) Pain and the sympathetic nervous system. Kluwer, London, pp 17–89
48. Jerrells TR, Marietta CA, Bone G, Weight FF, Eckardt MJ (1988) Ethanol-associated immunosuppression. In: Bridge TP et al (eds) Psychological, neuropsychiatric and substance abuse aspects of AIDS. Raven, New York, pp 173–185

49. Joris JL, Dubner R, Hargreaves KM (1987) Opioid analgesia at peripheral sites: a target for opioids released during stress and inflammation? Anest Analg 66:1277–1281
50. Kawamura M, Kuraishi Y, Minami M, Satoh M (1989) Antinociceptive effect of intrathecally administered antiserum against calcitonin gene-related peptide on thermal and mechanical noxious stimuli in experimental hyperalgesic rats. Brain Res 497:199–203
51. Kessler JP, Beaudet A (1989) Association of neurotensin binding sites with sensory and visceromotor components of the vagus nerve. J Neurosci 9:466–472
52. Kimball ES, Persico FJ, Vaught JL (1988) Substance P, neurokinin A, and neurokinin B induce generation of IL-1-like activity in P388D1 cells. J Immunol 141:3564–3569
53. Kimberly CL, Byers MR (1988) Inflammation of rat molar pulp and periodontium cause increased calcitonin gene-related peptide and axonal sprouting. Anat Rec 222:289–300
54. Kusugami K, Youngman KR, West GA, Fiocchi C (1989) Intestinal immune reactivity to interleukin 2 differs among Crohn's disease, ulcerative colitis, and controls. Gastroenterol 97:1–9
55. Landis SC (1988) Neurotransmitter plasticity in sympathetic neurons and its regulation by environmental factors in vitro and in vivo. In: Björklund A, Hökfelt T, Owman C (eds) Handbook of chemical neuroanatomy, Vol 6: The peripheral nervous system. Elsevier, Amsterdam New York Oxford, pp 65–115
56. Lindholm D, Heumann R, Meyer M, Thoenen H (1987) Interleukin 1 regulates synthesis of nerve growth factor in non-neuronal cells of rat sciatic nerve. Nature 330:658–659
57. Lindsay RM, Harmar AJ (1989) Nerve growth factor regulates expression of neuropeptide genes in adult sensory neurons. Nature 337:362–364
58. Lotz M, Vaughan JH, Carson DA (1988) Effect of neuropeptides on production of inflammatory cytokines by human monocytes. Science 241:1218–1221
59. Madden ME, Sarras Jr MP (1989) The pancreatic ductal system of the rat: cell diversity, ultrastructure, and innervation. Pancreas 4:472–485
60. Maggi CA, Meli A (1988) The sensory-efferent function of capsaicin-sensitive sensory neurons. Gen Pharmacol 19:1–11
61. Malfertheiner P, Büchler M, Stanescu A, Ditschuneit H (1987) Pancreatic morphology and function in relationship to pain in chronic pancreatitis. Int J Pancreatol 1:59–66
62. Mantyh CR, Gates TS, Zimmerman RP, Welton ML, Passaro Jr EP, Vigna SR, Maggio JE, Kruger L, Mantyh PW (1988) Receptor binding sites for substance P, but not substance K or neuromedin K, are expressed in high concentrations by arterioles, venules, and lymph nodules in surgical specimens obtained from patients with ulcerative colitis and Crohn disease. Proc Natl Acad Sci USA 85:3235–3239
63. Mantyh PW, Mantyh CR, Gates T, Vigna SR, Maggio JE (1988) Receptor binding sites for substance P and substance K in the canine gastrointestinal tract and their possible role in inflammatory bowel disease. Neuroscience 25:817–837
64. Mantyh PW, Catton MD, Boehmer CG, Welton ML, Passaro EP, Maggio JE, Vigna SR (1989) Receptors for sensory neuropeptides in human inflammatory diseases: implications for the effector role of sensory neurons. Peptides 10:627–645
65. Millan MJ (1986) Multiple opiod systems and pain. Pain 27:303–347
66. Millan MJ, Stein C, Weihe E, Nohr D, Höllt V, Czlonkowski A, Herz A (1988) Dynorphin and K-receptors in the control of nociception: response to peripheral inflammation and the pharmacology of K-antinociception. In: Besson JM, Guilbaud G (eds) The arthritic rat as a model of clinical pain? Excerpta Medica, Amsterdam, pp 153–171
67. Millan MJ, Weihe E, Czlonkowski AC (1989) Endogenous opioid systems in the control of pain. In: Almeida OFX, Schippenberg TS (eds) Opioid peptides and receptors: biochemistry, physiology and pharmacology. Springer, Berlin Heidelberg New York (in press)
68. Morton CR, Hutchinson WD (1989) Release of sensory neuropeptides in the spinal cord: studies with calcitonin gene-related peptide and galanin. Neuroscience 31:807–815
69. Mulderry PK, Ghatei MA, Spokes RA, Jones PM, Pierson AM, Hamid QA, Kanse S, Amara SG, Burrin JM, Legon S, Polak JM, Bloom SR (1988) Differential expression of α-CGRP and β-CGRP by primary sensory neurons and enteric autonomic neurons of the rat. Neuroscience 25:195–205
70. Müller S, Weihe E, Büchler M, Friess H, Beger HG (1989) Peptiderge Innervation bei chronischer Pankreatitis des Menschen. Verh Anat Ges (in press)

71. Nakamura M, Ferreira SH (1987) A peripheral sympathetic component in inflammatory hyperalgesia. Eur J Pharmacol 135:145–153

71a. Nakamura M, Ferreira SH (1988) Peripheral analgesic action of clonidine: mediation by release of endogenous enkephalin-like substances. Eur J Pharmacol 146:223–228

72. Nakamura-Craig M, Smith TW (1989) Substance P and peripheral inflammatory hyperalgesia. Pain 38:91–98

73. Nordmann JJ, Dayanithi G (1988) Release of neuropeptides does not only occur at nerve terminals. Biosci Rep 8:471

74. Nyberg F, Legrevos P, Terenius L (1988) Modulation of endopeptidase activity by calcitonin gene-related peptide: a mechanism affecting substance P action? Biochimie 70:65–68

75. Otten U (1984) Nerve growth factor and the peptidergic sensory neurons. TIPS 5:307–310

76. Otten U, Ehrhard P, Peck R (1989) Nerve growth factor induces growth and differentiation of human B lymphocytes. Proc Natl Acad Sci USA (in press)

77. Parnham MJ, Brune K (1989) Therapeutic control of inflammatory diseases. Agents Actions 27:236–238

78. Pert A (1987) Cholinergic and catecholaminergic modulation of nociceptive reactions. Pain Headache 9:1–63

79. Przlewlocki R, Gramsch C, Pasi A, Herz A (1983) Characterization and localization of immunoreactive dynorphin, α-neoendorphin, Met-enkephalin and substance P in human spinal cord. Brain Res 280:95–103

80. Roberts WJ, Foglesong ME (1988) II. Identification of afferents contributing to sympathetically evoked activity in wide-dynamic-range neurons. Pain 34:305–314

81. Russell NJW, Schaible HG, Schmidt RF (1987) Opiates inhibit the discharge of fine afferent units from inflamed knee joint of the cat. Neurosci Lett 76:107–112

82. Sachar DB (1989) Cyclosporine treatment for inflammatory bowel disease. New Engl J Med 321:894–896

83. Schultzberg M, Svenson SB, Unden A, Bartfai T (1987) Interleukin-1-like immunoreactivity in peripheral tissues. J Neurosci Res 18:184–189

84. Sharkey KA, Williams RG, Dockray GJ (1984) Sensory substance P innervation of the stomach and pancreas. Demonstration of capsaicin-sensitive sensory neurons in the rat by combined immunohistochemistry and retrograde tracing. Gastroenterology 93:852–862

85. Sibinga NE, Goldstein A (1988) Opioid peptides and opioid receptors in cells of the immune system. Annu Rev Immunol 6:219–249

86. Sinkovics JG (1988) Oncogenes and growth factors. Critical reviews in immunology 8:217–298

87. Stefano GB, Cadet P, Scharrer B (1989) Stimulatory effects of opioid neuropeptides on locomotory activity and conformational changes in invertebrate and human immunocytes: Evidence for a subtype of δ receptor. Proc Natl Acad Sci USA 86:6307–6311

88. Stein C, Millan MJ, Yassouridis A, Herz A (1988) Antinociceptive effects of μ- and kappa-agonostis in inflammation are enhanced by a peripheral opioid receptor-specific mechanism. Eur J Pharmacol 155:255–264

89. Stein C, Millan MJ, Shippenberg TS, Peter K, Herz A (1989a) Peripheral opioid receptors mediating antinociception in inflammation. Evidence for involvement of mu, delta and kappa receptors. J Pharmacol Exp Ther 248:1269–1275

90. Sternini C, Reeve JR, Brecha N (1987) Distribution and characterization of calcitonin gene-related peptide immunoreactivity in the digestive system of normal and capsaicin-treated rats. Gastroenterology 93:852–862

91. Steranka LR, Manning DC, DeHaas CJ, Ferkany JW, Borosky SA, Connor JR, Vavrek RJ, Stewart JM, Snyder SH (1988) Bradykinin as a pain mediator: receptors are localized to sensory neurons, and antagonists have analgesic actions. Proc Natl Acad Sci USA 85:3245–3249

92. Su HC, Bishop AE, Power RF, Hamada Y, Polak JM (1987) Dual intrinsic and extrinsic origins of CGRP- and NPY-immunoreactive nerves of rat gut and pancreas. J Neurosci 7:2674–2687

93. Suffys P, VanRoy R, Fiers W (1988) Tumor necrosis factor and interleukin 1 activate phospholipase in rat chondrocytes. FEBS Lett 232:24–28

94. Sundler F, Håkanson R (1988) Peptide hormone-producing endocrine/paracrine cells in the gastro-entero-pancreatic region. In: Björklund A, Hökfelt T, Owman C (eds) Handbook of chemical neuroanatomy, Vol 6: The peripheral nervous system. Elsevier, Amsterdam New York Oxford, pp 219–295

95. Taiwo YO, Levine JD (1988) Characterization of the arachidonic acid metabolites mediating bradykinin and noradrenalin hyperalgesia. Brain Res 458:402–406
96. Taylor PE, Byers MR, Redd PE (1988) Sprouting of CGRP nerve fibers in response to dentin injury in rat molars. Brain Res 46:371–376
97. Thoenen H, Bandtlow C, Heumann R, Lindholm D, Meyer M, Rohrer H (1988) Nerve growth factor: cellular localization and regulation of sythesis. Cell Molec Neurobiol 8:35–40
98. Tiffany CW, Burch RM (1989) Bradykinin stimulates tumor necrosis factor and interleukin-1 release from macrophages. FEBS Lett 247:189–192
99. Tiscornia OM, Dreiling DA, Yacomotti J, Kurtzbart R, LaTorre A, Farache S (1987) Neural control of the exocrine pancreas: an analysis of the cholinergic, adrenergic and peptidergic pathways and their positive and negative components. 1: Neural mechanisms. The Mount Sinai J Med 54:366–383
100. Varndell IM, Polak JM (1988) The ultrastructure of peptide-containing neurons. In: Björklund A, Hökfelt T, Owman C (eds) Handbook of chemical neuroanatomy, vol 6. The peripheral nervous system. Elevier, Amsterdam New York Oxford, pp 143–159
101. Wallace JL, MacNaughton WK, Morris GP, Beck PL (1989) Inhibition of leukotriene synthesis markedly accelerates healing in a rat model of inflammatory bowel disease. Gastroenterology 96:29–36
102. Weihe E, Hartschuh W, Weber E (1985) Prodynorphin opioid peptides in small somatosensory primary afferents of guinea-pig. Neurosci Lett 58:347–352
103. Weihe E, Leibold A, Nohr D, Fink T, Gauweiler B (1986) Coexistence of prodynorphin opioid peptides and substance P in primary sensory afferents of guinea-pig. Proc Int Narcotic Res Conf, San Francisco. NIDA Res Mon 75:295–298
104. Weihe E, Hartschuh W (1988) Multiple peptides in cutaneous nerves: regulators under physiological conditions and a pathogenetic role in skin disease? Sem Dermatol 7 (4):284–300
105. Weihe E, Nohr D, Hartschuh W (1988) Immunohistochemical evidence for a co-transmitter role of opioid peptides in primary sensory neurons. Prog Brain Res 74:189–199
106. Weihe E, Nohr D, Hartschuh W, Gauweiler B, Fink T (1988) Multiplicity of opioidergic pathways related to cardiovascular innervation: differential contribution of all three opioid precursors. In: Sumpe KO, Kraft K, Faden AI (eds) Opioid peptides and blood pressure control. Springer, Berlin Heidelberg New York, pp 27–49
107. Weihe E, Nohr D, Gauweiler B, Fink T, Nowak E, Konrad S (1988) Immunohistochemical evidence for a diversity of opioid coding in peripheral sympathetic, parasympathetic and sensory neurons: a general principle of prejunctional opioid autoinhibition? In: Illes P, Farsang C (eds) Regulatory role of opioid peptides. Symposium to the second world congress of neuroscience, Budapest. VCH, Weinheim, pp 16–32
108. Weihe E, Nowak E, Gauweiler B, Stuppi S, Nohr D (1988) Proenkephalin-derivatives are co-messenger candidates in cranial postganglionic parasympathetic neurons: opioid control of exocrine function? Adv Biosci 75:623–626
109. Weihe E, Nohr D, Millan MJ, Stein C, Müller S, Gramsch C, Herz A (1988) Peptide neuroanatomy of adjuvant-induced arthritic inflammation in rat. Agents Actions 25:255–259
110. Weihe E, Nohr D, Millan MJ, Stein C, Gramsch C, Höllt V, Herz A (1988) Experimental mono- and polyarthritis differentially intensify immunostaining of multiple proenkephalin- and prodynorphin-opioid peptides in rat lumbosacral neurons. Adv Biosci 75:359–362
111. Weihe E, Millan MJ, Leibold A, Nohr D, Herz A (1988) Colocalization of proenkephalin- and prodynorphin-derived opioid peptides in laminae IV/V spinal neurons revealed in arthritic rats. Neurosci Lett 85:187–192
112. Weihe E (1990) Neuropeptides in primary sensory neurons. In: Zenker W, Neuhuber W (eds) The primary afferent neuron – a survey of recent morpho-functional aspects. Plenum, New York (in press)
113. Weihe E, Müller S, Fink T, Zentel HJ (1989) Tachykinins, calcitonin gene-related peptide and neuropeptide Y in nerves of the mammalian thymus: interactions with mast cells in autonomic and sensory immunomodulation? Neurosci Lett 100:77–82
114. Weihe E, Millan MJ, Höllt V, Nohr D, Herz A (1989) Induction of the gene encoding prodynorphin by experimentally induced arthritis enhances staining for dynorphin in the spinal cord of the rats. Neuroscience 31:77–95

115. Weihe E, Müller S, Zentel HJ, Fink T (1989) Peptide in autonomen und sensiblen Nerven des Immunsystems: Signalüberträger der Neuroimmunmodulation? Verh Anat Ges (in press)
116. White DM, Ehrhard P, Hardung M, Meyer DK, Zimmermann M, Otten U (1987) Substance P modulates the release of locally synthesized nerve growth factor from rat saphenous nerve neuroma. Naunyn Schmiedeberg's Arch Pharmacol 336:587–590
117. White TT (1982) Pain. In: Bradley EL (ed) Complications and pancreatitis. Saunders, Philadelphia, pp 203–222
118. Wood JN, Coote PR, Minhas A, Mullaney I, McNeill M, Burgess GM (1989) Capsaicin-induced ion fluxes increase cGMP but not cAMP levels in rat sensory neurons culture. J Neurochem (in press)
119. Yaksh TL (1988) Substance P release from knee joint afferent terminals: modulation by opioids. Brain Res 458:319–324
120. Yaksh TL, Bailey J, Roddy DR, Harty GJ (1988) Peripheral release of substance P from primary afferents. In: Dubner R, Gebhart GF, Bond MR (eds) Proceedings of the Vth world congress on pain. Elsevier, Amsterdam
121. Zimmerman RP, Gates TS, Mantyh CR, Vigna SR, Welton ML, Passaro Jr EP, Mantyh PW (1989) Vasoactive intestinal polypeptide receptor binding sites in the human gastrointestinal tract: localization by autoradiography. Neuroscience 31:771–783

Is There a Link Between Chronic Pancreatitis and Pancreatic Cancer?*

P. M. POUR[1]

Introduction

There are difficulties in studying etiologic factors of pancreatic cancer. Considering the short survival time of the patients after the initial diagnosis, the population-based studies have been based to some extent on proxy interviews. For this reason, most published studies of pancreatic cancer have been small, based on 100 or less cases, and the available data are conflicting. Considering the published reports, almost everybody seems to be at risk for pancreatic cancer, including those who consume margarine on a slice of bread [1] or a large amount of pasta [2], beauticians and those who use professional makeup, such as actors [3], and those who live at certain geographical latitudes [4], consume sugar, eggs, milk, and diary products or undergo a tonsillectomy or spontaneous abortion [5], just to name a few. Chronic pancreatitis also has been mentioned among these risk factors. The purpose of this report is to focus on whether there is any link between chronic pancreatitis and pancreatic cancer based on review of the epidemiologic data and clinical and experimental experiences.

Epidemiologic Data

The epidemiologic data relative to possible association between chronic pancreatitis and pancreatic cancer are conflicting. Only a few studies have considered "chronic pancreatitis" as a confounding risk, whereas more reports do not include chronic pancreatitis as an etiologic factor for pancreatic cancer. However, some of the latter studies may not have focused on chronic pancreatitis as a risk factor. Clearly there are some problems with epidemiologic data which are based on retrospective studies on registered information, particularly owing to the small number of cases examined, the lack of appropriate control groups, and the apparent difficulties in distinguishing a primary from a secondary (obstructive) chronic pancreatitis. According to Höpker [6], the clinical data are incomplete or even wrong about the presence of pancreatic carcinoma. Schultz and Finkler [7] found insufficient followup data of chronic pancreatitis cases to preclude a link between the two diseases. Mainz and Webster [8], who studied epidemiologic data, reached the same conclusion.

* Supported by the Laboratory Cancer Research Center Support Grant No. CA36727, from the National Cancer Institute, NIH
[1] The Eppley Institute for Research in Cancer and Allied Diseases and Department of Pathology and Microbiology, University of Nebraska Medical Center, 42nd & Dewey Avenue, Omaha, NE 68105, USA

Chronic Pancreatitis
Ed. by Beger, Büchler, Ditschuneit, and Malfertheiner
© Springer-Verlag Berlin Heidelberg 1990

Considering the number of factors that have been claimed to play a role in pancreatic cancer etiology, we can admit that our knowledge on the efficacy of epidemiologically detectable factors responsible for pancreatitis and pancreatic cancer is fragmentary [8]. Correlation statistics between inflammatory and malignant exocrine pancreatic disease have shown that pancreatic cancer differs from acute and chronic pancreatitis in some clinical presentations [6]. Although cholelithiasis and cholecystitis may be present in all three diseases, other conditions seem to be more common in one or other diseases. For example, duodenal ulcer has been diagnosed commonly in pancreatitis cases whereas stomach ulcer occurs primarily in pancreatic cancer patients [6]. Moreover, other observations point to distinct differences in the pathogenesis of these two diseases. Alcohol is one of the major etiologic factors in chronic pancreatitis, whereas most case control studies do not show any significant association between alcohol and pancreatic cancer [9]. Lowenfels [10] followed 245 patients with chronic pancreatitis and found a significant excess of pancreatic cancer among this group. He did not, however, find a risk difference between outcome of cancer in alcohol-induced and non-alcohol-induced pancreatitis. (Readers are referred to Becker [11] for additional literature).

These differences may point to a divergence in the etiology of these diseases. But despite this, we cannot ignore the possibility that chronic pancreatitis provides a suitable environment for pancreatic cancer development similar to the role of colitis in the etiology of colon cancer. Histomorphologic observations lead in this direction.

Pathologic-Morphologic Data

In chronic pancreatitis, at least in the initial stage, regeneration and proliferation of ductal epithelium is a well recognized event [11]. This condition is regarded generally as a risk factor in carcinogenicity of many tissues, including the pancreas [12]. Some alterations seen in chronic pancreatic cases are hard to differentiate from premalignant or even malignant lesions [13]. Duplication or irregular cystic distention of ducts and ductules and fibrotic and sclerotic processes in the interstitium associated with distortion of ductal/ductular epithelium (Figs. 1, 2) are not uncommon in chronic pancreatitis [11], findings that could be misdiagnosed as malignant by pathologists who are not familiar with pancreatic diseases. The case illustrated in Figs. 1 and 2 was diagnosed as malignant and was sent to us for a second opinion. We believe that these lesions are degenerative, reparative and metaplastic in nature and differ from "true" hyperplastic changes seen in other pancreatic diseases, such hyperinsulinemic hypoglycemia of infancy. In the latter condition, endocrine cell hyperplasia (nesidioblastosis) may be associated with exocrine cell hypertrophy and hyperplasia, including acinar, ductal and ductular cells, which at times show atypical patterns (Figs. 3, 4). These cases are good examples of diagnostic difficulties and possible obfuscation, particularly in frozen sections or needle biopsy material. According to Becker [11] only the autodigestive cryptic pancreatitis with its prolonged tissue irritation and perpetual cell regeneration could be considered as a predisposing condition for pancreatic cancer. Although among 100 chronic pancreatitis cases 14% demonstrated pancreatic cancer [11], a distinction between the primary pancreatitis, as the cause, and the secondary pancreatitis, as the consequence of pancreatic cancer (see below),

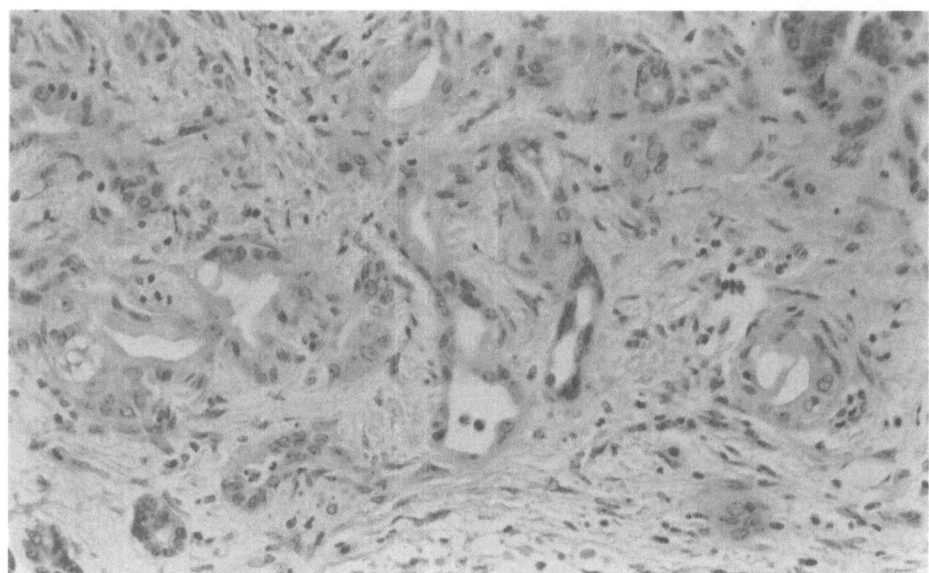

Fig. 1. This is a section from the pancreas of a 60-year-old man, who was hospitalized with upper abdominal discomfort, nausea, weight loss, and jaundice. After pancreaticoduodenectomy, examination of a pancreatic specimen and regional lymph nodes proved to be negative for tumor. There was a common duct stone. Several sections taken from the head of the pancreas revealed disseminated fibrosis superimposed with acute inflammation. Bile pigment was detectable in the pancreatic duct, the side branches of which showed epithelial hyperplasia virtually in every section of the pancreas. In fibrotic areas, there was degeneration of acinar and ductular cells, and duplication of ductules, some of which showed atypical patterns. In this photomicrograph, focal fibrosis with distorted ductules (glands) covered by pleomorphic epithelial cells is seen. H&E, × 200

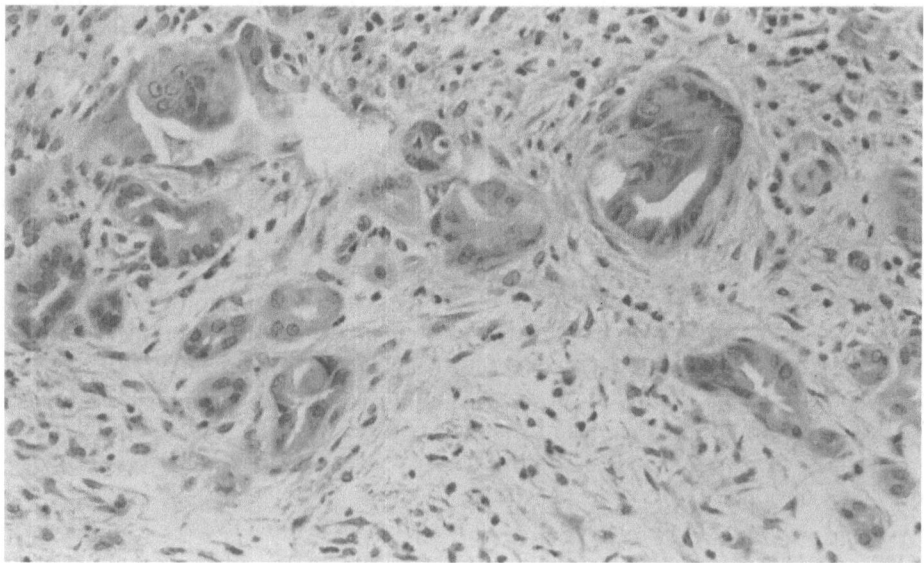

Fig. 2. Another area of the same pancreas in Fig. 1, depicting an area of fibrosis, inflammation, and atypical glandular structures. Note irregularity in size and polarity of the epithelial cells. H&E, × 200

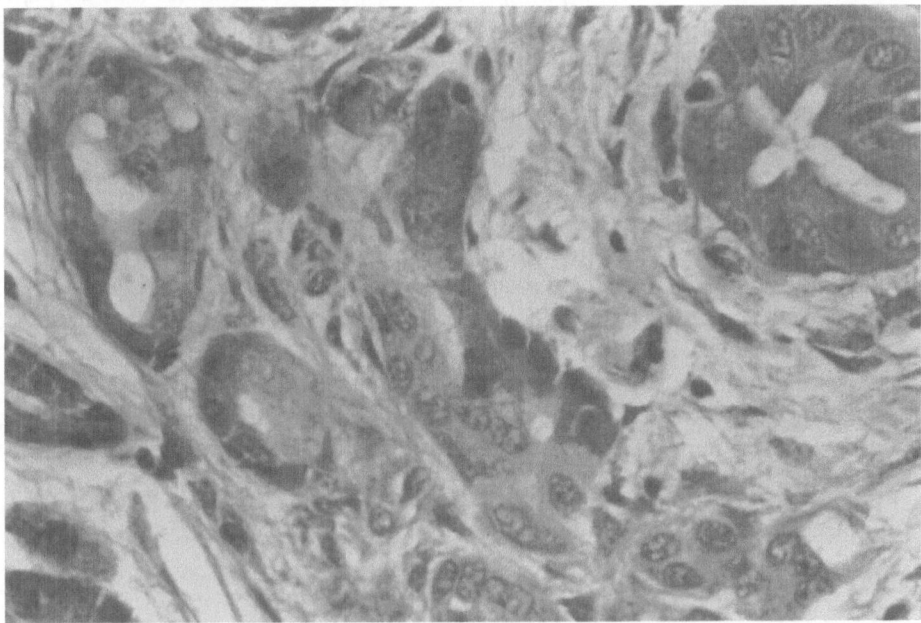

Fig. 3. A section from the pancreas of a child with hyperinsulinemic hypoglycemia. There was diffuse hyperplasia of centroacinar, islet, acinar, ductal, and ductular cells. This photomicrograph depicts an area of ductular cell proliferation with irregularity in appearance and cellular size. H&E, × 400

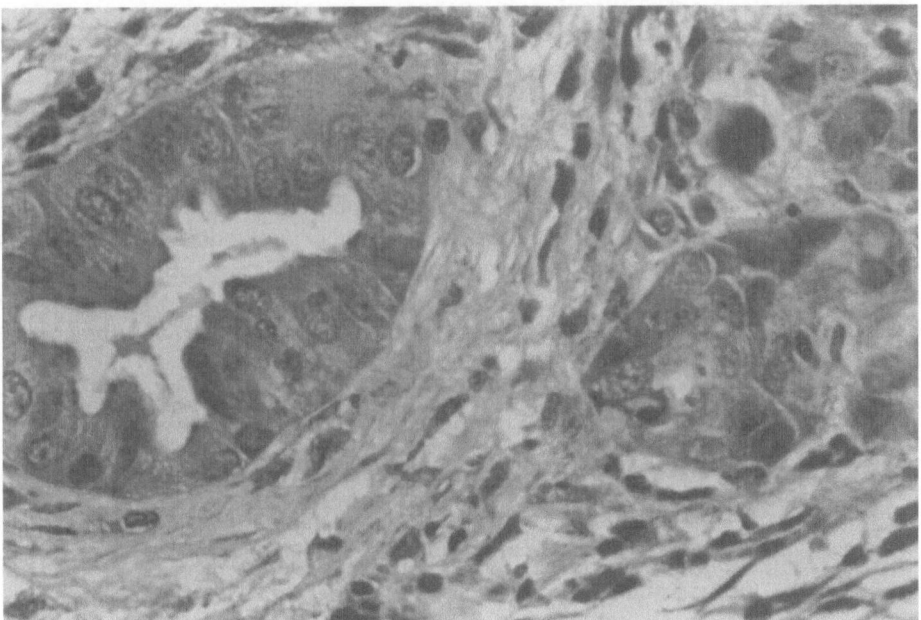

Fig. 4. Another area of the same pancreas in Fig. 3. Note the atypical duct with multilayered cells showing irregular nuclear size. Focal proliferation of (centroacinar) cells showing cell pleomorphims and nuclear hyperchromasia is seen *on the right*. H&E, × 400

was hard to make. To role of tropical pancreatitis in pancreatic cancer (see the paper of Pitchumoni in this issue) requires further studies to elucidate whether or not the observed high incidence of pancreatic cancer in these patients are merely the result of the tissue inflammation or other factors, including nutritional deficiency.

Diagnostic Criteria

If the diagnosis of chronic pancreatitis were based on the clinical history, the reported incidence of pancreatic cancer would range between 1% and 6% [14–22]. However, if calcification were used as criterion for chronic pancreatitis, a much higher incidence (between 9.4% and 24%) would result [23, 24], although Schulz and Finkler could not find any calcification in pancreatic cancer patients in contrast to the 18% incidence in chronic pancreatitis cases [7]. This indicates that calcification alone is not a reliable criterion for chronic pancreatitis, as recently has been demonstrated by Lankisch et al. [25].

Cause and Effect

A cause-and-effect is another consideration relative to an association between pancreatic cancer and chronic pancreatitis. Chronic pancreatitis may not be the cause but rather the consequence of pancreatic cancer. Pancreatic cancer develops in more than 60% of the cases in the head of the organ and leads gradually to ductal occlusion. This results in development of chronic (obstructive) pancreatitis, which can make symptoms much earlier than does the actual primary disease. In Japan, alterations of pancreatic enzyme levels, as seen in chronic pancreatitis, along with the ERCP findings are used to diagnose pancreatic cancer. This critical issue was overlooked apparently in the past, probably because of the lack of criteria for distinguishing a primary from a secondary (obstructive) chronic pancreatitis. The distinction between a primary and secondary pancreatitis on a histologic basis may be difficult. However, according to one of our recent studies with the monoclonal antibody CO17-1A, a distinction between a primary and secondary chronic pancreatitis seems possible [26]. Based on the result of this study, chronic pancreatitis, if present, was always of a secondary nature in all of our patients with pancreatic cancer. However, the number of our cases was not large enough to draw a definitive conclusion.

Incidence Data

Despite the above data, the likelihood that chronic pancreatitis precedes pancreatic cancer cannot be ruled out. Chronic pancreatitis, which is unrelated to age, can develop early in life. Pancreatic cancer, usually a disease of the elderly, develops later. If pancreatitis were a predisposing factor for the cancer of the pancreas, a higher rate of pancreatic cancer would be expected in these individuals than in the general population. This does not seem to be the case, however. The pancreatic cancer incidence in patients with chronic pancreatitis averages about 3%. This figure corresponds exactly with the expected pancreatic cancer incidence among the general population [27]. The conclusion is obvious. Individuals with chronic pancreatitis run the same risk of developing pancreatic cancer as those without chronic pancreatitis. A study by Ammann et al. [28] has shown that this situation is true also for other types of cancer. These investigators found that 11% of patients with chronic pancreatitis develop malignancies in various tissues. Only about 2.5% of the cancers originated from the pancreas and the rest from extrapancreatic tissues, including bronchus (3.2%), oral cavity (2.4%), larynx (1.2%), and other gastrointestinal tissues (1.5%). Consequently, it seems that the risk for cancer development in patients with chronic pancreatitis does not differ from the general population. This as has been shown also by autopsy data [6]. The possibility that the early death of patients with chronic pancreatitis may obscure the relationship between chronic pancreatitis and pancreatic cancer can only be hypothetical.

Experimental Data

Unavailable experimental models for human chronic pancreatitis and limits on models for pancreatic cancer have hampered experimental studies to examine any causal relationship between chronic pancreatitis and pancreatic cancer. In the hamster pancreatic cancer model, bile-induced acute pancreatitis did not enhance the incidence of pancreatic cancer. But relapsing pancreatitis, induced in hamsters by repeated induction of bile pancreatitis, did enhance pancreatic cancer incidence [29]. However, these results should be considered with caution. In our experiment, the induced relapsing (chronic) pancreatitis was morphologically and clinically far from being similar to human disease. Therefore, it is safe to say that our experimental results are irrelevant to the human situation.

Conclusion

Using these data, we have to agree with Appel [30] that there is no relationship between pancreatic cancer and chronic pancreatitis. The rare condition of familial relapsing pancreatitis, an autosomal dominant disorder with incomplete penetrance, is the exception. About 20 families have been reported with hereditary chronic pancreatitis, of which half developed pancreatic cancer (for literature see [31]). However, in some families the pancreatic cancer victims do not have a history of pancreatitis [32]. Therefore, we can assume that the same genetic defect might manifest itself differently.

In summary, based on epidemiologic, morphologic, and experimental data, no link between pancreatic cancer and chronic pancreatitis seems to exist.

References

1. Norell SE, Ahlbom A, Erwald R, Jacobson G, Lindberg-Navier, Olin R, Törnberg B, Wiechel K-L (1986) Diet and pancreatic cancer: a case-control study. Am J Epidemiol 124:894–902
2. Raymond L, Infante F, Tuyns AJ, Voirol M, Lowenfels AB (1987) Alimentation et cancer du pancréas. Gastroenterol Clin Biol 11:488–492

3. Depue RH, Kagey BT, Heid MF (1985) A proportional mortality study of the acting profession. Am J Ind Med 8:57–66
4. Kato I, Tajima K, Kuroishi T, Tominaga S (1985) Latitude and pancreatic cancer. Jpn J Clin Oncol 15:403–413
5. Lin RS (1981) A multifactorial model for pancreatic cancer in man. Epidemiologic evidence. JAMA 245:147–152
6. Höpker WW (1988) Epidemiology of pancreatic diseases. In: Becker U, Hübner K (eds) The pancreas in connection with the epigastric unit. Fischer, Stuttgart, pp 81–97
7. Schulz RE, Finkler NJ (1980) Pancreatic calcification and pancreatic carcinoma: the relationship reconsidered. Mt Sinai J Med (NY) 47:622–626
8. Mainz D, Webster PD (1974) Pancreatic carcinoma. A review of etiologic considerations. Dig Dis 19:459–464
9. Boyle P, Hsieh C-C, Maisonneuve P, La Vecchia C, Macfarlane GJ, Walker AM, Trichopolos D (1989) Epidemiology of pancreatic cancer. Int J Pancreatol (in press)
10. Lowenfels AB (1984) Letter to the editor. Gastroenterology 7:744
11. Becker V (1984) Chronische Pancreatitis. Klinische Morphologie. Georg Thieme Verlag, Stuttgart New York, pp 118–155
12. Pour PM, Donnelly K, Stepan K, Muffly K (1983) Modification of pancreatic carcinogenesis in the hamster model. II. The effect of partial pancreatectomy. Am J Pathol 110:75–82
13. Oertel JE (1989) The pancreas. Nonneoplastic alterations. Am J Surg Pathol [Suppl] 13:50–65
14. Alexander JH, Levard H, Camilleri JP (1981) Cancer du pancréas sue pancréatite chronique. Revue générale. Chirurgie 107:459–466
15. Bartholomew LG, Gross JB, Comfort MW (1958) Carcinoma of the pancreas associated with chronic relapsing pancreatitis. Gastroenterology 35:374–377
16. Gambill EE (1971) Pancreatitis associated with pancreatic carcinoma: a study of 26 cases. Mayo Clin Proc 26:174–177
17. Gray L, Crook JN, Cohn I (1973) Carcinoma of the pancreas. Gastrointestinal Cancer Proc Natl Cancer Conf 7:503–510
18. Johnson JR, Zintel HA (1963) Pancreatic calcification and cancer of the pancreas. Surg Gynecol Obstet 117:585–588
19. Kendig TA, Johnson RM, Shackford BC (1966) Calcification in pancreatic carcinoma. Ann Intern Med 65:122–124
20. Lundh G, Nordenstam H (1970) Pancreas calcification and pancreatic cancer. Acta Chir Scand 136:493–496
21. Robinson A, Scott J, Rosenfeld DD (1970) The occurrence of carcinoma of the pancreas in chronic pancreatitis. Radiology 94:289–290
22. Tucker DH, Moore IB (1963) Vanishing pancreatic calcification in chronic pancreatitis. Med Intell 268:31–33
23. Howard JM, Jordon RL (1960) Surgical disease of the pancreas. Lippincott, Philadelphia, p 216
24. Paulino-Netto A, Dreiling DA, Baronofsky ID (1960) The relationship between pancreatic calcification and cancer of the pancreas. Ann Surg 151:530–537
25. Lankisch PG, Otto J, Löhr A, Schirren C-A, Schuster R (1989) Pancreatic calcification in patients with normal pancreatic function. Int J Pancreatol (in press)
26. Takiyama Y, Tempero MA, Takasaki H, Onda M, Tsuchiya R, Büchler M, Ness M, Colcher D, Schlom J, Pour PM (1989) Reactivity of CA17-1A and B72.3 in benign and malignant pancreatic diseases. Hum Pathol (in press)
27. Silverberg E, Lbera JA (1989) Cancer statistics 1989. Ca-A cancer Journal for clinicians. American Cancer Society 39:2–20
28. Ammann RW, Knoblach M, Mohr P, Deyhle P, Largiader F, Akobiantz A, Schuler G, Schneider J (1980) High incidence of extrapancreatic carcinoma in chronic pancreatitis. Scand J Gastroenterol 15:395–399
29. Pour PM, Takahashi M, Donnelly T, Stepan K (1983) Modification of pancreatic carcinogenesis in the hamster model. X. Effect of pancreatitis. INCI 71:607–613
30. Appel MF (1974) Hereditary pancreatitis – review and presentation of an additional kindred. Arch Surg 108:63–65
31. Conrath SM (1986) The use of epidemiology, scientific data, and regulatory authority to determine risk factors in cancers of some organ of the digestive system. VI. Pancreatic cancer. Regul Toxicol Pharmacol 6:193–210
32. Levison DA (1979) Carcinoma of the pancreas. J Pathol 129:203–223

Pathophysiology

Chronic Pancreatitis: Search for Animal Models

M. V. Singer, P. Layer, and H. Goebell[1]

An experimental model of chronic pancreatitis probably does not exist. Whereas various experimental models of acute pancreatitis have been described (Table 1), chronic pancreatitis has not been consistently produced in experimental animals. Extensive overviews on the experimental models and concepts in acute pancreatitis [1–25, 26] have been published; international workshops on acute experimental pancreatitis have been held [24]. In addition, experimental models of exocrine pancreatic tumor have been developed [8]. As yet, however, no reproducible animal models of chronic pancreatitis have been reported.

Table 1. Some models of acute experimental pancreatitis

Invasive models

Retrograde ductal injection (of, e.g., bile)
Intraparenchymal injection
Closed duodenal loop
Duct ligation and stimulation of secretion

noninvasive models

Exposure to anticholinesterase insecticides
Secretagogue-induced (e.g., hyperstimulating doses of cerulein)
Diet-induced (e.g., choline-deficient ethionine-supplemented diet)
Administration of immune serum

The crucial question whether these experimental models of acute pancreatitis have any relevance to the clinical disease is unanswered for most of these animal models. But even if a relationship between experimental pathophysiological work and clinical pancreatitis is not direct, progress at such a basic level constitutes the foundation upon which the clinical and patho-anatomical understanding rests.

The ideal experimental model of acute or chronic pancreatitis would resemble the clinical disease in all features such as precipitating event or agent, pattern of progression, molecular biology and pathophysiology, response to therapy, and/or sequelae. Such models are available for only a relatively few, mostly infectious, diseases.

---

[1] Division of Gastroenterology Department of Medicine, University of Essen, Hufelandstrasse 55, D-4300 Essen 1, FRG

Chronic Pancreatitis
Ed. by Beger, Büchler, Ditschuneit, and Malfertheiner
© Springer-Verlag Berlin Heidelberg 1990

Two major *etiological factors* can be differentiated in *human chronic* (calcifying) *pancreatitis*. In the *Western World* and *Europe chronic pancreatitis* is an *alcohol-related disease*. In the *tropics, nonalcoholic nutritional disease predominates*. Other causes of pancreatitis (e.g., idiopathic, hereditary, trauma, hypercalcemia) are rare. Both in alcohol related and tropical nutritional chronic pancreatitis, calcified pancreatic stones are found.

For unknown reasons, it is very difficult to find an agent or tool to develop chronic alcoholic or nutritional pancreatitis in animals which resembles human chronic pancreatitis. Four major animal models for chronic pancreatitis have been published (Table 2):

1. Experimental pancreatolithiasis in the dog [6, 27].
2. Alcoholic chronic pancreatitis in rats and dogs fed ethanol for up to 2 years [18, 19].
3. Alcohol-induced chronic pancreatitis in rats after temporary occlusion of biliopancreatic ducts with Ethibloc [17].
4. Feeding of rats with a protein-deficient diet [for review see 13, 14, 18].

Table 2. Animal models for chronic pancreatitis

1. Experimental pancreatolithiasis in the dog
2. Alcoholic pancreatitis in rats and dogs fed ethanol for up to 2 years
3. Alcohol-induced chronic pancreatitis in rats after temporary occlusion of biliopancreatic ducts with Ethibloc
4. Feeding of rats with a protein-deficient diet

However, it has to be pointed out that none of these experimental models is really strictly comparable to the human disease. None of them has succeeded in producing the disease with typical *morphological* or *functional* changes of the pancreas. In addition, the term "chronic" has been used for periods of 2 weeks to 2 years. These time intervals are much shorter than those seen in humans in whom it takes usually more than 10 years of chronic alcoholism to develop chronic (calcifying) pancreatitis.

Experimental Pancreatolithiasis in the Dog

One of the earliest attempts to produce chronic pancreatitis in animals has been to ligate the major pancreatic duct. A careful review of this early work has been given by Floyd and Christophersen [4]. Today it is well established that ductal ligation with total obstruction to pancreatic drainage results in acinar atrophy and fibrosis. One of the earliest attempts to produce chronic pancreatitis by injection of a fibroblastic agent into the wall of the major pancreatic duct has been made by Floyd and Christophersen [4]. These authors observed chronic interstitial pancreatitis with ductal dilatation in dogs by injecting the wall of the major pancreatic duct with sodium dicetyl phosphate and placing a polyethylene collar around the site of injection. The pathologic process produced by this method appeared sufficiently comparable to that seen in man.

Since total ligation of the pancreatic duct produces no chronic pancreatitis, Japanese scientists have tried to develop a model of chronic pancreatitis and pancreatolithiasis by partial (incomplete) ligation of the major pancreatic duct in dogs. Takayama [27] and Konishi et al. [6] surgically created partial or complete pancreatic duct obstruction in dogs. Pancreatic calculi were demonstrated in almost 50% of the dogs with partial outflow obstruction for 4 months [6] or up to 1 year [17]. No pancreatic calculi were found in any of the dogs with complete pancreatic duct obstruction. All calculi produced were localized in the ductal system. The organic and inorganic composition of canine and human pancreatic calculi were quite similar. Connective tissue proliferation and mucous cell metaplasia of the ductal epithelium, often seen in association with clinical pancreatolithiasis, were also detected in the pancreata of dogs that had partial obstruction of pancreatic excretion.

Noda et al. [9] have shown that the antiepileptic agent, trimethadione, is capable of dissolving the pancreatic stones in that animal model.

Sakakibara et al. [17] reported on the *ultrastructural changes in the exocrine pancreas in this model*. Light micrographs demonstrated pancreatic lesions similar to those in humans. Electron micrographs revealed dilated lumens of small ducts and degenerated ducted cells 3 months after the ligation. These changes became more severe and appeared more often when the period of ligation was prolonged up to 1 year. Acinar cells demonstrated dilatation of the rough endoplasmic reticulum and the Golgi apparatus, swelling of the mitochondria, and increase in the number of prezymogen granules. Microfilamentous substance appeared in markedly dilated rough endoplasmic reticulum and in the intercellular space as acinar cell lesions progressed and the basal membrane became disrupted. The authors speculated that this substance might be involved in calculous formation, the incidence of which reached a plateau after 6 months of ligation, coinciding with the peak in appearance of the substance.

In dogs with incomplete ligation of the major pancreatic duct *advanced insufficiency of the exocrine* pancreas, evaluated by caerulein/secretin test was observed after 6 months [27].

Endocrine dysfunction observed in this model of pancreatolithiasis was substantially the same as that seen in the human disease, although less severe in the dogs [10]. Endocrine function was serially examined by intravenous glucose tolerance test and insulin tolerance test before and 3, 6, and 12 months after the duct ligation. Neither α-/ nor β-cell dysfunction became apparent until 12 months after the ligation. The disappearance rate of glucose in an intravenous glucose tolerance test decreased and the plasma insulin response to glucose was also reduced significantly. Although hypoglycemia induced during an intravenous insulin tolerance test was maximal in the 12th month, the distinct response of plasma pancreatic glucagon to the hypoglycemia disappeared.

Alcoholic Chronic Pancreatitis in Rats and Dogs Fed Ethanol for up to 2 Years

Sarles et al. [18–20] have tried for many years to induce chronic alcoholic pancreatitis in dogs and rats. The pancreas in *dogs* receiving alcohol at 2 g/kg per day for 1–3 years was frequently normal. In some cases it was possible to find intraductal plugs, periductal fibrosis, duct proliferation, and, less frequently, perilobular and intralobular fibrosis [18].

Changes in *pancreatic exocrine function* were observed in these alcoholic dogs which also received a diet rich in fat and protein. From the 16th week they began to excrete protein precipitates through the pancreatic cannula. After 2 years of alcohol administration, pancreatic biopsies showed lesions which were comparable with the early stages of human calcifying chronic pancreatitis, obstruction of the ducts by protein precipitates, some of which were calcified or atrophied or, on the other hand, hyperplasia and duplication of ducts, pericanalicular fibrosis, and atrophy of acinar cells [18, 20].

So far the histological observations by Sarles et al. [19] have not been confirmed or contradicted, since no other investigators have done similar experiments in dogs.

In 1971, Sarles et al. [19] described *lesions* in alcoholic Wistar *rats* which resembled those in human chronic alcoholic pancreatitis. Focal areas with reduction in number of acini, duct multiplication, protein plugs (sometimes calcified) in the ducts and sclerosis were observed in more than half of animals given a 20% solution of ethanol as the sole source of fluid for 20–30 months. These morphological changes were associated with protein hypersecretion in pancreatic juice. Sarles et al. [19] postulated that these calcified protein plugs play a major role in the pathogenesis of chronic pancreatitis.

Some control rats, however, spontaneously developed pancreatic lesions characterized by a spotty distribution and a frequency of intraductal, sometimes calcified, plugs. It was pointed out that Wistar rats develop such changes spontaneously probably due to arteriosclerotic changes in the vessels [5].

Other investigators using similar ethanol-feeding protocols were unable consistently to produce alcoholic pancreatitis in rats [3, 15, 16, 21].

Singh [22] tried to develop a model of chronic alcoholic pancreatitis in Sprague-Dawley rats fed a nutritionally adequate diet. Three groups of 15 animals each were fed Wayne Rodent-Blox ad libitum, Lieber-DeCarli diet with 40% of carbohydrate calories replaced by ethanol ad libitum and isocaloric amounts of Lieber-DeCarli diet respectively for a period of 18 months. All of the ethanol-fed animals developed morphological changes akin to human chronic pancreatitis. There were focal areas of parenchymal degeneration with fibrosis, protein plug formation, and tubular complexes. Based upon biochemical data, Singh [22] suggested that focal degenerative changes may be due to trypsin generated by intracellular activation of digestive enzymes by lysosomal enzyme cathepsin B.

Alcohol-Induced Chronic Pancreatitis in Rats After Temporary Occlusion of Biliopancreatic Ducts with Ethibloc

Pap and Boros [11] and Pap et al. [12] provoked chronic obstructive pancreatitis-like histological and biochemical alterations in male Wistar rats with Ethibloc occlusion of the common bile duct and the main pancreatic ducts. After the disappearance of the glue from the ducts, a gradual and almost total recovery was demonstrated during a 2-month observation period. About 12 g/kg alcohol (20% vol/vol) given daily by gastric intubation and ad libitum intake inhibited the recovery of pancreatic weight and enzyme contents in the occluded rats, and within a 2-month period chronic calcifying-type pancretitis became evident with some signs of remaining obstructive pancreatitis-like lesions. Cessation of alcohol administration after 2 months resulted in a recovery of pancreatic weight and enzyme contents, although morphological regeneration was less pronounced and calcification remained visible in some rats. A 50% raw soy flour diet provoked some further changes in the proportion of enzymes without any supplementary increases of pancreatic weight and protein content. The authors concluded that chronic obstructive and calcifying pancreatitis can appear together and earlier if the etiological factors act in combination. Suppression of pancreatic regeneration by alcohol seems to be necessary to maintain chronic pancreatitis-like lesions and to develop calcification [11].

Models for Tropical (Nutritional) Pancreatitis

In humans, the tropical type of chronic calcific pancreatitis is characterized by pancreatic calculi and diabetes mellitus occurring in children and young adults in India and some other third world countries. The occurrence of this syndrome, almost exclusively in the poorest sections of the population groups of developing countries, implicated malnutrition as the most likely etiological factor. This type of pancreatitis, "nutritional" or "tropical," is clinically and pathologically almost similar to the alcoholic variety seen in the West and fits in with the definition of chronic pancreatitis of the Marseille classification (for review see [13, 14]).

Protein malnutrition may be the most important and obvious etiological factor of tropical pancreatitis but additional pathogenetic factors are needed to cause chronic pancreatitis. A potential toxic effect of cyanogenetic glycosides (linamarin and linamarase) in cassava (the tuber of *Manihot esculenta)* and of micronutrient deficiencies on the pancreas has recently been reported [14]. Clinical and experimental studies have substantiated that the *pancreas* is *quite vulnerable* to *protein deprivation*. A generalized reduction in the size of the pancreas, atrophy, fibrosis, disorganization, and loss of acinar pattern are characteristic of pancreatic injury seen in kwashiorkor. Pancreatic function is markedly depressed in protein malnutrition. Experimental studies designed to study the effect of protein malnutrition on animals have confirmed the clinical observations. After 10 days of a protein-free diet, the acinar cells of the rat pancreas showed a coarsening of nuclear matrices, depletion of zymogen granules, loss of chromosomal material, and separation of the tubules of the endoplasmic reticulum [14].

Despite the availability of good experimental models of pancreatic insufficiency secondary to protein deficiency reproducing kwashiorkor, no existing model reproduces the lesions of human chronic pancreatitis, with its progressive development and high incidence of calcium-protein precipitates in the ducts. Although protein deficiency is responsible for acinar atrophy, it does not cause inflammatory lesions of the pancreas – and is therefore not "pancreatitis" – nor does it result in the development of calcium-protein deposits in the ducts as in chronic calcifying pancreatitis.

In *summary,* acinar atrophy produced at all ages in animals and man by protein deficiency does not at all resemble the lesions of chronic pancreatitis, lacking, in

particular, protein precipitates in the ducts and inflammatory lesions (sclerosis). There are three possible hypotheses:
a) other factors statistically related to protein deficiency are the source of the disease;
b) protein deficiency must be more longlasting than the common form of kwashior-kor, and in experimental protocols, and
c) one can still contemplate the idea that, as in alcoholism, there exist different constitutional susceptibilities which explain why certain individuals develop pancreatitis with minimal nutritional defect, while others do not develop pancreatitis with important nutritional defects because their pancreas is more resistant, or because they die meanwhile of lesions affecting other organs.

Concluding Comments

Despite the fact that partial obstruction of the major pancreatic duct and feeding alcohol to dogs and rats with and without temporary occlusion of the biliopancreatic ducts have been found to produce functional and morphological changes in the pancreas, none of these models is very close to the human disease. The results obtained in rats have been inconsistent, being dependent on many variables, such as strain, age, diet, and duration of ethanol administration.

The term "chronic" has to be questioned since it varies from study to study. Two months and 2 years of ethanol intake in animals might be not sufficient to induce pancreatic lesions similar to the human disease. The most interesting finding of the rat studies is the combined effects of ductal obstruction and alcohol on the pancreas.

Experimental models of ethanol dependence and liver injury have been described in rats and baboons [7]. It might well be that – for the pancreas – the wrong animmal species have been studied. Studies in the pig, an animal whose pancreatic exocrine function is quite similar to the human condition, might be more promising.

Although molecular biology promises to enhance greatly our understanding of human chronic pancreatitis, the search for the right animal model of chronic pancreatitis still seems to be necessary since in vitro studies alone will not help to solve the riddle of human chronic pancreatitis. Thus, young imaginative researchers and senior investigators are asked to use their creative imagination in a practical way and to develop an animal model of chronic pancreatitis similar to the human disease. There is still much work to be done.

References

1. Adler G, Kern HF, Scheele GA (1986) Experimental models and concepts in acute pancreatitis. In: Go VLW, et al. (eds) The exocrine pancreas: biology, pathobiology, and diseases. Raven, New York, pp 407–421
2. Boros L, Pap A, Varró V (1986) Recovery of the pancreatic enzyme content in Ethibloc®-induced obstructive pancreatitis can be inhibited by alcohol administration (Abstr). Digestion 35:10
3. Darle N, Ekholm R, Edlund Y (1970) Ultrastructure of the rat exocrine pancreas after long term intake of ethanol. Gastroenterology 58:62–67
4. Floyd CN, Christophersen WM (1956) Experimental chronic pancreatitis. Arch Surg 73:701–709

5. Kendrey G, Roe FJC (1969) Histopathological changes in the pancreas of laboratory rats. Lab Anim 3:207–220
6. Konishi K, Izumi R, Kato O, Yamaguchi A, Miyazaki I (1981) Experimental pancreatolithiasis in the dog. Surgery 89:687–691
7. Lieber CS, DeCarli LM (1976) Animal models of ethanol dependence and liver injury in rats and baboons. Fed Proc 35:1232–1236
8. Longnecker DS (1986) Experimental models of exocrine pancreatic tumors. In: Go VLW, et al. (ed). The exocrine pancreas: biology, pathobiology, and diseases. Raven, New York, pp 443–458
9. Noda A, Shibata T, Ogawa Y, Hayakawa T, Kameya S, Hiramatsu E, Watanabe T, Horiguchi Y (1987) Dissolution of pancreatic stones by oral trimethadione in a dog experimental model. Gastroenterology 93:1002–1008
10. Okumura N, Sakakibara A, Hayakawa T, Noda A (1982) Pancreatic endocrine function in experimental pancreatolithiasis in dogs. Am J Gastroenterol 77:392–396
11. Pap A, Boros L (1989) Alcohol-induced chronic pancreatitis in rats after temporary occlusion of biliopancreatic ducts with Ethibloc®. Pancreas 4:249–255
12. Pap A, Boros L, Berger Z, Varró V (1985) Chronic pancreatitis-like lesions provoked by duct occlusion with Ethibloc® in rats can be maintained by alcohol administration (Abstr). Digestion 32:210
13. Pitchumoni CS (1984) "Tropical" or "nitritional pancreatitis" – an update. In: Gyr KE, Singer MV, Sarles H (eds) Pancreatitis – concepts and classification. Elsevier, Amsterdam, pp 359–363
14. Pitchumoni CS, Scheele G, Lee PC, Lebenthal E (1986) Effects of nutrition on the exocrine pancreas. In: Go VLW, et al. (eds) The exocrine pancreas: biology, pathobiology, and diseases. Raven, New York, pp 387–406
15. Reber HA, Johnson FE, Montgomery CK, Carl WR, Wong MF (1977) The effect of chronic alcohol ingestion on rat pancreas (Abstr). Gastroenterology 72:94/1117
16. Roze C, Chariot J, de la Tour J, Camilleri JP, Sourchard M, Vaille C (1979) Effets de l'ingestion prolongée d'alcool (3 à 18 mois) sur le pancréas du rat. Gastroenterol Clin Biol 3:657–666
17. Sakakibara A, Okumura N, Hayakawa T, Kanzaki M (1982) Ultrastructural changes in the exocrine pancreas of experimental pancreatolithiasis in dogs. Am J Gastroenterol 77:498–503
18. Sarles H, Laugier R (1981) Alcoholic pancreatitis. Clin Gastroenterol 10:401–415
19. Sarles H, Lebreuil G, Tasso F, Figarella C, Clemente F, Devaux MA, Fagonde B, Payan H (1971) A comparison of alcoholic pancreatitis in rat and man. Gut 12:377–388
20. Sarles H, Figarella C, Tiscornia O, Colomb E, Guy O, Verine H, de Caro A, Multigner L, Lechene P (1980) Chronic calcifying pancreatitis (CCP). Mechanism of formation of the lesions. New data and critical study. In: Fitzgerald PJ, Morrison AB (eds). The pancreas. Williams and Wilkins, Baltimore, pp 48–66
21. Singh M (1983) Effect of chronic ethanol feeding on pancreatic enzyme secretion in rats in vitro. Dig Dis Sci 28:117–123
22. Singh M (1987) Alcoholic pancreatitis in rats fed ethanol in a nutritionally adequate liquid diet. Int J Pancreatol 2:311–324
23. Singh M, LaSure MM, Bockman DE (1982) Pancreatic acinar cell function and morphology in rats chronically fed an ethanol diet. Gastroenterology 82:425–434
24. Steer ML (1979) Workshop on experimental pancreatitis. Dig Dis Sci 30:575–581
25. Steer ML, Meldolesi J (1984) Experimental acute pancreatitis: relevance of models to clinical disease. In: Gyr KE, Singer MV, Sarles H (eds) Pancreatitis – concepts and classification. Elsevier, Amsterdam, pp 137–141
26. Steer ML, Meldolesi J (1987) The cell biology of experimental pancreatitis. N Engl J Med 316:144–150
27. Takayama T (1979) Pathophysiological study of experimental pancreatolithiasis in the dog. Nippon Shokakibyo Gakkai Zasshi 76:1325–1336

Pancreatic Adaptation, Growth, and Regeneration in Experimental Chronic Pancreatitis

A. Pap[1]

Previous Findings

There are several rat models of acute pancreatitis [1], but chronic pancreatitis-like lesions similar to the human disease are difficult to provoke in rats [8, 24, 25, 27, 29].

In a recent paper, we have demonstrated that occlusion of the biliopancreatic duct with Ethibloc resulted in temporal chronic pancreatitis-like alterations in rats [15], but some weeks after proteolytic disintegration of the glue the morphological and biochemical signs of chronic obstructive pancreatitis totally disappeared. Administration of high doses (about 12 g/kg per day) of alcohol prevented rapid regeneration and after 2 months even calcification occurred, in about 50% of animals. Thus histological signs of chronic obstructive and calcifying pancreatitis were observed in combination in this animal model, and the two etiological factors acting together accelerated the development of chronic pancreatitis as alcohol alone was without effect. Cessation of alcohol administration resulted in rapid biochemical and, less importantly, morphological recovery; thus alcohol seems to inhibit pancreatic regeneration and not directly provoke chronic pancreatitis-like lesions.

Pancreatic regeneration was widely examined after distal resection in rats [11, 23]. A 60% distal resection was followed by slow regeneration after a 1-month latency period, when some CCK release was also demonstrated (Table 1). CCK treatment accelerated; the CCK-antagonist CR 1409 inhibited pancreatic regeneration [2]. Alcohol administration totally prevented regeneration and CCK release after distal resection [21]. It seems, therefore, that the CCK has a central role in the pancreatic regeneration and the alcohol can influence the effect of CCK on the regeneration.

The mechanisms of action of alcohol administration on the trophic effect of endogenous [14] and exogenous [19] CCK were examined in rats. Two-week alcohol administration diminished the hypertrophy that is the typical, nonparallelly increased enzyme synthesis [5], but not the hyperplasia seen after CCK treatment, and eliminated the hyperplasia, as well as the hypertrophy provoked by soybean trypsin inhibitor (SBTI) administration. The alcohol alone did not influence the spontaneous growth and enzyme composition of the pancreas. Thus, the quiescent pancreas was not influenced, but the protein synthesis of the hyperplastic one became suppressed by alcohol. It was concluded [22] that the alcohol administration inhibited the enzyme synthesis in the CCK-stimulated, dividing, and/or newly formed acinar cells. As not

---

[1] First Department of Medicine, Albert Szent-Györgyi Medical University, H-6701, Szeged POB 469, Hungary

---

Chronic Pancreatitis
Ed. by Beger, Büchler, Ditschuneit, and Malfertheiner
© Springer-Verlag Berlin Heidelberg 1990

Table 1. Changes of plasma CCK levels after 60% distal resection. Effect of alcohol administration. (Bioassay on dispersed acini)

Time after operation	Without alcohol	With alcohol (12 g/kg per day)
1 day	0.69 ± 0.22	
2 weeks	1.23 ± 0.27	–
4 weeks	1.55 ± 0.78	–
6 weeks	2.00 S ± 0.39	0.93 s ± 0.08
8 weeks	1.26 ± 0.19	

x̄ ± SEM of seven rats; S, significant differences between 1-day and 6-week groups; s, significant differences between alcoholic and nonalcoholic rats

only the hypertrophy but also the hyperplasia of the pancreas in response to the 2-week SBTI administration was eliminated in alcoholic rats, further inhibiting mechanisms of alcohol have been supposed. Indeed, secretory studies and CCK measurements in conscious rats demonstrated that the endogenous CCK release in response to SBTI had already become disturbed after 3-day alcohol administration, whereas the secretory response to exogenous CCK had not yet changed significantly during this early period [22]. It seems, therefore, that among other mechanisms [26] the CCK-stimulated hypertrophy of regenerating acinar cells as well as the endogenous CCK release can be almost totally eliminated by alcohol administration in rats.

A central role of CCK in the pancreatic regeneration after distal resection [2, 20] and during development or progression of chronic pancreatitis in humans [16, 18] as well as in rats [15, 27] was supposed by us and others. Susceptibility of dividing or regenerating acinar cells [4] and the endogenous CCK release to alcohol may explain contradictory results of soy flour and CCK treatments in alcoholic patients [6, 17, 18]. Only long-lasting total abstinence can ensure that pancreatic regeneration stimulated by endogenous CCK results in functional and some morphological recovery in chronic pancreatitis.

Regeneration in Intraductal Oleic Acid Induced Pancreatic Atrophy

Intraductal oleic acid injection results in severe pancreatic atrophy in rats [13]. We have examined the time course of pancreatic regeneration of oleic acid induced chronic pancreatitis with and without alcohol administration or CCK treatment.

A quantity of 50 µl oleic acid was injected slowly into the common biliopancreatic duct near the duodenum during temporal occlusion of the biliary duct at laparotomy. Pancreatic histology, weight, protein, trypsin, and chymotrypsin content of the whole pancreas was examined 3, 15, 30, 60, and 90 days after operation.

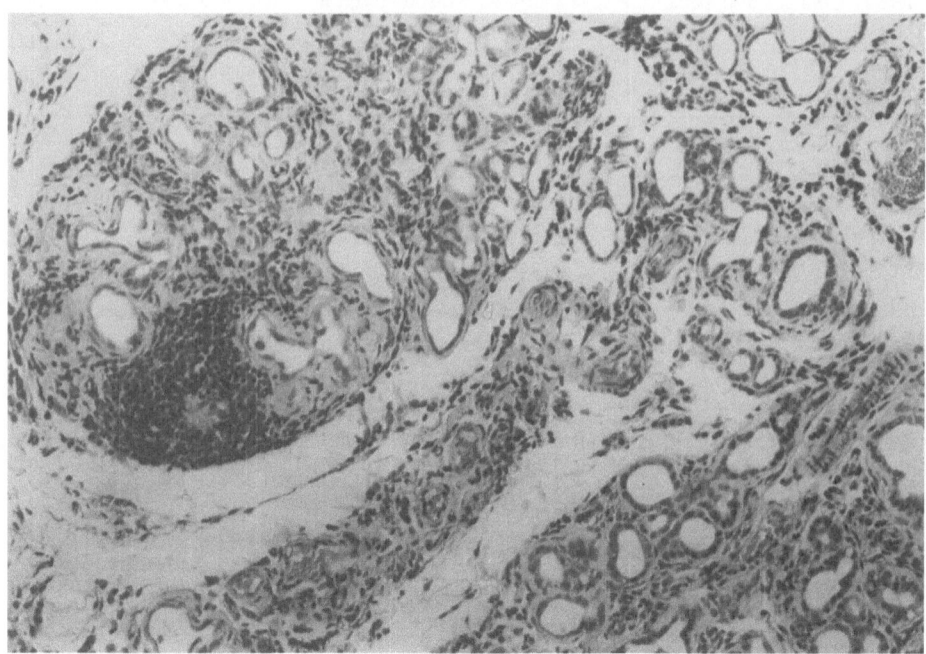

Fig. 1. Acute necrotizing pancreatitis 3 h after intraductal oleic acid injection. Pseudoductular complexes with acute inflammatory cell infiltration. H & E, × 40

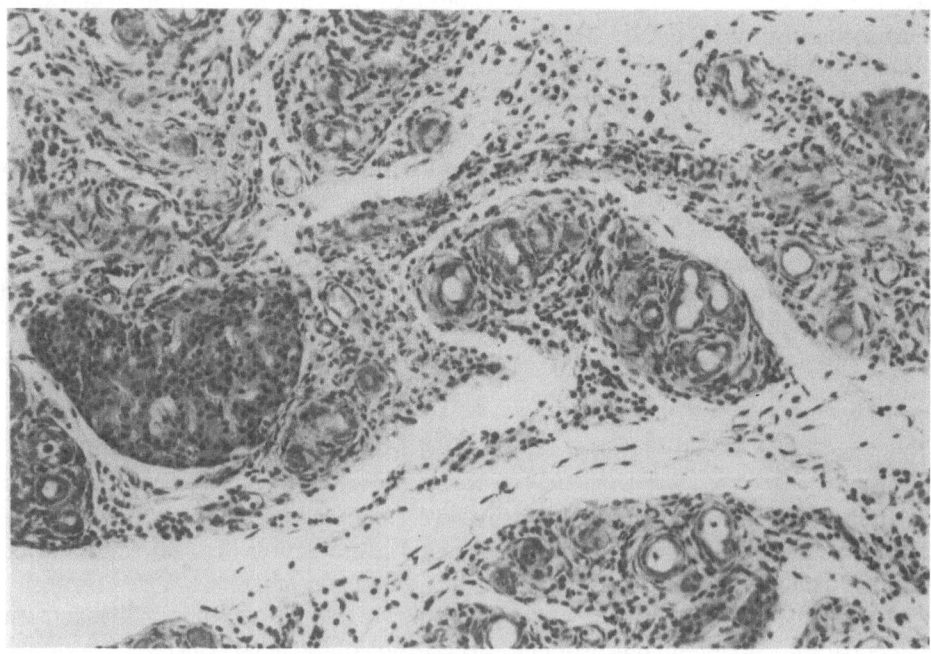

Fig. 2. Diffuse necrotizing pancreatitis 3 days after intraductal oleic acid injection. Acute inflammation with fibroblasts and pseudoductular lesions. H & E, × 40

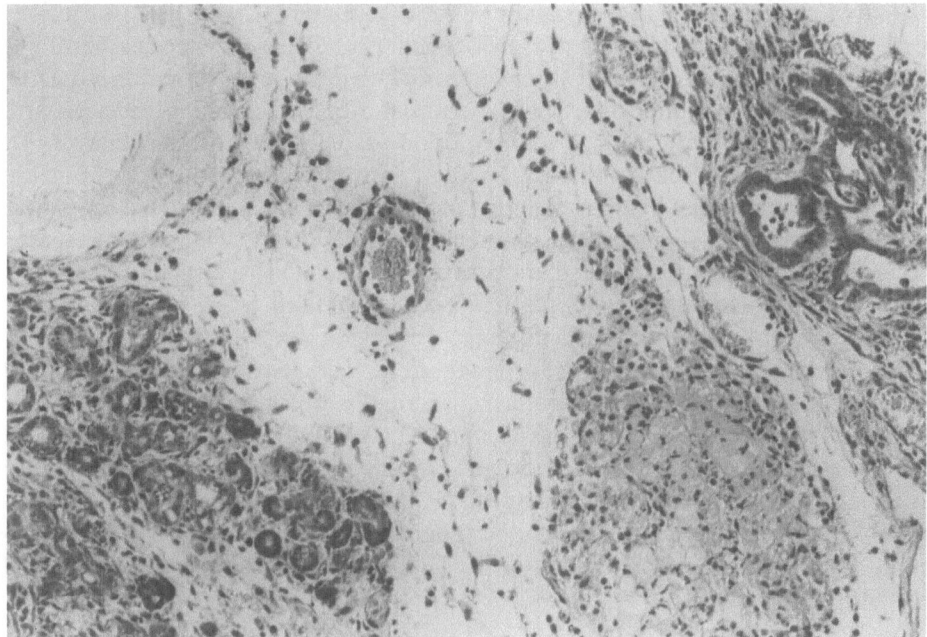

Fig. 3. Pancreatic atrophy 2 months after intraductal oleic acid injection. Necrotized and fibrotic areas with ductular proliferation and some necrobiotic acinar cells. H & E, × 40

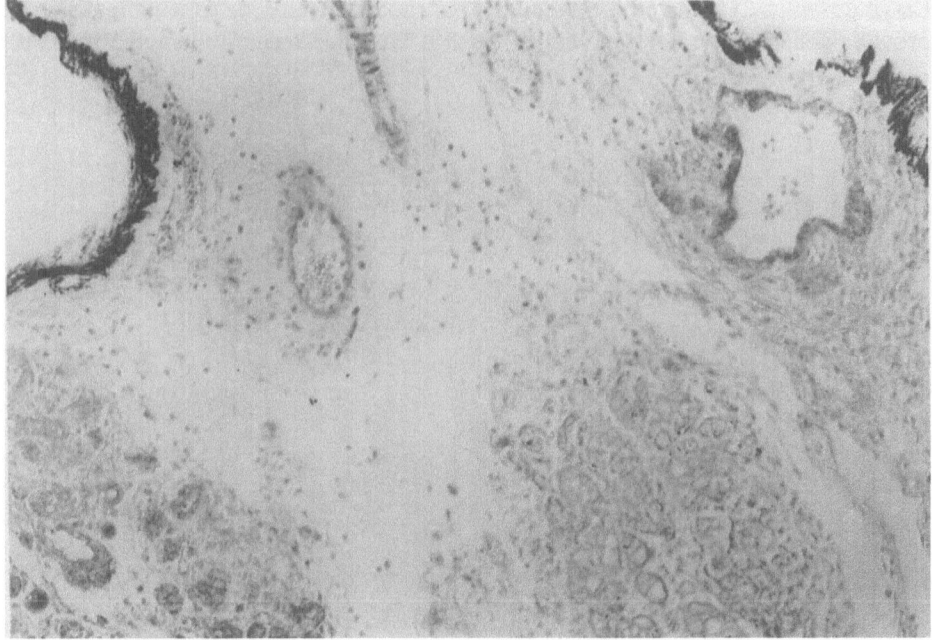

Fig. 4. Same area as Fig. 3 with special staining for calcium. Fine calcification around the necrotic areas. Kossa staining, × 40

Oleic acid injection resulted in severe necrotizing pancreatitis in every rat. Mortality rate was the same (about 40%) as after Ethibloc occlusion [15] but the acute lesions were more diffuse and fibrosis with pseudoductular complexes occurred earlier (Figs. 1, 2). The diffuse acinar cell atrophy and fibrosis with ductular proliferation remained stable during the 3-month observation period and fine calcification occurred at 2 months with or without alcohol administration in 70%–80% of rats (Figs. 3, 4). Nonconsistent biochemical recovery was demonstrated during this time, but the trypsin content increased earlier than that of protein and alcohol administration was able to eliminate this slight recovery; moreover at the 90th day significant differences occurred in all measured parameters between the alcoholic and nonalcoholic rats (Figs. 5–7). Cessation of alcohol resulted in only slight functional regeneration but CCK treatment accelerated biochemical recovery significantly during 1 month (Figs. 5–7). It seems, therefore, that the pronounced membrane toxic effect of oleic acid [13] can provoke severe acute necrotizing pancreatitis which can progress to chronic calcifying pancreatitis also without alcohol administration, although the alcohol somewhat inhibited pancreatic regeneration in this rat model too. Thus the diffuse acute lesions and less remaining acinar cell mass seem also to influence the effectiveness of pancreatic regeneration, and the progression after acute pancreatitis. However, regeneration can be accelerated by CCK even in this severe experimental chronic pancreatitis [27].

Effect of Alcohol on the Regeneration of Pancreatitis Provoked by Repeated CCK Overstimulation

Large doses of CCK given intravenously, intraperitoneally, or subcutaneously can provoke acute interstitial pancreatitis [9, 28]. We have recently demonstrated [10]

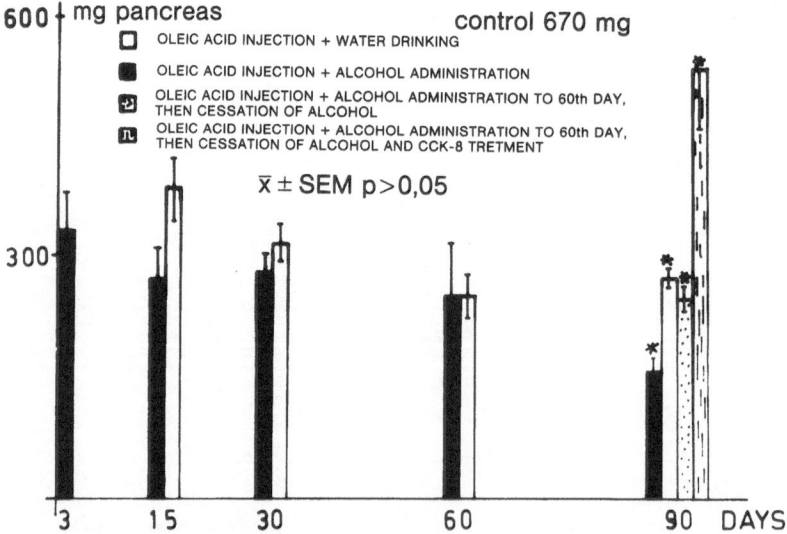

Fig. 5. Changes of pancreas weight after intraductal oleic acid injection with or without alcohol administration and CCK-8 (3 × 1 µg/kg per day) treatment

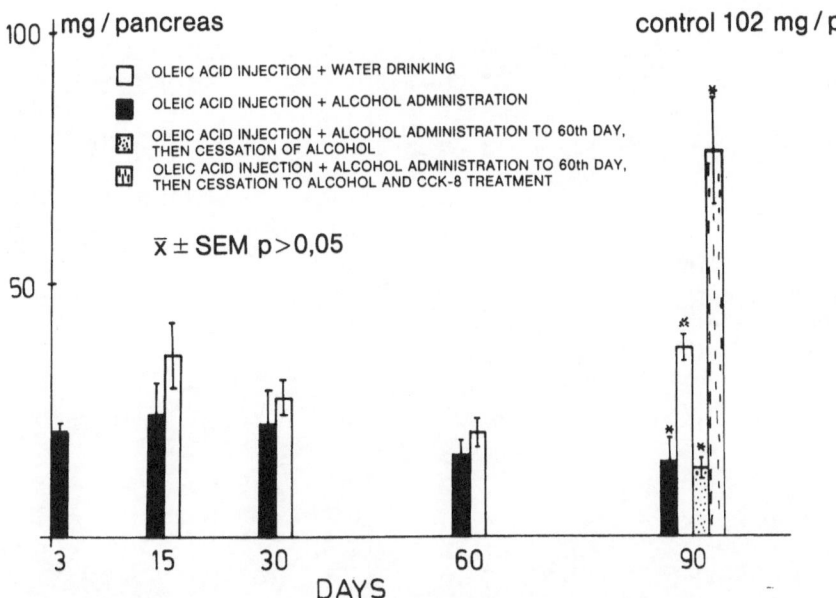

Fig. 6. Changes of pancreatic protein content after intraductal oleic acid injection with or without alcohol administration and CCK-8 (3 × 1 µg/kg per day) treatment

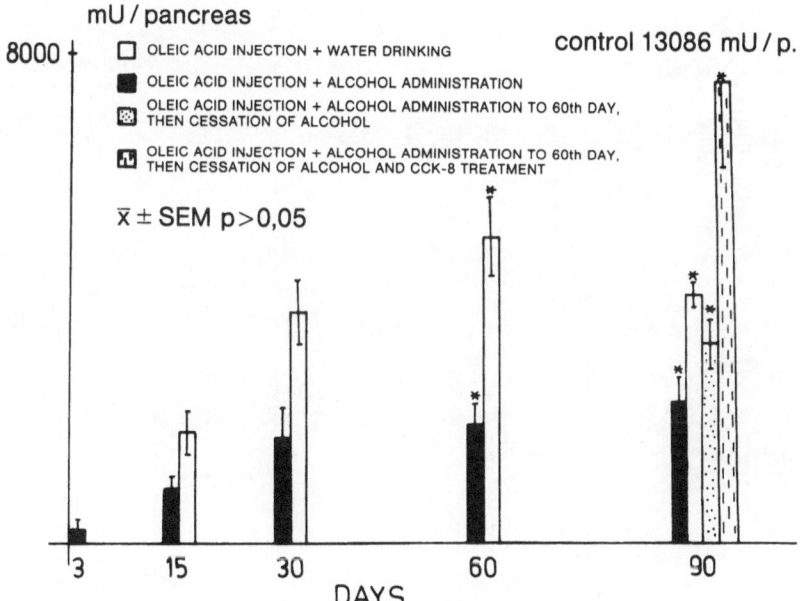

Fig. 7. Changes of pancreatic trypsin content after intraductal oleic acid injection with or without alcohol administration and CCK-8 (3 × 1 µg/kg per day) treatment

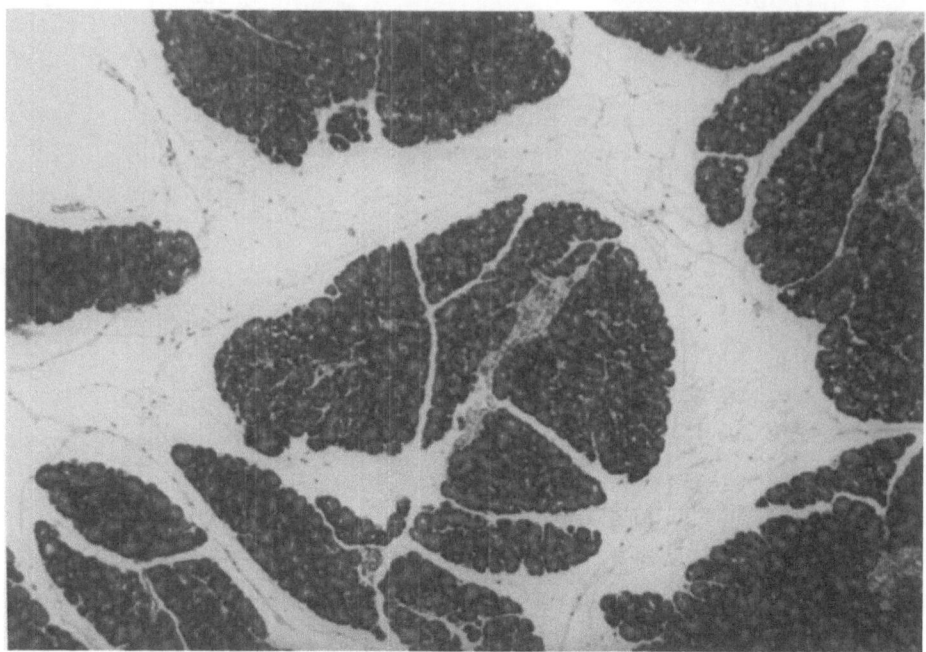

Fig. 8. Acute interstitial pancreatitis 3 h after serial CCK-8 (6 × 60 µg/kg s.c. hourly) overstimulation. Severe interlobular edema. H & E, × 16

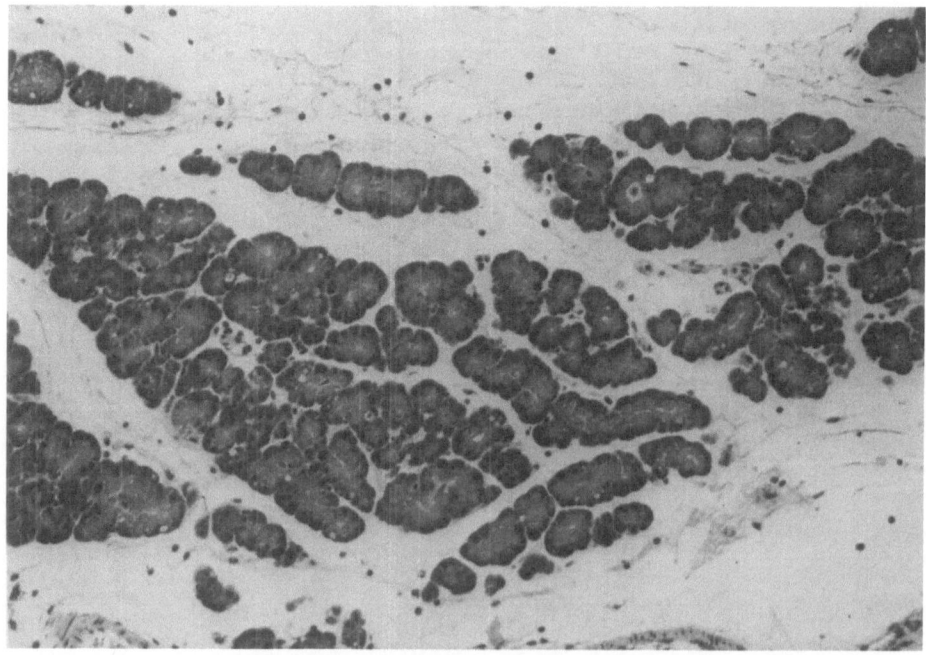

Fig. 9. Acute interstitial pancreatitis 3 h after serial CCK-8 (6 × 60 µg/kg s.c. hourly) overstimulation. Pronounced intralobular edema, almost intact acinar cells. H & E, × 40

that repeated, serial CCK injections (6 × 60 µg/kg per day) given subcutaneously for 7 days did not cause the acute pancreatitis to progress to a chronic process but at the 5th day a significant morphological and biochemical regeneration occurred in spite of the serial injections of toxic doses of CCK. Adaptation to the high doses of CCK seems to involve receptor mechanisms [3, 12], resulting in even faster regeneration with than without CCK injections.

In this study, we have administered high doses of alcohol (about 12 g/kg per day) beginning at the first CCK treatment and it was continued until the end of the observation period. Morphological (Figs. 8, 9) and biochemical signs of acute interstitial pancreatitis did not differ in alcoholic and nonalcoholic rats, but pancreatic regeneration was delayed during and some days after the end of CCK treatment (Figs. 10–15; Table 2).

Recovery of trypsin content (Fig. 12) was more effectively influenced by alcohol that that of amylase (Fig. 14) and lipase (Fig. 15).

Thus in this experiment, too, the alcohol administration influenced only the typical, nonparallelly increased enzyme synthesis of the CCK stimulated dividing and/or newly formed acinar cells, inhibiting just slightly and temporally the regeneration itself.

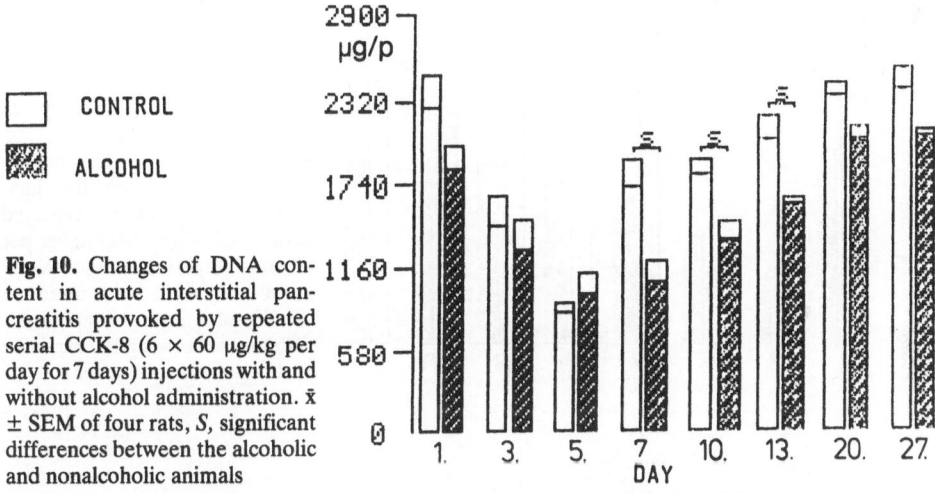

Fig. 10. Changes of DNA content in acute interstitial pancreatitis provoked by repeated serial CCK-8 (6 × 60 µg/kg per day for 7 days) injections with and without alcohol administration. x̄ ± SEM of four rats, S, significant differences between the alcoholic and nonalcoholic animals

Table 2. Mitotic index in CCK overstimulation pancreatitis with and without alcohol administration

Time	Mitosis/1000 acinar cells	
	Without alcohol	With alcohol (12 g/kg per day)
1st day	0.16	0.2
3rd day	0.66	0.33
5th day	2.0	1.66
7th day	4.6	1.66
10th day	3.3	2.0
13th day	0.2	1.66
20th day	0.33	0.16

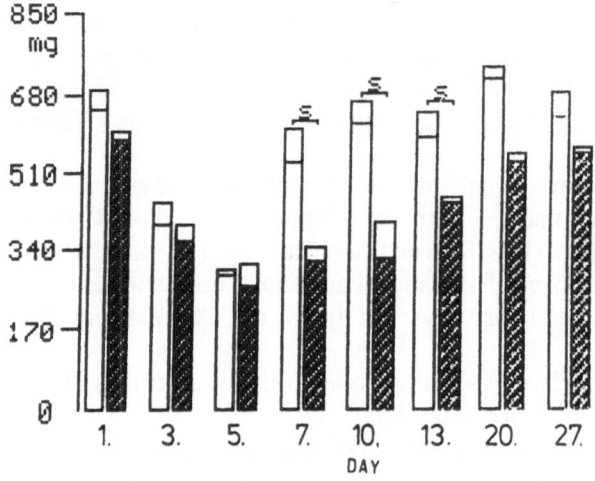

Fig. 11. Changes of pancreatic weight in acute interstitial pancreatitis provoked by repeated serial CCK-8 (6 × 60 μg/kg per day for 7 days) injections with and without alcohol administration. x̄ ± SEM of four rats, *S*, significant differences between the alcoholic and nonalcoholic animals

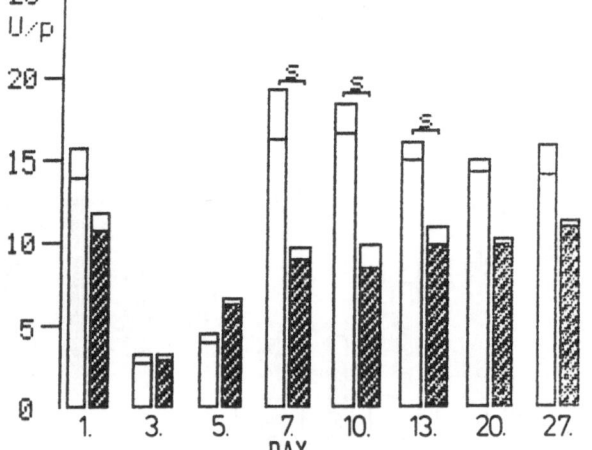

☐ CONTROL

▨ ALCOHOL

Fig. 12. Changes of trypsin content in acute interstitial pancreatitis provoked by repeated serial CCK-8 (6 × 60 μg/kg per day for 7 days) injections with and without alcohol administration. x̄ ± SEM of four rats; *S*, significant differences between the alcoholic and nonalcoholic animals

The acute pancreatitis was mild and the regeneration was not inhibited but even triggered by the repeated CCK injections, and it was only insufficiently influenced by alcohol administration. These facts together may explain why repeated CCK overstimulation cannot provoke chronic pancreatitis in rats.

Conclusions

Acute necrotizing pancreatitis can progress to chronic pancreatitis in rats if the acute pancreatitis was severe enough and the remaining acinar cell mass diminished sufficiently. The intraductal oleic acid provoked pancreatitis fulfills these conditions alone; the Ethibloc occlusion must be combined with alcohol administration, while

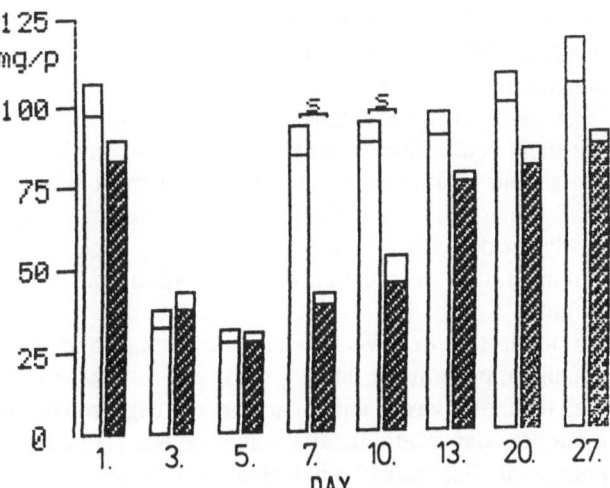

Fig. 13. Changes of protein content in acute interstitial pancreatitis provoked by repeated serial CCK-8 (6 × 60 µg/kg per day for 7 days) injections with and without alcohol administration. $\bar{x}$ ± SEM of four rats; *S*, significant differences between the alcoholic and nonalcoholic animals

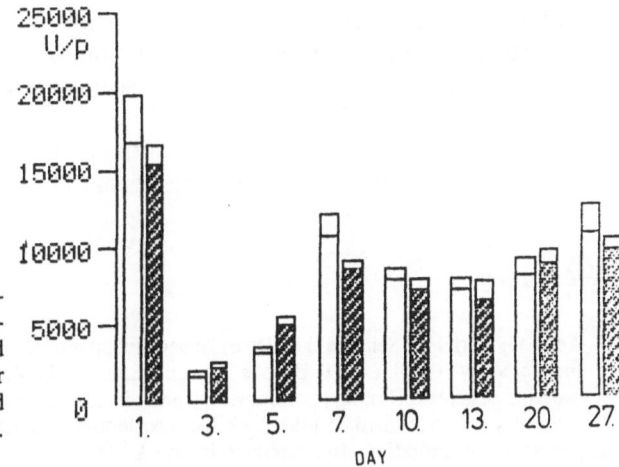

Fig. 14. Changes of amylase content in acute interstitial pancreatitis provoked by repeated serial CCK-8 (6 × 60 µg/kg per day for 7 days) injections with and without alcohol administration. $\bar{x}$ ± SEM of four rats

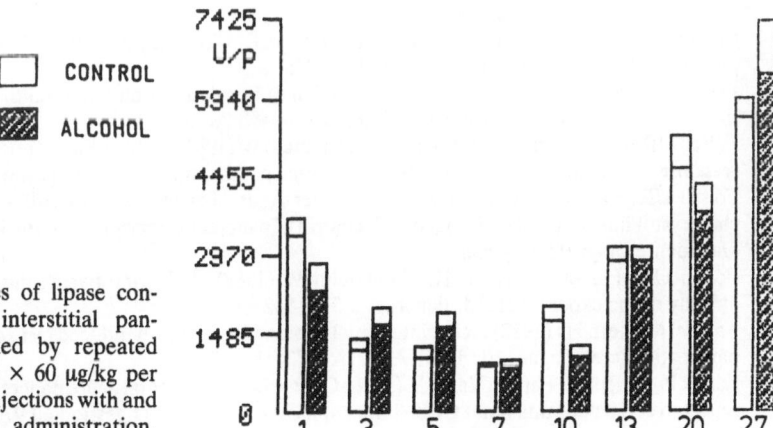

Fig. 15. Changes of lipase content in acute interstitial pancreatitis provoked by repeated serial CCK-8 (6 × 60 µg/kg per day for 7 days) injections with and without alcohol administration. $\bar{x}$ ± SEM of four rats

the repeated CCK overstimulation is unable to produce chronic pancreatitis even together with alcohol. Endogenous and/or exogenous CCK has an essential role in pancreatic regeneration at least in rats.

Endogenous CCK release seems to be insufficient for pancreatic regeneration in the oleic acid induced pancreatitis but not in the Ethibloc occlusion pancreatitis. Exogenous CCK proved to be effective in most models. Inhibition of the endogenous CCK release as well as the protein synthesis of the CCK-stimulated dividing and/or newly formed acinar cells by alcohol can explain the deleterious effect of alcohol administration on pancreatic regeneration and in the progression of chronic pancreatitis.

Long-lasting or severe pancreatic damage and delayed regeneration seem to be equally important for development and progression of chronic pancreatitis. In rats, high regenerative capacity of acinar cells triggered by endogenous CCK release due to a duodenopancreatic feedback mechanism [7] makes it difficult to provoke chronic pancreatitis-like morphological and functional alterations.

Signs of chronic obstructive and calcifying pancreatitis can appear together if the etiological factors act in combination as in the Ethibloc occlusion model treated by alcohol. However, calcification occurred frequently in the oleic acid induced chronic pancreatitis also without alcohol administration. Thus, the severe and prolonged pancreatic damage or delayed regeneration seem to be more important for calcification than the alcohol itself.

Results of experimental chronic pancreatitis models may have some relationship to the human disease but species differences seem to be important.

References

1. Adler G, Kern HF, Scheele GA (1986) Experimental models and concepts in acute pancreatitis. In: Go VLW, Gardner JD, Brooks FP, Lebenthal E, DiMagno EP, Scheele GA (eds) The exocrine pancreas. Biology, pathiobiology and diseases. Raven, New York, pp 407–421
2. Boros L, Pap Á, Varró V (1988) CCK-8 accelerates, the CCK-antagonist CR 1409 inhibits pancreatic regeneration after resection in rat (A-11). Digestion 40:71
3. Bussenot J, Balas D, Senegas-Balas F, Bertrand C, Ribet A (1987) Premières perturbations cellulaires lors d'une pancréatite par hyperstimulation à la céruleine chez le rat. 3rd Reunion of the Club Francais du Pancreas, Paris
4. Cumming ICR, Wood RA, Cushieri A, McGuiness E, Wormsley KG (1983) Effect of alcohol on pancreatic regeneration in the rat. Gut 24:A-479
5. Dagorn JC, Mongeau R (1977) Different action of hormonal stimulation on the biosynthesis of three pancreatic enzymes. Biochim Biophys Acta 498:76–82
6. Fölsch UR, Oldendörg A, Lankisch PG, Creutzfeld W (1984) Exocrine and endocrine function in response to raw soy flour in patients with chronic pancreatitis (A-57). Digestion 30:96
7. Fölsch UR, Cantor P, Wilms HM, Schafmayer A, Becker HD, Creutzfeldt W (1987) Role of cholecystokinin in the negative feedback control of pancreatic enzyme secretion in conscious rats. Gastroenterology 92:449–458
8. Fölsch UR, Fussek M, Ebert R, Creutzfeldt W (1988) Endocrine pancreatic function during atrophy of the exocrine gland. Pancreas 3:536–542
9. Lampel M, Kern HJ (1977) Acute interstitial pancreatitis in the rat induced by excessive doses of a pancreatic secretagogue. Virchows Arch [A] 373:97–117
10. Lászik Z, Berger Z, Pap Á, Varró V (1988) Course of experimental acute pancreatitis induced by repeated serial supramaximal CCK-8 injections in rats (A-72). Digestion 40:97

11. Lev MC, Fitzgerald PJ (1968) Pancreatic acinar cell regeneration. IV. Regeneration after surgical resection. Am J Pathol 53:513–535
12. McQuaid K, Wiliams J, Grendell J (1987) CCK-receptor binding affinity changes in diet-induced acute pancreatitis (Abstr). Dig Dis Sci 32:1176
13. Mundlos S, Adler G, Shaar M, Koop I, Arnold R (1986) Exocrine pancreatic function in oleic acid-induced pancreatic insufficiency in rats. Pancreas 1:29–36
14. Nagy I, Pap Á, Varró V (1986) Alcohol eliminates the trophic effect of soybean trypsin inhibitor (SBTI) administration (A-95). Digestion 35:42
15. Pap Á, Boros L (1989) Alcohol induced chronic pancreatitis in rats after temporary occlusion of biliopancreatic ducts with Ethibloc. Pancreas 4:249–256
16. Pap Á, Berger Z, Varró V (1981) Trophic effect of cholecystokinin-octapeptide in man. A new way in the treatment of chronic pancreatitis? Digestion 21:163–168
17. Pap Á, Berger Z, Varró V (1983) Beneficial effect of a soy flour diet in chronic pancreatitis. Mt Sinai J Med (N4) 50:208–212
18. Pap Á, Berger Z, Varró V (1984) Complementary effect of cholecystokinin octapeptide and soy flour treatment in chronic pancreatitis. Mt Sinai J Med (N4) 51:254–257
19. Pap Á, Nagy I, Tóth G, Varró V (1985) Alcohol diminishes the trophic effect of cholecystokinin-octapeptide (CCK-8) (A-116). Digestion 32:209–210
20. Pap Á, Flautner L, Karácsony S, Szécsény A, Varró V (1987) Recovery of pancreatic function after distal resection for chronic pancreatitis: regeneration or merely functional amelioration? Mt Sinai J Med (N4) 54:409–412
21. Pap Á, Boros L, Berger Z, Varró V (1988) Alcohol inhibits the regeneration after pancreatic resection in rats (A-98). Digestion 40:106–107
22. Pap Á, Nagy I, Takács T, Hajnal F, Varró V (1989) Mechanisms of action of alcohol administration on the trophic effect of soybean trypsin inhibitor and cholecystokinin-octapeptide in rat. Int J Pancreatol 5:263–272
23. Pearson KW, Scott D, Torrance B (1977) Effect of partial surgical pancreatectomy in rats. I. Pancreatic regeneration. Gastroenterology 72:469–473
24. Rao MS, Subbarao V, Yeldandi AV, Reddy JK (1987) Pancreatic acinar cell regeneration following cooper deficiency induced pancreatic necrosis. Int J Pancreatol 2:71–85
25. Sarles H, Laugier R (1981) Alcoholic pancreatitis. Clin Gastroenterol 10:401–415
26. Singh M (1986) Ethanol and the pancreas. In: Go VLW, Gardner JD, Brooks FP, Lebenthal E, DiMagno EP, Scheele GA (eds) The exocrine pancreas. Biology, pathobiology and diseases. Raven, New York, pp 423–442
27. Steinberg WM, Burns MK, Henry JP, Nochomovizt LE, Anderson KK (1987) Cerulein induces hyperplasia of the pancreas in a rat model of chronic pancreatic insufficiency. Pancreas 2:176–180
28. Tani S, Otsuki M, Itoh H, Fujii M, Nakamura T, Oka T, Baba S (1987) Histologic and biochemical alteration in experimental acute pancreatitis induced by supramaximal cerulein stimulation. Int J Pancreatol 2:337–348
29. Tomita T, Rhodes J, Falscroft J, Doull V, Kimmel JR, Polloch GG (1988) Endocrine pancreas in the rat model of exocrine pancreatic insufficiency. Pancreas 3:568–575

Lysosomal Enzyme Activation of Digestive Enzymes During Chronic Pancreatitis?

C. Figarella[1], D. Basso[2], and O. Guy-Crotte[1]

Introduction

Human pancreatic acinar cells synthesize and store numerous proteins whose intracellular processing has been extensively studied in its homologous guinea-pig cell [1]. Digestive enzymes which constitute most of the pancreatic proteins and lysosomal hydrolases are both synthesized by ribosomes attached to the rough endoplasmic reticulum. The nascent polypetide chains elongate within the cisternae of the reticulum, migrate through this compartment, and are transported to the Golgi complex where the pathways of the two classes of enzymes diverge. Secretory digestive proteins are accumulated into granules and when necessary are discharged into the acinar lumen by fusion-fission of the zymogen granule limiting membrane and the luminal plasmalemma whereas lysosomal hydrolases are usually targeted for inclusion into lysosomes.

Physiological Activation of Human Pancreatic Zymogens

Human digestive enzymes are a mixture of enzymes necessary for intraluminal digestion of diets which contain essentially proteins, lipids, and carbohydrates. All the classes of enzymes are present, but, for evident reason of safeguards against cell autolysis, most of the digestive enzymes are secreted as inactive forms called zymogens [2].

At their entrance into the duodenum, zymogens including trypsinogen 1 (which constitutes 18% of total proteins of human pancreatic juice) and trypsinogen 2 (which constitutes 9% of total proteins of the same juice) meet enterokinase, a brush border enzyme which is the key enzyme of digestion since it is responsible for trypsinogen's activation into trypsins. The generated trypsins, in turn activate their own zymogens, and we have shown in previous studies that, if enterokinase is the starter of trypsinogen activation, the predominant subsequent mechanism becomes the activation of trypsinogens by trypsins [3]. All other zymogens, proteolytic (chymotrypsinogens, proelastases, and procarboxypeptidases) and lipolytic (prophospholipase A2 and procolipase) are converted by trypsins into active enzymes.

---

[1] Groupe de Recherche sur les Glandes Exocrines, 27 Boulevard Lei Roure, 13009 Marseille, France
[2] Instituto di Medicini Interna, Università di Padova, Padova, Italy

---

Chronic Pancreatitis
Ed. by Beger, Büchler, Ditschuneit, and Malfertheiner
© Springer-Verlag Berlin Heidelberg 1990

Evidence of a Premature Zymogen Activation in Chronic Pancreatitis

Our previous studies on the pancreatic juice of patients suffering from chronic pancreatitis have enabled several signs of premature zymogen activation to be characterized:
- High frequency of free proteolytic activity
- Decrease in the potential activity of trypsinogens
- Presence of an alpha 1 proteinase inhibitor-chymotrypsin complex due to the concomitant presence in the juice of the seric inhibitor and of some active chymotrypsin. Such a complex does not exist in normal juice.

More importantly, we could demonstrate that the protein of 14000 molecular weight isolated from protein precipitates present in the pancreatic juice of patients suffering from chronic pancreatitis was a proteolysis product [4]. This proteolysis product may be purified from normal or pathological pancreatic juice slightly activated and we called this protein, whose the origin and function were unknown, protein X. As schematically shown in Fig. 1, this protein, which precipitates at pH 8, is produced by the proteolytic cleavage of a soluble glycoprotein of 19000 molecular weight with liberation of a small glycopeptide [4, 5]. It is now well established that the pancreatic protein X is identical to the pancreatic thread protein isolated later from human pancreas by Gross et al. [7] and to a form of pancreatic stone protein isolated from pancreatic calculi actually described [8].

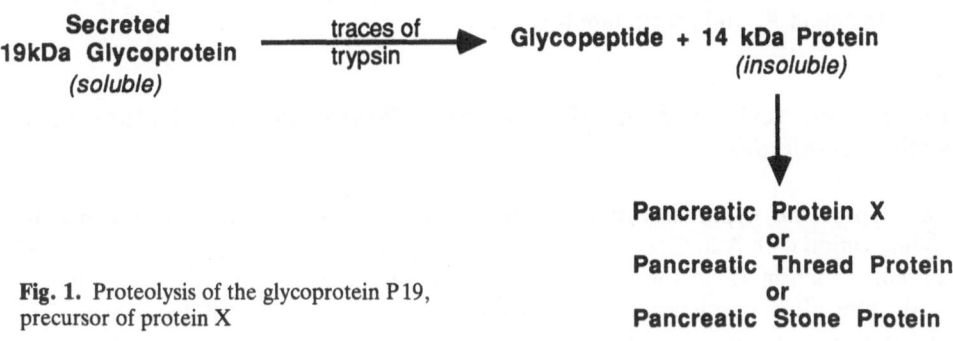

Fig. 1. Proteolysis of the glycoprotein P 19, precursor of protein X

Other characteristics have been found in the pancreatic juice of patients with chronic pancreatitis such as an increased level of acinar lactoferrin and an increase in the specific activities of acid phosphatase and other lysosomal enzymes showing a stimulation of the lysosomal system in the disease where the role played by lactoferrin remains to be elucidated [9]. All these data led us to propose, some years ago, a hypothesis on the pathogenesis of chronic pancreatitis [6, 10], which is presented in Fig. 2. This hypothesis is settled on several observations of the literature which have shown an overstimulation of pancreatic acinar cell in the disease [reviewed in 6, 11]. This overstimulation could likely provoke a deranged intracellular transport of secretory proteins leading to an abnormal admixture of digestive enzymes and lysosomal

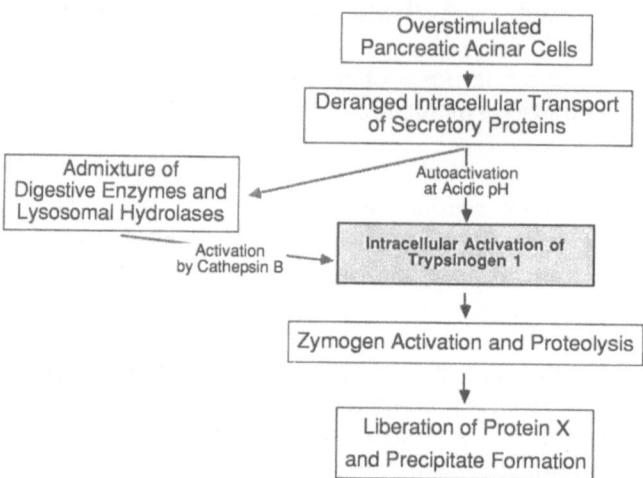

Fig. 2. Proposed hypothesis for the pathogenesis of chronic pancreatitis

hydrolases and/or a storage of pancreatic zymogens in acid compartments which in turn could provoke an intracellular activation of trypsinogen 1 by cathepsin B and/or acidic pH. Such a premature activation could be responsible for the described modifications of the pathological secretion: activation of zymogen and proteolysis, generation of protein X, and precipitate formation.

Possible Intracellular Activation of Human Trypsinogens by Cathepsin B and at Acidic pH

To support the hypothesis of intracellular activation of human trypsinogens, in collaboration with Alan Barrett (Cambridge, England) we have studied the effects of human cathepsin B on the two human trypsinogens. In an initial experiment we studied the effect of the lysosomal proteinase on the total proteins of the juice at 25°C and at pH 3.5 by measuring the generated tryptic activity. Full activation of trypsinogens was progressively attained, whereafter the trypsin activity rapidly decreased. This decrease could be attributed to the degradation of the newly formed trypsin by the other activated proteolytic enzymes present in the juice. At 37°C, both activation and proteolysis were faster but in all cases controls without cathepsin B were not activated. These results indicate that at acidic pH the secretory trypsin inhibitor present in pancreatic juice is unable to prevent the activation of the proteolytic zymogens contained in the juice.

We then repeated the experiments with the two human trypsinogens purified from pancreatic juice and the results are shown in Fig. 3. When trypsinogens were incubated by cathepsin B at pH 3.8 and 25°C, there was a progressive increase in trypsin activity for both zymogens. However, whereas human trypsinogen 1 reached the maximal specific activity as obtained in the standard conditions of enterokinase

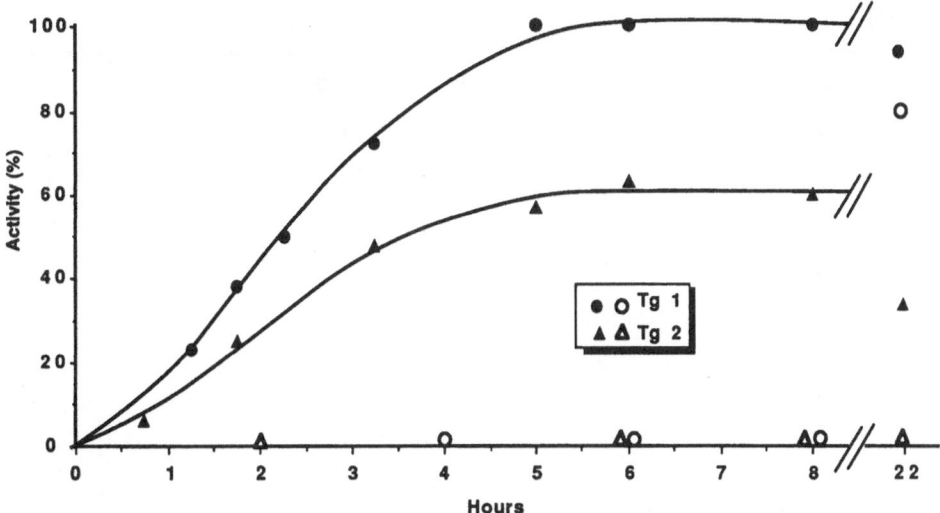

Fig. 3. Kinetics of activation of the two human trypsinogens by cathepsin B at pH 3.8 and 25°

activation, only 60% of trypsinogen 2 was converted into active trypsin. This phenomenon was due to the previously described instability of human trypsinogen 2 at acidic pH [2].

Controls without cathepsin B showed no activation after 8 h, but surprisingly 70% of the purified trypsinogen 1 was converted into active trypsin after 24 h in the absence of added lysosomal proteinase.

We therefore explored the spontaneous autoactivation of human trypsinogen 1 at different pH and we have chosen to report here (Fig. 4) the results obtained at pH 5, which is a pH very close to the pH of lysosomes. It can be seen that, in the absence of any added proteinase, human trypsinogen 1 can be fully converted into active trypsin. In the presence of cathepsin B, activation is faster.

The phenomenon was further explored with different concentrations of cathepsin B and the results are reported in Fig. 5, where only the early beginnings of trypsinogen 1 activations are shown. The ratios of cathepsin B to trypsinogen increase threefold from right to left of the diagram and the rate of activation increases with cathepsin B concentration. It is interesting to note the biphasic shape of the three kinetics. In the first part of the curve the activation follows the course of a monomolecular reaction and the rate is proportional to the concentration of cathepsin added. In the second part of the curve the activation is accelerated by the presence of the converted trypsin and the reaction becomes autocatalytic. Finally, it must be noticed that the phenomenon is much faster at 37°C than at 25°C and in the presence of high concentrations of pancreatic zymogens and cathepsin B (data not shown). These conditions could occur in vivo in the case of abnormal admixture of digestive enzymes and lysosomal hydrolases.

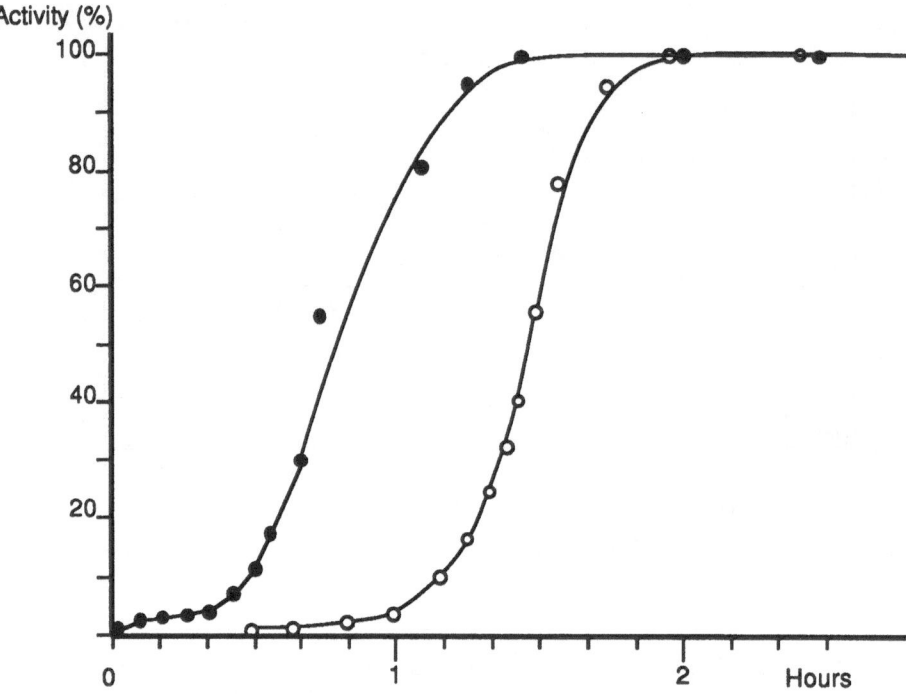

Fig. 4. Kinetics of autoactivation of human trypsinogen 1 at pH 5 in the presence (●) and in the absence (○) of cathepsin B

Conclusion

In conclusion, since the concentration of cathepsin B in lysosomes is high and evaluated to 1 mmol, and the intralysosomal pH between 4.5 and 5.5 [cited in 12], intracellular trypsinogen activation may occur in vivo in pathological conditions and be responsible for the early events leading to chronic pancreatitis.

References

1. Palade GE (1975) Intracellular aspects of the process of protein synthesis. Science 189:347–358
2. Figarella C, Guy-Crotte O, Barthe C, Amouric M (1987) Les protéines pancréatiques humaines à l'état normal et pathologique. Gastroenterol Clin Biol 11:891–897
3. Colomb E, Figarella C (1979) Comparative studies on the mechanism of activation of the two human trypsinogens. Biochim Biophys Acta 571:343–351
4. Guy-Crotte O, Amouric M, Figarella C (1984) Characterization and N-terminal sequence of a degradation product of 14000 molecular weight isolated from human pancreatic juice. Biochem Biophys Res Commun 125:516–523
5. Guy-Crotte O, Barthe C, Basso D, Fornet B, Figarella C (1988) Characterization of two glycoproteins of human pancreatic juice; P35 a truncated protease E and P19, precursor of protein X. Biochem Biophys Res Comm 156:318–322
6. Figarella C (1980) La lactoferrine dans les pancréatites chroniques calcifiantes. Hypothèse pour le rôle biologique de la lactoferrine. Gastroenterol Clin Biol 4:631–635

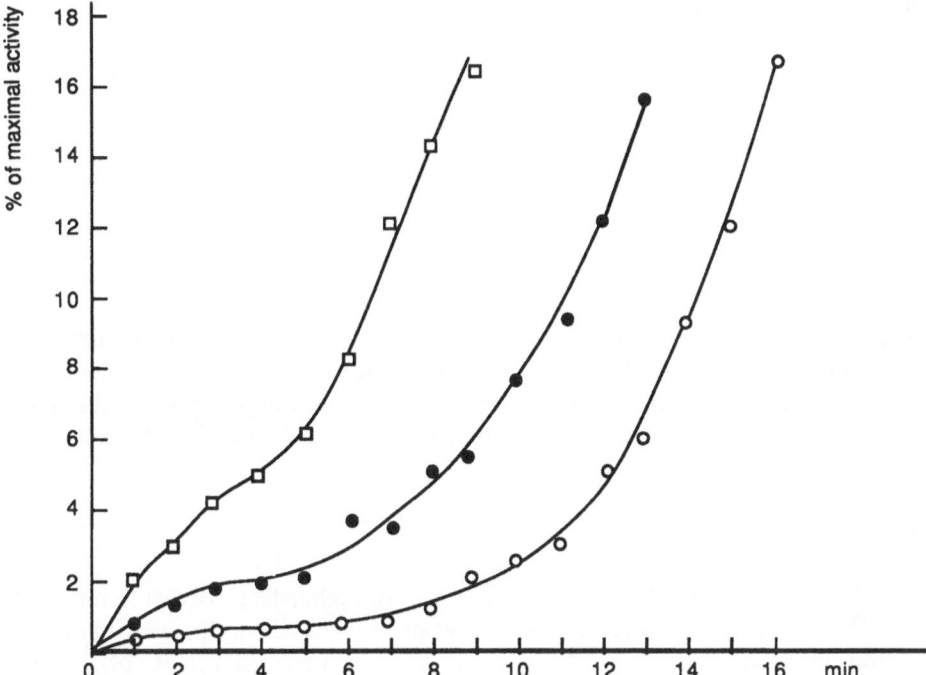

Fig. 5. Kinetics of activation of human trypsinogen 1 at pH 5 by increasing concentrations of cathepsin B

7. Gross J, Carlson RL, Brauer AW, Margolies MN, Warshaw AL, Wands JR (1985) Isolation, characterization, and distribution of an unusual pancreatic human secretory protein. J Clin Invest 76:2115–2126
8. De Caro AM, Adrich Z, Fournet B, Capon C, Bonicel JJ, de Caro JD, Rovery M (1989) N-Terminal sequence extension in the glycosylated form of human pancreatic stone protein. The 5-oxoproline N-terminal chain is O-glycosylated on the 5th amino acid residue. Biochim Biophys Acta 994:281–284
9. Figarella C, Vogt E, Hosli P (1982) Alkaline phosphatase and acid lysosomal hydrolases in pancreatic juice and fibroblast cell cultures of patients with chronic calcifying pancreatitis. Eur J Clin Invest 12:145–149
10. Steer ML, Meldolesi J, Figarella C (1981) Pancreatitis. The role of lysosomes. Dig Dis Sci 80:461–473
11. Braganza JM (1986) The pancreas. In: Pounder RE (ed) Recent advances in gastroenterology, vol 6. Livingstone, Edinburgh, pp 251–280
12. Figarella C, Miszczuk-Jamska B, Barrett AJ (1988) Possible lysosomal activation of pancreatic zymogens. Activation of both human tryspinogens by cathepsin B and spontaneous acid activation of human trypsinogen 1. Biol Chem Hoppe Seyler 369:293–298

Role of Alcohol in the Development of Chronic Pancreatitis

M. Singh[1]

Introduction

Ethanol is rapidly absorbed and metabolized in the liver by a complex mixture of isoenzymes (alcohol dehydrogenase) that oxidize it to acetaldehyde. Acetaldehyde may be formed in the pancreas or released from albumin complexes with subsequent preferential binding to target cells including pancreatic acinar and ductal cells.

Discussion

We fed ethanol as 36% of total calories as a part of Lieber-DeCarli diet to rats for 6, 12, and 18 months. Biochemical studies revealed increased specific activity of trypsinogen, chymotrypsinogen, and lipase and decreased specific activity of amylase. Trypsin-inhibiting activity was decreased in the tissue and the medium in a progressive fashion. In the ethanol-fed animals, basal secretion of trypsinogen and chymtrypsinogen was increased at 6, 12, and 18 months. In addition basal secretion of amylase and lipase was increased and that of trypsin inhibitor decreased at 12 and 18 months. Secretion of pancreatic secretory trypsin inhibitor was stimulated by a cholinergic agent whereas secretion of digestive enzymes was not stimulated in the ethanol-fed versus control group. Electron microscopic studies revealed progressive accumulation of lipid droplets in the acinar and ductal cells [15]. In the state of chronic alcoholism, others observed increased responsiveness of the pancreas to CCK stimulation in dogs [7] and humans [5] and increased protease zymogens in the pancreatic secretion [6].

To determine if constituents of diet altered the effect of ethanol on pancreatic macromolecular content and secretion, we studied the effect of a combination of AIN 76 diet containing 12% of total calories as fat with 36% of carbohydrate calories replaced with 5% concentration of ethanol. Unlike the results reported earlier, no changes in the total content, specific acitivities, concentration, and secretion of proteases, lipase, and amylase were observed [13]. This was in contrast to increased specific activity of proteases and lipase and increased secretion of digestive enzymes in animals fed ethanol with high fat content in the diet [15].

To determine the modification by sex of diet and ethanol effect on rat pancreas, we compared female rats with male rats fed ethanol as 36% of total carbohydrate calories

---

[1] Medical Research Service (509/151), VA Medical Center, Augusta, Georgia 30912, USA

Chronic Pancreatitis
Ed. by Beger, Büchler, Ditschuneit, and Malfertheiner
© Springer-Verlag Berlin Heidelberg 1990

replaced in Lieber-DeCarli diet with ethanol for a period of 3 months. Ethanol fed female rats had a significant increase in secretion of trypsinogen and amylase (and a proportional but statistically not significant increase in lipase) compared with male rats. These data indicated that chronic feeding of ethanol resulted in a nonparallel secretion of digestive enzymes in both sexes but with a greater discordance between the trypsinogen secretion and trypsin inhibitor in the female rats [11]. Since our studies demonstrated perturbation in the pancreatic protease and lipase content and secretion due to ethanol and its modification by diet, we next studied, under similar conditions, the perturbations in the lysosomal enzymes. To that intent, we fed Lieber-DeCarli diet with ethanol replacing 40% of carbohydrate calories for 18 months. The pancreatic glands were isolated and divided into portions for biochemical analyses, cell fractionation, and histology. In the pancreatic tissue of animals fed ethanol total protein, trypsinogen, and free trypsin were increased. In the cell fractionation studies, acid phosphatase was increased in all cell fractions and cathepsin B was increased in the mitochondrial-lysosomal fraction and the zymogen granule fractions of the ethanol-fed animals [14]. All of the ethanol-fed animals developed morphological changes akin to human chronic pancreatitis with focal parenchymal degeneration with fibrosis. Protein plugs of light and stratified nature were observed. Tubular complexes were observed. These were composites of ductular elements which were present in the normal parenchyma and of acinar cells which had dedifferentiated or undergone phenotypic modulation. They had lost zymogen granules and endoplasmic reticulum. There was concomitant loss of cell volume and therefore cell height. They presented as a collection of tubules showing proportions of normal or dilated ducts [14]. To determine the nature of fat accumulation and the effect of long-term ethanol intake on pancreatic lipid metabolism, we studied the effect of feeding Lieber-DeCarli diet with or without alcohol for 21 months. Compared to controls, ethanol-fed animals had a lower level of triglycerides, a higher level of cholesterol ester and moderate elevation in phospholipids, lower incorporation of ^{14}C palmitoyl in triglycerides, and increased ^{14}C activity in phospholipids and cholesterol esters. Chronic ethanol intake, therefore, caused marked changes in pancreatic lipid metabolism due to altered enzyme activities involved in the lipid pathways. It was suggested that increased cholesterol ester was responsible for intracellular fat accumulation and membrane disordering causing pancreatic injury [8].

Alcoholism causes deficiency of several micronutrients including zinc, selenium, magnesium, vitamin C and multiple B vitamin factors including folate, B12, B6, thiamin, riboflavin, niacin, pantothenic acid, and biotin. We, therefore, studied the effect of deficiency of some of these micronutrients on pancreatic acinar cell function. Specific changes due to zinc deficiency included decreased body weight and increase in the content and specific activity of lipase. Both the size and volume fraction of zymogen granules was reduced in zinc deficiency. The lumina of acinar and small ducts were collapsed with paucity of secretion products [3]. In the marginal zinc-deficient group, there was further reduction in the volume fraction of zymogen granules associated with increased secretion of serine proteases [4]. This indicated an accelerated discharge mechanism simulating ethanol-induced secretory alterations that we reported earlier. When marginal zinc nutriture was combined with ethanol, we observed that zinc and ethanol led to a specific injury independent of each other. However, marginal zinc nutriture in concert with ethanol resulted in impaired RNA synthesis and secretion of nascent proteins and increased secretion of serine proteases. Vitamin B_6 deficiency resulted in DNA injury, decreased RNA turnover, and increased protein turnover resulting in decreased amylase content and secretion [9]. Folate deficiency resulted in impaired DNA synthesis without any change in amylase secretion [1]. Thiamin deficiency resulted in reduced body weight, total protein, and amylase, but both basal and bethanechol-stimulated secretion were increased [10]. Niacin-tryptophan deficiency resulted in decreased body weight, pancreas weight, DNA, protein, amylase, lipase, and serine proteases. Secretion of amylase and trypsinogen were increased whereas lipase was not changed [12]. In riboflavin deficiency, both basal and bethanechol-stimulated secretion of chymotrypsinogen were increased [2].

Therefore, our working hypothesis is that the prolonged abuse of ethanol probably in combination with an unbalanced diet produces pancreatitis by interfering with the intracellular transport and discharge of digestive enzymes, causing colocalization of digestive and lysosomal hydrolases probably producing an augmented responsiveness of the exocrine pancreas to endogenously released CCK. Future directions of our research effort include investigation in alcoholism events such as autophagocytosis, crinophagy, blockade of exocytosis or evidence of ectopic discharge with electron microscopy and immunocytochemical labeling using antibodies to serine proteases and cathepsin B. The intracellular processing of prepropeptides of digestive and lysosomal enzymes, protein synthesis, and selective gene expression at transcriptional and translational level after chronic ethanol feeding need investigation. We need to localize the site of endogenous cathepsin B activation by studying lysosomal and nonlysosomal activation of endogenous trypsinogen with isolated subcellular elements and cytosol. To extend our observations on the secretory profiles of rat pancreatic juice, we need to study the sera and pancreatic juice of alcoholic rats for in vitro proteolytic activities.

References

1. Elseweidy M, Singh M (1984) Folate deficiency and pancreatic acinar cell function. Proc Soc Exp Biol Med 177:247–252
2. Gomez RL, Nichoalds GE, Singh M, Simsek H, LaSure MM (1988) In vitro assay of pancreatic acinar cell function of rats made chronically riboflavin deficient. Am J Clin Nutr 48:626–631
3. Perez-Jimenez F, Bockman DE, Singh M (1986) Pancreatic acinar cell function and morphology in rats fed zinc-deficient and marginal zinc-deficient diets. Gastroenterology 90:946–957
4. Perez-Jimenez F, Singh M, Bockman DE, Hahn HKJ (1986) Interaction between marginal zinc deficiency and chronic alcoholism: pancreatic structure and function in rats in vitro. Pancreas 1:254–263
5. Renner IG, Rinderknecht H, Valenzuela JE, Douglas AP (1980) Studies of pure pancreatic secretions in chronic alcoholic subjects without pancreatic insufficiency. Scand J Gastroenterol 15:241–244
6. Rinderknecht H, Stace NH, Renner IG (1985) Effects of chronic alcohol abuse on exocrine pancreatic secretion in man. Dig Dis Sci 30:65–71
7. Sarles H, Tiscornia O, Palasciano G, Brasca A, Hage G, Deveaux MA, Gullo L (1973) Effects of chronic intragastric ethanol administration on canine exocrine pancreatic secretion. Scand J Gastroenterol 8:85–96
8. Simsek H, Singh M (1989) Effect of chronic ethanol feeding on pancreatic lipid metabolism. Gastroenterology 96:A473

9. Singh M (1980) Effects of vitamin B_6 deficiency on pancreatic acinar cell function. Life Sci 26:715–724
10. Singh M (1982) Effect of thiamin deficiency on pancreatic acinar cell function. Am J Clin Nutr 36:500–504
11. Singh M (1986) Modification by sex of diet and ethanol effect on rat pancreatic acinar cell metabolism. Pancreas 1:164–171
12. Singh M (1986) Effect of niacin and niacin-tryptophan deficiency on pancreatic acinar cell function in rats in vitro. Am J Clin Nutr 44:512–518
13. Singh M (1987) Effect of chronic feeding of ethanol diet of "average" fat content on rat pancreas. Dig Dis Sci 32:57–64
14. Singh M (1987) Alcoholic pancreatitis in rats fed ethanol in a nutritionally adequate liquid diet. Int J Pancreatol 2:311–324
15. Singh M, LaSure MM, Bockman DE (1982) Pancreatic acinar cell function and morphology in rats chronically fed an ethanol diet. Gastroenterology 82:425–434

Fate of Pancreatic Enzymes During Gastrointestinal Transit

E. P. DiMagno[1]

In human studies, the fate of pancreatic enzymes during small-intestinal aboral transit has been a controversial issue. There are few data available. Borgstrom et al. [1] found that activities of all pancreatic enzymes decreased progressively and at similar rates as they moved from the proximal to the distal small bowel. In contrast, others have found in patients with ileostomies that the ileostomy effluent contained a large amount of trypsin and chymotrypsin activity [2, 3]. Recently we performed a study to determine how much pancreatic enzyme activity survives during small-intestinal aboral transit in healthy human volunteers by measuring the cumulative amount of lipase, trypsin, and amylase activities and lipase and trypsin immunoreactivities delivered postprandially (50 g, 400 ml semiliquid pure rice starch pudding) to the duodenum, mid-jejunum, and terminal ileum [4]. We found that as enzymes moved from the duodenum to the ileum 74% of amylase activity, 22% of trypsin activity, and 1% of lipase activity survived transit. Enzymatic activity and immunoreactivity of trypsin and lipase disappeared at different rates, suggesting that for these enzymes the sites of enzymatic activity and immunorecognition are not identical.

Several hypotheses might explain the cause of loss of pancreatic enzymes during aboral transit:
a) acidic inactivation of the enzymes,
b) conservation of pancreatic enzymes by reabsorption and subsequent intrapancreatic recirculation of intact enzymes,
c) enzymatic proteolysis of pancreatic enzymes, and
d) bile and other intraluminal contents (nutrients) affecting the rate of loss of enzyme activity during aboral gastrointestinal transit.

Our data from the above study [4] support the hypothesis that pancreatic enzymes disappear from the small-intestinal lumen because they are inactivated and/or destroyed by mechanisms that are independent of acidic pH. We previously have shown that, if the pH in the proximal small intestine (and in the stomach if enzymes are ingested) is less than 4, lipolytic activity is lost [5, 6]. In our study [4], the pH of all intestinal samples was at least 6, and at this pH acidic enzymatic inactivation of pancreatic enzymes does not occur.

Secondly, our data do not support the hypothesis that the absorption of intact enzymes is a major pathway for the removal of enzymes from the intestinal lumen. If this hypothesis were correct, we should have observed parallel decreases in enzymatic

---

[1] Gastroenterology Research Unit, Mayo Clinic, 200 First Street SW, Rochester, MN 55905, USA

Chronic Pancreatitis
Ed. by Beger, Büchler, Ditschuneit, and Malfertheiner
© Springer-Verlag Berlin Heidelberg 1990

and immunoreactive activity. Since the enzymatic immunoreactive activities of both lipase and trypsin disappeared at widely different rates [4], we concluded that intestinal absorption of intact enzymes is not quantitively important and cannot explain the loss of intraluminal lipase and trypsin during small-intestinal transit in humans.

As the first two hypotheses did not explain the loss of the activity or radioactivity of pancreatic enzymes, we recently conducted a series of experiments in both in vitro and in vivo. In in vitro experiments [7] we obtained duodenal aspirates from 22 human subjects and incubated samples in a 37°C water bath for 2 h after an inhibitor of trypsin or chymotrypsin or more of one of these enzymes was added to a test sample. We found that loss of lipase activity was totally abolished by inhibiting chymotrypsin, was partly prevented by inhibiting trypsin, was slightly accelerated by adding bovine trypsin, and markedly accelerated by addition of bovine chymotrypsin. We also found that after inhibiting chymotrypsin (to maintain lipase activity), lipolytic activity did not decrease by increasing trypsin activity after adding a single or repeated doses. Conversely, lipolytic activity was markedly decreased by the addition of a single dose of chymotrypsin after inhibiting trypsin activity. We concluded that chymotrypsin is a more potent inactivator of human lipase than trypsin, and that chymotrypsin inactivates lipase in the absence of trypsin, but that trypsin inactivation of lipase requires chymotrypsin.

We extended these studies to investigate the hypothesis that proteases in the human intestinal lumen cause the loss of lipolytic activity during duodenoileal transit. We varied the level of intraluminal protease activity by perfusing chymotrypsin, trypsin, or their inhibitors into the duodenum of healthy volunteers and found that the level of intraluminal chymotrypsin, but not trypsin, correlates with the loss of lipolytic activity during aboral transit. The most significant loss of lipolytic activity occurred during duodenojejunal transit [8–10].

Additionally, in a series of preliminary in vitro experiments in which duodenal contents were incubated with various concentrations of bile acids and nutrients (in concentrations that simulate usual postprandial concentrations of these substances), we found that bile and nutrients protect against the loss of proteolytic and lipolytic activity [9, 11, 12]. The protective effect of bile occurs in the absence and presence of nutrients (protein and triglyceride) but is more pronounced in the absence of nutrients. We have also found [11] that fat (triolein) and protein (casein), but not starch, significantly increase the survival of lipolytic and proteolytic activity.

Taken together, these data suggest that the loss of enzymatic activity during aboral intestinal transit may have important physiologic and pathophysiologic implications. Loss of enzymatic activity during aboral intestinal transit may be enhanced by ingesting high-carbohydrate diets and in conditions in which intraluminal bile acid concentrations are low. In normal human subjects these conditions could lead to increased amounts of undigested nutrients entering the distal small bowel and colon, which in turn could alter proximal gastrointestinal function. For example, others have shown that fat and protein perfused into the ileocolonic segment decreases gastric emptying and inhibits pancreatic enzyme secretion. We have recently found, in addition, that carbohydrate in the ileum slows gastric emptying [13] and bile entry into the duodenum and increases the rate of amylase secretion [14–17]. In patients with malabsorption of carbohydrate these alterations of upper gastrointestinal function should increase the digestion of carbohydrate. In patients with pancreatic insufficiency, increasing carbohydrate intake at the expense of fat and protein (a diet commonly ingested by patients with pancreatic insufficiency) and the presence of decreased intraluminal concentrations of bile secondary to acid precipitation may enhance lipase inactivation and result in a poor response to orally ingested pancreatic enzymes.

References

1. Borgstrom B, Dahlqvist A, Lundh G, Sjovall J (1957) Studies of intestinal digestion and absorption in the human. J Clin Invest 36:1521–1536
2. Goldberg DM, Campbell R, Roy AD (1969) Fate of trypsin and chymotrypsin in the human small intestine. Gut 10:477–483
3. Roy AD, Campbell R, Goldberg G (1967) Effect of diet on the trypsin and chymotrypsin output in the stools of patients with an ileostomy. Gastroenterology 53:584–589
4. Layer P, Go VLW, DiMagno EP (1986) Fate of pancreatic enzymes during small intestinal aboral transit in humans. Am J Physiol 251:G475–G480
5. DiMagno EP, Malagelada J-R, Go VLW, Moertel CG (1977) Fate of orally ingested enzymes in pancreatic insufficiency: comparison of two dosage schedules. N Engl J Med 296:1318–1322
6. Regan PT, Malagelada J-R, DiMagno EP, Glanzman SL, Go VLW (1977) Comparative effects of antacids, cimetidine, and enteric coating on the therapeutic response to oral enzymes in severe pancreatic insufficiency. N Engl J Med 297:854–858
7. Thiruvengadam R, DiMagno EP (1988) Inactivation of human lipase by proteases. Am J Physiol 255:G476–G481
8. Thiruvengadam R, Zinsmeister AR, DiMagno EP (1987) Can lipase activity be preserved during aboral intestinal transit in humans? Gastroenterology 92:1669
9. Thiruvengadam R, DiMagno EP (1987) Does bile affect survival of human lipase during intestinal transit? Gastroenterology 92:1669
10. Thiruvengadam R, Zinsmeister AR, DiMagno EP (1987) Is human lipase survival during aboral intestinal transit dependent upon intraluminal chymotrypsin (CT) activity and bile acid concentrations (BAC)? Dig Dis Sci 32:1189
11. Kelly DG, Bentley KJ, Sandberg RJ, Zinsmeister AR, DiMagno EP (1988) Do nutrients and bile in human duodenal juice affect the survival of lipase activity? Possible clinical implications. Gastroenterology 94:222
12. Kelly DG, Bentley KJ, Sandberg RJ, Twomey CK, Zinsmeister AR, DiMagno EP (1989) Bile improves survival of human lipolytic activity and trypsin during aboral small intestinal transit. Gastroenterology 96:A252
13. Jain NK, Boivin M, Zinsmeister AR, Brown ML, Malagelada JR, DiMagno EP (1989) Effect of ileal perfusion of carbohydrates and amylase inhibitor on gastrointestinal hormones and emptying. Gastroenterology 96:377–387
14. Jain N, Boivin M, Zinsmeister AR, Go VLW, DiMagno EP (1986) Carbohydrate (CHO) mediated feedback regulation of postprandial pancreatic enzyme secretion in normal humans. Dig Dis Sci 31:1135
15. Tohno H, Bentley KJ, Sandberg RJ, Sarr MG, DiMagno EP (1988) Is postprandial regulation of amylase secretion (A) by carbohydrate (CHO) in the ileum a response to gastric emptying (GE) of solids or liquids? Pancreas 3:620
16. Tohno H, Bentley KJ, Sandberg RJ, Sarr MG, DiMagno EP (1989) Carbohydrate (CHO) in the ileum slows canine postprandial jejunoileal transit (the CHO brake): an effect of peptide YY (PYY)? Gastroenterology 96:513
17. Tohno H, Nelson DK, Sarr MG, DiMagno EP (1989) Does peptide YY (PYY) mediate postprandial feedback regulation of amylase secretion induced by carbohydrate (CHO) perfusion into the ileum? Gastroenterology 96:513

The Carbon and Oxygen Isotope Composition of Pancreatic Stones

J. Hoefs[1]

Introduction

Human pancreatic stones consist predominantly of calcium carbonate. In this note I report on a study of the carbon and oxygen isotope composition of pancreatic calculi from three different geographic areas (India, Italy, Federal Republic of Germany). The objectives were
a) to relate isotopic variations to geographic enrivonment,
b) to evaluate the extent to which biochemical isotopic fractionations are significant in stone formation, and
c) to compare the carbon isotopic composition of pancreatic stones with that of kidney stones.

Materials and Methods

A total of 26 pancreatic stones (2 from India, courtesy of Dr. Pitchumoni; 14 from Italy, courtesy of Dr. Bassi; and 10 from the FRG, courtesy of Dr. Büchler) were analyzed in this study. Stone material (10–15 mg) was reacted with 100% phosphoric acid, according to the method described by McCrea (1950). The liberated CO_2 is then measured in a mass spectrometer (Finnigan MAT 251). Its isotopic composition is reported in δ values, which are defined as usually:

$$\delta^{13}C \text{ in } \permil = \frac{{}^{13}C/{}^{12}C(\text{sample}) - {}^{13}C/{}^{12}C(\text{standard})}{{}^{13}C/{}^{12}C(\text{standard})} \times 1000$$

$$\delta^{18}O \text{ in } \permil = \frac{{}^{18}O/{}^{16}O(\text{sample}) - {}^{18}O/{}^{16}O(\text{standard})}{{}^{18}O/{}^{16}O(\text{standard})} \times 1000$$

δ values are given relative to the international PDB standard. The total error of measurement is $\pm$ 0.2‰.

---

[1] Geochemisches Institut der Universität, Goldschmidtstrasse 1, 3400 Göttingen, FRG

Chronic Pancreatitis
Ed. by Beger, Büchler, Ditschuneit, and Malfertheiner
© Springer-Verlag Berlin Heidelberg 1990

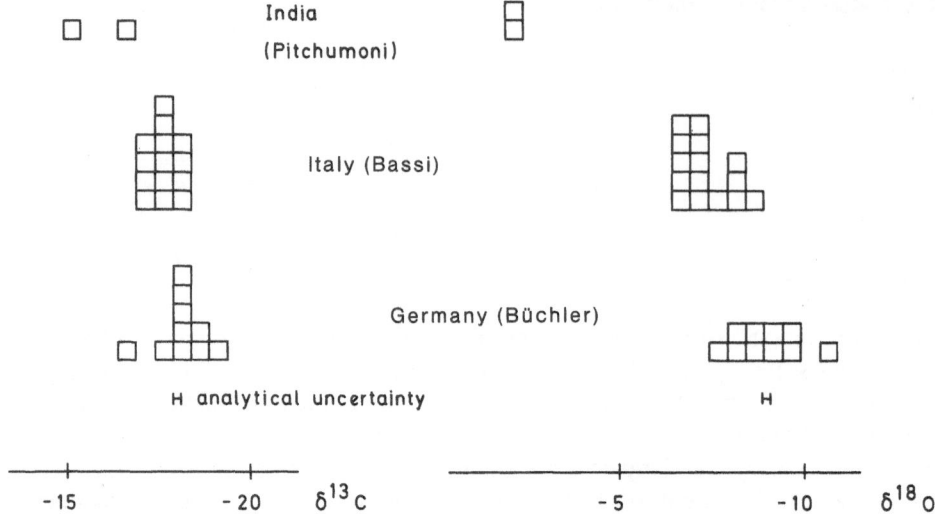

Fig. 1. $\delta^{13}C$ and $\delta^{18}O$ variations of pancreatic stones from India, Italy, and the FRG

Results

Figure 1 presents a histogram of the $\delta^{13}C$ and $\delta^{18}O$ values of the measured pancreatic stones. With respect to carbon, the majority of stones have $\delta^{13}C$ values between $-17‰$ and $-18‰$. There are, however, slight differences between the three different areas, with the two stones from India being the most ^{13}C enriched. $\delta^{18}O$ variations are larger than those for carbon. Especially noteworthy are the distinct ^{18}O enrichments of the two stones from India relative to the European ones. Calculi from Italy are on average slightly heavier than those from Germany.

Discussion

^{18}O Variations

Longinelli (1984) demonstrated that the oxygen isotope composition of water in blood and in the whole body depends on the isotopic composition of the ingested water. Due to a fast isotope equilibration between H_2O and CO_2 and its predominance over CO_2, the isotope composition of water determines that of carbon dioxide and respective carbonates. Therefore, pancreatic stones from a tropical country like India must be more enriched in ^{18}O than stones from Europe, and it is also understandable why the stones from Italy are on average more ^{18}O enriched than stones from Germany.

^{13}C Variations

The main question is whether the carbon isotope composition depends solely on exogenic sources (nutrition), or whether endogenic processes (within body biochemi-

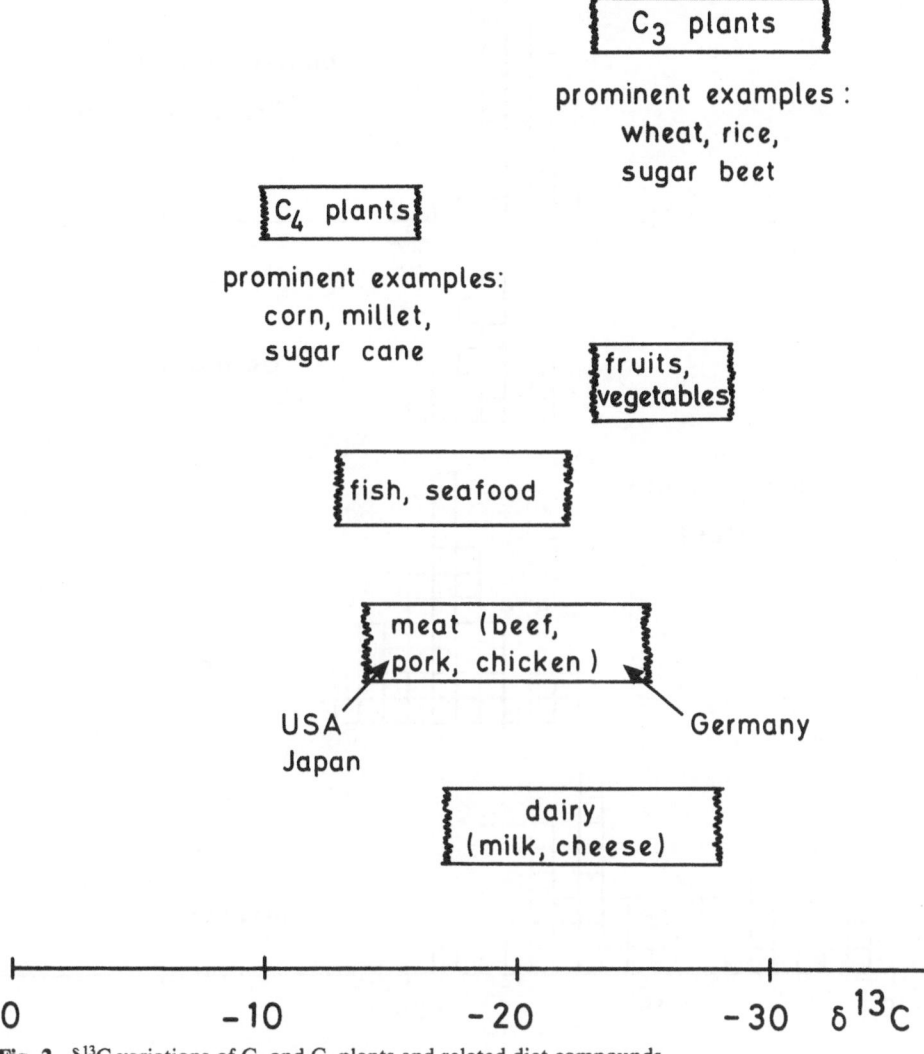

Fig. 2. $\delta^{13}C$ variations of C_3 and C_4 plants and related diet compounds

cal fractionations) also play a role. I begin with a discussion of $\delta^{13}C$ variations of some important natural diet compounds (Fig. 2).

The bulk of the plant kingdom fixes CO_2 during the so-called C_3 pathway with characteristic $\delta^{13}C$ values between $-22\permil$ and $-30\permil$. Most basic food stuffs, except corn, sugar cane, and millet, belong to this category. In contrast to C_3 plants the C_4 pathway discriminates ^{12}C to a much smaller extent, with $\delta^{13}C$ values between $-10\permil$ and $-15\permil$. Thus, C_4 and C_3 plants do not overlap in their carbon isotope ratios and represent an ideal tracer for deciphering different diet compounds in animals and humans (De Niro and Epstein, 1978; Minson et al., 1975; Nakamura et al. 1982 and others). De Niro and Epstein (1978) have convincingly demonstrated that the whole body of an animal reflects the carbon isotope composition of its diet, but the animal is

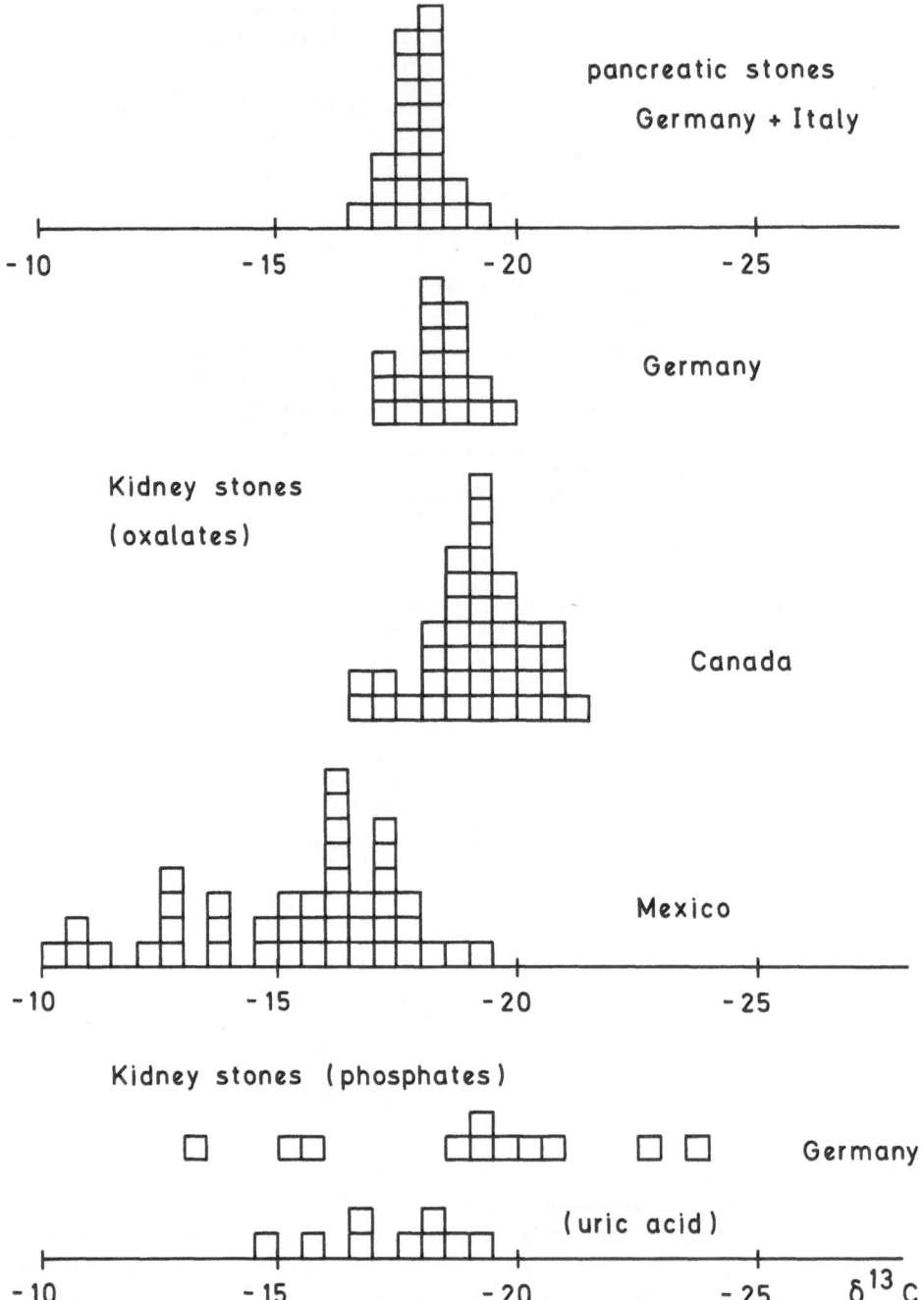

Fig. 3. $\delta^{13}C$ variations of kidney stones from different areas in comparison with pancreatic stones. (Data source on kidney stones [3, 4])

on average enriched in ^{13}C by about 1‰ relative to the diet. This ^{13}C enrichment of the body is balanced by a ^{13}C depletion of the respired CO_2. The same relationship is also found in humans (Nakamura et al. 1982 and other).

In summary, it can be stated that "we are what we eat (plus a few ‰)" (De Niro and Epstein, 1976). Besides this straight-forward correlation, within-body biochemical fractionations also occur. De Niro and Epstein (1978) demonstrated that $\delta^{13}C$ values of whole bodies of individuals of a species raised on the same diet may differ by up to 2‰. Lyon and Baxter (1978) have analyzed different human tissues from one individual, which may vary by more than 4‰ (Table 1). Even larger variations are observed when blood is analyzed.

Table 1. $\delta^{13}C$ values of human tissues and other materials from a single individual (from [6])

Thymus	−25.59
Pancreas	−25.25
Kidney	−24.00
Muscle	−23.56
Heart	−22.79
Liver	−22.72
Lung	−22.38
Brain	−21.05
Blood	−18.22
Bone carbonate	−13.50

I now turn to the carbon isotope composition of pancreatic stones, concentrating on the stones from Europe because little is known about the two Indian patients and their diets. Pancreatic stones from Europe are richer in ^{13}C than average European food and show a close similarity with the isotopic composition of blood. Nevertheless, diet may play a major role in determining the isotopic composition. This can be postulated by comparing kidney stones with pancreatic stones. Figure 3, summarizing data in the literature on kidney stones, demonstrates that oxalate stones from Germany have about the same composition as pancreatic stones. Oxalate stones from Mexico, however, differ from those of Germany, which can be interpreted as indicating a higher proportion of C_3 plants (corn). Such a dependence upon geographical location is an argument for the influence of diet. Specific diet compounds cannot, however, be linked to the formation of stones.

Acknowledgements. This study would not have been possible without the generous help of Drs. Bassi (Verona), Büchler (Ulm), and Pitchumoni (New York), who donated the pancreatic stones. To all three of them I owe my deepest thanks.

References

1. De Niro MJ, Epstein S (1976) You are what you eat (plus a few ‰): the carbon isotope cycle in food chains. Geol Soc Am Abstr Progr 8:834–835

2. De Niro MJ, Epstein S (1978) Influence of diet on the distribution of carbon isotopes in animals. Geochim Cosmochim Acta 42:495–506
3. Hoefs J, Armbruster T (1978) $^{13}C/^{12}C$-Verhältnisse in menschlichen Harnkonkrementen. Naturwissenschaften 65:586–589
4. Krouse HR, Levinson AA (1984) Geographical trends of carbon and sulphur isotope abundances in human kidney stones. Geochim Cosmochim Acta 48:187–191
5. Longinelli A (1984) Oxygen isotopes in mammal bone phosphate: a new tool for paleohydrological and paleoclimatological research. Geochim Cosmochim Acta 48:385–390
6. Lyon TD, Baxter MSC (1978) Stable carbon isotopes in human tissues. Nature 273:750–751
7. McCrea JM (1950) The isotopic chemistry of carbonates and a paleotemperature scale. J Chem Phys 18:849–857
8. Minson DJ, Ludlow MM, Throughton JH (1975) Differences in natural carbon isotope ratios of milk and hair from cattle grazing tropical and temperature pastures. Nature 256:602
9. Nakamura K, Schoeller DA, Winkler FJ, Schmidt HL (1982) Geographical variations in the carbon isotope composition of the diet and hair in contemporary men. Biomed Mass Spectrometry 9:390–394

A Fresh Look at Autoantibodies in Chronic Pancreatitis

W. A. Scherbaum[1], A. Fetzer[1], H. Friess[2], P. Malfertheiner[3], and M. Büchler[2]

Introduction

Several lines of evidence suggest that autoimmune phenomena may underlie a sub-group of cases with chronic pancreatitis (CP). In particular, autoantibodies (AB) to pancreatic acinar cells and ductal antigens have been described [7, 8, 11, 20], and lymphocytes specifically sensitized to crude pancreatic antigens have been detected in patients with CP [15, 21]. Lymphocytic infiltrates with activated cells can be detected in the exocrine pancreas, and besides hyperexpression of HLA class I molecules, aberrant expression of HLA-DR molecules on exocrine pancreatic cells has been described in CP [3, 6].

Thus far, only small numbers of patients with CP have been tested for pancreas-specific AB. In the most important previous studies, those in which adequate controls were used, Lendrum and Walker (1975) described 14 patients, Rumessen and coworkers (1985) reported on 23, and Lankisch and coworkers (1981) on 62 patients with this disease. These authors were unable to find an increase in circulating AB as compared to controls. However, only in one of the above studies [7], was an attempt made to subdivide the cases according to the origin of the disease. Complement-fixing AB to the exocrine pancreas, which may be relevant to the pathogenesis of CP, have been investigated in only one of the previous reports [8], and there are only limited data on the presence of AB to the endocrine pancreas and their correlation to diabetes mellitus in patients with CP [11, 16, 22].

The present study addressed the above questions on the basis of AB testing in a large series of well-defined patients with CP of known or undefinable origin.

Patients and Methods

The sera from 103 patients with an unequivocal diagnosis of CP were tested (median age 50.6 years; range 23–81 years; male/female ratio 3.7 : 1). Patients were selected on the basis of at least two methods among the following:
a) computed tomography,
b) endoscopic retrograde pancreatography (ERCP)

[1] Department of General Medicine I, University of Ulm, Robert-Koch-Strasse 8, 7900 Ulm, FRG
[2] Department of Surgery, University of Ulm, Steinhövelstrasse 9, 7900 Ulm, FRG
[3] Department of General Medicine II, University of Ulm, Robert-Koch-Strasse 8, 7900 Ulm, FRG

Chronic Pancreatitis
Ed. by Beger, Büchler, Ditschuneit, and Malfertheiner
© Springer-Verlag Berlin Heidelberg 1990

c) pancreolauryl test, and

d) laparotomy.

The origin of CP was secondary to chronic alcohol consumption in 59, biliary tract disease in 14, and other known causes in 15 cases. In 15 patients idiopathic CP was diagnosed. Thirty of the patients with CP had diabetes mellitus secondary to pancreatic disease, and one had type 1 diabetes.

Controls included 40 patients in whom CP had been suspected on the basis of signs and symptoms as well as elevated serum amylase and/or lipase levels, but in whom the diagnosis was then rejected on the basis of missing further criteria (median age 50.8 years; range 21–77 years; male/female ratio 1.7:1). Two of these had type 1, and four had type 2 diabetes. Furthermore, 21 patients with a carcinoma of the pancreas (median age 59.5 years; range 29–95 years; male/female ratio 1.6:1) and 50 mixed hospital controls without gastrointestinal or known autoimmune disease were investigated (median age 48.3 years; range 22–84 years; male/female ratio 1.1:1). No patient in the latter two groups had diabetes.

For the detection of the following AB the standard indirect immunofluorescence (IFL) test was employed on unfixed 4-μm cryostat sections of the respective fresh human tissues: AB to acinar cells of the exocrine pancreas (acinar AB), AB to cytoplasmic components of pancreatic ducts, AB to ductal connective tissue, AB to gastric parietal cells (PCA), AB to single endocrine cells of the pancreas (somatostatin cell AB, glucagon cell AB), and islet cell AB (ICA). For antinuclear antibody (ANA), smooth-muscle AB (SMA), and anti-mitochondrial (mito-AB) antibody testing, rat liver kidney and stomach were used. Undiluted sera were applied to test for antibodies to the endocrine pancreas, and ¹⁄₁₀ dilutions in PBS were taken to screen for mito-AB, PCA, ANA, SMA, and antibodies to the exocrine pancreas. PCA and mito-AB were judged as positive only when they also reacted at retesting on human stomach. Positive sera were titrated to end point. ICA results were evaluated using the standard serum of the Juvenile Diabetes Foundation and expressed in JDF units. The test quality in our assay has been judged 100% for all, validity, consistency, sensitivity, and specificity (International Diabetes Workshop ICA Proficiency Program, Lab ID Number 116). For the differentiation of AB to the exocrine pancreas and ANA, the immunoglobulin (Ig) class was determined by the use of specific anti-human IgG, IgA, and IgM antibodies as a conjugate. The complement-fixing ability of antibodies was detected by IFL testing using normal human sera as a source of complement, and an anti-human C3 conjugate [14]. Thyroid microsomal and thyroglobulin antibodies were determined using a commercial ELISA test kit (ELIAS, Freiburg, FRG).

Results

The overall results of organ-specific and non-organ-specific AB in patients with CP are given in Table 1. ANA were rarely of high titer; six patients with CP but none of the other patients had an ANA titer equal to or above ¹⁄₈₀. Other non-organ-specific AB did not differ in the four groups of patients tested.

Table 1. Prevalence of organ-specific and non-organ-specific autoantibodies in patients with chronic pancreatitis and controls

Antibodies to	Chronic pancreatitis ($n = 103$)	Chronic pancreatitis rejected ($n = 40$)	Carcinoma of pancreas ($n = 21$)	Mixed controls ($n = 50$)
Acinar cells				
⅟₁₀	46 (44.7%)	17 (42.5%)	2 (9.5%)	0
⅟₂₀	7 (6.8%)	1 (2.5%)	0	0
⅟₄₀	1 (1%)	0	0	0
Ductal, cytoplasmatic	1 (1%)	0	1 (4.8%)	0
Ductal, connective, tissue	25 (24.3%)	9 (22.5%)	7 (33.3%)	9 (18%)
Islet cells	10 (9.7%)	2 (5%)	0	0
Somatostatin cells	4 (3.9%)	0	0	0
Glucagon cells	0	0	0	0
Thyroglobulin	14 (13.6%)	3 (7.5%)	*nt*	*nt*
Thyroid microsomes	1 (1%)	2 (5%)	*nt*	*nt*
Parietal cells	0	0	0	0
Nuclear antigens	12 (11.7%)	8 (20%)	1 (4.8%)	1 (2%)
Smooth muscle	2 (2%)	2 (5%)	1 (4.8%)	0
Mitochondria	3 (2.9%)	0	1 (4.8%)	1 (2%)

nt, Not tested; the prevalence of thyroglobulin and thyroid microsomal antibodies in another group of 200 normal controls of similar age was 7.5% and 4%, respectively

Autoantibodies to the Exocrine Pancreas. The staining of acinar cell antibodies was cytoplasmatic and coarsely granular, except for a portion of exocrine cells. This pattern was enhanced by the complement fixation test (Fig. 1). The prevalence of antibodies to pancreatic acinar cells was not significantly different in patients with CP and the control groups. However, titers of ⅟₂₀ and above were significantly increased in CP patients as compared to controls. Titers above ⅟₄₀ were not observed. A homogenous cytoplasmic staining of pancreatic duct epithelium was seen in only one patient with CP (Fig. 2) and one with a carcinoma of the pancreas, but the ductal connective tissue pattern was quite common in all groups tested.

Subclass Distribution and Complement-Fixing Ability of Acinar Cell Antibodies. The determination of the immunoglobulin subclasses of acinar cell antibodies did not allow serological discrimination between patients with CP and the other patients. The prevalence of complement-fixing acinar cell antibodies was similar in the various groups of CP patients tested (Table 2).

Correlation of Antibodies with the Origin of CP. The results of AB to acinar cells, ICA, and ANA were correlated with the different groups of CP patients according to their etiology (Table 3). None of these groups exhibited an increased prevalence of one of these antibodies.

Islet Cell Antibodies in Chronic Pancreatitis. ICA were detected in 10 of the 103 patients with CP, in 2 (5%) of the 40 patients in whom the diagnosis was later rejected,

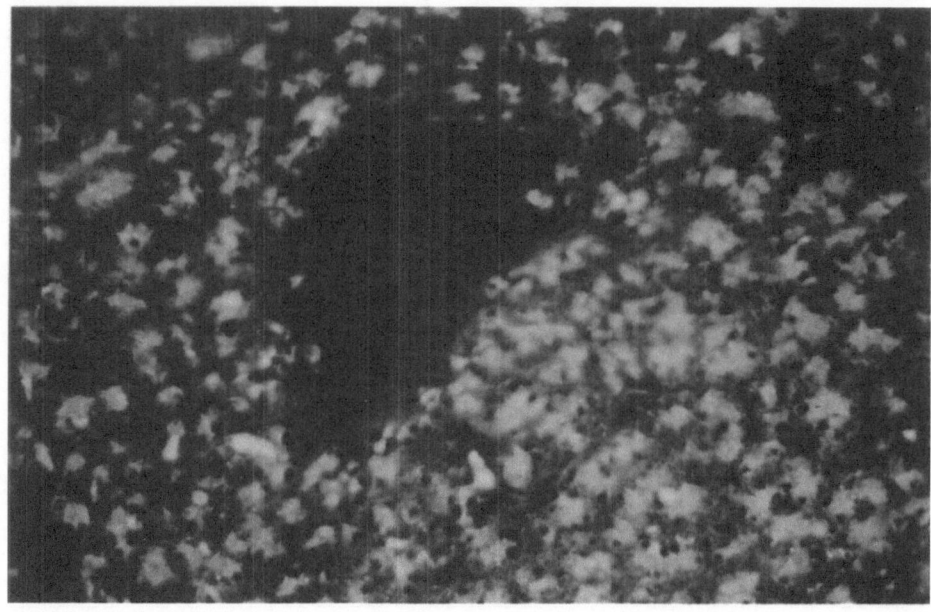

a

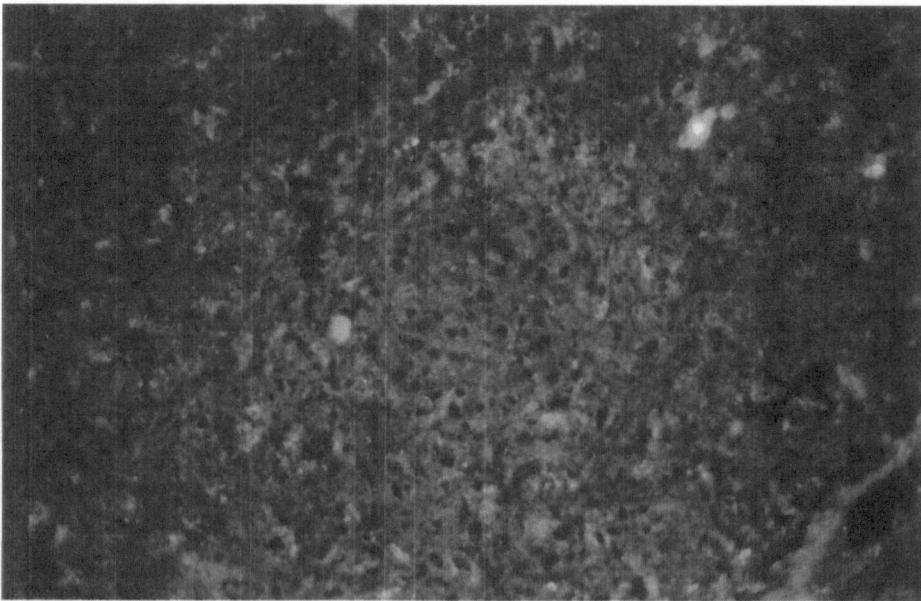

b

Fig. 1a,b. a Autoantibodies to acinus cells of the pancreas, detected in the serum of a patient with chronic pancreatitis. The serum was applied at dilution ½₀. Indirect immunofluorescence test with complement fixation on a cryostat section of human pancreas from a donor with blood group 0. A coarse granular cytoplasmatis staining is seen on most, but not all the acinus cells. **b** Normal human serum aplied to the same procedure as in **a.** (× 100)

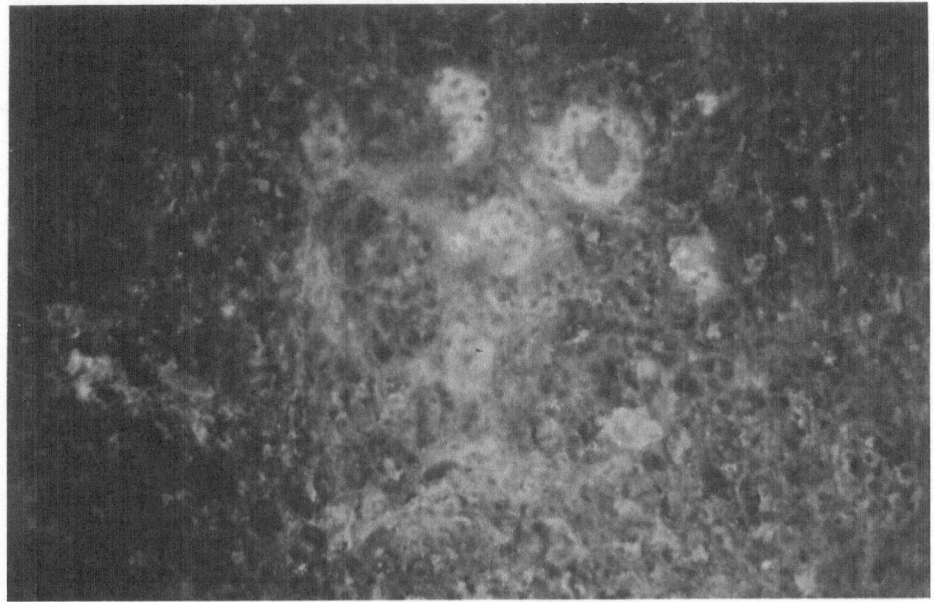

Fig. 2. Diffuse cytoplasmic staining of ductal epithelial cells of the exocrine pancreas. This antibody is rare in chronic pancreatitis ($\times$ 100)

Table 2. Immunoglobulin subclass distribution and complement-fixing ability of autoantibodies to pancreatic acinus cells in chronic pancreatitis and controls

Ig subclass of acinus cell AB	Chronic pancreatitis	Chronic pancreatitis rejected	Carcinoma of pancreas	Mixed controls
IgG positive	15 (14.3%)	3 (7.5%)	1 (4.8%)	0
IgM positive	28 (27.2%)	10 (25%)	0	0
IgA positive	37 (35.9%)	12 (30%)	1 (4.8%)	0
Total IgG and/or IgM and/or IgA	53 (51.4%)	19 (47.5%)	2 (9.5%)	0
Complement-fixation positive	41 (39.8%)	15 (37.5%)	5 (2.4%)	0

and in none of the other controls. The titers were low throughout: in the 10 cases they were at 20, and in the 2 instances at 42 JDF units. None of these ICA fixed complement. It is also important to note that all the CP patients with diabetes mellitus were ICA negative.

Discussion

Although most of the cases of CP in central Europe are due to chronic alcohol consumption and some to less frequent causes, there exist forms with unknown origin.

Table 3. Presence of acinus cell antibodies, islet cell antibodies, and antinuclear antibodies in chronic pancreatitis subdivided according to etiology

Antibodies to	Alcoholic ($n = 59$)	Biliary ($n = 14$)	Others ($n = 15$)	Idiopathic ($n = 15$)	Total ($n = 103$)
Acinus cells					
IgG	7 (11.9%)	2 (14.3%)	3 (20%)	1 (6.7%)	13 (12.6%)
IgM	21 (35.6%)	1 (7.1%)	2 (13.3%)	2 (13.3%)	26 (25.2%)
IgA	23 (39%)	8 (57.1%)	2 (13.3%)	5 (33.3%)	38 (36.9%)
Total	32 (54.2%)	9 (64.3%)	6 (40%)	5 (33.3%)	52 (50.5%)
CF	21 (35.6%)	7 (50%)	4 (26.7%)	5 (33.3%)	37 (35.9%)
Islet cells					
(ICA)	6 (10.2%)	1 (7.2%)	0	3 (20%)	10 (9.7%)
CF-ICA	0	0	0	0	0
Nuclear antigens					
ANA-IgG	3 (5.1%)	2 (14.3%)	0	1 (6.7%)	6 (5.8%)
ANA-IgM	2 (3.4%)	2 (14.3%)	0	2 (13.3%)	6 (5.8%)
ANA-IgA	0	0	0	0	0
Total	5 (8.5%)	4 (28.6%)	0	3 (20%)	12 (11.7%)

CF, Complement-fixing

In our cohort of patients from a specialized center for gastroenterology and pancreas surgery, 15 (14.5%) of the cases were classified as idiopathic. In analogy with other organ-specific chronic inflammatory diseases such as idiopathic Addison's disease [12] or idiopathic diabetes insipidus [13], we reassessed the possibility that AB may also play a role in the determination of the etiology of CP.

Using a selected human pancreas from a donor with blood group 0, AB to pancreatic acinus cells were detected in the sera from 44.7% of patients with CP, but also in 34% of patients in whom the initial symptoms suggested CP, but in whom the diagnosis was rejected on the basis of further investigations. These figures are much higher than those reported by Lendrum and Walker (1975), who found none out of 14 cases, or Rumessen and coworkers (1985), who found them in 4% of CP patients and 5% of controls. However, when only titers of ½₀ were considered in our assay, the results were comparable to those of other investigators. Mixed hospital controls were constantly negative for acinus cell antibodies.

No international standardization or exchange program exists thus far to compare the results of antibodies to the exocrine pancreas. It may well be that previous investigators felt uneasy about interpreting this staining as antibody-mediated. However, a multitude of antigens are present on exocrine pancreatic cells, and we now know that low levels of antibodies to naturally occurring antigens can also be detected in healthy individuals [9, 10, 18]. Therefore, with each source of antigen or individual organ, the antibody threshold must be considered and compared between patients and controls. Except for pancreatic acinus cell antibodies, none of the antibodies tested here was significantly increased in CP patients as compared to normal controls.

The complement fixation enhances the brightness of immunofluorescence, which allowed us to depict the general pattern observed in the sera of CP patients and controls. The demonstration of the complement-fixing ability of antibodies has been shown to correlate with the disease status in Addison's disease [12] and in type 1 diabetes [19]. However, in our series of patients there was no increase in complement-fixing acinus cell antibodies in CP patients as compared to the disease control group. Neither complement fixation testing of acinus cell antibodies nor the determination of immunoglobulin subclasses allowed subdivision of patients with CP. In particular, patients with idiopathic forms of the disease did not behave differently in this regard.

Islet cell antibodies are considered as a hallmark of type 1 (insulin-dependent) diabetes mellitus, which is known to have an autoimmune origin [2]. The incidence of diabetes in CP is reported to be around 10% [16, 22], which is many times the incidence in a normal population. Our data are in accordance with the above-mentioned reports. In cystic fibrosis ICA were even detected in 39% of the cases [17]. One explanation may be that CP leads to progressive fibrosis of the pancreas [1], including changes in the pancreatic nerve fibers [4] and a possible disruption of islet cells. However, no strict correlation can be found between the severity and duration of CP and the occurrence of diabetes, suggesting that other etiological factors may contribute to the development of diabetes in CP. One may speculate that infiltrating macrophages and other mononuclear cells present islet cell antigens to the immune system and finally induce ICA formation. In our study, only one out of 31 patients with CP who had diabetes was positive for ICA, and the ICA in nondiabetics with CP were of low titer, and they failed to fix complement. In a limited study on 19 patients with CP, Colman and coworkers (1987) found that in contrast to type 1 diabetes, ICA were absent in patients with diabetes secondary to CP, and that HLA-DR types were similar to control subjects and patients with CP without diabetes. These data suggest that diabetes secondary to CP is unrelated to autoimmunity.

In conclusion, our findings regarding AB in CP do not support the notion that this disease or its idiopathic subgroup is due to an autoimmune reaction directed to pancreatic tissue. However, the possibility still exists that antibodies to soluble antigens may play a role, which cannot be excluded on the basis of the methods used thus far.

References

1. Becker V, Stolte M (1976) Klinische Pathologie des Pankreas. Med Welt 27:901
2. Bottazzo GF, Pujol-Borrell R, Gale EAM (1986) Autoimmunity in diabetes: progress, consolidation and controversy. In: Alberti KGMM, Krall LP (eds) The diabetes annual/2. Elsevier, Amsterdam, pp 13–29
3. Bovo P, Mirakian R, Merigo F, Angelini G, Cavallini G, Rizzini P, Bottazzo GF, Scura LA (1987) HLA molecule expression on chronic pancreatitis specimens: is there a role for auto-immunity? A preliminary study. Pancreas 2:350–356
4. Büchler M, Bockman D, Bittner R, Beger HG (1988) Ultrastruktur der Nerven im menschlichen Pankreas: morphologische Belege zur Schmerzpathogenese bei chronischer Pankreatitis. Lang Arch Chir (Chirurgisches Forum) 187–192
5. Colman PG, Roberts-Thomson JC, Begley CG, Harrison LC, Tait BD (1987) Evidence against an immunogenetic basis for diabetes in chronic pancreatitis. Aust NZ J Med 17:392–395
6. Foulis AK, Farquharson MA, Hardman R (1987) Aberrant expression of class I major histocompatibility complex molecules by B cells and hyperexpression of class II major histocompatibility complex molecules by insulin containing islets in type 1 (insulin-dependent) diabetes mellitus. Diabetologia 30:333–343

7. Lankisch PG, Koop H, Seelig R, Seelig HP (1981) Antinuclear and pancreatic acinar cell antibodies in pancreatic diseases. Digestion 21:65–68
8. Lendrum R, Walker G (1975) Serum antibodies in human pancreatic disease. Gut 16:365–371
9. Logtenberg T, Melissen PMB, Kroon A, Gmelig-Meyling FHJ, Ballieux RE (1988) Autoreactive B cells in normal humans. Autoantibody production upon lymphocyte stimulation with autoantigen-xenoantigen conjugates. J Immunol 140:446–450
10. Richter W, Eiermann TH, Graf G, Glück M, Scherbaum WA, Pfeiffer EF (1989) Isolation of IgG islet cell antibody-producing B lymphocytes from the peripheral blood of type 1 diabetic patients and an ICA-positive non-diabetic individual. Horm Metab Res 21:686–688
11. Rumessen JJ, Marner B, Thorsgaard Pedersen N, Permin H (1985) Autoantibodies in chronic pancreatitis. Scand J Gastroenterol 20:966–970
12. Scherbaum WA, Berg PA (1982) Development of adrenocortical failure in non-addisonian patients with antibodies to adrenal cortex. A clinical follow-up study. Clin Endocrinol 16:345–352
13. Scherbaum WA, Bottazzo GF (1983) Autoantibodies to vasopressin cells in idiopathic diabetes insipidus. Evidence for an autoimmune variant. Lancet 1:897–901
14. Scherbaum WA, Mirakian R, Pujol-Borrell R, Dean BM, Bottazzo GF (1986) Immunochemistry in the study and diagnosis of organ-specific autoimmune diseases. In: Polak JM, Van Noorden S (eds) Immunocytochemistry. Modern methods and applications. Wright, Bristol, pp 456–476
15. Schütt C, Friemel H, Schulze HA, Zubaidi G (1975) Specific lymphocyte sensitization in chronic pancreatitis. Digestion 13:308–311
16. Scuro LA, Bovo P, Sandrini T, Angelini G, Cavallini G, Mirakian R (1983) Autoimmunity and diabetes associated with chronic pancreatitis. Lancet 1:424 (Letter)
17. Stutchfield PR, O'Halloran SM, Smith CS, Woodrow JC, Bottazzo GF, Heaf D (1988) HLA type, islet cell antibodies, and glucose intolerance in cystic fibrosis. Arch Dis Child 63:1234–1239
18. Tao T-W, Leu S-L, Kriss JP (1985) Peripheral blood lymphocytes from normal individuals can be induced to secrete immunoglobulin G antibodies against self-antigen thyroglobulin in vitro. J Clin Endocrinol Metab 60:279–282
19. Tarn AC, Thomas JM, Dean BM, Ingram D, Schwarz G, Bottazzo GF, Gale EAM (1988) Predicting insulin-dependent diabetes. Lancet 1:845–850
20. Thal AP, Murray MJ, Egner W (1959) Isoantibody formation in chronic pancreatic disease. Lancet 1:1128–1129
21. Velbri S, Nutt H (1973) Über die Rolle immunologischer Mechanismen bei Pankreaserkrankungen. Z Inn Med 28:222–227
22. Vialettes B, Lassmann V, Vague P (1983) Autoimmunity, diabetes, and chronic pancreatitis. Lancet 1:879 (Letter)

Feedback Regulation of Exocrine Function

Gastrointestinal Hormones in Chronic Pancreatitis

V. L. W. Go[1]

Introduction

The human pancreas consists of both exocrine and endocrine components, is responsible for the proper digestion of specific food nutrients, and regulates the metabolism of absorbed nutrients. The exocrine and endocrine pancreas are linked not only anatomically and embryologically but also vascularly and functionally. The gastrointestinal hormones regulate the secretion and synthesis of all digestive enzymes in the pancreatic acini (enteroacinar axis) and the secretions of pancreatic islet hormone, particularly insulin (enteroinsular axis). Recently, many islet vascular studies in experimental animals have provided evidence of a coexisting parallel and serial (insuloacinar) angioarchitecture [38]. This arrangement of the islet capillary blood flow to the periinsular acinar plexus has led to the proposal that exocrine pancreatic function is partly regulated by the endocrine islets and their hormones [16]. This functional relationship, enteroacinar axis, enteroinsular axis, and insuloacinar axis are all affected in chronic pancreatitis and can lead to pancreatic exocrine and endocrine defficiency.

My current presentation will focus on our laboratory work on the normal and abnormal states of the enteropancreatic axis, to set the stage for other contributors who will be discussing topics including: the enteroacinar feedback mechanism in the control of exocrine pancreatic function; the role of intestinal protease inhibitor and CCK receptor antagonists on pancreatic feedback regulation; and the abnormal pancreatic endocrine function (enteroinsular axis) in patients with chronic pancreatitis. The use of gastrointestinal hormones as diagnostic and therapeutic agents for pancreatic diseases will be covered by other authors of this volume.

Distribution of Gastrointestinal Hormones and Regulatory Peptides

The gastrointestinal tract, believed to have the largest mass of endocrine cells in the human body, releases a variety of hormones each of which is predominantly found at one location. Gastrin is primarily a gastric hormone. Cholecystokinin (CCK), secretin, gastric inhibitory polypeptide (GIP), and motilin are found mainly in the upper small intestine. Neurotensin and enteroglucagon (GLI) are lower small bowel hor-

[1] Department of Medicine, University of California, Los Angeles, Center for the Health Sciences, 10833 Le Conte Avenue, Los Angeles, CA 90024-1736, USA

Chronic Pancreatitis
Ed. by Beger, Büchler, Ditschuneit, and Malfertheiner
© Springer-Verlag Berlin Heidelberg 1990

mones, and peptide YY (PYY) is a colon hormone. Each endocrine cell secretes a specific peptide hormone which is scattered throughout the gut mucosa and dispersed among the epithelial absorptial cells. The intrastructure of gastrointestinal endocrine cells somewhat resembles that of other endocrine cells – the base of each cell contains secretory granules with hormone peptides that discharge into the adjacent capillaries – but they are different than other endocrine cells in that the apical portion of each cell contains microvilli in contact with gastrointestinal lumen. The gut endocrine cell has been suggested by Fujita [10] as part of a sensory system that senses the content of the lumen and releases the hormone that regulates gastrointestinal function, including the endocrine pancreas. Many of the gut hormones possess an incretin effect, influencing the secretion of insulin, glucagon, and human pancreatic polypeptide (HHP), which are present in the pancreatic islets [12, 22], and are now considered as components of the gastrointestinal endocrine system. In addition, nonhormonal regulatory peptides are found in the neurons, ganglia, and nerve fibers of the gut intrinsic plexus. These include vasoactive intestinal polypeptide (VIP), substance P, bombesin-like peptide, somatostatin, the enkephalins, peptide histidine-isoleucine (PHI), calcitonin gene-related peptide, galanin, and neuropeptide Y. These neuropeptides also have regional distributions similar to the gut hormone and can influence the release of gut hormones in each region. Their physiological role in the enteropancreatic axis, and their abnormality in pancreatic disease, remains to be investigated in humans.

The embryological origin of the gut neuroendocrine system, derived from the ectoderm and neural crest, is similar to that of the cerebral cortex, hypothalamus, pituitary, and sympathetic nervous system. Gut regulatory peptides and hormones, with the exception of secretin, GIP, and GLI, are also found in nervous tissue. Regional differences in distribution of these substances have been demonstrated in the gut, spinal cord, and brain [12, 4o]. These regulatory peptides influence the release of gut hormones and can also directly affect the functions of both exocrine and endocrine pancreas. In addition, gut hormones and regulatory peptides, along with the intrinsic and extrinsic nervous system, regulate digestive, absorptive, motor, secretory and immune function, and growth and adaptation of the gastrointestinal tract [11, 13].

Specificity and Potency of Intraluminal Nutrients on the Release of Gastrointestinal Hormones

The substances in the gastrointestinal lumen provide the most important stimuli for release of gastrointestinal hormones. Release of these hormones is stimulated by products of protein, fat, and carbohydrate digestion, by adjacent nerves, and by other hormones and ions in the circulation. Each nutrient has a different specificity for each peptide hormone as well as a different potency to stimulate its release. Similarly, each hormone released by the different nutrients has different actions, either stimulatory or inhibitory, on pancreatic acinar and duct cells (Table 1).

Peptides and amino acids have a potent effect on release of proximal gut hormones, particularly gastrin, CCK, and GIP, and a lesser effect on release of HPP and other distal gut hormones such as neurotensin, GLI, and PYY. In contrast, fat hydrolysates are potent releasers of distal gut hormones, as are CCK and GIP, while products of

Table 1. Release of gut hormones: specificity and potency of intraluminal nutrients and their action on the exocrine pancreas

Hormone	Stimuli			Exocrine pancreas	
	Proteine	Carbohydrate	Fat	Acinar cell	Duct cell
Gastrin	++++			++	+
CCK	+++		++++	+++++	+
Secretin			+	+	+++++
GIP	+++	++++	++	+	+
Motilin			++	+	+
HPP	+++	+	++	–	–
GLI		+	++++	–	–
Neurotensin	+	+	++++	+	+
PYY			++++	–	–

(+), stimulatory; (–), inhibitory

carbohydrate digestion are important in stimulating GIP release, and its insulino-trophic effect, with minimal effect on the release of other gastrointestinal hormones. The specificity and potency of each of these nutrients on the release of particular hormones has been reviewed in detail [5, 37]. I will focus only on some unique characteristics of each hormone, released after a meal, that might be relevant in pancreatic disease.

Gastrin

The release of gastrin to the circulation is gastric pH dependent. A gastric luminal pH below 3 inhibited gastrin release in the presence of amino acids or protein; the magnitude and duration of gastrin release were increased by maintaining the pH above 3. This feedback inhibition modulated the amount of gastrin normally released after a meal [37]. The amino acids phenylalanine and tryptophan stimulated gastrin release when perfused intraluminally but had no effect on gastrin release when administered intravenously [33].

Cholecystokinin

Cholecystokinin (CCK) stimulates pancreatic enzyme secretion and gallbladder con-traction, both of which require intraluminal protein digestion. In bioassays using intestinal perfusion systems on human subjects, phenylalanine and tryptophan had a potent effect on CCK release when perfused intraduodenally [14]. We have also investigated the effects of intraduodenal glycerol perfusion, fatty acid chain length, and fatty acid load on pancreatic gallbladder function, which are thought to be related to CCK release [27]. Although glycerol had no effect, pancreatic and gallbladder responses were augmented by increasing fatty acid chain length and fatty acid load until the maximum capacity for pancreatic secretion and gallbladder emptying were attained. These results have now been confirmed by using various radioimmunoassays of cholecystokinin [5, 37].

Recently, cholecystokinin has been found to mediate the feedback regulation of pancreatic enzyme secretion [25]. The intestinal feedback regulation of the pancreas was first theorized by Green and Lyman [15], suggesting that intraluminal trypsin can regulate pancreatic enzyme secretion. The removal of trypsin from the intestine is hypothesized to increase enzyme secretion, in part due to increased CCK release. This trypsin-sensitive CCK-releasing peptide has now been isolated [17], and this theory formed the basis for the use of trypsin inhibitors or CCK antagonists in the management of pancreatitis.

Gastric Inhibitory Polypeptide

Glucose is a potent stimulator of gastric inhibitory polypeptide (GIP) release. Studies in humans have shown that a perfusion of glucose into the upper gut increased GIP release [28], whereas inhibition of carbohydrate digestion by purified amylase inhibitor or by acarbose, a mucosal disaccharidase inhibitor, diminished GIP release [4, 7]. Glucose does not stimulate the release of gastrin, CCK, or secretin and only weakly stimulates release of the distal gut hormones GLI, neurotensin, and PYY. GIP is the leading candidate as the gut hormone responsible for augmenting insulin release. This insulinotrophic effect, which occurs only after plasma glucose reaches 17–20 mg/dl, is linearly related to plasma glucose levels [28]. The autonomic nervous system does not seem to directly affect glucose-stimulated GIP secretion in humans [30].

A mixed amino acid solution stimulated GIP release in humans when perfused intraduodenally but not when perfused intravenously [34]. Intraduodenal infusion of a mixture containing arginine, histidine-isoleucine, leucine, lysine, and threonine caused significant GIP release, whereas a mixture of phenylalanine, tryptophan methionine, and valine produced no response. These findings suggest that GIP release is stimulated by a different group of amino acids than those causing pronounced release of CCK and gastrin. In later investigations using a glucose-insulin clamp technique, we found that oral fat increased GIP release in humans and that insulin did not inhibit fat-stimulated GIP secretion under normal glycemic conditions [35]. We observed a higher GIP response to oral fat in the hypoglycemic clamp and a lower GIP response in the hyperglycemic clamp. These results suggest a glycemic effect on GIP secretion in the presence of hyperinsulinemia.

Distal Gut Hormones

Fat hydrolysates are potent stimuli for release of the distal gut hormones neurotensin, GLI, and PYY [37]. The effect of fatty acids on the release of these hormones is both dose and carbon chain length dependent. For example, oleic acid is a more powerful stimulator of hormone release than short- or medium-chain fatty acids. In humans, the inhibition of gastric emptying and intestinal transit in response to ileal fat has been called the "ileal brake" [26]. This phenomenon may be mediated by ileal and colonic hormones. All three distal gut hormones may function as enterogastrones – hormones that mediate the inhibition of gastric acid secretion after fat ingestion. The presence of pancreatic juice in the duodenal lumen enhances the fat-stimulated release of the distal gut hormones [23]. Protein and carbohydrate hydrolysates are not as potent as fat in the releasing of neurotensin, GLI, and PYY, and perhaps play a minimal role in the regulation of the secretions of these hormones.

Human Pancreatic Polypeptide and Motilin

The release of HPP and motilin is more dependent on neural cholinergic influence than on luminal nutrient composition and concentration. Ingestion of a protein meal and cholinergic reflexes cause release of HPP into the circulation, whereas anti-cholinergic agents markedly inhibit HPP and motilin release [9]. On the other hand, intravenous infusion of amino acids produced an even smaller release of HPP than an ingestion of fat. The secretions of HPP and motilin cycle with phase III of the interdigestive motor activity [20]. These two hormones are truly unique and have been considered interdigestive hormones, in contrast to the other GI hormones such as gastrin, CCK, GIP, neurotensin, PYY, GLI and insulin, which are considered digestive hormones released after a meal.

The Enteropancreatic Axis

The interrelationship between gut hormones and pancreatic islets has been referred to as the "enteroinsular axis" [6]. An exciting new hypothesis suggests that different gut hormones may function as incretins for different foodstuffs. Thus, CCK released by oral amino acids might potentiate their action on pancreatic islet insulin release, or GIP released by oral glucose might potentiate the action of glucose on insulin release. Recent findings indicate that GIP and insulin may potentiate CCK-stimulated secretion of pancreatic exocrine enzymes [29] and that gut hormones may potentiate maturation of both endocrine and exocrine pancreatic cells [39]. The secretions of pancreatic enzymes from pancreatic acini is therefore dependent on both gut and islet hormones and forms the so-called enteroacinar and insuloacinar axis. These axes, in turn, are dependent on the digestive function of panreatic enzymes on the foodstuff in intestinal lumen – the removal of pancreatic juice altered both gut endocrine and pancreatic endocrine functions [23].

Alteration of Gastrointestinal Hormone Release in Chronic Pancreatitis

Although recent advances have been made in understanding the enteropancreatic relationship in health, minimal studies have been conducted on this relationship in pancreatic diseases. Most investigations on gut hormones in cronic pancreatitis have been limited to use as part of a diagnostic test, such as CCK, secretin, and/or bombesin stimulation tests on the pancreatic secretory function. The measurement of fasting plasma or serum level of gastrointestinal hormones has no value in the management of chronic pancreatitis.

The alterations of gut hormone release can be demonstrated following the ingestion of a test meal (Table 2). This subject matter was reviewed by Long et al. [24] and Vinik and Jackson [36]. The finding can be summarized as follows: (1) most of the proximal gut hormones (gastrin, secretin, and GIP) are normal or diminished postprandially with the exception of plasma CCK, which is elevated [2]. The elevated CCK level can be explained by the lack of feedback inhibition due to pancreatic insufficiency [18, 32]. The diminished GIP secretions can be corrected by pancreatic enzyme replacement therapy. (2) The distal gut hormones, such as PYY, neurotensin, and GLI, are markedly elevated after a meal, primarily due to excessive nutrient load to the ileum and colon secondary to malabsorption [3]. (3) The interdigestive hormone HPP level does not cycle with the phase III of the interdigestive motor activity in patients with chronic pancreatitis. This result will be reported by P. Malfertheiner and coworkers in this volume. The postprandial HPP level, as well as CCK-stimulated HPP response, are diminished in patients with chronic pancreatitis, particularly those associated with pancreatic insufficiency [21, 31]. Curiously, plasma motilin has been reported to be elevated in patients with chronic pancreatitis [24]. Similarly, patients with diabetic gastroparesis failed to exhibit antral phase III activities and had significantly higher fasting motilin levels compared to healthy subjects [1]. (4) All islet hormone secretions are also altered in patients with chronic pancreatitis. A good correlation was found [19] between insulin responses to oral glucose and exocrine pancreatic function measured as the concentration of pancreatic enzymes in duodenal juice after intravenous injection of CCK. Furthermore, Domschke et al. [8] found that acquired diabetes mellitus in chronic pancreatitis is found when the pancreatic protease output is, on an average, reduced to about 10% of the mean maximal protease output of normal subjects. This means that a great majority of chronic pancreatitis patients with steatorrhea should have concomitant diabetes mellitus. All these abnormalities (Table 2), on postprandial gastrointestinal hormone release, are secondary to anatomical destruction of both exocrine and endocrine tissue which leads to malabsorption that alters the enteropancreatic axis.

Table 2. Gastrointestinal hormone level in chronic pancreatitis

Hormones	Level
Gastrin	N
CCK	↑
Secretin	N
GIP	↓
Motilin	↑
GLI	↑
Neurotensin	↑
PYY	↑
HPP	↓
Insulin	↓
Glucagon	↓

Summary

We have now understood that the enteropancreatic relationship is bidirectional. Gut hormone release is dependent on pancreatic enzymatic digestion of protein, fat, and carbohydrate. Gut hormones, in concert with the nervous system, regulate the pancreatic endocrine function, and pancreatic exocrine secretions. This interrelationship between the gut and the pancreas is well illustrated during pancreatic insufficiency, secondary to chronic pancreatitis. We hope our better understanding of this enteropancreatic axis will contribute to our investigations of the role of gut hormones in the pathogenesis and management of pancreatic disorders.

References

1. Achem-Karam SR, Funakoshi A, Vinik Al, et al. (1985) Plasma motilin concentration and interdigestive MMC in diabetic gastroparesis: effect of metoclopramide. Gastroenterology 88:492–499
2. Adrian TE, McKiernan J, Johnstone DI, et al. (1980) Hormonal abnormalities of the pancreas and gut in cystic fibrosis. Gastroenterology 79:460–465
3. Adrian TE, Savage AP, Bacarese-Hamilton AJ, Wolfe K, Besterman HS, Bloom SR (1986) Peptide YY abnormalities in gastrointestinal diseases. Gastroenterology 90:379–384
4. Boivin M, Zinsmeister AR, Go VLW, DiMagno EP (1987) Effect of a purified amylase inhibitor on carbohydrate metabolism after a mixed meal in healthy humans. Mayo Clinic Proc 62:249–255
5. Chey WY, Chang TM, Lee KY, You CH (1988) Gastrointestinal hormone in current gastroenterology. In: Yearbook Medical Publishers, Chicago, pp 161–234
6. Creutzfeldt W, Ebert R (1986) The enteroinsular axis. In: Go VLW, Gardner JD, Brooks FP, Lebenthal E, DiMagno EP, Scheele GA (eds) The endocrine pancreas. Raven, New York, pp 333–342
7. Dimitriadis G, Tessari P, Go VLW, Gerich J (1982) Effects of acarbose on metabolic and hormonal responses to meal ingestion and intravenous glucose in normal man. In: Creutzfeldt W (ed) Proceedings of the first international Symposium on Acarbose. Excerpta Medica, Amsterdam, pp 216–222
8. Domschke S, Stock KP, Pichl J, Schneider MU, Domschke W (1985) Beta-cell reserve capacity in chronic pancreatitis. Hepatogastroenterology 32:27–30
9. Floyd J, Fajan S, Chance RE (1977) A newly recognized pancreatic polypeptide: plasma levels in health and disease. Recent Prog Horm Res 33:519–570
10. Fujita T (1988) The cellular mechanism of gut hormone secretion. Proc Chin Acad Med Sci [Suppl 2] 3:40–41
11. Go VLW (1989) Role of gastrointestinal hormones in adaptation. In: Halsted CH, Rucker RB (eds) Nutrition and the origins of disease. Academic, San Diego, pp 321–329
12. Go VLW, Koch TR (1989) Distribution of gut peptides. In: Makhlouf GM (ed) Neuroendocrinology of the gut, vol 1. American Physiological Society, Bethesda (Handbook of physiology) (in press)
13. Go VLW, Miller LJ (1983) The role of gastrointestinal hormones in the control of postprandial and interdigestive gastrointestinal functin. Scand J Gastroenterol 18:135–142
14. Go VLW, Hofmann AF, Summerskill WHJ (1970) Pancreozymin bioassy in man based on pancreatic enzyme secretion: potency of specific amino acids and other digestive products. J Clin Invst 49:1558–1564
15. Green GM, Lyman RL (1972) Feedback regulation of pancreatic enzyme secretion as mechanism for trypsin inhibitor induced hypersecretion in rats. Proc Soc Exp Biol Med 14:6–12
16. Henderson JR, Daniel PM, Fraser PA (1981) The pancreas as a single organ: the influence of the endocrine upon exocrine part of the gland. Gut 22:158–167
17. Iwa K, Fushiki T, Fukuoka SI (1988) Pancreatic enzyme secretion mediated by novel peptide: monitor peptide hypothesis. Pancreas 3:720–728

18. Jansen JB, Hopman WP, Lamers CB (1984) Plasma cholecystokinin concentrations in patients with pancreatic insufficiency measured by sequence-specific radioimmunoassays. Dig Dis Sci 29:1109–1117
19. Kalk WJ, Vinik AI, Jackson WPU, Bank S (1979) Insulin secretion and pancreatic exocrine function in patients with chronic pancreatitis. Diabetologia 16:355–358
20. Keane FB, DiMagno EP, Dozois RR, Go VLW (1980) Relationship among canine interdigestive exocrine pancreatic and biliary flow, duodenal motor activity, plasma pancreatic polypeptide and motilin. Gastroenterology 78:310–316
21. Koch MB, Go VLW, DiMagno EP (1985) Can plasma human PP be used to detect diseases of the exocrine pancreas? Mayo Clin Proc 60:259–265
22. Koch TR, Carney JA, Go VLW (1987) Distribution and quantitation of gut neuropeptides in normal intestine and inflammatory bowel diseases. Dig Dis Sci 32:369–376
23. Lluis F, Gomez G, Hashimoto T, Fujimura M, Greeley G, Thompson JC (1989) Pancreatic juice enhances fat-stimulated release of enteric hormones in dogs. Pancreas 4:23–30
24. Long RG, Adrian TE, Bloom SR (1981) Gastrointestinal hormones in pancreatic disease. In: Mitchell CJ, Kelleher J (eds) Pancreatic disease in clinical practice. Pitman, New York, pp 223–239
25. Louie DS, May D, Miller P, Ouyang C (1986) Cholecystokinin mediated feedback regulation of pancreatic enzyme secretion in rats. Am J Physiol 250:G250–259
26. MacFarlane A, Kinsman R, Read NW, Bloom SR (1983) The ileal brake: ileal fat slows bowel transit and gastric emptying in man. Gut 24:A471–472
27. Malagelada J-R, DiMagno EP, Summerskill WHJ, Go VLW (1976) Regulation of pancreatic and gallbladder functions by intraluminal fatty acids and bile acids in man. J Clin Invest 58:493–499
28. McCullough AJ, Miller LJ, Service FJ, Go VLW (1983) Effect of graded intraduodenal glucose infusions on the release and physiological action of gastric inhibitory polypeptide. J Clin Endocrinol Metab 56:234–241
29. Mueller MK, Scheck T, Dressman V, Miodonski A, Goebell H (1987) GIP potentiates CCK stimulated pancreatic enzyme secretion: correlation of anatomical structures with the effect of GIP and CCK on amylase secretion. Pancreas 2:106–113
30. Nelson RL, Go VLW, McCullough AJ, Ilstrup DM, Service FJ (1986) Lack of a direct effect of the autonomic nervous system on glucose-stimulated gastric inhibitory polypeptide (GIP) secretion in man. Dig Dis Sci 31:929–935
31. Nousia-Arvanitakis S, Tomita T, Desai N, et al. (1985) Pancreatic polypeptide in cystic fibrosis. Arch Pathol Lab Med 109:722–726
32. Slaff JI, Wolfe MM, Toskes PP (1985) Elevated fasting cholecystokinin levels in pancreatic exocrine impairment: evidence to support feedback regulation. J Lab Clin Med 105:282–285
33. Taylor I, Byrne W, Christie D, Ament M, Walsh J (1982) Effect of individual L-amino acids on gastric secretion and serum gastrin and pancreatic polypeptide release in humans. Gastroenterology 83:273–278
34. Thomas F, Sinar D, Mazzaferri E, Cataland S, Makhjian H, Caldwell J, Fromkes J (1978) Selective release of gastric inhibitory polypeptide by introduodenal amino acid perfusion in man. Gastroenterology 74:1261–1265
35. Verdonk CA, Rizza RA, Nelson RL, Go VLW, Gerich JE, Service FJ (1980) Interaction of fat-stimulated gastric inhibitory polypeptide on pancreatic alpha and beta cell function. J Clin Invest 65:1119–1125
36. Vinik AI, Jackson WPU (1980) Endocrine secretions in chronc pancreatitis. In: Podolsky S, Viswanathan M (eds) Secondary diabetes: the spectrum of the diabetic syndromes. Raven, New York, pp 165–189
37. Walsh JH (1987) Gastrointestinal hormones. In: Johnson LR, Christensen J, Jackson MJ, Jacobson ED, Walsh JH (eds) Physiology of the gastrointestinal tract. Raven, New York, pp 181–253
38. Weaver C, Sorenson RL (1989) Islet vasculature in atrophic pancreas: evidence for coexisting parallel and serial (insuloacinar) angioarchitecture. Pancreas 4:10–32
39. Williams JA (1987) Gut-islet-pancreatic acinar interaction. Pancreas 2:240–241
40. Yaksh TL, Michener SR, Bailey JE, Harty GJ, Lucas DL, Nelson DK, Roddy DR, Go VLW (1988) Survey of distribution of substance P, vasoactive intestinal polypeptide cholecystokinin, neurotensin, met-enkephalin, bombesin and PHI in the spinal chord of cat, dog, sloth and monkey. Peptides 9:357–72

Feedback Mechanisms in the Control of Exocrine Pancreatic Function*

CH. OWYANG[1]

Recent physiological studies indicate that both cholecystokinin (CCK) and the cholinergic enteropancreatic reflexes are important to stimulate pancreatic enzyme secretion. Little is known, however, about regulating these pathways. In this study we investigated the mechanisms responsible for feedback modulation of CCK release and the enteropancreatic reflexes.

Feedback Regulation of Release of Cholecystokinin

Animal studies have demonstrated that pancreatic enzymes in the duodenum exhibit a feedback control of pancreatic exocrine secretion. Investigations in rats [1–3] have demonstrated that raw soybean or an isolated soybean trypsin inhibitor (SBTI) markedly stimulates the exocrine pancreas. Furthermore, Green and Lyman [4] found that, in rats with bile-pancreatic duct fistulas, removing pancreaticobiliary juice (PBJ) from the intestine resulted in a large increase in pancreatic enzyme secretion. Return of pancreaticobiliary juice or infusion of the PBJ components trypsin or chymotrypsin suppressed pancreatic enzyme secretion. Therefore, feedback inhibition of pancreatic enzyme secretion in the rat is mediated by trypsin in the intestine. Trypsin inhibitors stimulate pancreatic enzyme secretion indirectly, by binding or neutralizing trypsin and thereby removing its feedback inhibition.

A similar feedback control system was shown in chickens [5], pigs [6], and humans [8, 9]. In man, intraduodenal perfusion of trypsin inhibited phenylalanine-, oleic acid-, and meal-stimulated chymotrypsin and lipase outputs [8]. This inhibitory effect was protease specific since suppression was not observed with intraduodenal perfusion of lipase or amylase. A similar phenomenon was observed in patients with chronic pancreatitis [7]. In contrast, Dlugosz et al. [10] and Hotz et al. [11] intraduodenally infused aprotinin, a trypsin inhibitor, and found no effect on pancreatic enzyme secretion. Similar findings were reported using the new trypsin inhibitor FOY-305 [12]. Neither compound strongly inhibits human chymotrypsin, however. On the other hand, Liener et al [13] demonstrated that Bowman-Birk soybean trypsin inhibitor, an inhibitor of chymotrypsin and elastase, markedly stimulated pancreatic enzyme secretion in humans. These observations suggest that not only trypsin but also

* This investigation was supported in part by US Public Health Service Grants R01 DK 32838 and P30 DK 35933
[1] Department of Internal Medicine, Division of Gastroenterology, The University of Michigan Medical Center, Ann Arbor, Michigan 48109, USA

Chronic Pancreatitis
Ed. by Beger, Büchler, Ditschuneit, and Malfertheiner
© Springer-Verlag Berlin Heidelberg 1990

other proteases such as chymotrypsin and elastase should be removed to evoke stimulation of pancreatic enzyme secretion in humans.

Several studies suggest that feedback regulation of pancreatic enzyme secretion is mediated by a hormone secreted by the proximal small intestine. Khayambashi and Lyman [14] demonstrated that perfusion of an isolated rat pancreas with plasma from an animal fed over a short period with SBTI produced a threefold increase in amylase output, and addition of atropine to the perfusate did not inhibit the secretory response. Furthermore, resection of the duodenum and jejunum in rats abolished the increase in pancreatic enzyme secretion produced by administration of SBTI [15]. The characteristics of the SBTI-induced stimulating material observed in the rat studies reported by Khayamabashi and Lyman [14] are consistent with those of cholecystokinin (CCK). Both the stimulatory material and CCK originate from the upper gut and stimulate pancreatic enzyme secretion independent of a cholinergic mechanism. These observations are compatible with the hypothesis that trypsin in the duodenum inhibitis the release of CCK, and SBTI promotes the release of CCK by binding or neutralizing trypsin. In subsequent studies it has been demonstrated that diversion of bile pancreatic juice or duodenal infusion of SBTI in the rat increased plasma CCK levels and pancreatic enzyme secretion [16]. Duodenal infusion of trypsin abolished the increase in plasma CCK. Intravenous infusion of proglumide or L364,718, a specific CCK antagonist, abolished the increase in pancreatic secretion following diversion of bile pancreatic juice [16, 17]. These observations indicate that feedback regulation of pancreatic secretion by trypsin is mediated by release of CCK.

Evidence for the Presence of a Trypsin-Sensitive "CCK-Releasing Peptide"

The mechanism through which trypsin suppresses the release of CCK is unknown. We hypothesized that the increased pancreatic enzyme secretion following pancreatic juice diversion is mediated by a trypsin-sensitive peptide secreted by the small intestine which stimulates release of CCK. To test this hypothesis, rats were surgically prepared with bile-pancreatic fistulae and intestinal cannulae. Diversion of bile-pancreatic juice increased amylase output fivefold above basal and increased plasma CCK from a basal value of $0.5 + 0.08$ pM to $14 + 4$ pM. Rapid perfusion (3 ml/min) of the duodenum with phosphate-buffered saline reversed the increase in amylase output and lowered the plasma CCK to $3 + 0.7$ pM. Administration of intestinal perfusate (3 ml/min) collected from a "donor" rat into the duodenum of a "recipient" rat with diversion of bile pancreatic juice increased amylase output threefold above basal and increased plasma CCK [18]. Treatment of intestinal perfusate with trypsin abolished the stimulatory effect, but was unaffected by pretreatment with amylase, lipase, or boiling. Perfusion of intestinal perfusate from donor rats pretreated with atropine did not stimulate amylase output in recipient rats. Using molecular membrane exclusion filters, stimulatory activity was retained between 1K-5K daltons. These results indicated that feedback regulation of pancreatic enzyme secretion is mediated by a CCK-releasing peptide (CCK-RP), whose secretion from the duodenum is cholinergically mediated. This peptide is trypsin sensitive and has a molecular weight between 1K and 5K.

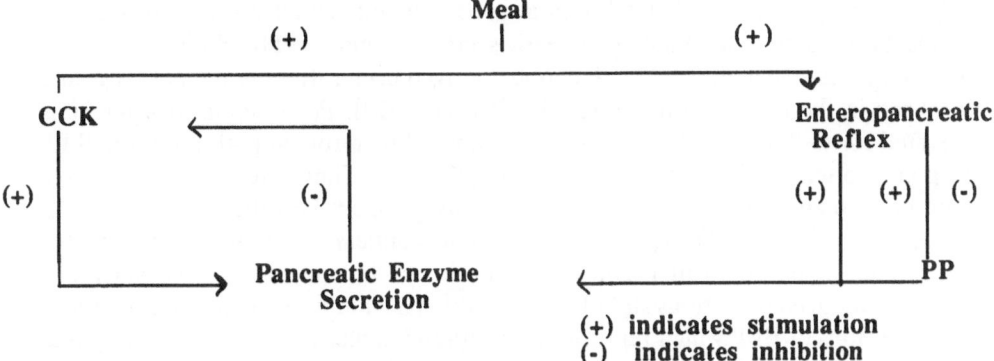

Fig. 1. Proposed pathways for feedback regulation of pancreatic enzyme secretion. Ingestion of a meal stimulates pancreatic enzyme secretion through release of CCK and activation of the enteropancreatic reflex. Intraluminal proteases inhibit CCK release whereas PP secreted in response to stimulation by an enteropancreatic reflex inhibits cholinergic transmission

Extraction and Purification of "CCK-Releasing Peptide" from Procine Intestinal Mucosa

To characterize the "CCK-releasing peptide" we extracted and partially purified this peptide from porcine intestinal mucosa. The duodenum was excised and washed with $1M$ acetic acid. The mucosa (1 kg) was scraped directly into liquid nitrogen, pulverized in a Waring blender and extracted in boiling $1M$ acetic acid and 4% TFA for 10 min followed by cooling in liquid nitrogen and the addition of 10 mM EDTA, 1 mM benzamidine hydrochloride, and 0.01% dithiothreitol (DDT). The extract was ultracentrifuged and the supernatant applied onto a C18 Sep Pak and eluted with 50% acetonitrile and 50% 0.1% TFA. Active fractions were pooled, centrifuged, and applied to a C2/C18 Pep RPC HR 5/5 FPLC column and eluted with a gradient of 0%–60% acetonitrile. The area demonstrating CCK-releasing peptide activity was rechromatographed employing a shallower acetonitrile gradient of 0%–25%. A single large peak predominated and demonstrated CCK-releasing peptide activity. We are currently purifying this material to homogeneity for sequencing.

Feedback Regulation of the Enteropancreatic Reflex

It is known that digestive products [19], duodenal distension [9, 20] and osmolality [9, 20] of the chyme can stimulate pancreatic secretion via the cholinergic enteropancreatic reflex, independent of CCK release. This mechanism may account for half of the postprandial secretory response [9]. Little is known about feedback modulation of the enteropancreatic reflex. We have shown in man that intraduodenal trypsin inhibits pancreatic enzymes stimulated by phenylalanine but not by volume or osmolarity [9]. This is expected since the presence of trypsin appears to suppress CCK release, whereas pancreatic secretion in response to volume or osmolarity is mediated via the enteropancreatic reflex.

Pancreatic polypetide (PP), a hormone predominantly under vagal control [21], is an ideal candidate to modulate pancreatic secretion stimulated by cholinergic transmission. PP is a 36 amino acid polypeptide derived primarily from the pancreas and localized in the islets and in scattered acinar cells [22]. Postprandial plasma PP is elevated for 6–8 h [23]. This response is abolished by atropine [24], but a small PP response often remains after vagotomy [23, 24]. Therefore, the responsible enteropancreatic signals may involve both a long vagovagal reflex and short local cholinergic pathways. These same pathways also appear to stimulate postprandial pancreatic secretion. In man and dogs, infusion of bovine PP inhibits pancreatic secretion induced by various stimulants [25–27]. The inhibitory action was observed with infusions of BPP which reproduced postprandial plasma levels, suggesting that PP is physiologically important to regulate pancreatic function.

Pancreatic polypeptide secretion is mainly governed by a cholinergic mechanism. In isolated perfused pancreas, PP output is four to ten times larger during acetylcholine stimulation than during stimulation with peptide hormones, arginine, isoproterenol, or Ca^{2+} ions [28, 29]. In anesthetized pigs, electrical stimulation of the vagus causes a rapid massive release of PP [30] and is abolished by hexamethonium or atropine. CCK [31], cerulein [32], bombesin [33] and neurotensin [34] also stimulate PP secretion. The action of these peptides of PP release can be abolished by atropine, suggesting they either act through a cholinergic mechanism or on the background of permissive cholinergic tone [35]. Thus PP is an ideal candidate to modulate pancreatic secretion stimulated by cholinergic enteropancreatic reflex.

Release and Physiological Role of Pancreatic Polypeptide in Canine Pancreatic Slices

To further examine the role of PP in the regulation of pancreatic amylase secretion we performed immunoneutralization experiments using PP antiserum (Ab S11) to neutralize endogenously released PP in canine pancreatic slices. Depolarization by K^+ (75 mM) caused a threefold increase in amylase output and a fourfold increase in PP secretion compared to basal values. Both the amylase release and PP response to K^+ depolarization were inhibited by atropine (10^{-6} M), suggesting K^+ stimulates exocrine and endocrine secretion by a cholinergic pathway. In subsequent studies, one half of the pancreatic slices were incubated for 3 h in Krebs Ringer buffer with control rabbit serum added and the other half in PP antiserum (final dilution 1:100). The incubation medium was replaced with buffer containing 75 mM KCl for 10 min, followed by collection and repletion of buffer every 10 min for a total of 60 min. In slices pretreated with PP antiserum, K^+ depolorization resulted in a five- to sixfold increase in amylase secretion whereas K^+ caused only a twofold increase in control slices. In contrast, slices treated with control rabbit serum responded to K^+ stimulation in a manner identical to the responses observed in control slices. Therefore, endogenously released PP plays an important role in modulating pancreatic enzyme secretion.

Inhibitory Action of Pancreatic Polypeptide Is Directed at Cholinergic Stimulation

Pancreatic polypeptide has been shown to inhibit meal and CCK-stimulated exocrine pancreatic secretion. However, its mechanism of action is unclear. We compared the effects of PP_6 on pancreatic enzyme secretion stimulated by vagal stimulation and CCK in conscious rats with bile pancreatic fistulae. Vagal stimulation was achieved by intravenous injection of 2-deoxy-D-glucose (2-DG, 75 mg/kg), which stimulated pancreatic protein output 320% $\pm$ 43% above basal ($n = 6$). Atropine completely blocked the action of 2-DG, suggesting mediation by a cholinergic pathway. Intravenous infusion of CCK8 (50 pmol/kg per hour) increased pancreatic protein output by 290% $\pm$ 31%. PP_6 (100 pmol/kg per hour) completely inhibited pancreatic protein output stimulated by 2-DG, but only partially (30%) reduced that stimulated by CCK8. Dose inhibition studies indicated that half maximal inhibitory concentrations for PP on pancreatic protein outputs stimulated by 2-DG and CCK8 were 60 and 1740 pmol/kg per hour respectively. These observations suggest that PP acts preferentially to inhibit pancreatic enzyme secretion stimulated by the vagal cholinergic pathway.

In Vitro Studies To Demonstrate Pancreatic Polypeptide Inhibits Pancreatic Enzyme Secretion Via Presynaptic Modulation of Acetylcholine Release

To investigate the mechanism of action of PP we examined the activity of PP on dispersed rat pancreatic acini. BPP (10^{-9}–10^{-6} M) did not suppress CCK8 (10^{-9} M) or carbachol (10^{-7} M)-stimulated amylase release from this preparation, suggesting that the inhibitory action of BPP on exocrine pancreatic secretion is mediated by an indirect mechanism. In isolated perfused rat pancreas, PP_6 (10^{-7} M) inhibited CCK8 (100 pM)-stimulated amylase secretion by 62% $\pm$ 9%. Treatment of the preparation with atropine abolished the inhibitory action of PP_6, suggesting that PP exerts its action through neural elements. To investigate this possibility, we demonstrated that in pancreatic lobules, which contain intrapancreatic nerve fibers, PP_6 (10^{-7} M) inhibited potassium-stimulated amylase release by 58% $\pm$ 6%. The inhibition was unaffected by addition of hexamethonium but blocked by atropine. In contrast, PP_6 had no effect on carbachol-stimulated amylase release. In addition, PP_6 (10^{-7} M) inhibited the K^+-evoked release of [^{3}H]acetylcholine by 42% $\pm$ 5% from pancreatic slices preloaded with [^{3}H]choline. Thus, PP inhibits pancreatic enzyme secretion via presynaptic modulation of acetylcholine release. This pathway provides a novel mechanism for hormonal inhibition of pancreatic enzyme secretion via modulation of classic neurotransmitter function.

Summary and Significance

Our studies demonstrated that feedback modulation of CCK release and the enteropancreatic reflexes are under separate control. We showed that the increased plasma CCK levels and pancreatic enzyme secretion following diversion of pancreatic juice is mediated by a trypsin-sensitive substance secreted into the proximal small intestine which we named "CCK-releasing peptide". This substance may serve as an important regulator for CCK release. We have isolated and partially purified this substance from porcine intestinal mucosa. Our studies also indicate that secretion of PP is under cholinergic control and this peptide acts by interfering with cholinergic transmission. This makes PP an ideal candidate to modulate pancreatic secretion stimulated by cholinergic enteropancreatic reflexes. This newly identified pathway provides a novel mechanism for hormonal inhibition of pancreatic enzyme secretion via modulation of the classic neurotransmitter function. Figure 1 shows the proposed feedback pathways.

References

1. Booth AND, Robbins WE, Ribelin WE, DeEds F (1960) Effect of raw soybean meal and amino acids on pancreatic hypertrophy in rats. Proc Soc Exp Biol Med 104:681–683
2. Lyman RL (1957) The effect of raw soybean meal and trypsin inhibitor diets on the intestinal and pancreatic nitrogen in the rat. J Nutr 62:285–294
3. Lyman RL, Lepkovsky S (1957) The effect of raw soybean meal and trypsin inhibitor diets on pancreatic enzyme secretion in rat. J Nutr 62:265–284
4. Green GM, Lyman RL (1972) Feedback regulation of pancreatic enzyme secretion as a mechanism for trypsin inhibitor-induced hypersecretion in rats. Proc Soc Exp Biol Med 140:6–12
5. Chernick SS, Lepkovsky S, Chaikoff IL (1948) A dietary factor regulating the enzyme content of the pancreas: changes induced in size and proteolytic activity of the chick pancreas by ingestion of raw soybean meal. Am J Physiol 155:33–41
6. Corring T (1973) Mechanisme de la secrétion pancréatique exocrine chez le porc: regulation par rétro inhibition. Ann Biol Anim Biochim Biophys 13:755–756
7. Slaff J, Jacobson D, Tillman CR, Curington C, Toskes P (1984) Protease-specific suppression of pancreatic exocrine secretion. Gastroenterology 87:44–52
8. Owyang C, Louie DS, Tatum D (1986) Feedback regulation of pancreatic enzyme secretion. J Clin Invest 77:2042–2047
9. Owyang C, May D, Louie DS (1986) Trypsin suppression of pancreatic enzyme secretion. Gastroenterology 91:637–647
10. Dlugosz J, Fölsch UR, Creutzfeldt W (1983) Inhibition of intraduodenal trypsin does not stimulate exocrine pancreatic secretion in man. Digestion 26:197–204
11. Hotz J, Ho SB, Go VLW, DiMagno E (1983) Short term inhibition of duodenal trypsin activity does not affect human pancreatic biliary or gastric function. J Lab Clin Med 101:488–495
12. Alder G, Mullenhoff A, Bozkurt T, Koop I, Göke B, Arnold R (1986) Effect of protease inhibitor (FOY 305) on pancreatic secretion and plasma CCK in human. Digestion 35:3
13. Liener IR, Goodale RL, Desmukh A, Satterberg TL, Ward G, DiPietro CM, Bankey PE, Borner JW (1988) Effect of trypsin inhibitor from soybeans (Bowman-Birk) on the secretory activity of the human pancreas. Gastroenterology 94:419–427
14. Khayambashi H, Lyman RL (1969) Secretion of rat pancreas perfused with plasma from rats fed soybean trypsin inhibitor. Am J Physiol 217:646–651
15. Ihse I (1976) Abolishment of oral trypsin inhibitor stimulation of the rat exocrine pancreas after duodenal resection. Scand J Gastroenterol 11:11–15
16. Louie DS, May D, Miller P, Owyang C (1986) Cholecystokinin mediates feedback regulation of pancreatic enzyme secretion in rats. Am J Physiol 250:G252–259
17. Louie DS, Liang JP, Owyang C (1988) Characterization of a new CCK antagonist L346,718: in vitro and in vivo studies. Am J Physiol 255:G261–G266
18. Lu L, Louie DS, Owyang C (1989) A cholecystokinin releasing peptide mediates feedback regulation of pancreatic secretion. Am J Physiol 256:G430–G435
19. Valenzuela JE, Lamers CB, Modlin IM, Walsh JH (1983) Cholinergic component in the human pancreatic secretory response to intraintestinal oleate. Gut 24:807–811
20. Dooley CP, Valenzuela JE (1984) Duodenal volume and osmoreceptors in the stimulation of human pancreatic secretion. Gastroenterology 86:23–27

21. Schwartz TW (1983) Pancreatic polypeptide: a hormone under vagal control. Gastroenterology 85:1411–1425
22. Larsson LI, Sundler F, Hakanson R (1976) Pancreatic polypeptide a postulated hormone: identification of its cellular storage site by light and electron-microscopic immunocytochemistry. Diabetologia 12:211–216
23. Schwartz TW, Rehfeld JF, Stadil F, Larsson LI, Chance RE, Moon M (1976) Pancreatic polypeptide response to food in duodenal ulcer patients before and after vagotomy. Lancet 1:1102–1105
24. Taylor IL, Impicciatore M, Walsh JH (1978) Effect of atropine and vagotomy on the pancreatic polypeptide response to a meal. Am J Physiol 235:E443–447
25. Greenberg GR, McCloy RF, Adrian TE, Chadwick VS, Baron JH, Bloom SR (1978) Inhibition of pancreas and gallbladder by pancreatic polypeptide. Lancet 2:1280–1282
26. Taylor IL, Solomon T, Walsh J, Grossman M (1979) Pancreatic polypeptide: metabolism and effect on pancreatic secretion in dogs. Gastroenterology 76:524–528
27. Greenberg GR, McCloy RF, Chadwick VS, Adrian TE, Baron JH, Bloom SR (1979) Effect of bovine pancreatic polypeptide on basal pancreatic and biliary outputs in man. Am J Dig Dis 24:11–14
28. Adrian TE, Bloom SR, Hermansen K, Iversen J (1978) Pancreatic polypeptide, glucagon and insulin secretion from the isolated perfused canine pancreas, Diabetologia 14:413–417
29. Hermansen K, Schwartz TW (1979) The influence of calcium on the basal and acetylcholine-stimulated secretion of pancreatic polypeptide. Endocrinology 105:1409–1474
30. Schwartz TW, Holst JJ, Fahrenkrug J, Jensen SL, Nielsen OV, Rehfeld JF, Schaffalitzkg DE, Muckadell OB, Stadil F (1978) Cholinergic vagal regulation of pancreatic polypeptide secretion. J Clin Invest 61:781–789
31. Guzman S, Lonovics J, Devitt PG, Heijtmancik KE, Rayford PL, Thompson JC (1981) Hormone-stimulated release of pancreatic polypeptide before and after vagotomy in dogs. Am J Physiol 240:G114–121
32. Adrian TE, Bloom SR, Besterman HS (1977) Mechanism of pancreatic polypeptide release in man. Lancet 1:161–163
33. Taylor IL, Walsh JH, Carter D, Wood J, Grossman MI (1979) Effect of atropine and bethanechol on bombesin-stimulated release of pancreatic polypeptide and gastrin in dog. Gastroenterology 77:714–718
34. Blackborn AM, Fletcher DR, Adrian TE, Bloom SR (1980) Neurotensin infusions in man: pharmacokinetics and effect on gastrointestinal and pituitary hormones. J Clin Endocrinol Metab 51:1257–1261
35. Adrian TE, Besterman HS, Bloom SR (1979) The importance of cholinergic tone in the release of pancreatic polypeptide by gut hormones in man. Life Sci 24:1989–1994

Influence of Intestinal Protease Inhibition on Pancreatic Feedback Regulation

G. Adler and M. Reinshagen[1]

Exocrine pancreatic secretion is dependent on the amount and activity of pancreatic enzymes released into the duodenum. This feedback regulation of exocrine pancreatic secretion was first described in the rat by Green and Lyman [1]. The exclusion of bile-pancreatic juice from the proximal small intestine of the rat caused a dramatic stimulation of pancreatic secretion. The exclusion of pancreatic juice alone had the same stimulatory effect. In a further study progressively increasing percentages of pancreatic juice were diverted from the intestine [2]. These experiments were performed to determine the relationship between the percentage of pancreatic secretion diverted from the intestine and pancreatic secretion. Return of only 5% of the secreted material into the duodenum caused a 50% reduction of pancreatic secretion. Pancreatic secretion was almost completely stopped when 10% of pancreatic juice secreted was returned to the intestine.

In this review we shall summarize the evidence that feedback regulation is specific to proteases and discuss the controversies on the mediators of this mechanism.

Effect of Protease Inhibition on Rat Pancreatic Secretion

In their original study, Green and Lyman [1] observed a significant stimulation of spontaneous pancreatic enzyme secretion after bile-pancreatic juice diversion in anesthetized rats. This stimulation was completely suppressed when either trypsin or chymotrypsin was instilled intraduodenally. The stimulatory effect of protein on pancreatic secretion was completely inhibited by trypsin and chymotrypsin. The specific role of trypsin and chymotrypsin in regulating pancreatic enzyme secretion was supported in further studies [3–6]. Even in the conscious rats trypsin suppressed the stimulation of pancreatic secretion after juice diversion [7, 8]. Furthermore elastase was shown to interfere with the feedback regulation, while amylase and lipase had no effect [9, 10]. The regulatory role of trypsin was dose dependent and restricted to the upper part of the small intestine [5]. When the proteases trypsin and chymotrypsin were inactivated by heat or with diisopropyl-fluorophosphate they showed no effect on pancreatic enzyme secretion [5]. The duodenal perfusion of a trypsin-like peptide from *Streptomyces griseus* which has no homology to pancreatic proteases inhibited pancreatic enzyme secretion [11]. These results indicate that the enzymatic activity of trypsin is needed for interference with the feedback regulation.

---

[1] Department of Internal Medicine, Division of Gastroenterology, Philipps University of Marburg, Baldingerstrasse, D-3550 Marburg, FRG

Chronic Pancreatitis
Ed. by Beger, Büchler, Ditschuneit, and Malfertheiner
© Springer-Verlag Berlin Heidelberg 1990

In the rat, intraluminal protein substrates caused a similar interruption of feedback regulation as protease inhibitors or diversion of pancreatic juice [12]. In contrast, protein hydrolysates had no effect. It was proposed that dietary proteins like protease inhibitors remove the proteases from the intestine, thereby abolishing their negative feedback on pancreatic enzyme secretion.

The role of intraluminal proteases in the regulation of pancreatic secretion in the rat was further proven in studies on the effects of protease inhibitors. The intragastric or intraduodenal administration of soybean trypsin inhibitor [1], potato chymotrypsin inhibitor [13], bovine lung trypsin inhibitor [4, 9], lima bean trypsin inhibitor [14], pancreatic secretory trypsin inhibitor [15], and nonprotein synthetic trypsin inhibitors [16] caused a significant stimulation of pancreatic enzyme secretion. In recent years, the powerful, synthetic serine protease inhibitor camostate mesilate (FOY-305) was used in several studies in rat and man. Camostate (MW, 494.5) is a guanidino acid ester [17]. After intestinal absorption, the molecule is degraded rapidly by esterases and pH-dependent nonenzymatic hydrolysis into FOY-251, which is still a potent protease inhibitor [18]. The degradation product of FOY-251, p-guinidinobenzoate (GBA), is inactive against proteases. After intravenous infusion and after oral feeding of camostate only the metabolites were detected in blood [19, 20]. However, in bile-pancreatic juice camostate and its metabolites were detected by HPLC [19]. These results point to penetration of the camostate molecule into the pancreatic tissue and pancreatic juice. In a recent study, we excluded a direct effect of camostate on the secretory process of rat pancreatic acini [21].

Application of a single dose of camostate via orogastric tube in rats caused a significant stimulation of pancreatic secretion. This effect became apparent at a dose of 25 mg/kg and was optimal at 100 mg/kg [22]. The stimulation of pancreatic enzyme secretion was paralleled by an increase in plasma CCK [22, 23]. A single dose of 100 mg/kg camostate revealed a threefold increase in enzyme output and a 70% depletion of pancreatic enzyme stores persisting for 6 h and reverting to control levels by 12 h. CCK plasma levels increased 15-fold within 30 min and declined to control levels by 9 h. Fine structural analysis of the pancreas demonstrated marked depletion of zymogen granules from acinar cells.

Feeding of camostate induced a remarkable growth of the pancreas. One single oral dose (100 mg/kg) caused a significant increase in mitotic activity of acinar cells [24]. After prolonged administration (15 days) pancreas weight doubled [23, 25]. This was paralleled by a significant increase in enzyme content and synthesis of trypsinogen and chymotrypsinogen, while amylase synthesis was decreased [23, 26].

The stimulation of enzyme secretion and pancreatic growth after protease inhibitor feeding or after diversion of pancreatic juice was ascribed to the increase of endogenous CCK [7, 8, 22, 23]. This concept was confirmed by studies which demonstrated a reversal of the stimulatory effect by potent CCK-receptor antagonists [8, 23, 27–29]. Furthermore, morphometric studies demonstrated a similar reduction of zymogen granules after diversion of pancreatic juice or intraduodenal instillation of a protease inhibitor as was observed after stimulation by exogenous CCK [30]. At this time, there is ample evidence that CCK is the mediator of feedback regulation of pancreatic secretion in the rat. The mechanism through which intestinal proteases regulate release of endogenous CCK is unknown. Two peptides have been proposed to account for this regulation: a trypsin-sensitive CCK-releasing peptide from the rat small intestine [31] and a pancreatic monitor peptide in rat pancreatic juice [32]. The evidence for these peptides will be extensively discussed in the contribution by Owyang in this volume.

Protease-specific feedback regulation exists in several species including pig, chicken, and chow. It was, however, not demonstrated in the dog [for review see 33].

Effect of Protease Inhibition on Human Pancreatic Secretion

In 1977, Ihse et al. [34] described a feedback regulation of pancreatic secretion in man. In a patient a tumor of the papilla of Vater completely prevented flow of bile-pancreatic juice into the duodenum. Bile and pancreatic juice were, therefore, exteriorized via a percutaneous transhepatic cholangiography catheter. The instillation of bile-pancreatic juice into the duodenum suppressed pancreatic enzyme secretion. A similar inhibition of enzyme output was observed during duodenal perfusion of trypsin. In contrast, in the presence of bile-pancreatic juice a trypsin inhibitor (aprotinin) caused a significant stimulation of pancreatic secretion. These results pointed to a feedback regulation of pancreatic secretion in man which is dependent on the activity of proteases in the duodenum. Three further studies could not demonstrate feedback regulation of pancreatic secretion in man. In these studies, intestinal perfusion of aprotinin or pancreatic enzymes had no effect on pancreatic secretion [35–37]. However, perfusion of trypsin suppressed enzyme output, which was stimulated by phenylalanine, oleic acid, or a meal [38–40]. In the study by Owyang et al., trypsin caused a dose-related inhibition [39].

The discrepancies in studies on feedback regulation in man could result from the use of different trypsin inhibitors. Hotz et al. [36] were the first to mention that this regulatory mechanism might depend on duodenal activity of several proteases including trypsin and chymotrypsin. Aprotinin, used in two studies [35, 36], is only a weak inhibitor of chymotrypsin. Soybeans contain two protease inhibitors that differ with respect to their specificity for chymotrypsin [41]. The Kunitz inhibitor inhibits trypsin, whereas the Bowman-Birk inhibitor is also capable of inhibiting chymotrypsin. In accordance with this concept, the Bowman-Birk inhibitor was shown to increase stimulated enzyme output [42]. The role of the different protease inhibitors in feedback regulation in man is still not completely understood. Holm et al. [43] demonstrated that different concentrations of protease inhibitors in soybean meals caused different enzyme secretion. Recently, we used the protease inhibitor camostate to analyze feedback regulation in man. The intraduodenal instillation of a single dose of camostate (600 mg) markedly inhibited the enzymatic activity of trypsin and chymotrypsin in duodenal juice for a period of 90 min [44, 45]. This prolonged inhibitory effect of camostate was explained by the formation of FOY-251, the active metabolite of camostate. FOY-251 was detected in plasma for up to 3 h after ingestion of camostate [17]. It reached its plasma peak after 40 min and had a half-life time of 70 min. In man, camostate and its metabolites were measured by HPLC (R. Müller, Sanol Schwarz, Monheim, FRG) in pure pancreatic juice and bile which were obtained from ERCP at different times (30–90 min) after ingestion of 600 mg camostate (Adler, unpublished data). In bile, camostate and its metabolites were detected 60 min after ingestion of camostate. In five out of eight investigations camostate and FOY-251 were found in pure pancreatic juice 60 min after ingestion of camostate. These data show that camostate and its active metabolite appear in pure pancreatic juice and bile. Thus, it is suggested that camostate and FOY-251 due to their low molecular weight enter the pancreatic acinar cell and are released into pancreatic juice. This mechanism, however, needs further confirmation. If the active protease inhibitor is secreted by the pancreas, inhibition of pancreatic proteases could occur within the duct system. When compared to controls the enzymatic activity of trypsin and chymotrypsin in pure pancreatic juice was significantly lower after ingestion of camostate. The concentration of trypsin as measured by RIA was not different between both groups. It is concluded that camostate and its metabolite reach the pancreas via the blood supply in sufficient concentrations to be transported to the acinar cell and released into pancreatic juice. These pharmacokinetic data explain why the duodenal activities of trypsin and chymotrypsin were inhibited for 90 min after ingestion of a single dose of camostate.

The inhibition of trypsin and chymotrypsin was paralleled by a significant increase of amylase and lipase secretion [44, 45]. When trypsin output was measured by RIA, a similar increase was observed. The peak enzyme output was reached 45–75 min after intraduodenal instillation of camostate. The output of all enzymes was elevated until the end of the 90-min observation period. The infusion of secretin (0.037 CU/kg per hour, stimulated enzyme output, which was further enhanced after the instillation of camostate [44]. When pancreatic secretion was stimulated by a Lundh test meal, the enzyme output was not altered by the ingestion of camostate.

Studies in rat using protease inhibitors have shown significant trophic effects on the pancreas. It is not exactly known whether protease inhibitors are able to exert trophic effects in man. Pap et al. administered 30 g raw soy flour three times daily for 1 month in patients with chronic pancreatitis [46]. In this uncontrolled study the protease inhibitor treatment caused an increase in enzyme output after endogenous (Lundh meal) and exogenous (CCK and secretin) stimulation. The effect lasted for 3 months after protease inhibitor treatment. In a controlled study Fölsch et al. could not demonstrate an amelioration of exocrine or endocrine pancreatic function after daily treatment with 90 g soy flour in patients with chronic pancreatitis [47]. We analyzed pancreatic function in healthy volunteers after ingestion of camostate for 5 days [48]. In this short-term study camostate had no effect on basal and stimulated pancreatic enzyme secretion.

Longer periods of protease inhibitor treatment are needed to clarify whether a trophic effect of protease inhibitors on the pancreas exists in man.

Owyang et al. [39] proposed CCK as mediator of feedback regulation of pancreatic secretion in man. A test meal and the intraduodenal perfusion of phenylalanine induced an increase in plasma CCK which was abolished by concomitant duodenal perfusion of trypsin. The role of CCK in feedback regulation in man was questioned in several studies [43, 44, 49, 50]. The induction of feedback regulation in man by the protease inhibitor camostate was not accompanied by an increase in plasma CCK [44, 45, 50].

While the role of CCK in feedback regulation in man is still a matter of controversy, significant evidence has accumulated for an important role of the cholinergic system. In a study by Owyang et al. [51], the duodenal perfusion of trypsin reduced stimulated enzyme output by only 37%. The addition of atropine, however, completely abolished the enzyme response to phenylalanine. In a recent study from our laboratory, atropine completely prevented the stimulation of enzyme secretion after treatment with the protease inhibitor camostate [45]. An important argument against the mediator role of CCK in feedback regulation in man comes from a recent study using the specific CCK antagonist loxiglumide [45]. In this study, the infusion of loxiglumide had no effect on protease inhibitor-induced stimulation of pancreatic secretion.

Conclusion

A protease-specific feedback regulation of pancreatic secretion exists in rat and in man. This was proven by the use of protease inhibitors and by the duodenal perfusion of trypsin and chymotrypsin. In the rat this mechanism is mediated by CCK. The role of CCK as mediator of feedback regulation in man is still controversial. A strong argument for the humoral regulation of feedback regulation in man comes from a recent study in patients with transplanted pancreas [52]. Enzyme secretion from the pancreatic allografts was significantly inhibited by orally administered pancreatic enzyme extracts. Since the transplanted pancreas is denervated, these results point to a hormonal regulation of feedback regulation in man.

References

1. Green GM, Lyman RL (1972) Feedback regulation of pancreatic enzyme secretion as a mechanism for trypsin inhibitor-induced hypersecretion in rats. Proc Soc Exp Biol 140:6–12
2. Miyasaka K, Green GM (1984) Effect of partial exclusion of pancreatic juice on rat basal pancreatic secretion. Gastroenterology 86:114–119
3. Green GM, Nasset ES (1977) Importance of bile in regulation of intraluminal proteolytic enzyme activities in the rat. Gastroenterology 79:695–702
4. Ihse I, Lilja P, Lundquist I (1979) Trypsin as a regulator of pancreatic secretion in the rat. Scand J Gastroenterol 14: 873–880
5. Schneeman BO, Lyman RL (1975) Factors involved in the intestinal feedback regulation of pancreatic enzyme secretion in the rat. Proc Soc Exp Biol Med 148:897–903
6. Lyman RL, Olds BA, Green GM (1974) Chymotrypsinogen in the intestine of rats fed soybean trypsin inhibitor and its inability to suppress pancreatic enzyme secretions. J Nutr 104:105–110
7. Louie D, May D, Miller P, Owyang C (1986) Cholecystokinin mediates feedback regulation of pancreatic enzyme secretion in rats. Am J Physiol 250:G252–G259
8. Fölsch UR, Cantor P, Wilms HM, Schafmayer A, Becker HD, Creutzfeldt W (1987) Role of cholecystokinin in the negative feedback control of pancreatic enzyme secretion in conscious rats. Gastroenterology 92:449–458
9. Lilja P (1980) Effects of intraduodenal amylase, lipase, trypsin, and bile on pancreatic enzyme secretion in the rat. Eur Surg Res 12:383–391
10. Green GM, Levan VH (1985) Inhibition of rat pancreatic secretion by elastase. IRCS Med Sci 13:153–154
11. Fushiki T, Fukuoka S, Iwai K (1984) Stimulation of rat pancreatic enzyme secretion by diet components. Agric Biol Chem 48:1867–1874
12. Green GM, Miyasaka K (1983) Rat pancreatic response to intestinal infusion of intact and hydrolyzed protein. Am J Physiol 245:G394–G398
13. Green GM, Lyman RL (1971) Chymotrypsin inhibitor stimulation of pancreatic enzyme secretion in the rat. Proc Soc Exp Biol Med 136:649–654

14. Levan VH, Green GM (1983) Role of gastric juice in feedback regulation of rat pancreatic secretion by luminal proteases. Gastroenterology 84:1228
15. Fushiki T, Fukuoka S, Iwai K (1984) Stimulatory effect of an endogenous peptide in rat pancreatic juice on pancreatic enzyme secretion in the presence of atropine: evidence for different mode of action of stimulation from exogenous trypsin inhibitors. Biochem Biophys Res Commun 118:527–532
16. Geratz JD (1969) Secretory stimulation of the rat pancreas by p-aminobenzamidine. Am J Physiol 216:812–817
17. Saithoh Y (1982) Clinical results with an oral protease inhibitor FOY-305 in chronic pancreatitis. In: Grozinger KH, Schrey A, Wabnitz RW (eds) Proteinasen-Inhibition. Wolf, Munich, pp 156–167
18. Göke B, Adler G (1986) Biochemische Grundlagen der Wirkung von Aprotinin und der synthetischen Proteinaseninhibitoren Gabexat-Mesilat und Camostate. In: Schmidt FW, Caspary WF (eds) Ergebnisse der Gastroenterologie 1986. Demeter, Grafelfing, pp 148–150
19. Göke B, Stöckmann F, Müller R, Lankisch PG, Creutzfeldt W (1984) Effect of a specific serine protease inhibitor on the rat pancreas: systemic administration of camostate and exocrine pancreatic secretion. Digestion 30:171–178
20. Beckh KH, Göke B, Müller R, Arnold R (1987) Elimination of the low molecular weight proteinase inhibitor camostate (FOY-305) and its degradation products by the rat liver. Res Exp Med 187:401–406
21. Göke B, Leferink J, Göke R, Adler G (1989) Effect of a low-molecular weight serine proteinase inhibitor (camostate) on amylase release from isolated pancreatic acini. Res Exp Med 189:33–38
22. Rausch U, Adler G, Weidenbach H, Weidenbach F, Rudolff D, Koop I, Kern HF (1987) Stimulation of pancreatic enzyme secretory process in the rat by low-molecular weight proteinase inhibitor. Cell Tissue Res 247:187–193
23. Göke B, Printz H, Koop I, Rausch U, Richter G, Arnold R, Adler G (1986) Endogenous CCK release and pancreatic growth in rats after feeding a proteinase inhibitor (camostate). Pancreas 1:509–515
24. Puplat P, Elsässer HP, Adler G, Kern HF. Autoradiographic study on the early trophic effect of camostate on rat pancreas. (submitted for publication)
25. Yonezawa H (1983) Secretory responses of hypertrophied rat pancreas induced by repeated oral administrations of a synthetic protease inhibitor. Jpn J Physiol 33:183–195
26. Keim V, Göke B, Adler G (1988) Changes in pattern of enzyme secretion by rat pancreas during repeated trypsin inhibitor treatment. Am J Physiol 255:G236–G241
27. Wisner JR, McLaughlin RE, Rich KA, Ozawa S, Renner IG (1988) Effects of L-364,718, a new cholecystokinin receptor antagonist, on camostate-induced growth of the rat pancreas. Gastroenterology 94:109–113
28. Niederau C, Liddle RA, Grendell JH (1986) Chronic camostate exerts a trophic effect on the pancreas which is blocked by a CCK inhibitor. Gastroenterology 90:1565
29. Louie DS, Liang JP, Owyang C (1988) Characterisation of a new CCK antagonist, L364,718: in vitro and in vivo studies. Am J Physiol 255:G261–G266
30. Kashima K, Sato T, Herman L (1988) Morphometric study of the rat exocrine pancreas after diversion of bile and pancreatic juice from the intestine. Gastroenterology 95:1607–1616
31. Lu L, Louie D, Owyang C (1989) A cholecystokinin peptide mediates feedback regulation of pancreatic secretion. Am J Physiol 256:G430–G435
32. Fushiki T, Iwai K (1989) Two hypotheses on the feedback regulation of pancreatic enzyme secretion. FASEB J 3:121–126
33. Schneeman BO, Gallaher D (1986) Pancreatic response to dietary trypsin inhibitor: variations among species. Adv Exp Biol Med 199:185–187
34. Ihse I, Lilja P, Lundquist I (1977) Feedback regulation of pancreatic enzyme secretion by intestinal trypsin in man. Digestion 15:303–308
35. Krawisz B, Miller L, DiMagno E, Go V (1980) In the absence of nutrients, pancreatic-biliary secretions in the jejunum do not exert feedback control of human pancreatic or gastric function. J Lab Clin Med 95:13–18
36. Hotz J, Ho S, Go V, DiMagno E (1983) Short term inhibition of duodenal trypsin activity does not affect human pancreatic biliary or gastric function. Lab Clin Med 101:488–495

37. Dlugosz J, Fölsch UF, Creutzfeldt W (1983) Inhibition of intraduodenal trypsin does not stimulate exocrine pancreatic secretion in humans. Digestion 26:197–204
38. Slaff J, Jacobson D, Tillman CR, Curington C, Toskes P (1984) Protease-specific suppression of pancreatic exocrine secretion. Gastroenterology 87:44–52
39. Owyang C, Louie D, Tatum D (1986) Feedback regulation of pancreatic enzyme secretion. J Clin Invest 77:2042–2047
40. Dlugosz J, Fölsch UR, Czajkowski A, Gabryelewicz A (1988) Feedback regulation of stimulated pancreatic enzyme secretion during intraduodenal perfusion of trypsin in man. Eur J Clin Invest 18:267–272
41. Liener IE (1986) Trypsin inhibitors: concern for human nutrition or not? J Nutr 116:920–923
42. Liener IE, Goodale R, Deshmukh A, Satterberg T, Ward G, di Pietro C, Bankey P, Borner J (1988) Effect of a trypsin inhibitor from soybeans (Bowman-Birk) on the secretory activity of the human pancreas. Gastroenterology 94:419–427
43. Holm H, Hanssen H, Krogdahl A, Florholmen J (1988) High and low inhibitor soybean meals affect human duodenal protease activity differently. J Nutr 118:515–520
44. Adler G, Müllenhoff A, Bozkurt T, Göke B, Koop I, Arnold R (1988) Stimulation of pancreatic secretion in man by a protease inhibitor. Eur J Clin Invest 18:98–104
45. Adler G, Reinshagen M, Koop I, Göke B, Schafmayer A, Rovati L, Arnold R (1989) Differential effects of atropine and a cholecystokinin receptor antagonist on pancreatic secretion. Gastroenterology 96:1158–1164
46. Pap A, Berger Z, Varro V (1983) Beneficial effect of a soy flour diet in chronic pancreatitis. M Sinai J Med (NY) 50:208–212
47. Fölsch UR, Öldendörp A, Siegel E, Lembcke B, Lankisch PG, Creutzfeldt W (1984) Wirkung einer Sojabohnendiät auf die exokrine und endokrine Pankreasfunktion des Menschen. Verh Dtsch Ges Inn Med 90:1062–1065
48. Adler G, Müllenhoff A, Bozkurt T, Göke B, Koop I, Arnold R (1988) Comparison of the effect of single and repeated administrations of a protease inhibitor (camostate) on pancreatic secretion in man. Scand J Gastroenterol 23:158–162
49. Olsen O, Schaffalitzky de Muckadell OB, Cantor P, Erlanson-Albertsson C, Palnaes Hansen C, Worning H (1988) Effect of trypsin on the hormonal regulation of the fat-stimulated human exocrine pancreas. Scand J Gastroenterol 23:875–881
50. Watanabe S, Shitatori K, Takeuchi T, Chey W (1986) Intrajejunal administration of a synthetic trypsin inhibitor (camostate) stimulates the release of endogenous secretin but not cholecystokinin in man. Gastroenterology 90:1685
51. Owyang C, May D, Louie D (1986) Trypsin suppression of pancreatic enzyme secretion. Gastroenterology 91:637–643
52. Burton FR, Garvin PJ, Shoba NJ (1989) Human pancreatic graft fistula exocrine suppresssion by oral pancreatic enzymes. Transplantation 47:888–891

Influence of Cholecystokinin-Receptor Antagonists on Feedback Regulation of Pancreatic Secretion*

C. Niederau, M. Niederau, R. Lüthen, and J. H. Grendell[1]

Development and Characterization of CCK-Receptor Antagonists

In 1981 proglumide and benzotript were shown to act as specific and competitive CCK-receptor antagonists in vitro [32]. However, these compounds had low potencies in antagonizing the action of CCK in the intact organ [62]. More recently, several new CCK antagonists have been described which are more potent in vitro compared to proglumide. First, C-terminal CCK fragments or analogs such as CCK-(27-32)-amide were shown to act as specific CCK antagonists up to 75 times more potent than proglumide [77]. CCK fragments, however, were shown to be rapidly degraded in physiological fluids [45]. Subsequently, peptide molecules with a proglumide-like structure were synthesized which were up to 500–5000 times more potent than proglumide in vitro and in vivo [53, 64–66] (Fig. 1). More recently, asperlicin, a nonpeptide substance isolated from *Aspergillus aliaceus* (Fig. 1) was shown to act as a specific CCK-antagonist which was 200 times more potent than proglumide in inhibiting CCK-stimulated secretion in vitro [11] (Fig. 2). Asperlicin, however, was poorly water soluble and, thus, difficult to use for in vivo experiments. In 1986, several nonpeptide substances, structurally similar to asperlicin, were described which were more water soluble than asperlicin. The most potent of these asperlicin derivatives, L-364,718, was shown to be 10000 to 3000000 times more potent than proglumide in inhibiting CCK's action and binding in vitro and in vivo [10, 12, 18, 66] (Figs. 1, 2). Both the new potent peptide and nonpeptide antagonist only inhibit the actions of those agonists which bind to the CCK receptor [66]. All antagonists exhibit the kinetics of competitive inhibition [66]. The rank order of potency of the compounds to antagonize cerulein-stimulated secretion in vivo agreed with their relative potencies to antagonize cerulein- or CCK-8-stimulated amylase secretion from pancreatic acini in vitro as well as with their affinity to bind to peripheral CCK receptors in vitro [66] (Fig. 2). Although the antagonists showed the same order of potency in vitro and in

* C. Niederau was supported by grants from the Deutsche Forschungsgemeinschaft (Ni 224/1-1, 224/2-1, and 224/2-2) and from the Ministerium für Wissenschaft und Forschung des Landes Nordrhein-Westfalen. J. H. Grendell was supported by grants from the Research Evaluation and Allocation Committee, the Committee on Research of the Academic Senate, School of Medicine, University of California, San Francisco, and the National Institute of Health (DK 38939)

[1] Medizinische Klinik und Poliklinik, Abteilung für Gastroenterologie, Heinrich-Heine-Universität Düsseldorf, FRG, Departments of Medicine and Physiology, University of California, San Francisco, CA 94143, and Medical Service, San Francisco General Hospital, San Francisco, CA 94110, USA

PROGLUMIDE

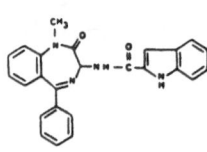

CR1392

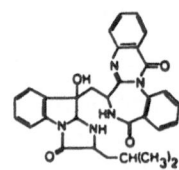

CR1409

CR1505

L-364,718

ASPERLICIN

Fig. 1. Structure of various CCK-receptor antagonists. Molecular weights are 334 for proglumide, 441 for CR1392, 483 for CR1505, 462 for CR1409, 535 for asperlicin, and 408 for L-364,718 (Modified from Niederau et al. [66])

vivo, in particular the most potent antagonists CR1409 and L-364,718 were in relation to proglumide 10–33 times less potent in vivo than in vitro [66] (Fig. 2).

Influence of CCK-Receptor Antagonists on Feedback Regulation

Secretory studies in the Experimental Animal

The diversion of pancreatobiliary secretions from the proximal small intestine produces a marked increase in pancreatic secretion in the rat [29, 30, 56, 57]. A similar increase in secretion is seen if rats are fed trypsin inhibitors [19], or after the infusion of trypsin inhibitors into the duodenum [38, 74]. This stimulation of secretion is thought to be due to feedback inhibition of pancreatic secretion which is suppressed when the protease activity in the duodenum is lowered. On the other hand, intraduodenal administration of proteases abolishes the increase in pancreatic secretion seen after diversion of pancreatobiliary juice. Feedback regulation has been demonstrated in the rat [29, 30, 38, 56, 57], chicken [4, 13], pig [14, 39], hamster [5], mouse [65], and calf [15], but appears to be absent in the dog [16, 72]. Several studies indicate that the increase in pancreatic secretion induced by diversion of pan-

IN-VITRO EXPERIMENTS

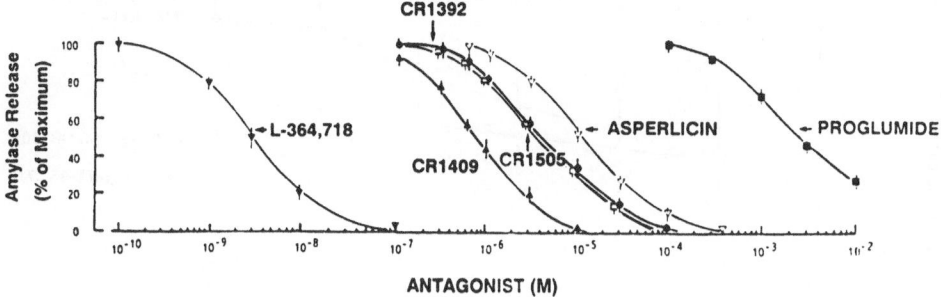

IN-VIVO EXPERIMENTS

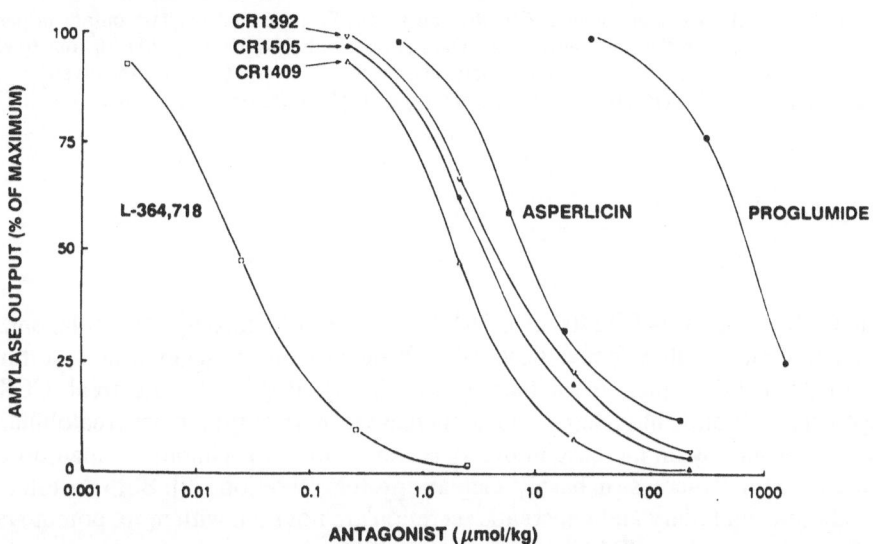

Fig. 2A, B. Comparative inhibitory potencies of various CCK-receptor antagonists. **A** In vitro experiments: Effects of antagonists on amylase release from isolated pancreatic acini stimulated by 60 pM CCK-8. In each experiment, basal release was subtracted and stimulated release was calculated as a percentage of maximal release in that experiment. Basal and maximal release in these experiments was 2%–5% and 24%–33%, respectively. **B** In vivo experiments: Effects of antagonists on ductal secretion of amylase in the anesthesized rat. Secretions were calculated as mean integrated 1-h responses to 0.25 μg/kg cerulein. Data are presented as percentages of the response to this cerulein dose in the absence of antagonists. Standard errors are omitted for illustrative reasons and were 1%–5% (n = 4–8). (Modified from Niederau et al. [66])

creatobiliary juice or administration of protease inhibitors is associated with an increase in endogenous CCK [22, 50, 75]. A similar increase in the fasting plasma concentration of CCK was also observed in the pancreatic duct-ligated rats [75].

Our own experiments show that in the anesthesized rat amylase output in pancreatobiliary secretion only slightly increased after diversion of pancreatobiliary juice (Fig. 3; as yet unpublished results). This increase was completely inhibited by both the CCK-antagonists CR1409 and L-364,718 (Fig. 3). Intravenous administration of the

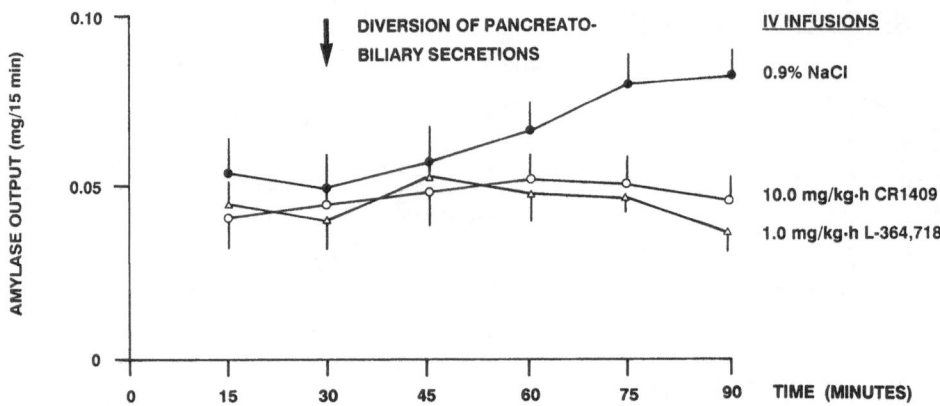

Fig. 3. Effects of the CCK antagonists CR1409 and L-364,718 on ductal amylase output in pancreatobiliary secretion in the anesthesized rat. Data are presented as means ± SD for four to six independent experiments. Amylase output only slightly increased 45–60 min after diversion of pancreatobiliary secretion ($P < 0.05$ by analysis of variance). This increase was abolished by both CR 1409 and L-364,718

potent CCK-antagonists CR1409 or L-364,718 at doses which completely antagonize the action of maximally effective doses of CCK did not alter basal enzyme secretion prior to diversion of pancreatobiliary juice (Fig. 3). Previously, the weak CCK-antagonist proglumide has been shown to increase protein output in pancreatobiliary secretion, mainly by an increase in biliary secretion [59]. Proglumide at high doses also caused a small increase in basal pancreatic protein secretion [59]. Both the effects of proglumide on biliary and pancreatic secretion are not seen with more potent and specific antagonists like CR1409 and L-364,718 [66].

In conscious rats equipped with pancreatic and biliary cannulas pancreatic protein output markedly increased after diversion of pancreatobiliary juice (Fig. 4; as yet unpublished results). The CCK antagonists CR1409 and L-364,718 significantly inhibited this increase in pancreatic protein secretion after diversion of pancreatobiliary juice. However, after diversion there was still some increase in protein output compared to prior basal values despite the administration of high doses of the potent CCK-antagonists (Fig. 4). Pancreatic protein secretion during recirculation of pancreatobiliary juice tended to be lower in the presence of CCK antagonists, although the differences compared to the infusion of 0.9% NaCl did not reach statistical significance (Fig. 4). The intravenous administration of atropine, however, markedly decreased basal pancreatic protein secretion during recirculation of pancreatobiliary juice when compared to control studies with NaCl infusion (Fig. 4). Atropine only partly inhibited the increase in pancreatic protein secretion after diversion of pancreatobiliary juice, similar to what was reported previously [56]. Only the simultaneous administration of atropine and the CCK-antagonist CR1409 completely inhibited the increase in pancreatic secretion after diversion of pancreatobiliary juice in conscious rats. The simultaneous administration of atropine and CR1409 also caused a

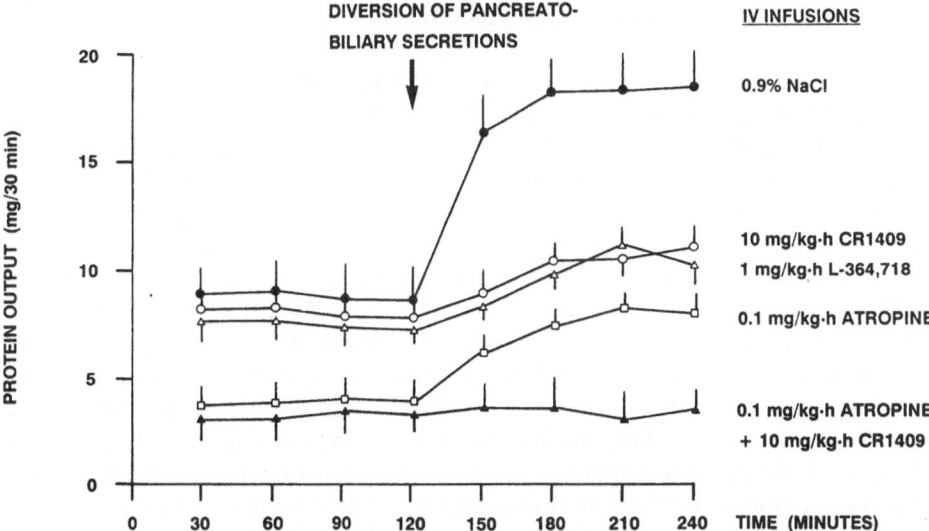

Fig. 4. Effects of the CCK antagonists CR1409 and L-364,718 and of atropine on ductal amylase output in pancreatic secretion in the conscious rat equipped with pancreatic and biliary cannulas. Data are presented as means ± SD for four to six independent experiments. Amylase output sharply increased 30 min after diversion of pancreatobiliary secretion ($P < 0.01$ by analysis of variance). This increase was markedly reduced but not completely abolished by the CCK antagonists CR1409 and L-364,718. Both CCK antagonists did not significantly alter pancreatic protein secretion under recirculation of pancreatobiliary secretion. Atropine, however, markedly reduced protein secretion under recirculation ($P < 0.01$) and partly reduced the increase in pancreatic protein secretion after diversion. Only the simulatenous administration of both atropine and CR1409 completely abolished the increase in pancreatic protein secretion after diversion of pancreatobiliary secretion

marked inhibition of basal pancreatic secretion (pancreatic juice recirculated). Thus, the basal tone of rat pancreatic secretion under the physiological conditions of drainage of pancreatic and biliary juice into the proximal small intestine appears to be mainly regulated by cholinergic mechanisms. In the rat, atropine had no effect on pancreatic enzyme output during intraduodenal infusion of a protease inhibitor [24]. The stimulation of pancreatic secretion after diversion of pancreatobiliary juice appears to be regulated mainly by CCK and to a lesser part also by cholinergic factors. In addition other factors like secretin might be involved in the mediation of feedback stimulation after diversion of pancreatobiliary juice [78]. Previous studies with the weak CCK- and gastrin-receptor antagonist proglumide also suggested that CCK blockade reduces the increase in pancreatic secretion seen after diversion of pancreatobiliary juice [22, 50, 59, 75]. Similar to the results obtained with specific CCK-receptor antagonists immunoneutralization of circulating free CCK with an anti-CCK serum also inhibited the increase in secretion induced by diversion in the rat [75].

In summary, several recent studies using specific CCK-receptor antagonists and anti-CCK serum support the original proposal of Green and Lyman [29] and Green et al. [30] that CCK plays an important role in the mechanism of exocrine pancreatic feedback inhibition in rats.

Studies on Pancreatic Growth in the Experimental Animal

It is well established that exogenous CCK and CCK analogs, like cerulein, as well as feeding of trypsin inhibitors stimulate pancreatic growth in the experimental animal [13, 19–21, 65]. Pancreatobiliary diversion also stimulates pancreatic growth in the rat [29, 55]. Both feeding of trypsin inhibitors and pancreatobiliary diversion may stimulate pancreatic growth by the same mechanism of decreasing intraduodenal activity of proteases. The inhibition of proteases by potent inhibitors, such as camostate, or their diversion from the duodenum is thought to cause an increase in plasma CCK which may mediate pancreatic growth [29, 55]. Recent studies have tried to establish the hormone responsible for pancreatic growth after pancreatobiliary diversion or feeding of a protease inhibitor by administration of the weak CCK- and gastrin-antagonist proglumide [26, 55]. Proglumide significantly inhibited pancreatic growth after pancreatobiliary diversion as well as after camostate feeding [26, 55]. However, in the previous studies proglumide only partly inhibited pancreatic growth due to these stimuli. Furthermore, proglumide at high doses exerted a trophic effect which was interpreted as a partial agonist activity [26, 82].

Recently, we have studied the effects of the potent and specific CCK-receptor antagonist CR1409 on pancreatic growth stimulated by exogenous CCK or by feeding of the protease inhibitor camostate in mice [65]. Feeding of camostate for 10 days not only stimulated growth of the mouse pancreas but also markedly increased plasma concentrations of CCK. The CCK antagonist CR1409 greatly reduced the stimulatory effect of camostate feeding and completely abolished the effect of exogenous CCK [65]. The antagonist CR1409, given without exogenous CCK or substances which release endogenous CCK, did not show any stimulation of pancreatic growth and, thus, no partial agonist activity. Feedback stimulation of pancreatic growth after inhibition of intraduodenal proteases, previously described in the rat [19, 20, 26, 55], also exists in the mouse. This camostate-induced feedback stimulation of mouse pancreatic growth is mainly mediated by release of CCK [65].

Secretory Studies in Healthy Humans

The nature of feedback regulation of pancreatic secretion in humans remains unclear. In patients whose pancreatic juice is excluded from the duodenum by tumor obstruction or diverted by fistulas, pancreatic secretion was decreased when trypsin or pancreatic juice was infused into the duodenum [6, 39, 83]. It was also reported that intraduodenal administration of trypsin decreases pancreatic enzyme secretion in healthy humans and in patients with chronic pancreatitis [68, 69, 76]. CCK has been suggested as a mediator of such feedback control in humans [68, 69, 73, 76]. Other workers, however, were unable to show that the inhibition of duodenal trypsin activity [17, 36, 46] or the infusion of pancreatic juice or trypsin into the small intestine affect basal pancreatic enzyme secretion or plasma concentrations of CCK [2, 35, 44]. The involvement of secretin in feedback regulation was shown in two studies [67, 80], but not observed in two other investigations [2, 35].

Most previous human studies were, however, associated with potential pitfalls. In humans it is difficult to quantitatively assess basal pancreatic secretion. It is even more difficult to completely collect or divert pancreatic secretion in healthy volunteers.

Furthermore, protease inhibitors used in most previous studies mainly inhibited trypsin activity, but did not to the same extent inhibit the activities of chymotrypsin and elastase. The regulatory mechanism might, however, depend not only on duodenal activity of trypsin, but also on the activity of other proteases like chymotrypsin or elastase [8, 28, 36]. At least in the rat, the latter enzymes are able to reduce the increase in pancreatic secretion due to loss of feedback inhibition [28]. In the rat recirculation of only 5% of the diverted pancreatic juice was able to markedly inhibit the feedback response after diversion of pancreatobiliary juice [57]. Most previous studies in humans, however, were not able to cause a 95% inhibition of trypsin and chymotrypsin by intraduodenal infusion of protease inhibitors. Recent studies also suggested a physiologic role of bile salts in the negative feedback regulation of release of CCK and pancreatic enzyme secretion in response to nutrients in dogs and humans [27].

Aprotinin, used in two previous human studies [17, 36], is only a weak inhibitor of chymotrypsin [54, 78]. The two protease inhibitors in soybeans differ in their specificity for chymotrypsin [48]. The Kunitz inhibitor mainly inhibits trypsin, whereas the Bowman-Birk inhibitor also inhibits chymotrypsin. In a recent study, the intraduodenal infusion of Bowman-Birk inhibitor-supplemented pancreatic juice increased pancreatic enzyme secretion stimulated by intraduodenal amino acids and secretin [49]. In this study both trypsin and chymotrypsin activities had been abolished and pancreatic secretion was collected by direct cannulation of the papilla.

Feeding of the synthetic protease inhibitor camostate to rats induced a marked increase in plasma CCK and in pancreatic secretion [26, 70]. In humans the intraduodenal administration of camostate stimulated pancreatic enzyme secretion, but did not increase plasma CCK [5, 14]. Furthermore, the infusion of the CCK antagonist loxiglumide did not alter camostate-induced stimulation of amylase and lipase secretion [3]. Atropine, however, completely inhibited the increase in pancreatic secretion after duodenal infusion of camostate [3]. Thus, in humans there appears to exist a cholinergic regulation of the pancreatic feedback mechanism without involvement of CCK. However, these results of the only study which as yet has evaluated the effects of a potent CCK antagonist on camostate-induced feedback regulation in humans do not conclusively answer the question whether feedback control of basal pancreatic secretion in humans is also mediated by other than cholinergic mechanisms such as CCK and secretin. Similar to most previous studies camostate inhibited chymotrypsin activity only by about 75% [3]. A stronger inhibition of intraduodenal proteases might have further increased pancreatic secretion and possibly also plasma CCK. In addition, it is unclear whether camostate only acts by inhibition of intraduodenal proteases or whether it may also directly stimulate pancreatic secretion by cholinergic or peptidergic mechanisms. Indeed, recent studies in the rat showed that the elimination of pancreatic enzymes from the intestine does not affect camostate-induced stimulation of pancreatic secretion nor the release of CCK [81]. On the other hand camostate did not stimulate amylase release from isolated rat pancreatic acini [1].

Cholinergic mechanisms are also involved in feedback regulation of stimulated pancreatic secretion in humans [68–69]. Intraduodenal infusion of trypsin inhibited phenylalanine-stimulated release of CCK in a dose-related manner. The minimal concentration of trypsin needed to reduce the rise in plasma CCK was comparable to the amount required to decrease pancreatic enzyme secretion [68]. These observations suggest that trypsin mediates feedback regulation of pancreatic enzyme secretion by inhibiting the release of CCK [68]. Although plasma CCK levels decreased to basal values during intraduodenal perfusion of phenylalanine and trypsin, there remained a significant increase in pancreatic enzyme secretion [68]. In addition, the duodenal perfusion of trypsin reduced phenylalanine-stimulated enzyme secretion by only 37%. Infusion of atropine plus perfusion of trypsin, however, completely abolished enzyme response to phenylalanine stimulation [68–69]. Thus, stimulated pancreatic enzyme secretion is probably regulated by both CCK and cholinergic mechanisms.

In summary, the human studies indicate that proteases are able to inhibit stimulated pancreatic secretion and that inhibition of proteases might increase stimulated secretion. In humans, such feedback mechanisms appear to be difficult to demonstrate for basal pancreatic secretion. It is unclear whether complete inhibition of intraduodenal proteases or complete diversion of proteases from the small intestine results in an increase in gastrointestinal hormones such as CCK and secretin. Feedback regulation of pancreatic secretion may differ between humans and rats. In the latter species administration of trypsin inhibitors markedly stimulates the exocrine pancreas, and trypsin in the duodenum inhibits pancreatic secretion [29, 30]. In humans, however, basal amounts of trypsin in the duodenum may be too small to exert an inhibitory effect [68–69].

This may explain the results of those studies which failed to show a significant feedback control of human pancreatic secretion in the absence of stimulatory nutrients or hormones [46]. Feedback inhibition in rats versus humans may also differ with respect to the involvement of CCK. Whereas, in the rat, studies with CCK antagonists clearly demonstrate an important role for CCK in feedback regulation, the only study which employed a CCK antagonist in humans was unable to corroborate the rat results [3]. Instead, the human study suggests that cholinergic mechanisms may mediate feedback regulation of basal pancreatic secretion in humans without involvement of CCK [3]. As yet a role of CCK in feedback regulation in humans has only been demonstrated for stimulated pancreatic secretion [68–69].

Studies in Patients with Chronic Pancreatic Insufficiency

The existence of a feedback regulation of pancreatic enzyme secretion in man may have important clinical implications. Chronic pancreatic insufficiency may be associated with elevated plasma CCK levels. This may reflect a failure in the feedback regulation of CCK release due to a deficiency of pancreatic enzyme secretion. The elevated CCK concentrations may stimulate the pancreatic secretion and intraductal pressure, and finally produce pain. Thus, effective enzyme replacement may reduce stimulation and pain. Indeed, large doses of pancreatic extract have been reported to produce relief of pain in a considerable number of patients with chronic pancreatitis [40, 76]. However, other studies in patients with chronic pancreatitis failed to show an increase in plasma concentration of CCK [7, 9, 44] as well as an effect of oral administration of enzymes on pain [33].

Mechanism of CCK Release

Until recently the increase in pancreatic secretion after diversion of pancreatobiliary juice and after intraduodenal infusion of a trypsin inhibitor was thought to be caused by the same mechanism. At least in the rat, both diversion of pancreatobiliary juice and intraduodenal administration of a trypsin inhibitor increase plasma CCK concentrations. Although release of CCK appears to be a common mechanism in the two treatments, the trigger for CCK release may not be the same. Atropine only inhibits pancreatic enzyme secretion induced by diversion of pancreatobiliary juice in the rat, but it does not affect enzyme secretion induced by intraluminal infusion of soybean trypsin inhibitors [23, 47]. This suggests that the mechanisms underlying the stimulation of enzyme secretion are not completely identical.

Recently, a new peptide, called "monitor peptide," was isolated from pancreatic secretions in the rat [41, 42]. This monitor peptide was suggested to cause the increase in pancreatic enzyme secretion after intraduodenal administration of trypsin inhibitors or food [23, 25, 43, 57]. The peptide, however, cannot be involved in the mechanism underlying diversion-induced hypersecretion because it is removed after diversion of pancreatobiliary juice. Thus, feedback regulation of pancreatic enzyme secretion appears to be controlled by two different systems, an atropine-sensitive mechanism and an atropine-insensitive one [24, 25, 43].

Also, recently, the existence of a trypsin-sensitive, CCK-releasing peptide has been reported in the small intestine [31, 51, 52]. The secretion of this small (1000 MW) CCK-releasing peptide from the small intestine has been proposed to be cholinergically mediated [31]. It has also been shown that its release may be inhibited by somatostatin [34].

Acknowledgment. The authors thank Ms. Christine Genz and Ms. Monika Ebbert for expert technical assistance.

References

1. Adler G, Rausch U, Weidenbach F, Arnold R, Kern HF (1984) General and selective inhibition of pancreatic enzyme discharge using a proteinase inhibitor (FOY-305). Klin Wochenschr 62:406–411
2. Adler G, Müllenhoff A, Koop I (1988) Stimulation of pancreatic secretion in man by a protease inhibitor (camostate). Eur J Clin Invest 18:98–104
3. Adler G, Reinshagen M, Koop I, Göke B, Schafmayer A, Rovati LC, Arnold R (1989) Differential effects of atropine and a cholecystokinin receptor antagonist on pancreatic secretion. Gastroenterology 96:1158–1164
4. Alumot E, Nitsan Z (1961) The influence of soybean antitrypsin on the intestinal proteolysis of the chicken. J Nutr 73:71–77
5. Andrén-Sandberg A, Ihse I (1983) Regulatory effect on the pancreas of intraduodenal pancreatic juice and trypsin in the Syrian golden hamster. Scand J Gastroenterol 18:697–706
6. Boyd EJS, Cumming JGR, Cuschieri A, Wormsley KG (1985) Aspects of feedback control of pancreatic secretion in man. Ital J Gastroenterol 17:18–22
7. Bozkurt T, Adler G, Koop I, Koop H, Türmer W, Arnold W (1988) Plasma CCK levels in patients with pancreatic insufficiency. Dig Dis Sci 33:276–281
8. Campbell DR, Potter ML, Curington CW, Toskes PP (1986) Evidence that elastase may be important in feedback control of pancreatic exocrine secretion (Abstr). Dig Dis Sci 31:1127

9. Cantor P, Petronijevic L, Worning H (1986) Plasma cholecystokinin concentrations in patients with advanced chronic pancreatitis. Pancreas 1:488–493

10. Chang RSL, Lotti VJ (1988) Biochemical and pharmacological characterization of an extremely potent and selective nonpeptide cholecystokinin receptor antagonist. Proc Natl Acad Sci USA 83:4923–4926

11. Chang RSL, Monaghan RL, Birnbaum J, Stapley AA, Goetz MA, Albers-Schonberg G, Patchett AA, Liesch JM, Hensens OD, Springer JP (1985) A potent nonpeptide cholecystokinin antagonist selective for peripheral tissues isolated from *Aspergillus aliaceus*. Science 230:177–179

12. Chang RSL, Lotti VJ, Chen TB, Kunkel KA (1986) Characterization of the binding of (^{2}H)-(±)-L364,718: a new potent, nonpeptide cholecystokinin antagonist radioligand selective for peripheral receptors. Mol Pharmacol 30:212–217

13. Chernick SS, Lepkovsky S, Chaikoff IL (1948) A dietary factor regulating the enzyme content of the pancreas: changes induced in size and proteolytic activity of the chick pancreas by ingestion of raw soybean meal. Am J Physiol 115:33–41

14. Corring T (1973) Mechanisme de la secrétion pancréatique exocrine chez le porc: regulation par rétro inhibition. Ann Biol Anim Biochim Biophys 13:755–756

15. Davicco MJ, Lefaivre J, Thivend P, Bartlet JP (1979) Feedback regulation of pancreatic secretion in the young milk-fed calf. Ann Biol Anim Biochim Biophys 19:1147–1152

16. Diaz GR, Devaux MA, Johnson CD (1981) Physiological condition for the study of basal and meal stimulated exocrine pancreatic secretion in the dog. Absence of feedback inhibition of basal secretion. Can J Physiol Pharmacol 60:1287–1295

17. Dlugosz J, Fölsch UR, Creutzfeldt W (1983) Inhibition of intraduodenal trypsin does not stimulate exocrine pancreatic secretion in man. Digestion 26:197–204

18. Evans BE, Block MG, Rittle KE, DiPardo RM, Whitter WL, Veber DF, Anderson PS, Freidinger RM (1986) Design of potent, orally effective, nonpeptidal antagonists of the peptide hormone cholecystokinin. Proc Natl Acad Sci USA 83:4918–4922

19. Fölsch UR, Creutzfeldt W (1985) Adaptation of the pancreas during treatment with enzyme inhibitors in rats and man. Scand J Gastroenterol [Suppl 112] 20:54–63

20. Fölsch UR, Winckler K, Wormsley KG (1974) Effect of soybean diet on enzyme content and ultrastructure of the rat exocrine pancreas. Digestion 11:161–171

21. Fölsch UR, Winckler K, Wormsley KG (1978) Influence of repeated administration of cholecystokinin and secretin on the pancreas of the rat. Scand J Gastroenterol 13:663–671

22. Fölsch UR, Cantor P, Wilms HM, Schafmayer A, Becker HD, Creutzfeldt W (1987) Role of cholecystokinin in the negative feedback control of pancreatic enzyme secretion in conscious rats. Gastroenterology 92:449–458

23. Fukuoka S, Tsujikawa M, Fushiki T, Iwai K (1986) Stimulation of pancreatic enzyme secretion by a peptide purified from rat bile-pancreatic juice. J Nutr 116:1540–1546

24. Fushiki T, Fukuoka S, Kajiura H, Iwai K (1978) Atropine-non-sensitive feedback regulatory mechanism of rat pancreatic enzyme secretion in response to food protein intake. J Nutr 117:948–954

25. Fushiki T, Fukuoka S, Iwai K (1984) Stimulatory effect of an endogenous peptide in rat pancreatic juice on pancreatic enzyme secretion in the presence of atropine: evidence for different mode of action of stimulation from exogenous trypsin inhibitors. Biochem Biophys Res Commun 18:532–537

26. Göke B, Printz H, Koop I (1986) Endogenous CCK release and pancreatic growth in rats after feeding a proteinase inhibitor (camostate). Pancreas 1:509–515

27. Gomez G, Upp JR, Louis F, Alexander RW, Poston GJ, Greeley GH, Thompson JC (1988) Regulation of the release of cholecystokinin by bile salts in dogs and humans. Gastroenterology 94:1036–1346

28. Green GM, Levan VH (1985) Inhibition of rat pancreatic secretion by elastase. IRCS Med Sci 13:153–154

29. Green GM, Lyman RL (1972) Feedback regulation of pancreatic enzyme secretion as a mechanism for trypsin inhibitor-induced hypersecretion in rats. Proc Soc Exp Biol Med 140:6–12

30. Green GM, Olds BA, Matthews G, Louis DS (1973) Protein as a regulator of pancreatic enzyme secretion in the rat. Proc Soc Exp Biol Med 142:1162–1167

31. Guan D, Ohta H, Tawil T, Liddle R, Green G (1988) Regulation of rat pancreatic secretion by a putative intraluminal CCK-releasing factor: effect of atropine. Gastroenterology 17:158

32. Hahne WF, Jensen RT, Lemp GF, Gardener JD (1981) Proglumide and benzotript: members of a different class of cholecystokinin receptor antagonists. Proc Natl Acad Sci USA 78:6304–6308
33. Halgreen H, Pedersen NT, Worning H (1986) Symptomatic effect of pancreatic enzyme therapy in patients with chronic pancreatitis. J Gastroenterol 21:104–108
34. Herzig KH, Lu L, May D, Owyng C (1989) Somatostatin inhibits feedback regulation of pancreatic enzyme secretion: activation of the inhibitory regulation protein (G1) to inhibit secretion of CCK releasing peptide. Gastroenterology 94:A207
35. Holm H, Hanssen LE, Krogdahl A, Florholmen J (1988) High and low inhibitor soybean meals affect human duodenal proteinase activity differently: in vivo comparison with bovine serum albumin. J Nutr 118:515–520
36. Hotz J, Ho SB, Go VLW, DiMagno EP (1983) Short-term inhibition of duodenal tryptic activity does not affect human pancreatic, biliary, or gastric function. J Lab Clin Med 101:488–495
37. Ihse I, Lilja P (1979) Effect of intestinal amylase and trypsin on pancreatic secretion in the pig, Scand J Gastroenterol 14:1009–1013
38. Ihse I, Lilja P, Lundquist I (1974) Trypsin as a regulator of pancreatic secretion in the rat. Scand J Gastroenterol 14:875–880
39. Ihse I, Lilja P, Lundquist I (1977) Feedback regulation of pancreatic enzyme secretion by intestinal trypsin in man. Digestion 15:303–308
40. Isaksson G, Ihse I (1983) Pain reduction by an oral pancreatic enzyme preparation in chronic pancreatitis. Dig Dis Sci 28:97–102
41. Iwai K, Fukuoka S, Fusiki T, Kodaira T, Ikai N (1986) Elevation of plasma CCK concentration after intestinal administration of a pancreatic enzyme secretion-stimulating peptide purified from rat bile-pancreatic juice, analysis with N-terminal region specific radioimmunoassay. Biochem Biophys Res Commun 136:701–706
42. Iwai K, Fukuoka S, Fushiki T (1987) Purification and sequencing of a trypsin-sensitive cholcystokinin releasing peptide from rat pancreatic juice. J Biol Chem 262:8950–8959
43. Iwai K, Fushiki T, Fukuoka S (1988) Pancreatic enzyme secretion mediated by novel peptide: monitor peptide hypothesis. Pancreas 3:720–728
44. Jansen J, Hopman W, Lamers C (1984) Plasma cholecystokinin concentration in patients with pancreatic insufficiency measured by sequence-specific radioimmunoassays. Dig Dis Sci 29:1108–1117
45. Koulischer DL, Moroder L, Deschodt-Lanckman M (1982) Degradation of cholecystokinin octapeptide, related fragments and analogs by human and rat plasma in vitro. Regul Pept 4:127–139
46. Krawitz BR, Miller LJ, DiMagno EP, Go VLW (1980) In the absence of nutrients, pancreatic-biliary secretions in the jejunum do not exert feedback control of human pancreatic or gastric function. J Lab Clin Med 95:13–18
47. Levan VH, Green GM (1986) Effect of atropine on rat pancreatic secretory response to trypsin inhibitors and protein. Am J Physiol 251:G64–69
48. Liener IE (1986) Trypsin inhibitors: concern for human nutrition or not? J Nutr 116:920–923
49. Liener IE, Goodale RL, Deshmukh A, Satterber TI, Ward G, DiPietro CM, Bankey PE, Borner JW (1988) Effect of a trypsin inhibitor from soybeans (Bowman-Birk) on the secretory activity of the human pancreas. Gastroenterology 94:419–427
50. Louie DS, May D, Miller P, Owyang C (1986) Cholecystokinin mediates feedback regulation of pancreatic enzyme secretion in rats. Am J Physiol 250:G252–259
51. Lu L, Louie DS, May D, Owyang C (1987) Regulation of pancreatic enzyme secretion by a trypsin sensitive intestinal peptide that stimulates cholecystokinin release. Dig Dis Sci 32:1175
52. Lu L, Louie DS, Wider M, May D, Owyang C (1989) Extraction and characterization of a CCK-releasing peptide mediating feedback regulation of pancreatic secretion. Gastroenterology 94: A 270
53. Makovec F, Christe R, Bani M, Pacini MA, Setnikar I, Rovati LA (1985) New glutaramic acid derivatives with potent competitive and specific cholecystokinin-antagonistic activity. Arznei-mittelforschung 35:1048–1051
54. Mallory PA, Travis J (1975) Inhibition spectra of the human pancreatic endopeptidases. Am J Clin Nutr 28:823–830
55. Miazza BM, Turberg Y, Guillaume P, Hahnen W, Chayvialle JA, Loizeau (1985) Mechanism of pancreatic growth induced by pancreatico-biliary diversion in the rat. Digestion 20:75–83

56. Miyasaka K, Green GM (1983) Effect of atropine on rat basal pancreatic secretion during return or diversion of bile-pancreatic juice. Proc Soc Exp Biol Med 174:187–192
57. Miyasaka K, Green GM (1984) Effect of partial exclusion of pancreatic juice of rat basal pancreatic secretion. Gastroenterology 86:114–119
58. Miyasaka K, Kitani K (1986) A difference in stimulatory effects on pancreatic exocrine secretion between ursodeoxycholate and trypsin inhibitor in the rat. Dig Dis Sci 31:978–986
59. Miyasaka K, Kurosawa H, Kitani K (1987) Proglumide stimulates basal pancreatic secretion in the conscious rat. Digestion 37:135–143
60. Miyasaka K, Nakamura R, Funakoshi A, Kitani K (1989) Stimulatory effect of monitor peptide and human pancreatic secretory trypsin inhibitor on pancreatic secretion and cholecystokinin release in conscious rats. Pancreas 4:139–144
61. Niederau C, Ferrell LD, Grendell JH (1985) Caerulein induced acute necrotizing pancreatitis in mice: Protective effects of proglumide, benzotript, and secretin. Gastroenterology 88:1192–1204
62. Niederau C, Grendell JH, Rothman SS (1985) Effects of proglumide on ductal and basolateral secretion of pancreatic digestive enzymes. Am J Physiol 249:G100–107
63. Niederau C, Ferrell LD, Liddle RA, Grendell JH (1986) Beneficial effects of cholecystokinin receptor blockade and inhibition of proteolytic enzyme activity in experimental acute hemorrhagic pancreatitis in mice. J Clin Invest 78:1056–1063
64. Niederau C, Niederau M, Williams JA, Grendell JH (1986) New proglumide analogue CCK-receptor antagonists: very potent and selective for peripheral tissues. Am J Physiol 251:G856–860
65. Niederau C, Liddle RA, Williams JA, Grendell JH (1987) Pancreatic growth: interaction of exogenous cholecystokinin, a protease inhibitor and a cholecystokinin receptor antagonist in mice. Gut 28:63–69
66. Niederau M, Niederau C, Strohmeyer G, Grendell JH (1989) Comparative effects of CCK receptor antagonists on rat pancreatic secretion in vivo. Am J Physiol 256:G1–8
67. Osnes M, Hanssen LE (1980) The influence of intraduodenal administration of pancreatic juice on the bile-induced pancreatic secretion and immunoreactive secretin release in man. Scand Gastroenterol 13:1041–1047
68. Owyang C, Louie DS, Tatum D (1986) Feedback regulation of pancreatic enzyme secretion: suppression of chelecystokinin release by trypsin. J Clin Invest 77:2042–2047
69. Owyang C, May D, Louie DS (1986) Trypsin suppression of pancreatic enzyme secretion. Gastroenterology 91:637–643
70. Rausch U, Adler G, Weidenbach H (1987) Stimulation of pancreatic secretory process in the rat by low-molecular weight proteinase inhibitor. Cell Tissue Res 247:187–193
71. Rowell WG, Curington CW, Toskes PP (1989) Studies indicating that other factors in addition to CCK mediate feedback regulation of pancreatic enzymes. Gastroenterology 94:A388
72. Sale JK, Goldberg DM, Fawcett N, Wormsley KG (1977) Chronic and acute studies indicating absence of exocrine pancreatic feedback inhibition in dogs. Digestion 15:540–555
73. Schafmayer A, Becker HD, Werner M, Fölsch UR, Creutzfeldt W (1985) Plasma cholecystokinin levels in patient with chronic pancreatitis. Digestion 32:136–139
74. Schneemann BO, Lyman RL (1975) Factors involved in the intestinal feedback regulation of pancreatic enzyme secretion in the rat. Proc Soc Exp Biol Med 148:897–903
75. Shiratori K, Chen YF, Chey WY, Lee KY, Chang TM (1986) Mechanism of increased exocrine pancreatic secretion in pancreatic juice-diverted rats. Gastroenterology 91:1171–1178
76. Slaff J, Jacobson D, Tillmann CR, Curington C, Toskes P (1984) Protease-specific suppression of pancreatic exocrine secretion. Gastroenterology 87:44–52
77. Sparnakel M, Martinez J, Briet C, Jensen RT, Gardener J (1983) Cholecystokinin-27-32-amide. A member of a new class of cholecystokinin receptor antagonists. J Biol Chem 258:6746–6748
78. Sun G, Lee KY, Chang T-M, Chey WY (1989) Effect of pancreatic juice diversion on secretin release in rats. Gastroenterology 96:1173–1179
79. Takasugi S, Toki N (1980) Inhibitory effects of native and synthetic protease inhibitors on plasma proteases in acute pancreatitis. Hiroshima J Med Sci 29:189–194
80. Watanabe S, Shiratori K, Takeuchi T, Chey WY (1986) Intrajejunal administration of a synthetic trypsin inhibitor (camostate) stimulates the release of endogenous secretin, but not cholecystokinin in humans. Gastroenterology 90:A1685

81. Watanabe S, Chang JH, Shiratori K, Moriyoshi Y, Shimizu K, Takeuchi T (1989) Effect of elimination of pancreatic enzymes on camostate-induced release of CCK and secretin in rats: evidence to support direct stimulation by camostate. Gastroenterology 94:A537
82. Yamaguchi T, Tabat K, Johnson LR (1985) Effect of proglumide on rat pancreatic growth. Am J Physiol 249:G294–298
83. Yasui A, Nimura Y, Hayakawa N, Hayakawa T, Shibata T, Kondo T, Naruse S, Shionoya S (1988) Feedback regulation of basal pancreatic secretion in humans. Pancreas 3:681–687

Does Feedback Regulation Exist in Chronic Pancreatitis*?

J. Mössner, H. P. Wresky, and T. Back[1]

Introduction

Regulation of pancreatic enzyme secretion by pancreatic proteases in the duodenum via negative feedback has been demonstrated in a number of studies on animals such as rats [12, 17, 30], chicken [5], and pig [6]. In rats this negative feedback control is clearly mediated via cholecystokinin (CCK) [9, 23, 28]. The findings in humans are more controversial [7, 14, 16, 21, 35, 38]. Studies on patients with chronic pancreatitis seemed to further support the hypothesis that negative feedback regulation exists in humans. In this disease, which leads sooner or later to a decrease of pancreatic protease secretion, elevated plasma CCK levels have been reported [11, 37]. It has been further reported that treatment with pancreatic enzymes causes a reduction of pain in some patients with chronic pancreatitis which was considered to be due to lowering of the pressure of pancreatic ducts by intraluminal trypsin [18]. Others, however, could neither confirm elevated CCK levels in advanced chronic pancreatitis nor could they confirm a reduction of pain when patients were treated with pancreatic enzymes [4, 13]. In the present study, we investigated, therefore, the effects of commercially available porcine pancreatic extracts on pancreatic enzyme secretion and on plasma CCK in healthy volunteers. Furthermore, we studied the effect of food given alone or together with porcine pancreatic extracts on plasma CCK in healthy controls and in patients with long-standing chronic pancreatitis. The aim was to clarify whether commercially available capsules of pancreatic enzymes, given in a dosage known to be effective in pancreatic insufficiency, are able to inhibit pancreatic secretion possibly by lowering plasma CCK.

Material and Methods

Materials

The following chemicals were purchased: N-2-hydroxyethyl-piperazine-N'-2-ethanesulfonic acid (HEPES), ethylenediaminetetraacetic acid, partially purified lyophilized enterokinase, porcine pancreatic lipase (type IV-S), porcine pancreatic amylase (type VI), porcine pancreatic trypsin (type IX), soybean trypsin inhibitor

* This study was supported by a grant from the Deutsche Forschungsgemeinschaft (Mo 372/3-1).
[1] Medizinische Poliklinik, University of Würzburg, Klinikstrasse 8, D-8700 Würzburg, FRG

(type I-S), cholecystokinin oactapeptide (CCK_8), gum arabic, bovine plasma albumin (fraction V) from Sigma Chemical, St. Louis, MO; chromatographically purified collagenase (type CLSPA) from Cooper Biomedical, Wiesbaden, FRG; polyethylene glycol 4000 (PEG), trichloroacetic acid, zinc sulfate, phenol red, indigo carmine, acetonitrile, tris(hydroxymethyl)aminomethane from Merck, Darmstadt, FRG; Bio-Rad protein assay from Bio-Rad Laboratories, Richmond, CA; octadecylsilylsilica (SEP-Pak C-18) cartridges from Water Associates, Milford, MA; synthetic secretin (Sekretolin) from Hoechst, Frankfurt, FRG; aprotinin (Trasylol) from Bayer, Leverkusen, FRG; Whatman 42 ashless filters from W & R Balston Ltd., UK; and minimal Eale's medium amino acid supplement from Biochrom KG, Berlin, FRG. Panzytrat 20000 was a gift from Nordmark Arzneimittel GmbH, Uetersen, FRG. All other reagents were of the highest purity grade commercially available.

Methods

Subjects

Twenty healthy male volunteers, 22–50 years old, participated in the studies. All subjects were within 10% of their ideal body weight. None were taking any medication, or had any history of gastrointestinal diseases. Furthermore 16 male patients with chronic pancreatitis known for more than 5 years were studied. All patients showed at the time they were studied no signs of acute relapses of their disease and were pain free. For further characteristics of their disease see Mössner et al. [33]. The studies were approved by the Commission for Ethics at the University of Würzburg.

Intraduodenal / Jejunal Perfusion Studies

Intraduodenal perfusion studies were only done in controls. All studies were performed after an overnight fast. A four-lumen polyvinyl tube was placed under fluoroscopic control. Gastric secretions were continuously aspirated via the first lumen with the tube situated at the gastric antrum using an automatic pump. PEG 4000 was infused via the second lumen just distal to the pylorus. Duodenal secretions were aspirated via the third tube by continuous suction with the aspiration holes of the tube 15–25 cm distal to the PEG infusion site. Pancreatic extracts were given distal to the ligament of Treitz via the fourth tube 30 cm distal to the last duodenal aspiration site.

We first investigated whether pancreatic extracts alone without simultaneous addition of food have any influence on endogenous pancreatic secretions. A new preparation of acid-protected commercially available porcine pancreatic enzymes was administered in a dosage commonly used for treatment of pancreatic insufficiency [22] (Panzytrat 20000, capsules with microtablets, containing the number per capsule according to the information provided by the manufacturer, triacylglycerollipase 20000 Ph. Eur.-U., amylase 18000 Ph. Eur.-U., proteases 1000 Ph. Eur.-U.). For our studies, three capsules of Panzytrat 20000 were homogenized in 20 ml buffer containing 10 mM HEPES, 140 mM NaCl, 4.7 mM KCl, 1 mM NaHPO$_4$, 1.13 mM MgCl$_2$, 1.28 mM CaCl$_2$, adjusted to pH 7.4. According to our own measurements, the activities of various pancreatic enzymes /20 ml buffer were as follows: trypsin 28.62 ±

1.63 U (in comparison, 20 mg pure porcine trypsin obtained from Sigma Chemicals had an activity of 33.83 ± 0.55 U); chymotrypsin 9.31 ± 0.40 U; lipase 198.25 ± 27.54 U; amylase 55900 ± 7738 U (mean ± SM for $n = 8$ separate determinations).

Polyethylene glycol 4000 was continuously perfused (15 g/l physiological saline, 3 ml/min) starting at time 0. Duodenal contents were recovered by constant suction, collected on ice, and pooled at 15-min intervals. Thirty minutes later a continuous intravenous low-dose infusion of secretin was started to achieve minimal pancreatic flow (Sekretolin, 0.5 U/min per kilogram body wt.). At the same time three capsules of Panzytrat 20000 homogenized in 20 ml HEPES-Ringer buffer were perfused via the fourth lumen within 5 min. After a further 5 min, duodenal contents were collected for 2×15 min (time 55 and 70 min). This schedule was repeated three times: pancreatic extracts were perfused at 70, 110, and 150 min, and duodenal contents were collected at 80–110, 120–150, and 160–190 min. At times 110 and 150 min, however, instead of perfusing active enzymes, the same amount of heat-denatured Panzytrat 20000 solution was used. In another five volunteers the same procedure was repeated, but instead of starting with active enzymes heat-denatured enzymes were given first, at times 30 and 70 min. In both groups 24 ml blood was collected at times −5, 10, 25, 35, 50, 65, 75, 90, 105, 115, 130, 145, 155, 170, 185 min for determination of CCK.

Influence of Food and Pancreatic Extracts on Plasma CCK

Volunteers and patients with chronic pancreatitis received after an overnight fast a mixed liquid meal (6 ml/kg body wt. of cream, milk, eggs, cocoa, and sugar (49.6% fat, 20.4% protein, 30% carbohydrates; 7.21 kcal/kg body wt.) which they had to drink within 2 min. Twenty milliliters of blood was drawn 15 and 1 min before and 7.5, 15, 30, 45, 60, and 90 min after feeding for determinations of CCK. This procedure was repeated with some of the same subjects the day after but with an additional administration of microtablets from six–ten capsules Panzytrat 20000.

Cholecystokinin Bioassay

Cholecystokinin was measured by bioassay as previously published using a modification of methods described by Liddle et al. [24–26], and Mössner et al. [31]. In summary plasma was diluted with icecold 2% trifluoroacetic acid (TFA) (1:4). CCK was extracted by adsorption on SEP-PAK cartridges previously washed with acetonitrile and 0.1% TFA. The cartridges were then washed again with 0.1% TFA and the CCK was eluted with acetonitrile/0.1% TFA (1:1). The eluates were collected in flat-bottomed incubation vials and dried under a nitrogen stream at 45°C and stored at −70°C. These vials were subsequently used for incubation with 1 ml of acini suspensions as previously published.

Preparation of Isolated Pancreatic Acini

Pancreatic acini were prepared from male Sprague-Dawley rats by digestion of pancreatic tissue with purified collagenase at 37°C in an agitating water bath as described in the literature [36, 39]. Isolated acini were then incubated with either plasma extracts or various concentrations of CCK_8 for 30 min at 37°C and the release of amylase monitored. Amylase release, expressed as percentage of total amylase activity, was compared to a dose-response curve for CCK_8 in order to calculate the CCK content of plasma expressed as CCK_8 equivalents. The threshold dose was between 1 and 3 pM and maximal secretion was seen at 30–100 pM.

Assays

Amylase activity for bioassays of CCK was assayed in pancreatic homogenates and supernatants using procion yellow as substrate [20]. Protein was measured according to the method of Bradford using the Bio-Rad reagent [3]. Measurement of pancreatic enzymes in duodenal contents: Trypsin activity was assayed using an enzymatic colorimetric test with benzoyl-arginine-*p*-nitroanilide as the substrate (test combination, Boehringer, Mannheim) [8]. Chymotrypsin activity was assayed using a colorimetric enzyme assay with *N*-(3-carboxypropionyl)-phenylalanine-*p*-nitroanilide as the substrate (Boehringer, Mannheim) [34]. Lipase and amylase activity were assayed using a nephelometric method with purified olive oil as the substrate for lipase and amylopectin for amylase [41, 42]. Bicarbonate was measured via back titration with 0.1 M NaOH with phenol red as indicator. PEG was measured turbidometrically according to the methods described by Hyden [15] and Malawer and Powell [29]. Statistical analysis was performed using analysis of variance (ANOVA) with the acceptance criteria of $p = 0.05$. All results were expressed as mean ± SE.

Results

Effect of Porcine Pancreatic Extracts on Human Pancreatic Secretion

Commercially available porcine pancreatic extracts, used for treatment of human pancreatic insufficiency, were administered to the upper jejunum and secretion of bicarbonate and endogenous pancreatic digestive enzymes measured. When compared with perfusion of the upper jejunum with HEPES-Ringer buffer alone, pancreatic enzymes caused a small but statistically significant increase of amylase and chymotrypsin secretion but not of trypsin and lipase (Fig. 1). The proteases contained in the enzyme capsules did not cause any decrease of endogenous non-food-stimulated enzyme secretion when compared with controls. When pancreatic extracts were heat denatured prior to their jejunal administration a small but significant increase of secretion of amylase and chymotrypsin was again seen but none for trypsin and lipase (Fig. 1). When the effect of active enzymes on pancreatic secretion was compared with the effect of inactive ones in the same volunteer, many subjects showed a lower enzyme secretion after the application of active enzymes. Trypsin for example was lower in eight out of ten subjects after the administration of active enzymes as compared to inactive ones, chymotrypsin in eight, amylase in six, and lipase in five subjects (data not shown). Due to considerable variations in pancreatic secretion between different subjects, however, neither the means of enzyme activities in each 15-min fraction (Fig. 2) nor of the pooled 15-min fractions (Fig. 1) showed any statistically significant difference.

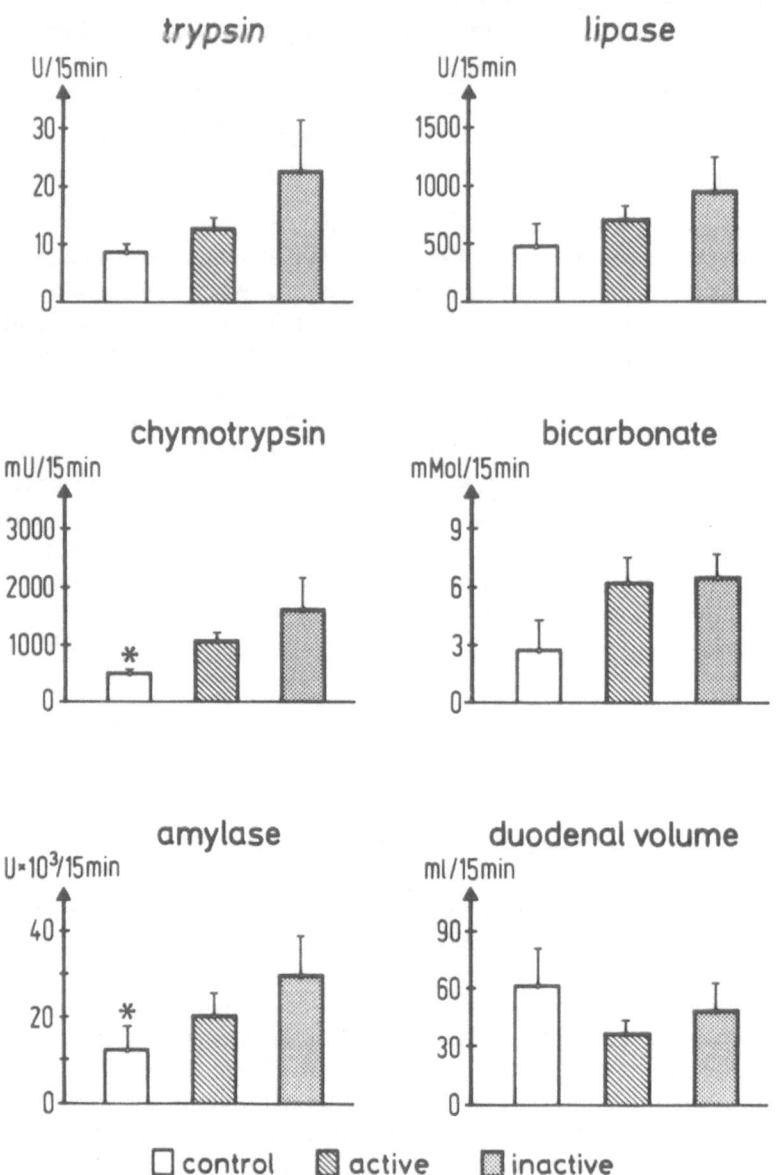

Fig. 1. Influence of porcine pancreatic extracts on pancreatic secretion. Five male volunteers received active pancreatic extracts intrajejunally two times within 80 min and duodenal contents were collected to measure output of pancreatic enzymes. This was followed by the administration of the same amount of heat-denatured inactive pancreatic extracts. In another five volunteers, the same procedure was performed with administration of inactive extracts prior to the active ones. Three volunteers received HEPES-Ringer buffer instead of pancreatic extracts (control). The mean of four 15-min duodenal fractions per subject was formed after either active or inactive extracts, as well as from eight 15-min fractions per control subject. *Bars* show the mean ± SE of the data from all subjects ($n = 10$ for those who received pancreatic extracts; $n = 3$ for controls). For further details see under "Methods". *Asterisk* indicates a statistically significant difference between control and both active and inactive extracts. (From [32])

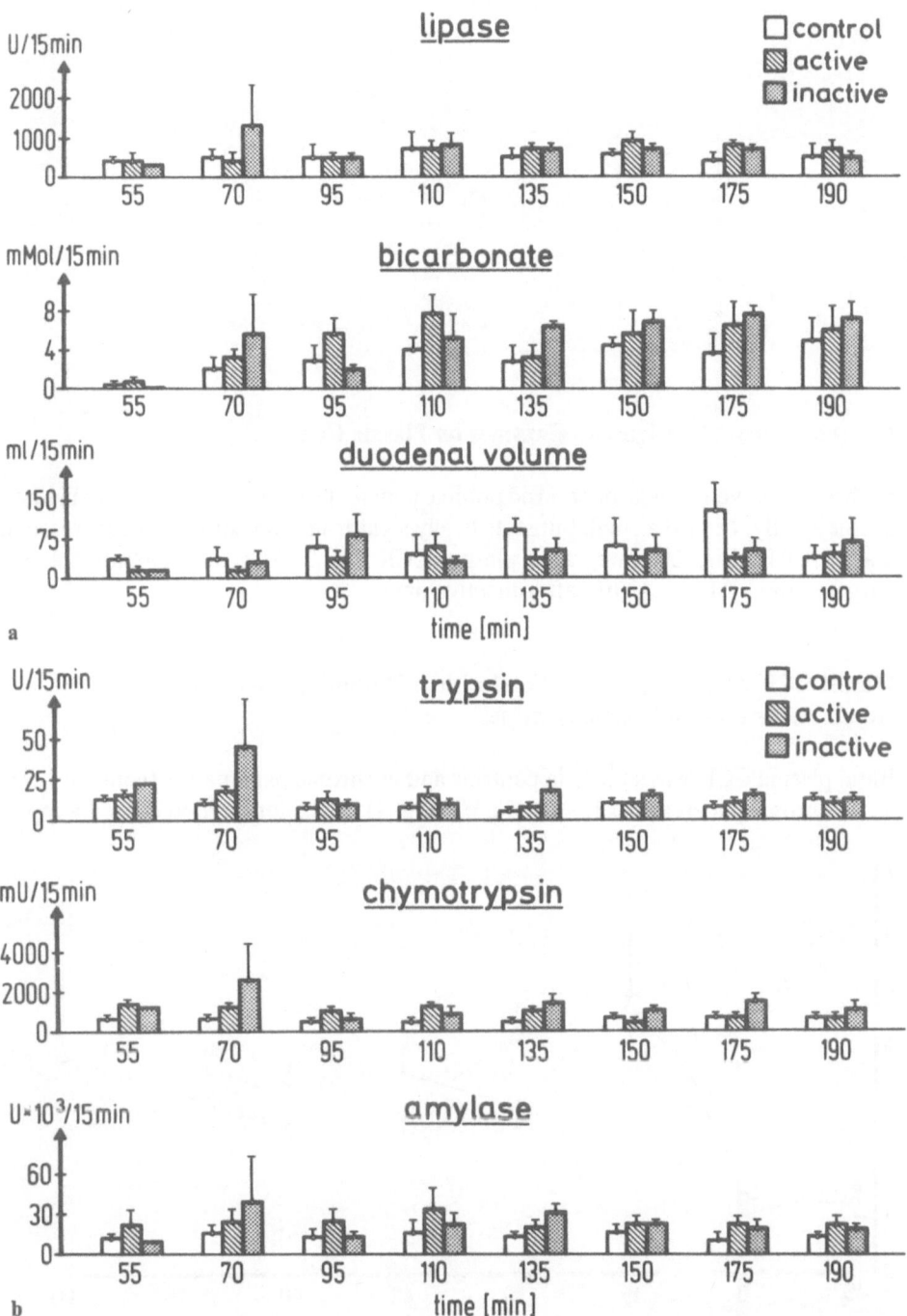

Fig. 2a, b. Influence of porcine pancreatic extracts on pancreatic secretion of digestive enzymes. *Bars* show the mean ± SE of enzyme output per pooled 15-min fraction from five subjects (same as in Fig. 1). Pancreatic extracts were administered intrajejunally at times 30, 70, 110, and 150 min. For further details see under "Methods"

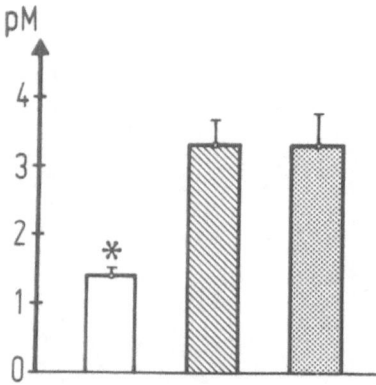

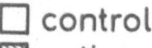

Fig. 3. Influence of active and inactive pancreatic extracts on plasma CCK. Plasma CCK was measured via bioassay. *Bars* show the mean ± SE of integrated plasma CCK values of subjects from Fig. 1. Asterisk displays a statistically significant difference between control and both active and inactive extracts. (From [32])

Effect of Pancreatic Digestive Enzymes on Plasma CCK

Both active as well as heat-denatured porcine pancreatic enzymes, when administered intrajejunally, caused a small but statistically significant and comparable increase in plasma CCK (Fig. 3). Integrated plasma CCK was 3.32 ± 0.34 pM after active enzymes and 3.31 ± 0.43 pM after inactive ones.

Plasma CCK After Ingestion of Food with or Without Simultaneous Administration of Pancreatic Enzymes

Basal plasma CCK was similar in controls and in chronic pancreatitis (control: 1.3 ± 0.2 vs chronic pancreatitis: 1.5 ± 0.3 pM) (Fig. 4). Ingestion of food caused a rapid,

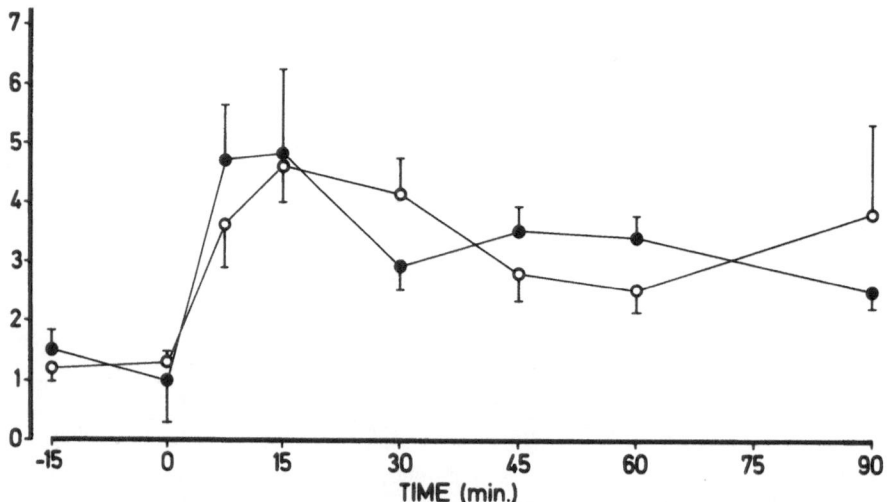

Fig. 4. Effect of food on plasma CCK in controls and patients with chronic pancreatitis. Plasma CCK was measured via bioassay before and after administration of a liquid test meal. Values are means ± SE. *Open circles*, controls ($n = 20$); *closed circles*, patients with chronic pancreatitis ($n = 16$). (From [33])

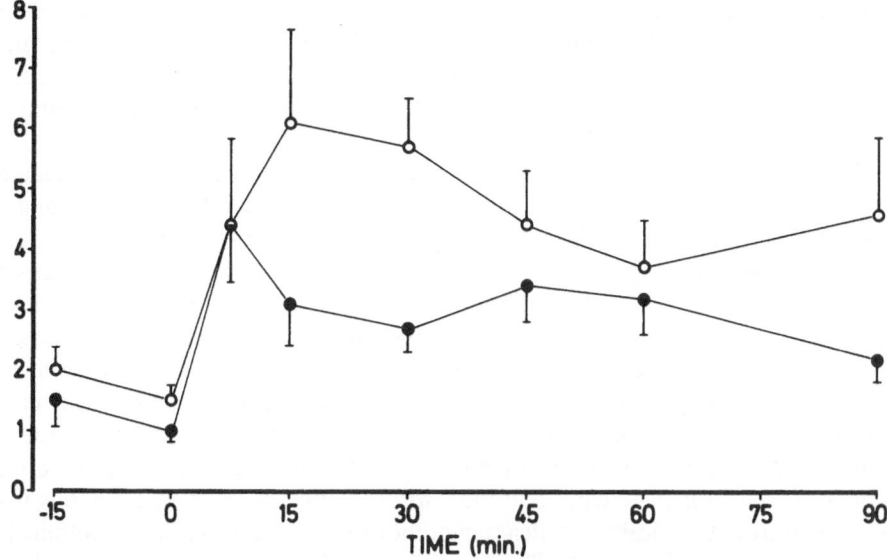

Fig. 5. Effect of food containing active pancreatic extracts on plasma CCK in patients with chronic pancreatitis. Ten patients with severely impaired pancreatic function due to chronic pancreatitis received a liquid test meal on day 1 *(closed circles)* and on the next day a similar test meal containing ten capsules of pancreatic extracts (Panzytrat 20000) *(open circles)*. (From [33])

sustained, and comparable increase of plasma CCK in both controls and patients with chronic pancreatitis (Fig. 4). There was no statistically significant difference between food-stimulated plasma CCK of controls and patients.

The addition of six capsules of Panzytrat 20000 to the liquid meal did not cause a different pattern of plasma CCK in controls (data not shown). In humans CCK is released predominantly by small peptides, amino acids, and fat. We evaluated, therefore, whether in patients with severely impaired digestive capacity the addition of pancreatic extracts to a test meal is able to inhibit pancreatic enzyme secretion due to the content of proteases or rather stimulate secretion due to improvement of maldigestion. The application of large amounts of pancreatic extracts (ten capsules) together with food caused in nearly all of the ten patients studied significantly higher CCK plasma levels as compared to food alone (Fig. 5).

Discussion

Treatment of pain in patients suffering from chronic pancreatitis is an important clinical issue. Pain may be due to an elevation of pressure in pancreatic ducts [40]. A reduction of pressure via an inhibition of pancreatic secretion could, therefore, reduce pain. There are now many studies supporting the hypothesis of negative feedback regulation of human pancreatic secretion by proteases [16, 35, 38]. With the administration of proteases, therefore, one should be able to inhibit pancreatic secretion. Patients with pancreatic insufficiency are usually treated with porcine pancreatic extracts. These commercially available pancreatic extracts contain a mixture of digestive enzymes. There are large variations according to the relative amount of each enzyme present in preparations from different manufacturers. Presently, acid-protected tablets with high amounts of lipase are preferred in the treatment of pancreatic insufficiency [22].

In this study, we have investigated whether acid-protected porcine pancreatic extracts alone are able to inhibit pancreatic secretion in healthy controls. Pancreatic extracts were used in a dosage known to be successful in the treatment of severe pancreatic insufficiency [22]. In the study reported by Owyang et al. [35] only pure enzymes, and not a combination of digestive enzymes, were perfused intraduodenally. However, it may be possible that the amount of other proteins present in pancreatic extracts overwhelms a potential inhibitory effect of proteases, which was demonstrated by our studies. Both active pancreatic extracts and heat-denatured enzymes caused a small increase in plasma CCK and an increase in secretion of chymotrypsin and amylase when compared with controls. Comparing the effect of active extracts on pancreatic secretion with inactive ones, it was not possible to demonstrate a statistically significant inhibition of pancreatic enzyme secretion. Thus, we could not demonstrate feedback regulation of enzyme secretion with doses of pancreatic extracts commonly used in clinical medicine. Since pancreatic extracts alone did not display inhibition of secretion, we next added those extracts to food. With this experimental design it is not possible to measure endogenous secretion since one cannot divert pancreatic secretions. We measured, therefore, plasma CCK assuming that the level of CCK displays a strong correlation to pancreatic secretion. However, again the addition of active pancreatic extracts to food did not cause a lower increase in plasma CCK.

Perfusing the duodenum with trypsin, Owyang et al. [35] clearly demonstrated an inhibition of phenylalanine-, oleic acid-, and meal-stimulated chymotrypsin and lipase output. The amount of trypsin they used to inhibit pancreatic secretion, however, was rather high. The trypsin activity per tablet of porcine pancreatic extracts available in the Federal Republic of Germany ranges between 800 and 2000 FIP units. According to our own measurements with regards to Panzytrat 20 000, which contains 1000 FIP, one capsule corresponds approximately to 6 mg trypsin (porcine type IX, Sigma). According to the data of Owyang et al. [35] one would have to use 25–50 capsules/meal to achieve inhibition of secretion. In the study reported by Slaff et al. [38], protease-specific suppression of pancreatic exocrine secretion was also seen only with very high doses of trypsin, finding a beneficial pain-relieving effect with 32 tablets pancreatin (Viokase). One may assume that trypsin binds to food. Thus high levels of trypsin were needed in the studies reported by Owyang et al. [35] and Slaff et al. [38] to overcome the binding of trypsin to food so that sufficient trypsin is present to exert negative feedback. In pancreatic function studies performed at our unit for diagnostic purposes, we stimulate patients intravenously with cerulein (Takus 100 ng/kg body wt./h, Farmitalia, Freiburg, FRG) in parallel with synthetic secretin (Sekretolin 1 U/kg body wt./h, Hoechst, Frankfurt, FRG). Employing such a maximal hormonal stimulation, we observed in 20 normal healthy male volunteers a trypsin secretion of 60–100 U/h (unpublished). This corresponds to the trypsin activity contained in six to ten capsules Panzytrat. We have used a similar dose of enzymes in our perfusion studies.

The existance of negative feedback regulation of pancreatic secretion in humans is still controversial. This may be due to differences in methodological approaches. Perfusion of the duodenum with phenylalanin caused stimulation of pancreatic secretion which could be inhibited by trypsin [35]. In these studies negative feedback was clearly mediated via CCK. In another study pancreatic secretion was measured directly by canulation of the main pancreatic duct via ERP. Reperfusion of the duodenum with the body's own pancreatic secretion reduced further secretions, which again could be reversed by the administration of Bowman-Birk soybean trypsin inhibitor [27]. Camostate, another protease inhibitor, stimulated interdigestive and secretin-stimulated pancreatic secretion [1]. However, negative feedback seemed not to be mediated by CCK in these studies. In our studies we were not able to demonstrate an inhibition of pancreatic secretion or CCK release by perfusion of the upper gut with pancreatic extracts in a dosage which one may expect to correspond to a maximal endogenous secretion of the pancreas. Thus, the biological and pathophysiological significance of putative negative feedback regulation of pancreatic secretion in humans remains a matter of debate.

Elevated plasma levels of CCK in chronic pancreatitis seemed to support the concept of negative feedback regulation [11, 37]. However, basal CCK levels measured by RIA reported by a Japanese group were ten times higher even in controls as compared to CCK levels measured by bioassay or RIA by other groups [4, 25, 26, 31, 35]. Thus, interpretation of their data of elevated CCK in patients with chronic pancreatitis and pain is difficult [11]. The same group reported an impaired CCK release after the addition of food in patients with severe pancreatic insufficiency, which is again in contrast to our results [10]. We found no elevated basal CCK plasma levels, measured by bioassay, in patients with chronic pancreatitis, which is in accordance with others who measured CCK by RIA [2, 4, 19]. Like another group we found a normal CCK release after the addition of food [2].

Two different groups observed an improvement of pain in patients with chronic pancreatitis under therapy with pancreatic extracts [18, 38]. This was considered as proof of negative feedback regulation. In our studies we cannot deny the possibility that treatment of patients with chronic pancreatitis with pancreatic extracts may relieve pain. However, we found that pancreatic extracts did not inhibit but rather stimulated pancreatic secretion. This may be due to the high protein content of extracts and to improvement of digestion. We do not deny that proteases in very high concentrations in the presence of food and in possibly lower concentrations in the absence of food are capable of inhibiting human pancreatic secretion. We conclude, however, that pancreatic extracts given in a dosage commonly used in clinical medicine may not exert their potential pain-relieving effect via an inhibition of pancreatic secretion.

Acknowledgements. We thank Dr. I. Haubitz, Rechenzentrum, University of Würzburg, for performing statistical analysis and Mss. G. Gebert and L. Kneis for expert technical assistance.

References

1. Adler G, Müllenhoff A, Koop I, Bozkurt T, Göke B, Beglinger C, Arnold R (1988) Stimulation of pancreatic secretion in man by a protease inhibitor (camostate). Eur J Clin Invest 18:98–102
2. Bozkurt T, Adler G, Koop I, Koop H, Türmer W, Arnold R (1988) Plasma CCK levels in patients with pancreatic insufficiency. Dig Dis Sci 33:276–281
3. Bradford M (1976) A rapid and sensitive method for the quantitation of microgram quantities of protein utilizing the principle of protein-dye binding. Anal Biochem 72:248–254
4. Cantor P, Petronijevic L, Worning H (1986) Plasma cholecystokinin concentrations in patients with advanced chronic pancreatitis. Pancreas 1: 488–493
5. Chernick SS, Lepkovsky S, Chaikoff IL (1948) A dietary factor regulating the enzyme content of the pancreas: changes induced in size and proteolytic activity of the chick pancreas by ingestion of raw soybean meal. Am J Physiol 155:33–41
6. Corring T (1973) Mechanisme de la secrétion pancréatique exocrine chez le porc: régulation par rétro inhibition. Ann Biol Anim Biochim Biophys 13:755–756
7. Dlugosz J, Fölsch UR, Creutzfeldt W (1983) Inhibition of intraduodenal trypsin does not stimulate exocrine pancreatic secretion in man. Digestion 26:197–204
8. Erlanger BF, Kokowsky N, Cohen W (1961) The preparation and properties of two new chromogenic substrates of trypsin. Arch Biochem Biophys 95:271–278
9. Fölsch UR, Cantor P, Wilms HM, Schafmayer A, Becker HD, Creutzfeldt W (1987) Role of cholecystokinin in the negative feedback control of pancreatic enzyme secretion in conscious rats. Gastroenterology 92:449–458
10. Funakoshi A, Nakano I, Shinozaki H, Ibayashi H, Tateishi K, Hamaoka T (1985) Low plasma cholecystokinin response after ingestion of a test meal in patients with chronic pancreatitis. Am J Gastroenterol 80:937–940
11. Funakoshi A, Nakano I, Shinozaki H, Tateishi K, Hamaoka T, Ibayashi H (1986) High plasma cholecystokinin levels in patients with chronic pancreatitis having abdominal pain. Am J Gastroenterol 81:1174–1178
12. Green GM, Lyman RL (1972) Feedback regulation of pancreatic enzyme secretion as a mechanism for trypsin inhibitor-induced hypersecretion in rats. Proc Soc Exp Biol Med 140:6–12
13. Halgreen H, Pedersen TN, Worning H (1986) Symptomatic effect of pancreatic enzyme therapy in patients with chronic pancreatitis. Scand J Gastroenterol 21:104–108
14. Hotz J, Ho SB, Go VLW, DiMagno EP (1983) Short-term inhibition of duodenal tryptic activity does not affect human pancreatic, biliary, or gastric function. J Lab Clin Med 101:488–495
15. Hyden S (1956) A turbidometric method for the determination of higher polyethylene glycols in biological materials. Kungl Lantbrukshögsk Ann 22:139–145
16. Ihse I, Lilja P, Lundquist I (1977) Feedback regulation of pancreatic enzyme secretion by intestinal trypsin in man. Digestion 15:303–308
17. Ihse I, Lilja P, Lundquist I (1979) Trypsin as a regulator of pancreatic secretion in the rat. Scand J Gastroenterol 13:873–880
18. Isaksson G, Ihse I (1983) Pain reduction by an oral pancreatic enzyme preparation in chronic pancreatitis. Dig Dis Sci 28:97–102
19. Jansen JBMJ, Hopman WPM, Lamers CBHW (1984) Plasma cholecystokinin concentrations in patients with pancreatic insufficiency measured by sequence-specific radioimmunoassays. Dig Dis Sci 29:1109–1113
20. Jung DH (1980) Preparation and application of procion yellow starch for amylase assay. Clin Chim Acta 100:7–10
21. Krawisz BR, Miller LJ, DiMagno EP, Go VLW (1980) In the absence of nutrients, pancreatic-biliary secretions in the jejunum do not exert feedback control of human pancreatic or gastric function. J Lab Clin Med 95:13–18
22. Lankisch PG, Lembcke B, Kirchhoff S, Hilgers R, Creutzfeldt W (1988) Treatment of pancreatogenic steatorrhea: a comparison of two acid-protected enzyme preparations. Dtsch Med Wochenschr 113:15–17
23. Lee PC, Newman BM, Praissman M, Cooney DR, Lebenthal E (1986) Cholecystokinin: a factor responsible for the enteral feedback control of pancreatic hypertrophy. Pancreas 1:335–340

24. Liddle RA, Goldfine ID, Williams JA (1984) Bioassay of plasma cholecystokinin in rats: effects of food, trypsin inhibitor, and alcohol. Gastroenterology 87:542–549
25. Liddle RA, Goldfine ID, Rosen MS, Taplitz RA, Williams JA (1985) Cholecystokinin bioactivity in human plasma. J Clin Invest 75:1144–1152
26. Liddle RA, Morita ET, Conrad CK, Williams JA (1986) Regulation of gastric emptying in humans by cholecystokinin. J Clin Invest 77:992–996
27. Liener IE, Goodale RL, Deshmukh A, Satterberg TL, Ward G, DiPietro CM, Bankey PE, Borner JW (1988) Effect of trypsin inhibitor from soybeans (Bowman-Birk) on the secretory activity of the human pancreas. Gastroenterology 94:419–424
28. Louie DS, May D, Miller P, Owyang C (1986) Cholecystokinin mediates feedback regulation of pancreatic enzyme secretion in rats. Am J Physiol 250:G252–259
29. Malawer SJ, Powell DW (1967) An improved turbidometric analysis of polyethylene glycol utilizing an emulsifier. Gastroenterology 53:250–256
30. Miyasaka K, Green GM (1984) Effect of partial exclusion of pancreatic juice on rat basal pancreatic secretion. Gastroenterology 86:114–119
31. Mössner J, Regner UF, Zeeh JM, Bruch H-P, Eberlein G (1989) Influence of food on plasma cholecystokinin and gastrin in patients with partial gastric resections and roux-en-Y anastomosis. Z Gastroenterol 27:94–98
32. Mössner J, Wresky H-P, Kestel W, Zeeh J, Regner U, Fischbach W (1989) Influence of treatment with pancreatic enzymes on pancreatic enzyme secretion. Gut 30:1143–1149
33. Mössner J, Back T, Regner U, Fischbach W (1989) Plasma-Cholecystokininspiegel bei chronischer Pankreatitis. Z Gastroenterol 27:401–405
34. Nagel W, Willig F, Peschke W, Schmidt FH (1965) Über die Bestimmung von Trypsin und Chymotrypsin mit Aminosäure-p-Nitroaniliden. Hoppe Seylers Z Physiol Chem 340:1–9
35. Owyang C, Louie DS, Tatum D (1986) Feedback regulation of pancreatic enzyme secretion. Suppression of cholecystokinin release by trypsin. J Clin Invest 77:2042–2047
36. Sankaran H, Iwamoto Y, Korc M, Williams JA, Goldfine ID (1981) Insulin action in pancreatic acini from streptozotocin-treated rats. II. Binding of ^{125}I-insulin to receptors. Am J Physiol 240:G63–68
37. Schafmayer A, Becker HD, Werner M, Fölsch UR, Creutzfeldt W (1985) Plasma cholecystokinin levels in patients with chronic pancreatitis. Digestion 32:136–139
38. Slaff J, Jacobson D, Tillman CR, Curington C, Toskes P (1984) Protease-specific suppression of pancreatic exocrine secretion. Gastroenterology 87:44–52
39. Williams JA, Korc M, Dormer RL (1978) Action of secretagogues on a new preparation of functionally intact, isolated pancreatic acini. Am J Physiol 235: E517–524
40. Wolfson P (1980) Surgical management of inflammatory disorders of the pancreas. Surg Gynecol Obstet 151:689–698
41. Zinterhofer L, Wardlaw S, Jatlow PJ, Seligson D (1973) Nephelometric determination of pancreatic enzymes. II Lipase. Clin Chim Acta 44:173–178
42. Zinterhofer L, Wardlaw S, Jatlow PJ, Seligson D (1973) Nephelometric determination of pancreatic enzymes. I. Amylase. Clin Chim Acta 44:5–12

Clinical Features

Pain in Chronic Pancreatitis: Pathomechanism and Clinical Presentation

P. A. BANKS[1]

The causes of abdominal pain in chronic pancreatitis remain elusive. Possible causes include acute inflammation of the pancreas, increased intrapancreatic pressure within ducts and/or parenchyma, and neural inflammation. Possible extrapancreatic causes include common bile duct stenosis and duodenal stenosis.

Pancreatic Causes

Acute Inflammation

Acute inflammation is readily apparent when there is severe abdominal pain and tenderness, elevation of serum amylase and lipase, and evidence of acute pancreatic inflammation on CT scan. The causes would presumably be the same as in inflammation associated with acute pancreatitis involving activated enzymes and other injurious substances.

Increased Intrapancreatic Pressure
Ducts

In chronic pancreatitis, there are a variety of ductal abnormalities that could increase intraductal pressure [2]. When dilatation of the pancreatic duct is on the basis of a ductal stenosis, focal obstruction, irregular dilatation, or the presence of occluding stones, increased intraductal pressure would be possible. On the other hand, when the duct is in general dilated without severely narrowed areas or when the duct is not dilated, the possibility of increased intraductal pressure is less certain. When a pseudocyst communicates with a stenotic duct, there could be increased intracyst pressure; if the pseudocyst does not communicate, increased pressure is less certain.

It is important to know whether any of these anatomic abnormalities is invariably associated with pain. The evidence thus far is that the presence of these anatomic derangements do not predict whether a patient is experiencing pain or has experienced pain [1-4]. Nonetheless, when a patient is experiencing pain and one or more of these abnormalities is present, we tend to hold them responsible. In support of this belief is the success in relieving pain following decompression of a dilated main

---

[1] Tufts University School of Medicine, Chief of Gastroenterology, St. Elizabeth's Hospital, 736 Cambridge Street, Boston, Massachusetts, USA

Chronic Pancreatitis
Ed. by Beger, Büchler, Ditschuneit, and Malfertheiner
© Springer-Verlag Berlin Heidelberg 1990

pancreatic duct by lateral pancreaticojejunostomy [5] and decompression of a pseudocyst, either surgically [5] or percutaneously [6].

What, then, is the evidence that intraductal pressure is increased in association with ductal abnormalities and that pain is relieved when the pressure decreases? Measurements of intraductal pressure have been made in patients without pancreatic disease and those with ductal abnormalities. Thus far, among patients without pancreatic disease, intraductal pressure has been found to be 7 mmHg by direct puncture at surgery in one patient [7] and 10–16 mmHg by ERCP among 33 patients without pancreatic disease [8–10]. By comparison, in three studies of intraductal pressure measured by direct puncture at surgery in 59 patients with a dilated duct, intraductal pressure ranged from 18–48 mmHg [7, 8, 11]. In general, precise descriptions of pain were lacking in these studies. In one [8], all 19 patients with a dilated main pancreatic duct asscociated either with a chain-of-lakes appearance or a pseudocyst has prompt relief of pain.

Additional pressure measurements will be very helpful, especially if generated by direct puncture rather than by ERCP. In one study that relied on ERCP measurements alone, no difference in ductal pressure could be found between normal controls and patients with chronic pancreatitis [12].

The impact of intraductal stones on intraductal pressure and pain is unclear. There is preliminary information that lithotripsy is capable of shattering stones, reducing the caliber of the main pancreatic duct and apparently also reducing the severity of pain [13]. More data are required to evaluate this approach.

Thus far, there is no information on intraductal pressure when the main pancreatic duct is not dilated. These measurements would be very difficult to make.

Finally, regarding the relationship between pancreatic pseudocysts and pressure, in two studies in which direct intracyst measurements were made during surgery in 15 patients, the intracyst pressure ranged from 10–48 mmHg [7, 8]. In one study [8], decompression of the pseudocyst was associated with relief of pain. The precise mechanism of pain associated with either ductal dilatation or pseudocyst remains unclear, but may be related to the generation of increased pressure within the parenchyma.

Parenchyma

Pancreatic tissue pressure measurements made at surgery in six patients with a normal pancreas was 3–11 mmHg [7]. In comparison, pancreatic tissue pressure among eight patients with a dilated pancreatic duct and six with a pancreatic pseudocyst ranged between 17 and 21 mmHg [14]. In all patients, pancreatic tissue pressure fell to levels of 7–10 mmHg following decompression of the duct or cyst. These lowered levels were similar to pressures among the six patients with a normal pancreas [7]. The reduction in pancreatic tissue pressure resulted in relief of pain among 12 of the 14 patients. Eventually, four patients again developed pain associated with either a reoccurrence of the pseudocyst or dilatation of the main pancreatic duct. No additional measurements were made to determine whether these abnormalities were once again associated with increased pancreatic tissue pressure. Accordingly, there is now evidence that there are increased intraductal and increased tissue pressures in association with ductal abnormalities and that decompression of the duct reduces tissue pressure and relieves pain. The pathophysiology of pain may be increased intraductal pressure leading to increased parenchymal pressure. The buildup of pressure in the parenchyma may be related to fibrosis of the gland and capsule, rendering it unable to expand. The way that increased tissue pressure causes pain is not clear.

Neural Inflammation

Evidence is accumulating through the work of Bockman et al. [15] that in chronic pancreatitis there are major disturbances in and around nerves. The most important of these is an alteration in the perineurial sheath that ordinarily shields nerves from surrounding connective tissue. In this regard, immunohistological studies have shown that the amount of neurotransmitters such as substance P is increased in afferent pancreatic nerves among patients with chronic pancreatitis [16]. Additional information will be required to determine whether these changes are restricted to those patients with pain.

There is also evidence that eosinophils are increased in the perineurial space among patients who have ingested alcohol recently [17]. The suggestion was made that degranulation of these eosinophils might be a factor in the generation of pain. Additional work will be required to determine the impact of alcohol on cellular aggregates in the perineurial area.

Extrapancreatic

Stenosis of the distal common bile duct has been noted to be associated with relatively severe abdominal pain. While this pain might be caused by distention of the common bile duct, pain might also be caused by an associated duodenal stenosis or by continued inflammation of the head of the pancreas [5, 18].

Stenosis of the descending duodenum [18] in chronic pancreatitis may be caused by extensive fibrosis that envelops the wall of the duodenum or by extension of active inflammation of the pancreatic tissue within the wall of the duodenum. In one patient, we found by histologic examination ectopic pancreatic tissue within the wall of the duodenum, and in another a small pseudocyst that had actually penetrated the muscular layer of the duodenum [18]. Pain associated with duodenal stenosis may also be caused by active inflammation of the head of the pancreas.

Clinical Presentation and Summary

In both alcoholic and idiopathic pancreatitis, abdominal pain is the most frequent presenting symptom [19, 20]. In chronic pancreatitis of the tropics, the presenting symptom derived from hospital experiences is either abdominal pain or symptoms related to diabetes mellitus [21]. In order to learn about the features of chronic pancreatitis of the tropics prior to hospital experience, a field survey has just been conducted in the state of Kerela in India. On the basis of this field survey of 28000 inhabitants, a total of 36 patients with chronic pancreatitis has been identified. Of these 36, 17 presented with abdominal pain, 15 with symptoms of diabetes mellitus, and 4 with evidence of malabsorption. Hence, abdominal pain is a frequent presenting symptom in chronic pancreatitis of the tropics.

We have much to learn about the causes of pain in chronic pancreatitis. In order to make progress in this area, we must plan future studies in a way that will generate meaningful data. These studies should be prospective, utilize standardized description of pain, and have uniform entry criteria with notations made as to etiology and extent of alcohol intake. At entry, there should be standardized tests of structure and function. The protocol itself should be uniform as to data collection, treatment, and evaluation of treatment. Finally, we need to generate new data including pressure measurements before and after treatment, histology in chronic pancreatitis, and newer techniques including immunohistochemical studies. If future studies do not include features such as these, progress in our understanding of pain in chronic pancreatitis is likely to be very slow.

References

1. Girdwood AH, Marks IN, Bornman PC, Kottler RE, Cohen M (1981) Does progressive pancreatic insufficiency limit pain in calcific pancreatitis with duct stricture or continued alcohol insult? J Clin Gastroenterol 3:241–245
2. Bornman PC, Marks IN, Girdwood AH, Clain JE, Narunsky L, Clain DJ, Wright JP (1980) Is pancreatic duct obstruction or stricture a major cause of pain in calcific pancreatitis? Br J Surg 67:425–428
3. Jensen AR, Matzen P, Malchow-Moller A, Christoffersen (The Copenhagen Pancreatitis Study Group) (1984) Pattern of pain, duct morphology, and pancreatic function in chronic pancreatitis. Scand J Gastroenterol 19:334–338
4. Malfertheiner P, Büchler M, Stanescu A, Ditschuneit H (1987) Pancreatic morphology and function in relationship to pain in chronic pancreatitis. Int J Pancreatol 1:59–66
5. Warshaw AL (1985) Conservation of pancreatic tissue by combined gastric, biliary, and pancreatic duct drainage for pain from chronic pancreatitis. Am J Surg 149:563–569
6. Banks PA, Gerzof SG (1985) Role of percutaneous aspiration in the treatment of pancreatic pseudocysts. In: Sato T, Yamauchi H (eds) Pancreatitis. University of Tokyo Press, Tokyo, pp 199–204
7. Ebbehoj N, Borly L, Madsen P, Svendsen LB (1986) Pancreatic tissue pressure and pain in chronic pancreatitis. Pancreas 1:556–558
8. Bradley EL III (1982) Pancreatic duct pressure in chronic pancreatitis. Am J Surg 144:313–316
9. Okazaki K, Yamamoto Y, Kagiyama S, Tamura S, Sakamoto Y, Morita M, Yamamoto Y (1988) Pressure of papillary sphincter zone and pancreatic main duct in patients with alcoholic and idiopathic chronic pancreatitis. Int J Pancreatol 3:457–468
10. Staritz M, zum Büschenfelde KHM (1988) Elevated pressure in the dorsal part of pancreas divisum: the cause of chronic pancreatitis? Pancreas 3:108–110
11. Madsen P, Winkler K (1982) The intraductal pancreatic pressure in chronic obstructive pancreatitis. Scand J Gastroenterol 17:553–554
12. Novis BH, Bornman PC, Girdwood AW, Marks IN (1985) Endoscopic manometry of the pancreatic duct and sphincter zone in patients with chronic pancreatitis. Dig Dis Sci 30:225–228
13. Cremer M, Vandermeeren A, Delhaye M (1988) Extracorporeal shock wave lithotripsy (ESWL) for pancreatic stones. Gastroenterol 94:A80
14. Ebbehoj N, Svendsen LB, Madsen P (1984) Pancreatic tissue pressure: techniques and pathophysiologic aspects. Scand J Gastroenterol 19:1066–1068
15. Bockman DE, Büchler M, Malfertheiner P, Beger HG (1988) Analysis of nerves in chronic pancreatitis. Gastroenterology 94:1459–1469
16. Büchler M, Weihe E (1988) Distribution of neurotransmitters in afferent human pancreatic nerves. Digestion 38:8

17. Keith RG, Keshavjee SH, Kerenyi NR (1985) Neuropathology of chronic pancreatitis in humans. Can J Surg 28:207–211
18. Makrauer FL, Antonioli DA, Banks PA (1982) Duodenal stenosis in chronic pancreatitis. Clinicopathological correlations. Dig Dis Sci 27:525–532
19. Hayakawa T, Kondo T, Shibata T, Sugimoto Y, Kitagawa M (1989) Chronic alcoholism and evolution of pain and prognosis in chronic pancreatitis. Dig Dis Sci 34:33–38
20. Ammann RW, Buehler H, Muench R, Freiburghaus AW, Siegenthaler W (1987) Differences in the natural history of idiopathic (nonalcoholic) and alcoholic chronic pancreatitis. A comparative long-term study of 287 patients. Pancreas 2:368–377
21. Balakrishnan V (ed) (1987) Chronic pancreatitis in India. St Joseph's Trivandium

Ductal Morphology and Pain in Chronic Alcohol-Induced Pancreatitis*

A. H. GIRDWOOD, P. C. BORNMAN, and I. N. MARKS[1]

The morphological changes of the pancreatic ductal system in chronic alcohol-induced pancreatitis (AIP) usually follow a progressive course with the development of pancreatic duct stones, strictures and obstructions, and dilatation of the pancreatic duct [11]. There is a perception that these changes cause obstruction to the flow of pancreatic juice, leading to pancreatic duct hypertension and pain. Available data on the correlation between these changes and pain, however, do not substantiate this seemingly logical hypothesis. Patients with pancreatic duct strictures or obstructions (PDSOs) may or may not have associated duct dilatation and, conversely, pancreatic duct dilatation (PDD) may be unassociated with PDSO.

The Cape Town group examined the possible correlation between pain and the presence of PDSO as seen on endoscopic retrograde pancreatography in a group of patients with calcific pancreatitis [3]. There was a high incidence of PDSO in patients with moderate to severe pain (15/19, 79%), but this was essentially similar to the incidence in those patients who were free of pain for > 1 year (13/20, 65%). The incidence of PDSO was significantly less in patients with pain in the less advanced, noncalcific form of the disease (7/35, 20%) [4]. Of further interest in this study was the finding of PDSO in no fewer than three of the six patients with painless disease. These studies were in keeping with the concept of progressive structural changes of the pancreatic duct and showed moreover that factors other than PDSO may also be strategic in the causation of pain in AIP.

The question of the correlation between pain and PDD is also largely unresolved. In three recent studies (Table 1) PDD was not the predominant finding in patients with severe pain [8, 10, 12]. The interpretation of these studies, however, is bedevilled by

Table 1. Correlation between severe pain and pancreatic duct size on ERCP in chronic alcohol-induced pancreatitis

	Number	Dilated (size)	Not dilated
Jensen et al. [8]	24	12 (≥ 5 mm)	12
Malfertheiner et al. [10]	15	6 (NR)	9
Nieuwoudt et al. [12]	30	12 (≥ 10 mm)	18

NR, not recorded

* Support from the South African Medical Research Council is acknowledged
[1] Gastrointestinal Clinic, and Surgical Gastroenterology, Groote Schuur Hospital, and Departments of Medicine and Surgery, University of Cape Town, Cape Town, South Africa

differences in the severity of disease in the patient material, the definition of duct dilatation, and the lack of information with regard to frequency of PDSO in patients with PDD. In any event, Table 1 suggests that PDD is absent in 50%–60% of patients with severe pain due to chronic AIP.

Furthermore, there is evidence that the majority of patients with PDD have little or no pain. Nieuwoudt et al. [12], in a retrospective assessment of ERCPs in 307 patients with documented chronic AIP, found 76 cases with a pancreatic duct greater than 10 mm. Of these, only 12 (16%) had pain sufficiently severe to warrant a pancreatic duct drainage procedure. This casts some doubt on the association of even gross PDD with pain and, moreover, raises the question as to the cause of PDD in chronic AIP. Is this due simply to outlet obstruction and resultant increased pancreatic duct pressure, or does the dilatation develop pari passu with ongoing parenchymal destruction, particularly in those patients without an obvious PDSO? The correlation between PDD and pancreatic insufficiency, as observed by Jensen et al. [8], may be reconciled with both possibilities.

Less controversial, perhaps, is the well-documented role of progressive pancreatic insufficiency and pain relief [1, 2] Ammann's thesis was supported by the findings of Girdwood et al. [5], who showed, in addition, that patients with pancreatic insufficiency had a reduced incidence of pain despite the presence of PDSO or, indeed, continued drinking. The reduced tendency toward pain in patients with gross pancreatic insufficiency is probably due to impaired pancreatic secretory pressure, even in patients with a PDSO. This does not imply that the pain in patients with lesser degrees of pancreatic insufficiency is not due to increased pressure – the pain relief achieved in 70%–80% of cases after a lateral pancreaticojejunostomy cannot be ignored [7, 9, 13, 14].

Available data suggest that the cause of pain in chronic AIP is a multifactorial one, and that morphological changes of the pancreatic duct reflect but one of them.

References

1. Ammann RW, Largiader F, Akovbiantz A (1979) Pain relief by surgery in chronic pancreatitis. Scand J Gastroenterol 14:209–215
2. Ammann RW, Akovbiantz, A, Largiader F, Schneier G (1981) Course and outcome of chronic pancreatitis. Gastroenterology 86:820–828
3. Bornman PC, Marks IN, Girdwood AH, et al. (1980) Is pancreatic duct obstruction or stricture a major cause of pain in calcific pancreatitis? Br J Surg 76:425–428
4. Bornman PC, Girdwood AH, Marks IN, Hatfield ARW (1982) The influence of continued alcohol intake, pancreatic duct hold-up and pancreatic insufficiency on the pain pattern in chronic non-calcific and calcific pancreatitis: a comparative study. Surg Gastroenterol 1:5–9
5. Girdwood AH, Marks IN, Bornman PC, Kottler RE, Cohen M (1981) Does progressive pancreatic insufficiency limit pain in calcific pancreatitis with duct stricture or continue alcohol insult? J Clin Gastroenterol 3:241–245
6. Girdwood AH, Bornman PC, Marks IN (1988) Intractable pain in alcohol induced pancreatitis. Can one wait for the pancreas to burn itself out? Int J Pancreatol [Suppl 2] 3:S244
7. Holmberg JT, Isaksson G, Ihse I (1985) Longterm results of pancreatico-jejunostomy in chronic pancreatitis. Surg Gynecol Obstet 160:339–346
8. Jensen AR, Matzen P, Malchow-Møller A, Christoffersen I (1984) The Copenhagen Pancreatitis Study Group. Pattern of pain, duct morphology, and pancreatic function in chronic pancreatitis. Scand J Gastroenterol 19:334–338

9. Leger L, Lenroit JP, Lemaigre G (1974) Five to twenty year follow-up after surgery for chronic pancreatitis in 148 patients. Ann Surg 180:185–191
10. Malfertheiner P, Büchler M, Stanescu A, Ditschuneit H (1987) Pancreatic morphology and function in relationship to pain in chronic pancreatitis. Int J Pancreatol 1:59–66
11. Nagata A, Homma T, Tamai K, et al. (1981) A study of chronic pancreatititis by serial endoscopic pancreatography. Gastroenterology 81:884–891
12. Nieuwoudt JHM, Girdwood AH, Bornman PC, Marks IN (1986) The correlation between pancreatic duct size and pain in chronic pancreatitis. S Afr J Surg 24:124
13. Prinz RA, Greenlee HB (1981) Pancreatic duct drainage in 100 patients with chronic pancreatitis. Ann Surg 194:313–318
14. White TT, Slavotinek AH (1979) Results of surgical treatment of chronic pancreatitis: report of 142 cases. Ann Surg 138:129–133

Relationship Between Function and Morphology in Chronic Pancreatitis

O. Pieramico[1], M. Büchler[2], and P. Malfertheiner[1]

Introduction

In the last two decades, the introduction of new imaging procedures and their technical refinement has profoundly changed the diagnostic iter in chronic pancreatitis (CP). Ultrasonography (US), computed tomography (CT), and endoscopic retrograde pancreatography (ERP) allow direct visualization of the parenchyma and ductular structures of the pancreas and an accurate assessment of pathological changes. Though less dramatically, pancreatic function tests have also strongly improved in quality due to the better standardization of test procedures. Patient tolerance has considerably increased with the introduction of indirect (tubeless) function tests. Today, the physician who is challenged to establish the diagnosis of CP can rely on a variety of functional and morphological techniques to assess and eventually grade pancreatic damage. The various investigation techniques offer different degrees of diagnostic accuracy; the more invasive procedures are more sensitive. Advanced stages of CP can be accurately assessed with each individual method, even with the less invasive methods such as US and indirect pancreatic function tests. In the early to moderate stages of the disease, where pain is the only symptom, CP continues to present a diagnostic problem and its accurate diagnosis requires the use of the most invasive techniques. The combination of function tests and imaging (ERP) appears to be most effective in these cases. In some cases, diagnosis can be established only by serial follow-up.

The present article updates the relationship between imaging procedures and direct and indirect function tests for the detection and grading of chronic pancreatitis.

Relationship Between Direct Function Tests and Imaging Procedures

Direct pancreatic function tests require gastroduodenal intubation and the collection of aspirates following intravenous stimulation with secretin and cholecystokinin (or ceruletide) or following a test meal. With this method, pancreatic secretion can be directly quantified by determining the amount of enzymes (amylase, trypsin, chymotrypsin, lipase) and bicarbonate. The sensitivity and specificity of direct pancreatic function tests vary between 97% [1] and 78% [2] according to the stage of the disease.

---

[1] Department of Gastroenterology, University of Ulm, Robert-Koch-Str. 8, D-7900 Ulm, FRG
[2] Department of General Surgery, University of Ulm, Steinhövelstrasse 9, D-7900 Ulm, FRG

Chronic Pancreatitis
Ed. by Beger, Büchler, Ditschuneit, and Malfertheiner
© Springer-Verlag Berlin Heidelberg 1990

Table 1. Comparison between Direct Function Tests (Duodenal Intubation) and Imaging Procedures in the Diagnosis of Chronic Pancreatitis

Imaging procedures			Direct function test	Reference
Ultra-sonography	Computed tomography	Endoscopic retrograde pancreato-graphy	Secretin-cerulein test	
78%			97%	[1]
75%			96%	[7]
	87%		94%	[1]
	78%		87%	[5]
		98%	93%	[1]
		89%	87%	[5]
		100%	83%	[20]
		85%	78%	[2]

The fact that the detection rate of CP varies during different stages of the disease explains why several different results have been reported in the literature concerning the sensitivity of various function tests and imaging procedures.

When the two most sensitive diagnostic methods, secretin-cerulein test (SC) and ERP are directly compared, a sensitivity ranging from 78% to 100% is confirmed for both (Table 1). When the degree of ductal abnormalities and the degree of functional impairment are compared, Braganza et al. [3] found a significant inverse correlation among pancreatic secretory volume, bicarbonate and enzyme outputs, and the ductal changes observed in ERP. On account of the wide interindividual range in this study, the degree of morphological changes in the ductal system cannot be predicted on the basis of functional data. In similar studies [1], we found a significant correlation among SC test, CT, and ERP. In agreement with other authors [4, 6], when using ERP, we found advanced ductal changes in the majority (75%) of patients with severe pancreatic insufficiency [5]. However, the association between the degree of pancreatic insufficiency and of pancreatic parenchymal damage as detected by CT was less strong (47%). Among the interindividual secretory parameters, bicarbonate output showed the highest negative correlation with the severity of ductal abnormalities detected by ERP, whereas amylase output correlated best with the degree of parenchymal changes shown in CT. In patients with moderate to mild pancreatic insufficiency, patterns of morphological damage vary from slight to marked and the correlation between function and imaging results is poor in these cases [5]. Elsborg et al. [6] reported in a prospective study on patients with alcoholic CP significantly decreased lipase activity in the duodenal juice of patients with ERP that showed advanced CP, but normal lipase activity in the duodenal juice of patients with minor to moderate changes shown in ERP. Twenty percent of the patients with mild to moderate pancreatic functional impairment had a normal CT picture in our studies [1].

No significant correlation was found when the degree of pancreatic functional impairment detected by SC was compared with the degree of abnormalities reported using US [1]. In this study, 20% of the patients with marked pancreatic insufficiency had a normal US picture, a fact which demonstrates the limits of US in the diagnosis of

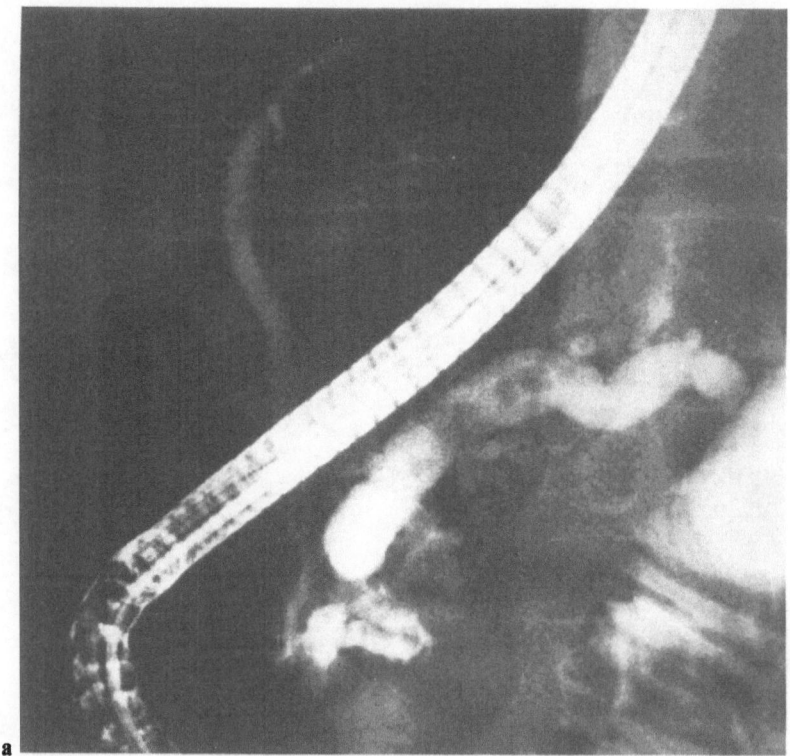

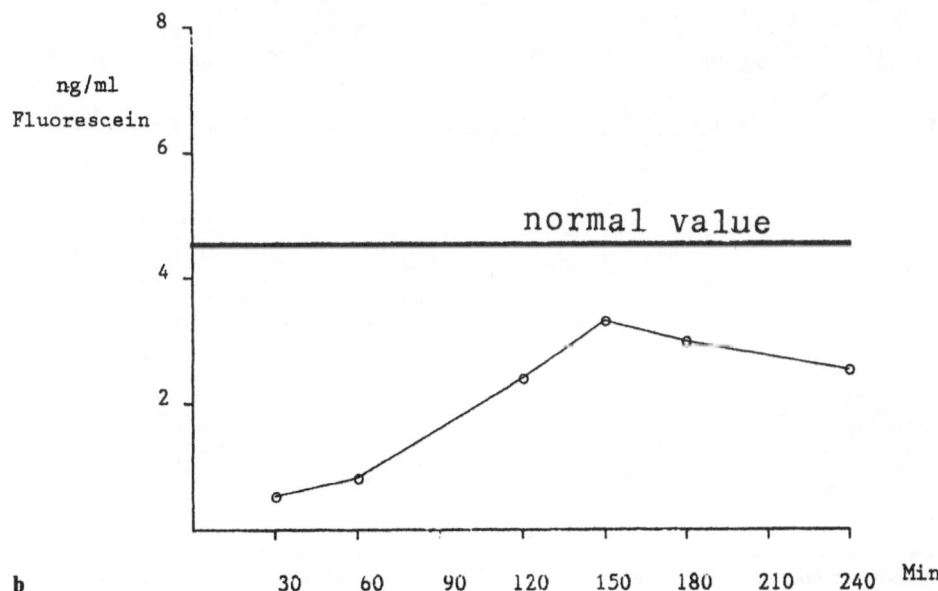

Fig. 1. A 39 year-old patient with severe chronic pancreatitis. ERP shows dilatation of the main pancreatic duct with ductal lithiasis. PLT serum test shows impairment of exocrine function

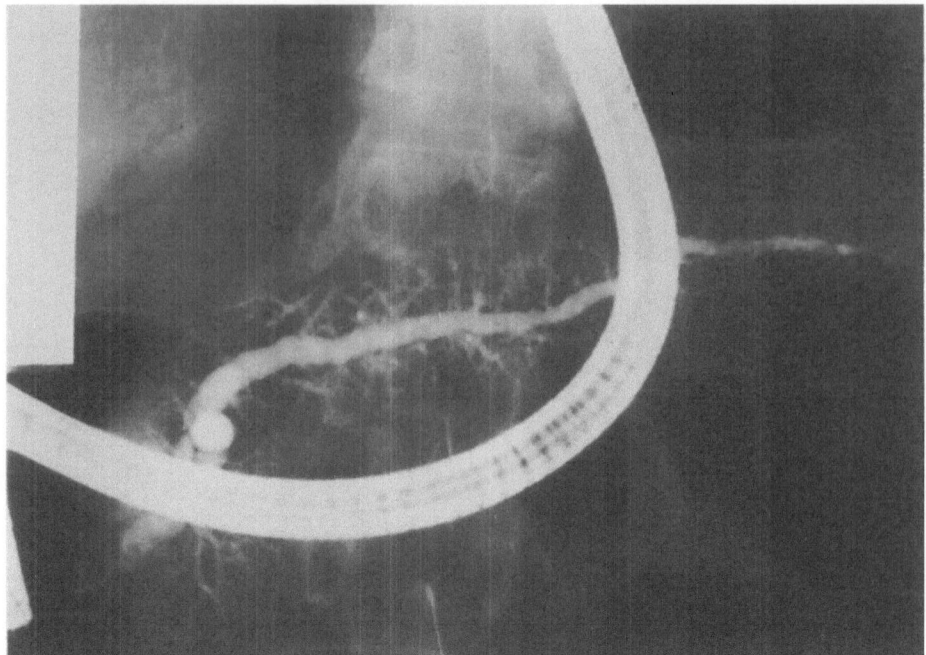

a

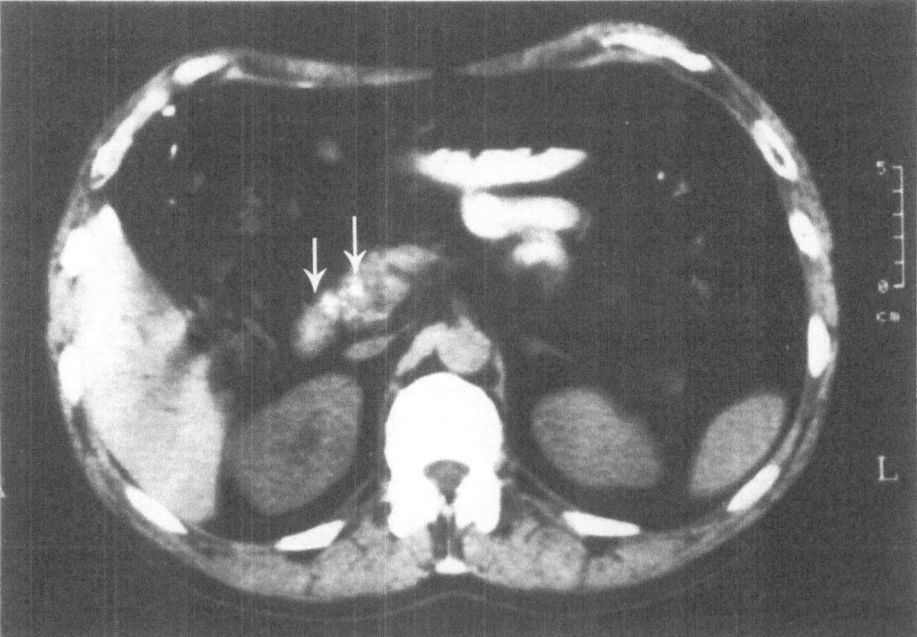

b

Fig. 2a-c. A 41-year-old patient with chronic pancreatitis. ERP shows moderate irregularity of the main pancreatic duct and of the side branches. CT shows the presence of parenchymal calcifications in the head region. Despite of these morphological alterations PLT serum test shows normal pancreatic function

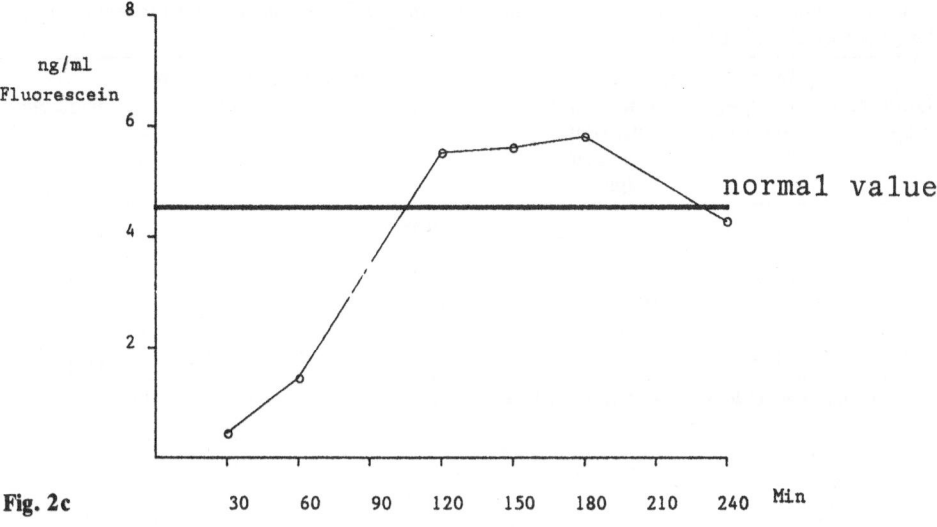

Fig. 2c

CP. Bolondi et al. [7] confirmed the SC test to have a higher sensitivity than US in detecting CP (96% vs 75%) because of several false-negative results in US in patients with moderate pancreatic functional impairment. These results emphasize that both direct pancreatic function tests and morphological techniques should be combined and may contribute to the diagnosis of less advanced stages of CP.

Relationship Between Indirect Function Tests and Imaging Procedures

In the last decade, several indirect (tubeless) function tests have become available and are now widely employed in clinical routine for the detection of pancreatic insufficiency [8]. These tests offer advantages over duodenal intubation tests because of better patients tolerance and less technical effort. Indirect pancreatic function tests are based on the ingestion of complex substrates containing markers liberated by specific pancreatic enzymes. The recovery of these marker substances in urine or serum provides qualitative information on pancreatic function [9–11]. The test procedures most commonly used are the pancreolauryl test (PLT) and the N-benzoyl-L-tyrosyl-*para*-aminobenzoic acid test (NBT-PABA) (Table 2). The specificity of the PLT and NBT-PABA tests is about 80%–90% [10–12], but anatomical alterations in the gastrointestinal tract ought to be considered separately [13]. The sensitivity of these tubeless function tests is highly dependent on the severity of CP. In the early to moderate stages of the disease, the sensitivity of PLT and NBT-PABA is less than 70% but increases to 85%–90% in more advanced stages of CP. In the presence of steatorrhea, both tests have a 100% sensitivity [10]. The sensitivity of PLT in the diagnosis of CP correlates better with the results of US and CT (sensitivity of PLT 75% and 72%) than with those obtained with ERP (63%) [14].

This study [14] shows that US, CT, and PLT have a similar sensitivity in detecting moderate to severe stages of CP and are also similarly accurate in evaluating the stage

Table 2. Comparison between Indirect Pancreatic Function Tests and Imaging Procedures in the Diagnosis of Chronic Pancreatitis

Imaging procedures			Noninvasive function tests		
Ultrasono-graphy	Computed tomography	Endoscopic retrograde pancreato-graphy	PLT	NBT-PABA	Reference
72%			80%		[1]
	78%		76%		[1]
	84%		74%		[15]
		96%	74%		[1]
		94%	77%		[15]
70%	71%			76%	[16]

PLT, pancreolauryl test; NBT-PABA, N-benzoyl-L-tyrosyl-*para*-aminobenzoic acid test

of CP. ERP and PLT findings can scarcely be correlated because ERP is more highly sensitive in the detection of early to moderate stages of CP when PLT still indicates normal function.

The additional application of PLT may be of diagnostic importance when US or CT scans are performed, since it could indicate that a patient has CP in spite of normal US and CT findings [15]. The PLT is of further value in patients with abnormal US and CT findings because it increases the specificity of the imaging findings and further helps to assess the stage of CP.

Previous reports [16] concerning the NBT-PABA test have shown no relationship between the NBT-PABA test and the stage of CP assessed by ERP although the sensitivity of the NBT-PABA test was good (70%). In a small group of patients with CP, Mitchell and Foster [17] found a similar degree of sensitivity in US (70%), CT (71%), and NBT-PABA (76%). Ventrucci et al. [18] compared the sensitivity of PLT, NBT-PABA, and SC in patients with prevalently mild to moderate CP and in controls. The overall degree of sensitivity of PLT and NBT-PABA was similar (55% and 43% respectively) but was only 29% when patients with an early stage of the disease were taken into account. The evaluation of fecal chymotrypsin activity (FCT) is another indirect method for assessing exocrine pancreatic function. The sensitivity and specificity of FCT are 78% and 84% respectively [12]. Although the degree of sensitivity is similar to that of PLT and NBT-PABA in severe CP, its reliability appears to be lower in moderate stages of the disease (60%) [9]. These results were not confirmed by Amman et al. [19] who found FCT to be markedly more sensitive than NBT-PABA, immunoreactive trypsin, and pancreatic isoamylase. No studies have reported a correlation between FCT and findings from imaging techniques. In summary, the clinical relevance of indirect pancreatic function tests is high in severe forms of CP but is of limited use in diagnosing earlier stages of CP. In these cases, a high rate of false-negative results does not reliably exclude CP. If CP is still suspected despite normal results from indirect function tests and US/CT findings, the use of more invasive function tests and imaging procedures such as SC and ERP should not be discouraged.

Conclusions

The technical improvement of imaging procedures and the introduction of new tests for assessing pancreatic function have reduced the cases of suspected CP. However, results available in the literature and our own experience clearly demonstrate that imaging procedures and function tests are not alternative methods for the diagnosis of CP but rather complementary methods for the assessing the presence and stage of the disease.

The sensitivity of the direct pancreatic function test using duodenal intubation, i. e., SC test in detecting CP is higher than that of US and CT and similar to that of ERP. ERP is much more reliable than indirect pancreatic function tests, but the sensitivity of these tests can be compared to CT and US with obvious limits in the detection of early to moderate pancreatic damage.

The combination of function tests and imaging procedures increases diagnostic accuracy in the early to moderate stages of CP and allows a better classification of advanced stages of CP.

References

1. Malfertheiner P, Büchler M, Beger HG, Ditschuneit H (1984) Exocrine pancreatic function in correlation to morphological findings (assessed by different imaging procedures) in chronic pancreatitis. In: Gyr KE, Singer MV, Sarles H (eds) Pancreatitis, concepts and classification. Excerpta Medica, Amsterdam, pp 291–299
2. Valentini M, Cavallini G, Vantini I, Farini R, Oselladore D, Fratton A, Ghidini O, Dobrilla G (1981) A comparative evaluation of endoscopic retrograde cholangiography and the Secretin-Cholecystokinin Test in the diagnosis of chronic pancreatitis: a multicentre study in 124 patients. Endoscopy 13:64–67
3. Braganza JM, Hunt LP, Warwick F (1982) Relationship between pancreatic exocrine function and ductal morphology in chronic pancreatitis. Gastroenterology 82:1341–1347
4. Reimer-Jensen A, Matzen P, Malchow-Moller A, Christoffersen I (1984) Pattern of pain, duct morphology, and pancreatic function on chronic pancreatitis. Scand J Gastroenterol 19:334–338
5. Malfertheiner P, Büchler M, Stanescu A, Ditschuneit H (1986) Exocrine pancreatic function in correlation to ductal and parenchymal morphology in chronic pancreatitis. Hepatogastroenterol 33:110–114
6. Elsborg L (1987) Endoscopic retrograde pancreatography and exocrine pancreatic function. Digestion 37 [Suppl 1]:18–24
7. Bolondi L, Gaiani S, Casanova P, Santi V, Labó G (1986) Critical evaluation and controversial points of ultrasound findings in chronic pancreatitis. In: Malfertheiner P, Ditschuneit H (eds) Diagnostic procedures in pancreatic disease. Springer-Verlag, Berlin Heidelberg New York Tokyo, pp 149–154
8. Gyr K, Toskes P (1984) Pancreatic function testing. In: Gyr K, Singer MV, Sarles H (eds) Pancreatitis, concepts and classification. Excerpta Medica, Amsterdam, pp 329–335
9. Lankisch PG, Schreiber A, Otto J (1983) Pancreolauryl test: Evaluation of a tubeless pancreatic function test in comparison with other indirect and direct tests for exocrine pancreatic function. Dig Dis Sci 28:490–493
10. Lankisch PG, Brauneis J, Otto J, Göke B (1986) Pancreolauryl and NBT-PABA tests: are serum tests more practicable alternatives to urine tests in the diagnosis of exocrine pancreatic insufficiency? Gastroenterology 90:350–354
11. Malfertheiner P, Büchler M, Müller M, Ditschuneit H (1987) Fluorescein dilaurate (FDL) serum test: a rapid tubeless pancreatic function test. Pancreas 2:53–60

12. Lang C, Gyr K (1986) Indirect pancreatic function test with NBT-PABA. In: Malfertheiner P, Ditschuneit H (eds) Diagnostic procedures in pancreatic disease. Springer-Verlag, Berlin Heidelberg New York Tokyo, pp 215–222
13. Lankisch PG (1986) The indirect pancreatic function test "Pancreolauryl" in chronic pancreatitis. In: Malfertheiner P, Ditschuneit H (eds) Diagnostic procedures in pancreatic disease. Springer-Verlag, Berlin Heidelberg New York Tokyo, pp 223–300
14. Freise J, Ranft U, Fricke K, Schmidt FW (1984) Chronische Pankreatitis: Sensitivität, Spezifizität und prädiktiver Wert des pankreolauryl Test. Z Gastroenterol 22:705–712
15. Malfertheiner P, Büchler M (1989) Correlation of imaging and function in chronic pancreatitis. Radiol Clin North Am 27:51–64
16. Stalder GA, Darmer C, Lang C (1984) The relationship between clinical diagnosis, ERCP and BT-PABA test in patients with pancreatitis. In: Gyr KE, Singer MV, Sarles H (eds) Pancreatitis – concepts and classification. Excerpta Medica, Amsterdam, pp 301–306
17. Mitchell CJ, Foster PN (1984) Ultrasound, computed tomography and an oral pancreatic function test in the diagnosis of pancreatic disease: A prospective comparison. In: Gyr KE, Singer MV, Sarles H (eds) Pancreatitis – concepts and classification. Excerpta Medica, Amsterdam, pp 317–322
18. Ventrucci M, Gullo L, Daniele C, Priori P, Labo G (1983) Pancreolauryl test for pancreatic exocrine insufficiency. Am J Gastroenterol 78:806–809
19. Amman RW, Bühler H, Pei P (1982) Comparative diagnostic accuracy of four tubeless pancreatic function tests in chronic pancreatitis. Scand J Gastroenterol 17:997–1002
20. Heij H, Obertop H, van Blankestein M, Nix GA, Westbroek DL (1987) Comparison of endoscopic retrograde pancreatography with functional and histologic changes in chronic pancreatitis. Acta Radiol 28:289–293

Gastrointestinal Motility in Chronic Pancreatitis

P. Malfertheiner[1], O. Pieramico[1], M. Büchler[2], D. K. Nelson[3],
and H. Ditschuneit[1]

Introduction

Chronic pancreatitis is characterized by an inflammatory process that begins with
focal lesions and later spreads throughout the pancreas, leading to progressive damage of the exocrine and endocrine compartments of the gland. The dominant symptom of chronic pancreatitis is pain, either due to outflow obstruction of pancreatic
secretions or to inflammation of neural structures [1, 2]. Motility disorders of the
gastrointestinal tract could also contribute to the abdominal discomfort, since in other
clinical conditions disorders such as antral hypomotility were found to be related to
dyspeptic symptoms [3].

Our current understanding of the involvement of gastrointestinal motor function in
chronic pancreatitis is incomplete [4, 5]. Based on the current physiological concepts
it could be speculated that interdigestive gastrointestinal motility is altered because of
a disturbed release of pancreatic polypeptide (PP) and motilin [6, 7]. Both these
hormones are altered in chronic pancreatitis [7–9] and both participate in the regulation of interdigestive motility [10–15] and interdigestive pancreatic secretion [12, 16].

To contribute to the understanding of these complex mechanisms, we investigated
gastroduodenal motility in the fasting and postprandial state in patients with chronic
pancreatitis. Particular attention was paid to the release of PP during phases of
interdigestive motility. Our findings on gastroduodenal motility in chronic pancreatitis are discussed here with regard to the available literature.

Interdigestive Motility

Few data are available concerning the influence of chronic pancreatitis on interdigestive gastrointestinal motility (Table 1). Brugge et al. [17] have shown that in chronic
alcoholic pancreatitis the interdigestive duodenal contraction rate is normal, while
trypsin and protein outputs are decreased. However, no information was available
from this study concerning the duration of the phases of the migrating motor complex
(MMC) since motility was recorded exclusively from the duodenum for a short
interval of time (30 min) during phase II. Moreover, these limited data are inconclu-

[1] Department of Internal Medicine II, University of Ulm, Robert-Koch-Str. 8, D-7900 Ulm, FRG
[2] Department of General Surgery, University of Ulm, Steinhövelstr. 9, D-7900 Ulm, FRG
[3] Gastroenterology Research Unit, Mayo Clinic, Rochester, MN 55905, USA

Chronic Pancreatitis
Ed. by Beger, Büchler, Ditschuneit, and Malfertheiner
© Springer-Verlag Berlin Heidelberg 1990

Table 1. Studies of gastrointestinal motility in chronic pancreatitis

Interdigestive motility	
Normal duodenal contraction rate	Brugge et al. [17]
Prolonged phase II in antrum	Malfertheiner et al. [18]
Post-prandial motility	
Rapid gastric emptying of liquid fatty meals in pancreatic insufficiency	Long and Weiss. [4]
Normal gastric emptying of a solid meal	Regan et al. [5]
Normal postprandial antral motility	Malfertheiner et al. [18]

sive because during phase II the motor activity is not constant, being low at the beginning and progressively increasing in frequency and amplitude.

Abnormal motilin and PP plasma values have been reported in chronic pancreatitis. Most studies have found increased plasma motilin levels [7, 8] and decreased PP plasma levels [8, 9], but these findings were not correlated to motility patterns. Since the release of these two peptides is coordinated with the interdigestive motor events of the upper gastrointestinal tract, disturbed fasting motor patterns might be expected in chronic pancreatitis.

To examine this hypothesis, we studied [18] the interdigestive and postprandial motor patterns and associated changes in plasma concentrations of PP in a group of eight patients with chronic pancreatitis and in seven healthy control subjects.

Interdigestive motility was studied by means of a low compliance manometric recording system measuring intraluminal pressures in antrum and duodenum. Motility was recorded for a period of at least 4 h after the fluoroscopic placement of the

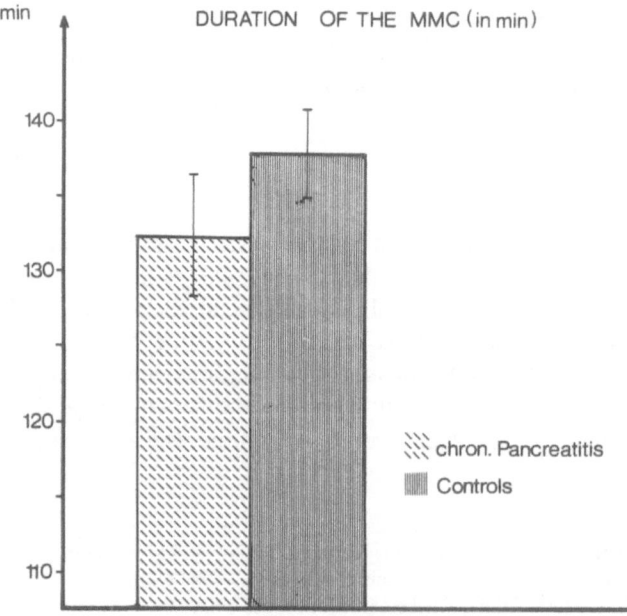

Fig. 1. Duration of the interdigestive migrating motor complex (MMC)

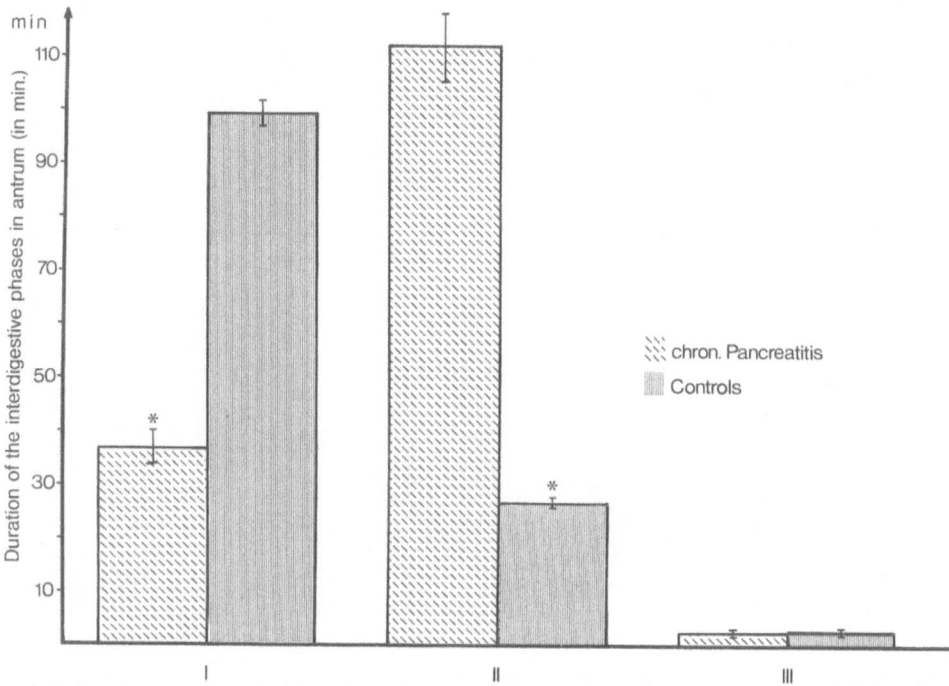

Fig. 2. Duration of the individual interdigestive phases in gastric antrum (asterix = p < 0.05)

catheter tip beyond the angle of Treitz. During the study plasma samples were taken every 15 min for the determination of PP [9].

Results from this study show that the periodicity (= duration of the total cycle) of the antroduodenal MMC is not different from normal in chronic pancreatitis (Fig. 1). *Antral* phase I appeared to be significantly shortened while phase II was prolonged in patients with chronic pancreatitis (Fig. 2). In contrast, *duodenal* interdigestive motor patterns were not altered. Plasma levels of PP were *not* abnormal during phases I and II in chronic pancreatitis. However compared to controls PP plasma concentrations showed no significant peak during phase III in chronic pancreatitis and were decreased. (Fig. 3).

From these findings we conclude that in chronic pancreatitis there is an increased fasting motor activity in the antrum. This phenomenon is associated with a loss of interdigestive cycling in PP plasma concentrations. As we have suggested from earlier experimental studies in dogs [14], PP is likely to play a role in controlling antral fasting motility. The decrease of plasma PP levels in chronic pancreatitis might be related to this motor disturbance in the interdigestive state.

Postprandial Motility

Two previous studies examining postprandial gastrointestinal motility in chronic pancreatitis focused on gastric emptying. Long and Weiss [4] reported abnormally

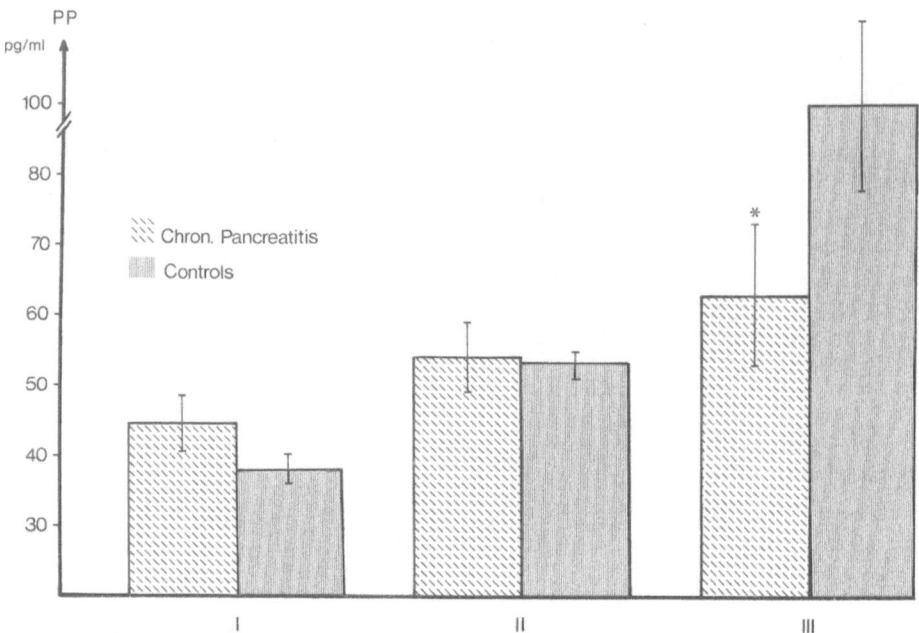

Fig. 3. Plasma levels of Pancreatic Polypeptide PP during the individual phases of interdigestive MMC (asterix = p < 0.05)

rapid gastric emptying of a liquid fatty meal in patients with pancreatic insufficiency. Although the autors speculated on the existence of a primary motor disorder, this was not confirmed by a later study by Regan et al. [5]. By simultaneous measurements of gastric emptying and gastric secretion before and following the ingestion of a solid meal, the latter group detected no abnormality in gastric emptying, but did note a decreased amount of gastric acid production. The administration of pancreatic enzyme preparations also did not modify the patterns of gastric emptying [5]. The authors concluded from these observations that the accelerated gastric emptying reported by Long and Weiss more likely reflected a normal adaptation to reduced total gastric juice volume.

In our group of patients with chronic pancreatitis, we investigated antroduodenal motility for 1–2 h following the ingestion of a standard meal. A postprandial antral motor index, based on the sum of amplitudes and frequency of the waves every 15 min, was calculated. This index was not different between patients and controls (Fig. 4). This is in support of the findings on gastric emptying reported by Regan et al. [5]. In spite of the normal motor pattern during the postprandial state, PP plasma levels were significantly lower in patients with chronic pancreatitis (Fig. 5). This suggests that PP has little if any role in the control of postprandial motility and that fed motility is not unduly altered in the face of pancreatic exocrine and endocrine insufficiency. Data on intestinal transit time following test meals are few in chronic pancreatitis and do not indicate major motor disturbances of the small bowel [19]. Colonic motility has not been investigated in patients with severe chronic pancreatitis and steatorrhea,

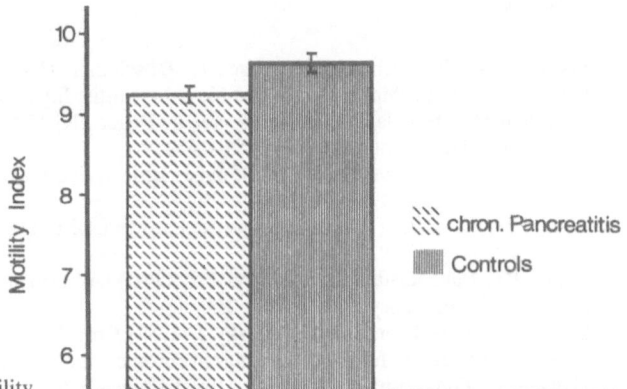

Fig. 4. Postprandial antral motility

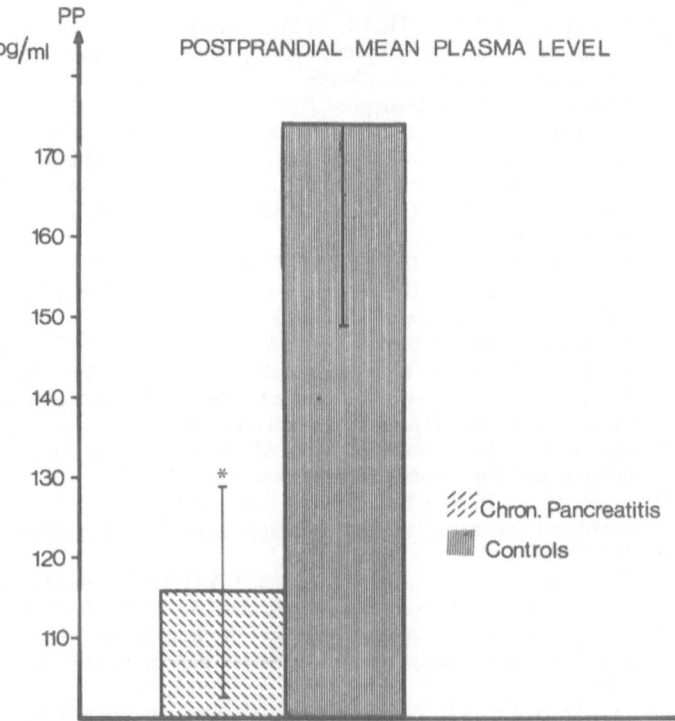

Fig. 5. Postprandial peak plasma concentration of PP (mean values, asterix = p < 0.05)

although it might be of clinical interest. Both postprandial and interdigestive motility are likely to be regulated by a redundancy of control factors, that are obviously sufficient to guarantee that no significant abnormality of gastrointestinal motility is observed in chronic pancreatitis.

An exacerbation of pain was never observed during any of the interdigestive and postprandial motility phases. Therefore it is unlikely that motor activities of the upper gastrointestinal tract may account for pain attacks in chronic pancreatitis.

References

1. Malfertheiner P, Büchler M, Stanescu A, Ditschuneit H (1987) Pancreatic morphology and function in relationship to pain in chronic pancreatitis. Int J Pancreatol 1:59–66
2. Bockman DE, Büchler M, Malfertheiner P, Beger HG (1988) Analysis of nerves in chronic pancreatitis. Gastroenterology 94:1459–1469
3. Malagelada JR, Stanghellini V (1985) Manometric evaluation of functional upper gut symptoms. Gastroenterology 88:1223–1231
4. Long WB, Weiss JB (1974) Rpaid gastric emptying of fatty meals in pancreatic insufficiency. Gastroenterology 67:920–925
5. Regan PT, Malagelada IR, DiMagno EP, Go WLW (1979) Postprandial gastric function in pancreatic insufficiency. Gut 20:249–254
6. Stern I, Roberts-Thomson IC, Hansky J (1982) Correlation between pancreatic polypeptide response to secretin and ERCP findings in chronic pancreatitis. Gut 23:235–238
7. Owyang C, Funakoshi A, Vinik AI (1983) Evidence for modulation of motilin secretion by pancreatico-biliary juice in health and in chronic pancreatitis. J Clin Endocrinol Metab 57:1015–1020
8. Besterman HS, Adrian TE, Bloom SR, Christofides ND, Mallinson CN, Ponti V, Lombardo L, Modigliani R, Guerin S, South M (1982) Pancreatic and gastrointestinal hormones in chronic pancreatitis. Digestion 24:195–208
9. Koch MB, Go WLW, DiMagno EP (1985) Can plasma human pancreatic polypeptide be used to detect diseases of the exocrine pancreas? Mayo Clin Proc 60:259–265
10. Rees WDW, Malagelada JR, Miller LJ, Go WLW (1982) Human interdigestive and postprandial gastrointestinal motor and gastrointestinal hormone patterns. Dig Dis Sci 27:321–329
11. Sarr MG, Kelly KA, Go WLW (1983) Motilin regulation of canine interdigestive intestinal motility. Dig Dis Sci 28:249–256
12. Keane FB, DiMagno EP, Dozois RR, Go WLW (1980) Relationship among canine interdigestive exocrine pancreatic and biliary flow, duodenal motor activity, plasma pancreatic polypeptide and motilin. Gastroenterology 78:310–316
13. Konturek SJ, Thor PJ, Bilski J, Bielanski W, Laskiewicz J (1986) Relationship between duodenal motility and pancreatic secretion in fasted and fed dogs. Am J Physiol 250:G570–574
14. Malfertheiner P, Sarr MG, DiMagno EP (1989) Role of pancreas in the control of interdigestive gastrointestinal motility. Gastroenterology 86:200–205
15. Owyang C, Achem-Karam SR, Vinik AI (1983) Pancreatic polypeptide and intestinal migrating motor complex in humans. Gastroenterology 84:10–17
16. Malfertheiner P, Sarr MG, Spencer MP, DiMagno EP (1989) Effect of duodenectomy on interdigestive pancreatic secretion, gastrointestinal motility and hormones in dogs. Am J Physiol 257:G415–422
17. Brugge WR, Burke CA, Brand DL, Chey WY (1985) Increased interdigestive pancreatic trypsin secretion in alcoholic pancreatic disease. Dig Dis Sci 30:431–439
18. Malfertheiner P, Pieramico O, Nelson DK, Büchler M, Ditschuneit H (1989) Interdigestive gastroduodenal motility and pancreatic polypeptide release in chronic pancreatitis. Pancreas 5:630
19. Lemcke B, Kraus B, Lankisch PG (1985) Small intestinal function in chronic relapsing pancreatitis. Hepatogastroenterol 32:149–151

Endocrine Pancreatic Function During Atrophy of the Exocrine Gland in Rats and Patients with Chronic Pancreatitis

U. R. Fölsch, F. Stöckmann, M. Nauck, and W. Creutzfeldt[1]

The association between diabetes mellitus and chronic pancreatitis has been debated for many years. It is known that the overall incidence of latent and overt diabetes mellitus secondary to chronic pancreatitis varies between 40% and 70% [1]. In patients with chronic calcifying pancreatitis the frequency of overt diabetes increases up to 90% [1].

More than 18 years ago a series of articles investigated the islet function of patients and rats with exocrine pancreatic insufficiency [2–4]. These studies, particularly in patients with chronic pancreatitis, indicated that the "incretin effect," i.e., the greater insulin secretion after an oral as compared to an intravenous glucose load, functions only in the presence of an intact exocrine gland. The authors claimed that this is due to an unresponsiveness of the β-cell to cholecystokinin (CCK) and secretin in the absence of acinar tissue.

However, in another study patients with chronic pancreatitis responded to crude exogenous CCK which contained significant amounts of gastric inhibitory polypeptide (GIP). Subsequently, we tried to investigate the presence or absence of the incretin effect in rats with an atrophy of the exocrine pancreas and in man with chronic pancreatitis and impaired glucose tolerance.

Materials and Methods

Studies in Animals

Male Wistar rats (150–300 g) were fed a choline- and copper-deficient diet (Altromin, Lage/Lippe, FRG) according to French [6] supplemented with 2% choline dehydrogen citrate and 300 mg D-penicillamine/kg body weight. Between 10 and 13 weeks after starting the diet, the acinar portion of the pancreas had almost completely disappeared and had been replaced by fatty and connective tissue, whereas the islets of Langerhans seemed to be intact [7] (Figs. 1a, b, 2). To substitute for pancreatic enzymes, the diet was supplemented with 300 mg pancreatin (Kali-Chemie Pharma GmbH, Hannover, FRG), daily. The control group received the copper-deficient diet without penicillamine. Under the latter conditions no morphological changes of the pancreas could be observed. All animals were pair-fed to obtain comparable metabolic conditions.

[1] Division of Gastroenterology and Endocrinology, Department of Medicine, Georg-August-Universität, Robert-Koch-Strasse, D-3400 Göttingen, FRG

Chronic Pancreatitis
Ed. by Beger, Büchler, Ditschuneit, and Malfertheiner
© Springer-Verlag Berlin Heidelberg 1990

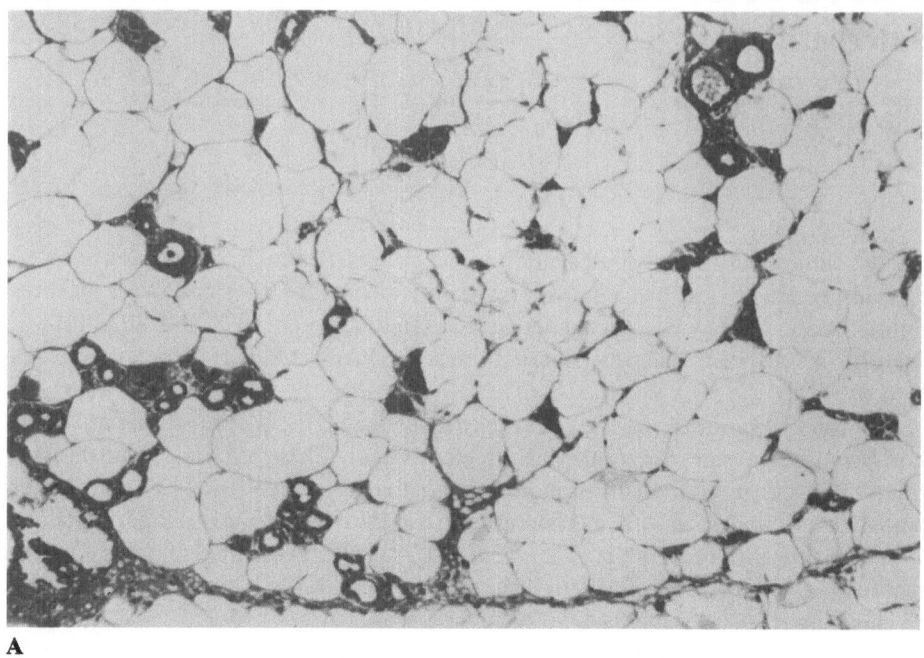

A

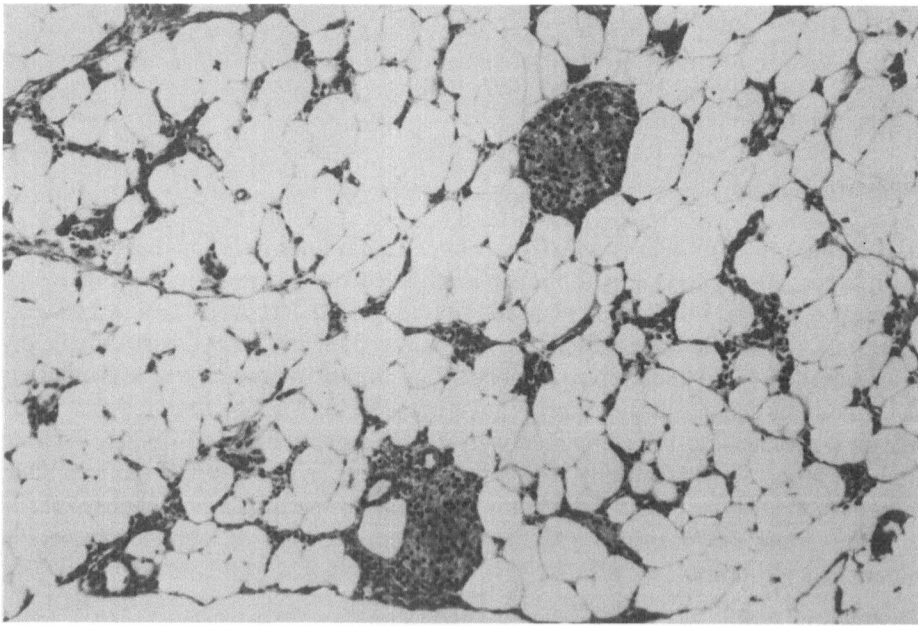

B

Fig. 1 A, B. Complete replacement of acinar tissue and well-preserved duct system **A** and islets of Langerhans **B**. Pancreas of a rat on a copper-deficient diet treated with *D*-penicillamine (300 mg/k daily for 13 weeks). Fixation in Bouin's fluid. H & E, × 40

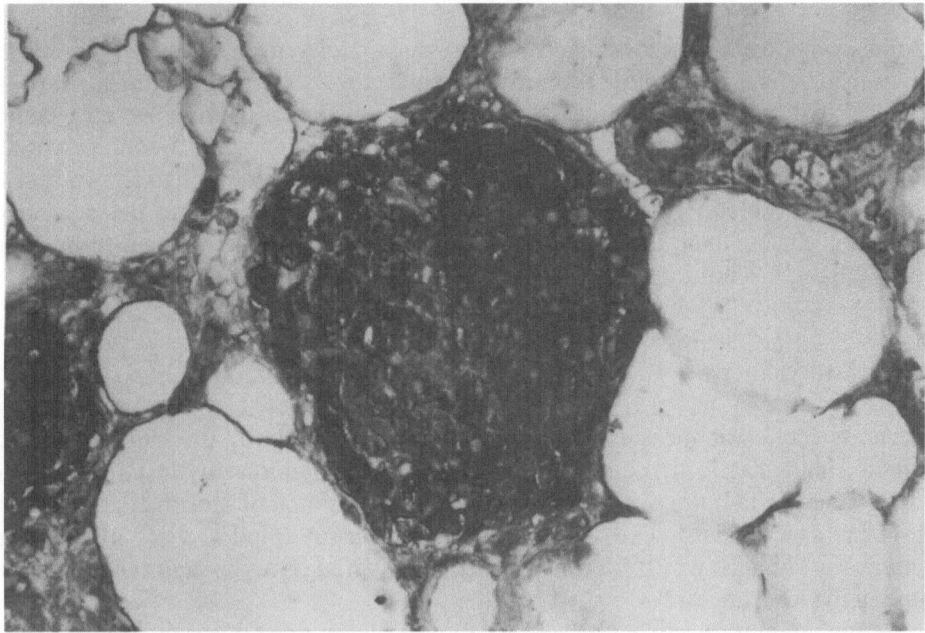

Fig. 2. Immunohistochemical staining of a single islet of Langerhans in the same atrophied pancreatic gland. Technique: fixation in Bouin's fluid. Embedding in paraffin: incubation of the deparaffinized sections with anti-insulin serum of guinea pigs in a 1:20 dilution. The sections were then washed and stained with anti-guinea pig serum of rabbits in a dilution of 1:20. Reaction to benzidine, × 400

Glucose Tolerance Test

Oral Glucose Load (n = 9 in Each Group)

After an overnight fast the animals were anesthetized. Rectal temperature of the animals was recorded continuously and the body temperature kept constant at 37°C. Through a midline incision the pylorus was exposed and ligated. A butterfly cannula was positioned in the duodenum just below the pylorus for the infusion of the glucose load.

A plastic catheter was placed into the left carotid artery. Just before the start of the experiments, another animal ("donor rat") that was fed a normal laboratory diet was provided with a catheter in the carotid artery, as described above, and heparinized with a saline solution containing 130 U heparin/100 g body weight. After each blood sampling, a corresponding volume of blood (0.6 ml) was transfused. Both rats with pancreatic atrophy and control animals received 2 g glucose/kg body weight as a 20% solution ($\cong$ 1 ml/100 g body weight) via the butterfly cannula into the duodenum within 8 min. Blood samples (0.6 ml) were withdrawn before and 30, 60, 90, and 120 min after the glucose load for determination of blood glucose, insulin, and GIP.

Intravenous Glucose Load

Animals that were used for the intravenous glucose tolerance tests were prepared as described before, but without performing laparotomy. Both the experimental rat and the pair-fed control animal received the glucose load as a continuous intravenous infusion at a rate of 1.2 g/kg per hour ($\cong 0.6$ ml/kg per hour) as a 20% solution within 120 min. This glucose load was used because preliminary studies had shown that it simulated the blood glucose concentrations reached in response to the described duodenal glucose load. Blood glucose, insulin, and GIP were determined at the same time intervals as indicated for the intraduodenal glucose load.

Analytical Methods

Serum glucose was measured in duplicate in each sample by the glucose oxidase method immediately after each experiment. Serum immunoreactive insulin (IRI) was determined by radioimmunoassay according to the method of Melani et al. [8] using rat insulin as standard. The detection limit of this assay amounted to 6 µU/ml. The interassay variance was 16%, and the intraassay variance in the high range was 6% and in the low range 12%.

Serum immunoreactive GIP (IR-GIP) was determined by radioimmunoassay according to the method of Kuzio et al. [9] with some modifications to improve the sensitivity of the assay system [10] using antiserum Gö 5/76/9 raised in rabbits. The interassay variance was 12.9% and the intraassay variance 7.4% (mean of 14 assays).

Evaluation of Data and Statistical Analysis

All values are presented as means $\pm$ SEM. $\triangle$ glucose, $\triangle$ IRI, and $\triangle$ IR-GIP are expressed as the values at time t minus the basal values. Integrated responses to corresponding loads (intraduodenal glucose, intravenous glucose) for IRI and IR-GIP were calculated according to the trapezoid rule.

For statistical evaluation the t test for unpaired groups was used (integrated values and values received from parameters measured in the pancreatic tissue such as pancreatic weight, protein, trypsin, and insulin). Results for absolute and relative values (blood glucose and serum IRI) were analyzed using the t test for unpaired groups adapted for multiple comparisons according to Holm [11].

Studies in Man

In these experiments it was investigated whether in patients with exocrine pancreatic insufficiency due to chronic pancreatitis the "incretin effect" is still functioning. Six patients with chronic pancreatitis proven by steatorrhea and pathological pancreatic function test were allocated to the study. All patients had normal fasting blood glucose levels but displayed an impaired glucose tolerance. They were asked to swallow 50 g glucose. Before and after the glucose digestion venous blood glucose, serum insulin (IRI) and gastric inhibitory polypeptide (GIP) were assessed over 180 min. In a second test glucose was infused intravenously in an amount which achieved blood glucose values identical to those observed after the oral load and again IRI and GIP were measured. Healthy volunteers served as controls.

Results

Pancreatic Protein, Trypsin, and Insulin

Protein content and trypsin concentration/mg protein were severely diminished in experimental animals as compared with controls (Table 1), proving the nearly complete destruction of the exocrine portion of the gland. On the other hand, the insulin content was only slightly diminished and did not significantly differ between the groups.

Table 1. Pancreatic weight and tissue content of protein, trypsin, and insulin in rats with an exocrine pancreatic atrophy and pair-fed controls ($\bar{x} \pm$ SEM)

Diet	n	Pancreatic weight (g)	Protein (mg)	Trypsin (mU/mg protein)	Insulin (mU/pancreas)
I Controls	18	1.06 ± 0.04	158 ± 6.5	86.0 ± 13.8	1.41 ± 0.11
II Experimental animals	18	0.56 ± 0.06	19.3 ± 1.7	0.17 ± 0.05	1.1 ± 0.10
		I/II $p < 0.001$	I/II $p < 0.001$	I/II $p < 0.001$	I/II n.s.

Blood △ Glukose Response to Intraduodenal and Intravenous Glucose Load

Following the intraduodenal glucose load (2.0 g/kg body weight), blood glucose levels of the animals with pancreatic atrophy increased steadily to a maximum of 17.5 ± 1.33 mmol/l at 120 min.

The control animals displayed a distinctly smaller blood glucose response to intraduodenal glucosc. A similar difference between experimental and control animals could be observed after intravenous glucose infusion. However, as can be seen in Fig. 3, blood glucose concentrations in response to intravenous glucose load approximated the corresponding blood glucose curve after intraduodenal glucose administration in the respective groups.

Serum IRI Response to Intraduodenal and Intravenous Glucose Load

The time courses of IRI concentrations after intraduodenal and intravenous glucose load are also depicted in Fig. 3. The insulin responses following an intraduodenal

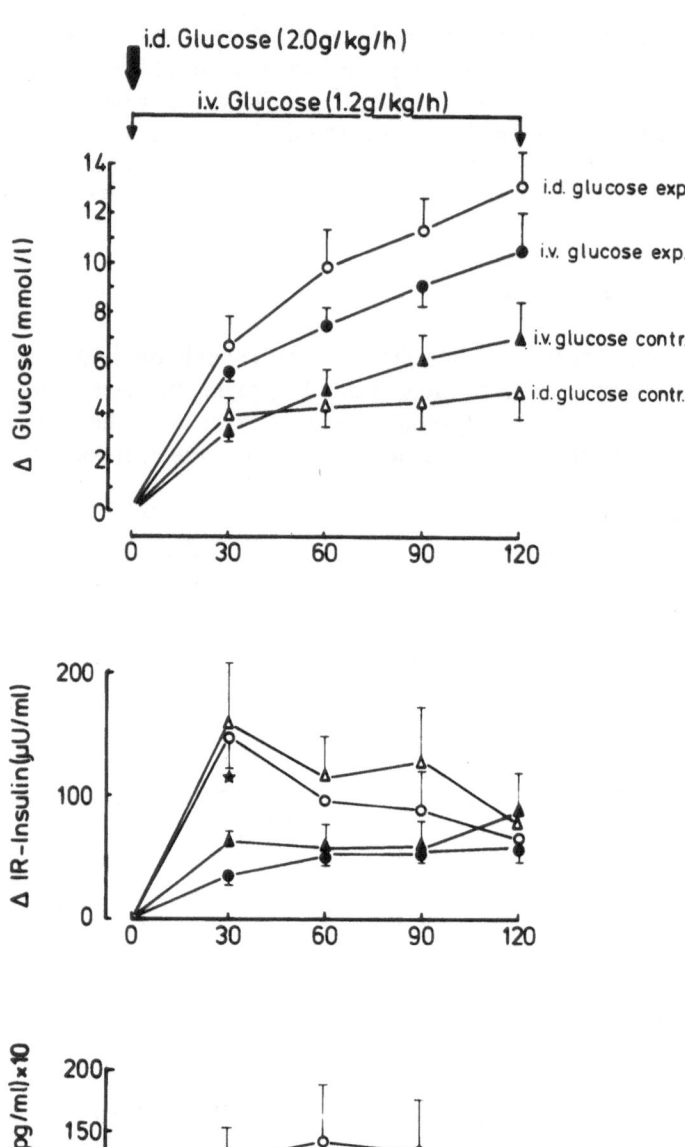

Fig. 3. Serum levels of △ glucose *(top)*, △ IRI *(middle)*, and △ IR-GIP *(bottom)* to intraduodenal and intravenous glucose administration in rats with exocrine pancreatic atrophy *(exp.)* and pair-fed controls *(contr.)*. All values are presented as means ± SEM ($n = 9$)

Table 2. Integrated values of serum levels of glucose, IRI, and IR-GIP ($\bar{x} \pm$ SEM) in response to an intraduodenal (i. d.; 2 g/kg b. wt.) or intravenous (i. v.; 2.4 g/kg b. wt./2 h) glucose load in rats with an exocrine pancreatic atrophy and pair-fed controls

Group	n	Glucose load	Glucose (g/dl/120 min)	IR insulin (mU/ml per 60 min)	IR insulin (mU/ml per 120 min)	IR-GIP (ng/ml per 120 min)
I Experimental animals	9	i. d. glucose	25.1 ± 2.8	8.2 ± 1.4	11.9 ± 3.0	136.2 ± 37.3
II Controls	9	i. d. glucose	9.2 ± 1.6	8.3 ± 2.0	14.5 ± 3.7	121.2 ± 22.6
III Experimental animals	9	i. v. glucose	17.5 ± 1.6	2.6 ± 0.3	5.9 ± 0.8	-23.2 ± 7.2
IV Controls	9	i. v. glucose	11.5 ± 1.9	3.6 ± 0.7	8.0 ± 2.2	-26.7 ± 8.3
				I/III $p < 0.005$	I/III n. s.	I/III $p < 0.001$
				II/IV $p < 0.05$	II/IV n. s.	II/IV $p < 0.001$

glucose load were higher than the corresponding values following an intravenous glucose infusion in the respective groups. At 30 min the difference between the insulin response after intraduodenal and intravenous glucose load was significant in the experimental animals ($p < 0.025$). The integrated insulin values calculated over 60 but not over 120 min were also significantly different (Table 2). Although IRI levels in the experimental animals were lower than those in the controls, the relative insulin responses ($\triangle$ IRI) displayed almost identical values, indicating an intact insulin-secretory mechanism in animals fed a copper-deficient diet supplement with **D**-penicillamine (Fig. 3).

IR-GIP Responses

In Fig. 3 the IR-GIP concentrations after intraduodenal glucose loads and during intravenous glucose infusion are also presented. Whereas during intravenous infusion no increase in IR-GIP could be observed, the administration of an intraduodenal glucose load was followed by a marked and identical increase in both groups (Fig. 3, Table 2).

"Incretin Effect" in Patients with Chronic Pancreatitis

Blood glucose concentrations after intravenous and oral glucose load reached similar levels both in patients with chronic pancreatitis (Fig. 4B) and in normal volunteers, respectively (Fig. 4A). However, blood glucose concentrations were higher in patients with chronic pancreatitis compared to controls. Clearly, the insulin response was significantly higher to the oral glucose load compared to an isoglycemic intravenous glucose administration both in patients with chronic pancreatitis and healthy volunteers. While the glucose concentrations were higher in the patients with chronic

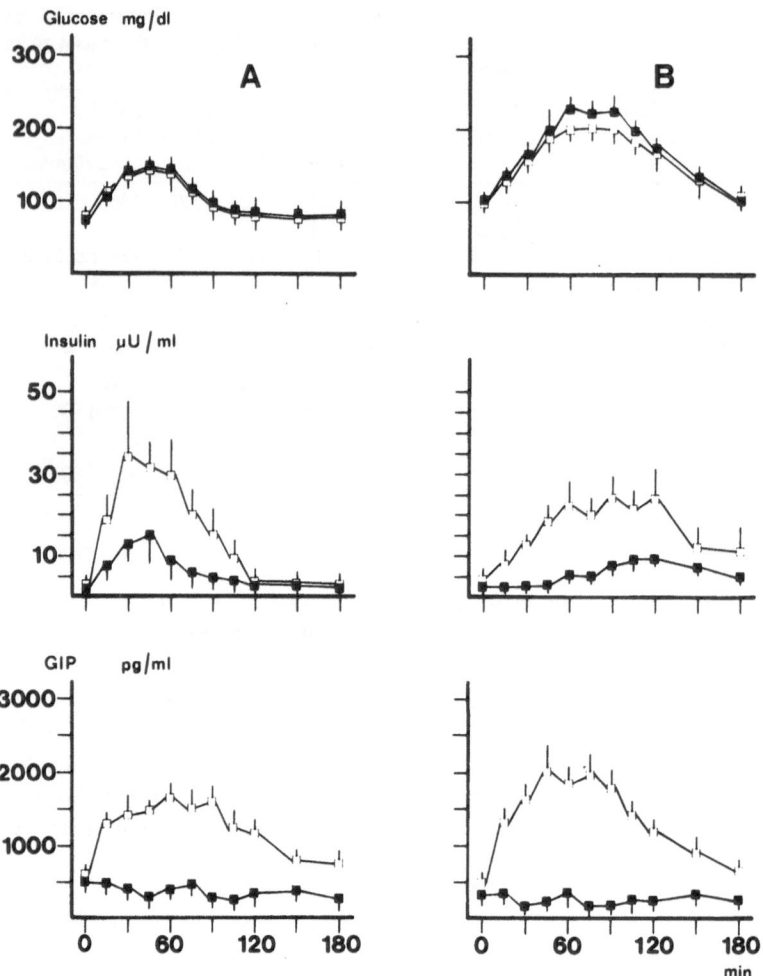

Fig. 4A, B. Serum levels of glucose, insulin, and GIP in response to an oral (50 g) or an isoglycemic intravenous glucose load in healthy volunteers **A** or in patients with chronic pancreatitis and impaired glucose tolerance ($n = 6$) **B** (□——□: oral glucose load; ■——■ intravenous glucose load)

pancreatitis the insulin response tended to be somewhat smaller, while the GIP responses were nearly identical.

Discussion

It has been claimed that in patients with chronic pancreatitis the "incretin effect," i. e., the greater insulin release in response to an oral as compared to an intravenous glucose load is missing [4]. Consequently, a so-called enteroreceptor at the islet cell has been postulated which functions only if the acinar tissue is intact [4].

In the present study using an experimental model with complete atrophy of the exocrine pancreas and investigating patients with chronic pancreatitis, an intact "incretin effect" could be demonstrated despite complete abolition or severe damage of the acinar tissue. Obviously the proper function of the enteroinsular axis is independent of an intact exocrine gland. The differences between the results of Raptis et al. [4] and the present investigation are difficult to explain. Considering the absolute insulin concentrations in plasma under basal and stimulated concentrations in the present study, it can be seen that rats with pancreatic atrophy had significantly lower values though the insulin content in the pancreatic gland was not significantly lower. In a histochemical study it has been demonstrated that a copper-deficient diet supplemented with **D**-penicillamine not only affects the exocrine part of the pancreas by lowering the activity of the copper-containing enzyme cytochrome C oxidase, but causes also a slight decrease in this enzyme in the endocrine cells [12]. Since this enzyme is a catalyst of oxidative phosphorylation, the slightly lowered insulin levels under basal and stimulated conditions might result from a disturbance of this enzyme in endocrine cells of the pancreas. On the other hand, Weaver et al. [13] described an identical insulin release in the perfused pancreas of copper-deficient penicillamine-treated rats during low (50 mg/dl) and high (300 mg/dl) glucose load. If exocrine pancreatic insufficiency was produced in rats by injection of oleic acid into the pancreatic duct, the insulin release and glucose tolerance were distinctly impaired [14]. However, since the intravenous glucose load was not isoglycemic (maximal blood glucose value after oral load 180 mg/dl and after intravenous load 500 mg/dl) no conclusions could be drawn regarding preservation of the "incretin effect" from these experiments.

Also in patients with chronic pancreatitis the insulin concentrations in plasma under basal and stimulated conditions were lower in comparison to healthy volunteers indicating that chronic pancreatitis frequently affects the islets [1]. On the other hand, these patients responded similarly to healthy subjects to an oral glucose load with greater insulin release than to an isoglycemic intravenous glucose infusion.

In conclusion, rats with exocrine pancreatic atrophy and patients with chronic pancreatitis and an impaired glucose tolerance retain the capacity to respond with an augmented insulin release after intraduodenal glucose as compared to an isoglycemic intravenous glucose load, i.e., showing an incretin effect. Thus, the contention that the B cells do not respond to an incretin in the absence of the exocrine pancreatic tissue [4] has not been confirmed.

Acknowledgment. This study was supported by the Deutsche Forschungsgemein-schaft, Bonn-Bad Godesberg (grant Fo 73/7–6).

References

1. Bank S, Marks IN, Vinik AI (1975) Clinical and hormonal aspects of pancreatic diabetes. Am J Gastroenterol 64:13–22
2. Hinz M, Katsilambros N, Schweitzer B, Raptis S, Pfeiffer EF (1971) The role of the exocrine pancreas in the stimulation of insulin secretion by intestinal hormones. I. The effect of pancreozymin, secretin, gastrin-pentapeptide and glucagon upon insulin secretion of isolated islets of rat pancreas. Diabetologia 7:1–5
3. Goberna R, Fussgänger RD, Raptis S, Telib M, Pfeiffer EF (1971) The role of the exocrine pancreas in the stimulation of insulin secretion by intestinal hormones. II. Insulin responses to

secretin and pancreozymin in experimentally induced pancreatic insufficiency. Diabetologia 7:68-72

4. Raptis S, Rau RM, Schröder KE, et al. (1971) The role of the exocrine pancreas in the stimulation of insulin secretion by intestinal hormones. III. Insulin responses to secretin and pancreozymin, and to oral and intravenous glucose, in patients suffering from chronic insufficiency of the exocrine pancreas. Diabetologia 7:160-167

5. Kalk WJ, Vinik AI, Botha JL, Keller P, Jackson WPU (1975) Insulin responses to crude cholecystokinin-pancreozymin in normal subjects, in patients with chronic pancreatitis and patients with mild maturity diabetes. J Clin Endocrinol 41:172-176

6. French SW (1966) Effect of chronic ethanol ingestion on liver enzyme changes induced by thiamine, riboflavine, pyridoxine or choline deficiency. J Nutr 88:291-302

7. Fölsch UR, Creutzfeldt W (1977) Pancreatic duct cells in rats: secretory studies in response to secretin, cholecystokinin-pancreozymin and gastrin in vivo. Gastroenterology 73:1053-1059

8. Melani F, Ditschuneit H, Bartlet KM, Friedrich H, Pfeiffer EF (1965) Über die radio-immunologische Bestimmung von Insulin im Blut. Klin Wochenschr 43:1000-1007

9. Kuzio M, Dryburgh JR, Malloy KM, Brown JC (1974) Radioimmunoassay for gastric inhibitory polypeptide. Gastroenterology 66:357-364

10. Ebert R, Finke U (1978) Gastric inhibitory polypeptide (GIP). Z Gastroenterol 16:311-316

11. Holm S (1979) A simple sequential rejection multiple test procedure. Scand J Statist 6:65-70

12. Fell BF, King TP, Davies NT (1982) Pancreatic atrophy in copper deficient rat; histochemical and ultrastructural evidence of a selective effect on exocrine tissue. Histochem J 14:665-680

13. Weaver FRC, Sorenson RL, Kaung H-LC (1986) An immunohistochemical, ultrastructural, and physiological study of pancreatic islets from copper-deficient, penicillamine-treated rats. Diabetes 35:13-19

14. Göke B, Elsebach K, Hausmann W, Schaar M, Arnold R, Adler G (1987) Endocrine pancreatic morphology and function in exocrine insufficiency in rats. Am J Physiol 253:G139-145

Pancreas Divisum and Pancreatitis: Implications and Rationale for Treatment

M. L. STEER[1]

Embryology

The pancreas develops during the 8th week of gestation when the dorsal pancreatic anlage emerges from the medial wall of the duodenum and the ventral pancreatic anlage emerges from the liver bud on the lateral side of the duodenum. As it enlarges, the dorsal pancreas extends medially across the mid-line anterior to the mesenteric vessels. Eventually, it gives rise to the tail, body, and cephalad portion of the head of the pancreas. The ventral pancreatic anlage extends from the bile duct and, as the stomach and duodenum enlarge, the bile duct and ventral pancreas rotate behind the duodenum to eventually lie along the medial wall of the duodenum. As a result of this rotation, the terminal bile duct is situated behind or within the dorsal pancreas and the ventral pancreas lies behind the mesenteric vessels. Eventually, the ventral pancreas develops into the uncinate process and caudal portion of the head of the pancreas. The ventral pancreas is drained by the duct of Wirsung which, along with the bile duct, enters the duodenum at the papilla of Vater. The dorsal pancreas, on the other hand, is drained by the duct of Santorini which enters the duodenum at the lesser papilla. When the dorsal and ventral pancreata fuse, the ductal systems usually communicate and, in most instances, drainage predominantly occurs via the papilla of Vater.

Pancreas divisum occurs when complete fusion of the dorsal and ventral pancreata does not occur. Usually, the two anlagen merge into a single structure and the failure of fusion involves only the ductal elements. As a result, completely separate ducts of Wirsung and Santorini are maintained. Thus, in pancreas divisum, the tail, body, and cephalad portion of the head of the pancreas are drained, by the duct of Santorini, into the duodenum at the lesser papilla while the uncinate process and caudal portion of the pancreatic head drain, via the duct of Wirsung, into the duodenum at the papilla of Vater. In some individuals partial pancreas divisum may occur if there is incomplete merger of the ductal systems.

Incidence

In autopsy studies, the incidence of pancreas divisum has been reported to vary between 4% and 14% while studies based on endoscopic retrograde pancreatography suggest that the incidence of pancreas divisum is 1%–7% (see [1] and references

---

[1] Harvard Medical School, Beth Israel Hospital, 330 Brookline Avenue, Boston, MA 02215, USA

Chronic Pancreatitis
Ed. by Beger, Büchler, Ditschuneit, and Malfertheiner
© Springer-Verlag Berlin Heidelberg 1990

therein). As a rough approximation, most workers consider the incidence of pancreas divisum to be 9%–10%.

Clinical Significance

Chronic pancreatitis

The clinical significance of pancreas divisum is unknown although considerable controversy surrounds this issue. A number of reports have suggested that the incidence of pancreatitis is increased in individuals with pancreas divisum (Table 1). For example, Cotton [3] noted that 16.4% of patients with recurrent pancreatitis and 25.6% of patients with idiopathic pancreatitis undergoing ERCP had pancreas divisum while only 3.6% of patients with biliary disease undergoing ERCP had pancreas divisum. Sahel et al. [4] found a 5% incidence of pancreas divisum among all patients undergoing ERCP but noted that the incidence of pancreas divisum among patients with acute pancreatitis was 21%. Richter [5] found pancreas divisum in 5% of their patients undergoing ERCP but noted that the incidence of pancreas divisum was 12% in patients with pancreatitis and 19% in patients with idiopathic pancreatitis. These observations suggested that pancreas divisum might be a cause for otherwise unexplained pancreatitis. This presumed cause-effect relationship was explained by the hypothesis that the orifice of the lesser papilla might be too small to permit flow of the large volume of pancreatic secretion which must empty into the duodenum by that route in pancreas divisum and, as a result, pancreas divisum might cause a form of obstructive pancreatitis.

Table 1. Incidence of pancreas divisum. (Adapted from [2])

Reason for study	Cotton [3] ($n = 47$)	Sahel et al. [4] ($n = 41$)	Richter [5] ($n = 26$)	Delhaye et al. [1] ($n = 304$)	Sugawa et al. [2] ($n = 41$)
Overall group	5.8	5	5	5.7	2.7
Pancreatitis	16.4	21	12	6.9	2.3
Idiopathic pancreatitis	25.6	–	19	5.3	2.4

More recently, however, several reports have indicated that the incidence of pancreatitis might, actually, not be increased in individuals with pancreas divisum (Table 1). Delhaye et al. [1] in Belgium reported the results of a study involving 6324 patients undergoing ERCP for biliopancreatic complaints. Successful pancreatography was obtained in 85% of the patients and pancreas divisum was diagnosed in 304 individuals (5.7% of subjects). Successful cannulation of the lesser papilla and dorsal duct pancreatography was achieved in 97 of the patients with pancreas divisum. Delhaye et al. noted that the incidence of pancreas divisum was similar in patients with chronic pancreatitis (6.4%), acute pancreatitis (7.5%), and non-pancreatic diseases (5.5%) (Table 2). Similar results were also reported by Sugawa et al. [2], who

Table 2. Incidence of pancreatic diseases in patients with and without pancreas divisum. (Adapted from [1])

Disease	(+) Pancreas divisum		(−) Pancreas divisum		
	No.	%	No.	%	P
Acute pancreatitis	25	8.2	310	6.1	NS
Acute idiopathic pancreatitis	4	1.3	56	1.1	NS
Chronic pancreatitis	26	8.6	380	7.5	NS
Pancreatic carcinoma	16	5.3	275	5.4	NS
Papillary carcinoma	2	0.6	66	1.3	NS
Nonpancreatic diseases	235	77.3	4022	79.6	NS
Total	304	–	5053	–	–

NS, not significant by x^2 analysis

found 41 patients with pancreas divisum among a group of 1529 undergoing ERCP (overall incidence = 2.7%). In their study, Sugawa et al. [2] found that the incidence of pancreas divisum among those with idiopathic pancreatitis was not increased. Sugawa et al. [2] also noted that the incidence of pancreas divisum was not increased in individuals with unexplained upper abdominal pain (Table 1). Thus, the results reported by Delhaye et al. [1] and by Sugawa et al. [2] suggest that pancreas divisum is not a frequent cause of either pancreatitis or upper abdominal pain. It is not entirely clear why the earlier studies, such as those of Cotton [3], Sahel et al. [4] and Richter [5] indicated an increased incidence of pancreas divisum among patients with pancreas divisum. It is possible that those earlier studies may have been misleading because they reflected the selection bias that can occur in centers with exceptional endoscopic skills. Patients with pancreas divisum and patients with unexplained pancreatitis are likely to be referred to such centers and, as a result, the incidence of pancreas divisum among patients with pancreatitis may appear to be increased when such an increase is not present in a more random sampling of patients.

In certain circumstances, the anatomic arrangement of pancreas divisum may actually serve to reduce the severity of pancreatitis. For example, in cases of gallstone pancreatitis, the anatomic variant of pancreas divisum could result in less severe episodes of pancreatic injury since only that portion of the pancreas drained via the papilla of Vater may be involved. Similarly, the pancreatitis associated with Vaterian or peri-Vaterian obstructing lesions or caused by lesions blocking the duct of Wirsung could be relatively mild and, as a result, go unrecognized in patients with pancreas divisum. In contrast, lesions interfering with drainage from the lesser papilla or obstructing the duct of Santorini may be more likely to produce severe pancreatitis and pancreatic insufficiency in patients with pancreas divisum. Indeed, several patients with pancreas divisum have been described whose changes of chronic pancreatitis were confined to the dorsal pancreas. It is clear, however, that patients with idiopathic chronic pancreatitis confined to the dorsal pancreas and associated with pancreas divisum are rare and that they constitute only a small fraction of those with pancreas divisum.

Attacks of Abdominal Pain

In contrast to the small group of patients with objective evidence of chronic pancreatitis (i. e., morphological and/or functional changes), there exists a much larger group of individuals with pancreas divisum who lack objective evidence of chronic pancreatitis but who are evaluated because of episodes of upper abdominal "pancreas-like" pain. These attacks of pain may or may not be accompanied by hyperamylasemia, hyperlipasemia, or other biochemical signs of pancreatic involvement. The epidemiological studies cited above do not indicate that pancreas divisum, alone, is a frequent cause of such attacks. Some clinicians, however, have suggested that patients with pancreas divisum might develop such attacks if they also had stenosis of the lesser papilla orifice. Warshaw [6] has claimed that sphincteroplasty of the lesser papilla benefits such patients. In a recent report, he noted that 75% of patients with discrete attacks of abdominal pain and 40% of patients with chronic otherwise unexplained upper abdominal pain and pancreas divisum were cured by that procedure. Furthermore, he has reported that 85% of those benefited by lesser papilla sphincteroplasty were found, at operation, to have a lesser papillary orifice which would not admit a 0.75-mm-diameter lacrimal probe and was, therefore, considered to be stenotic. Warshaw et al. [7] have reported that those patients who had stenosis of the lesser papilla orifice and who would be benefited by lesser papillotomy could be detected by preoperative ultrasonographic studies of pancreatic duct size before and after secretin stimulation. They noted that secretin stimulation caused prolonged ($\sim$ 30 min) ductal dilitation in such patients but not in control patients or in individuals with unexplained abdominal pain whose lesser papilla orifice was not found to be stenotic. Taken together, these observations if confirmed would strongly suggest that a significant group of patients with pancreas divisum and attacks of abdominal pain with or without hyperamylasemia develop these attacks because of outflow obstruction at the lesser papilla and that such patients will benefit from lesser papillotomy.

The issue, however, remains highly controversial primarily because most of the evidence supporting those conclusions has emanated from a single institution and because others working in this field have been unable to duplicate those findings. Several groups, for example, have found that most patients with pancreas divisum and abdominal pain with or without hyperamylasemia are not benefitted by either surgical or endoscopic lesser papillotomy [8]. Furthermore, many have found accurate calibration of the lesser papilla orifice to be difficult even at the time of surgical exposure. Finally, the reliability of the ultrasound-secretin test has been questioned. It had been previously noted that transient ($\sim$ 5 min) ductal dilitation following secretin stimulation occurred in most normal individuals [9] but, in pancreas divisum patients, the duration of secretin-induced dilitation was believed to be prolonged. Recently, however, Lowes et al. [10] have reported the results of an ultrasonographic study evaluating pancreatic duct caliber 5, 10, and 15 min after secretin stimulation (Table 3). Four groups of individuals were studied: 9 pain-free controls, 9 controls with nonpancreatic abdominal pain who did not have pancreas divisum, 17 patients with pancreas divisum and attacks of abdominal pain but no evidence of pancreatitis, and 9 patients with pancreas divisum plus either chronic or recurrent acute pancreatitis. The maximal ductal dilitation induced by secretin stimulation was similar in all four groups ($\sim$ 1 mm) and, if anything, tended to be greater in the normal controls. In addition, the

Table 3. Pancreatic duct diameter after secretin infusion. (Adapted from [10])

	Controls ($n = 9$)	Pain, no PD ($n = 9$)	PD, no CP ($n = 17$)	PD and CP ($n = 9$)
Maximum duct Dilitation ± SD (mm)	1.05 ± 0.77	0.74 ± 0.44	0.94 ± 0.58	0.83 ± 0.56
Number with positive test	5	3	5	3

frequency with which secretin was found to stimulate ductal dilitation was similar in each of the four groups. From these results, it would appear either that the pancreatic duct does not dilate after secretin stimulation in patients who have pancreatitis or pancreatic pain and pancreas divisum or, alternatively, that the secretin-ultrasound test is an unreliable indicator of pancreatic pathology in these patients.

Conclusions and Therapeutic Recommendations

A critical analysis of the currently available epidemiological data concerning pancreas divisum has led this reviewer to conclude that pancreas divisum is a frequently occurring developmental variant which, by itself, is of no clinical significance. Its presence may alter the presentation of pancreatic inflammatory disease by minimizing the severity of gallstone pancreatitis as well as pancreatitis resulting from peri-Vaterian obstructing lesions. In the presence of lesions obstructing the lesser papilla, chronic obstructive pancreatitis confined to the dorsal pancreas can develop. When, in such cases, the duct of Santorini becomes dilated, ductal decompressive procedures such as longitudinal pancreaticojejunostomy should be performed. When objective evidence of chronic pancreatitis of the dorsal pancreas is present but the duct is not dilated, lesser papillotomy or lesser papilla dilitation might be considered but prior experience with similar procedures performed at the papilla of Vater for patients whose chronic pancreatitis not associated with pancreas divisum would suggest that a successful outcome using this approach is unlikely. Thus, a resective procedure may eventually prove to be more appropriate in this setting.

The controversy surrounding treatment of patients who have abdominal pain with pancreas divisum but who lack objective evidence of pancreatitis continues [11, 12]. It is unlikely that pancreas divisum, alone, is the cause of this syndrome. Perhaps, lesser papillary stenosis combined with pancreas divisum may account for some of these patients' attacks and, if so, the critical issue remains that of accurately identifying such patients. Without such identification, the results of procedures designed to improve drainage from the lesser papilla are destined to remain poor. In fact, there have been deaths from such procedures and, in some, the manipulations (surgical as well as endoscopic) at the lesser papilla may have caused a stenosis when none had existed previously. Early hopes that preoperative ultrasound measurement of pancreatic duct dilitation after secretin stimulation or intraoperative calibration of the lesser papillary orifice could reliably identify patients likely to benefit from lesser papillotomy have not been supported by later studies. The value of these maneuvers must await confirmatory results from truly objective trials. In the absence of a clearly reliable objective method of identifying patients likely to benefit from lesser papillotomy, considerable caution should be exercised in the management of patients with abdominal pain but no objective evidence of pancreatitis. For those with pain associated with transient hyperamylasemia unresponsive to medical therapy, lesser papillotomy may prove to be the only available treatment option. In view of the considerable uncertainty regarding outcome, however, a randomized prospective trial of the therapy of such patients would seem reasonable. For those without even transient hyperamylasemia to incriminate the pancreas as the cause of abdominal pain, surgical or endoscopic procedures at the lesser papilla would seem unwarranted and possibly even dangerous.

References

1. Delhaye M, Engelholm L, Cremer M (1985) Pancreas divisium: congenital anatomic variant or anomaly? Gastroenterology 89:951–958
2. Sugawa C, Walt AJ, Nunez DC, Masuyama H (1987) Pancreas divisum: is it a normal anatomic variant? Am J Surg 153:62–67
3. Cotton PB (1980) Congenital anomaly of pancreas divisum as cause of obstructive pain and pancreatitis. Gut 21:105–114
4. Sahel J, Cros RC, Bourry J, Sarles H (1982) Clinicopathological conditions associated with pancreas divisum. Digestion 23:1–8
5. Richter JM (1981) Association of pancreas divisum and pancreatitis, and its treatment by sphincteroplasty of the accessory ampulla. Gastroenterology 81:1104–1010
6. Warshaw AL, Simeone JF, Schapiro RH, Flavin-Warshaw B (1990) Evaluation and treatment of the dominant dorsal duct syndrome (Pancreas divisum redefined). Am J Surg 159:59–66
7. Warshaw AL, Simeone J, Schapiro RH, Hedberg SE, Mueller PE, Ferrucci JT (1985) Objective evaluation of ampullary stenosis with ultrasonography and pancreatic stimulation. Am J Surg 149:65–72
8. Russell RCG, Wong NW, Cotton PB (1984) Accessory sphincterotomy (endoscopic and surgical) in patients with pancreas divisum. Br J Surg 71:954–957
9. Bolondi L, Gaiani S, Gullo L, Labo G (1984) Secretin administration induces a dilatation of main pancreatic duct. Dig Dis Sci 29:802–808
10. Lowes JR, Lees WR, Cotton PB (1989) Pancreatic duct dilatation after secretin stimulation in patients with pancreas divisum. Pancreas 4:371–374
11. Steer ML (1987) More doubts about the clinical significance of pancreas divisum. Gastroenterology 93:206–207
12. Warshaw AL (1987) Reply to selected summary: more doubts about the clinical significance of pancreas divisum. Gastroenterology 93:1140–1141

Complications

Complications in Chronic Pancreatitis

H. A. Reber[1]

The most common complications in chronic pancreatitis are pain and the development of pseudocysts. These, as well as obstruction of the common bile duct by the fibrotic pancreas, are discussed elsewhere in this volume. The present review will concern itself with the complications of pancreatic fistula and ascites, bowel obstruction, splenic vein thrombosis, and hemorrhage.

Pancreatic Fistula

External pancreatic fistula as a complication of chronic pancreatitis is unusual, and occurs most commonly after operative or percutaneous external drainage of a pseudocyst. It may also follow operative injury (e. g., pancreatic biopsy) or arise from a leak of a pancreatic anastomosis (e. g., pancreaticojejunostomy). The diagnosis is usually suspected when clear fluid drains from the cutaneous orifice, and it is confirmed when the amylase content of the fluid is shown to be elevated. Most of these fistulas close spontaneously, providing that the general guidelines for the management of external gastrointestinal fistulas are followed. Infection must be eradicated, nutritional support must be provided, fluids and electrolytes must be replaced, and the skin must be protected. The fistula volume may be as high as 1 l/day, but often it is considerably less. Most patients can be fed by mouth during the time that healing is taking place, greatly simplifying their management. There is no evidence that this prolongs the time until closure occurs. When the tract is well formed (usually 10–14 days after infection is controlled), a fistulogram should be obtained. If there is evidence of ductal obstruction between the site of the leak and the duodenum, then operative repair of the fistula may be necessary. This is most easily accomplished by a Roux-en-Y anastomosis with the jejunum over the opening where the leak originates.

Recently the gut hormone somatostatin has been used in patients with pancreatic fistula to decrease the volume of fistula drainage. This may simplify their management considerably. Claims that somatostatin also hastens the spontaneous closure of pancreatic fistulas have not yet been rigorously tested.

---

[1] Department of Surgery, UCLA School of Medicine, 10833 LeConte Avenue, Los Angeles, California 90024, USA

Chronic Pancreatitis
Ed. by Beger, Büchler, Ditschuneit, and Malfertheiner
© Springer-Verlag Berlin Heidelberg 1990

Pancreatic Ascites

Pancreatic ascites is a consequence of the leakage of pancreatic juice from a pseudo-cyst or the pancreatic duct. It occurs typically in alcoholic cirrhotics, with muscle wasting and extreme weight loss. They usually complain of mild to moderate abdominal pain as a result of the abdominal distension. Because of the clinical presentation, the diagnosis is often erroneously attributed to decompensated Laënnec's cirrhosis. However, paracentesis reveals that the ascitic fluid has a protein concentration in excess of 3 g/dl, and a high amylase concentration. These findings are diagnostic. If the fluid does not leak directly into the peritoneal cavity, it can track in the retroperitoneum before it accumulates a considerable distance from the pancreas (e. g., mediastinum, pleural space). Nevertheless the treatment is the same.

The patients are given nothing by mouth and placed on parenteral nutrition to prepare them for surgery. Somatostatin (see previous discussion) is probably also of value. Paracenteses may be useful if the abdominal distension is severe, but there is no evidence that the complete evacuation of the ascitic fluid is more likely to result in spontaneous sealing of the leak. Carbonic anhydrase inhibitors and diuretics, although used in the past, have no place in current management. During this period of preparation, which should last about 2 weeks, the ascites may resolve spontaneously in as many as one-third of patients, and surgery can be avoided. In some series as many as one-fourth of the patients have also died during this time. This has been attributed to their generally poor condition to begin with.

An ERCP must precede surgery in order to identify the precise site of the leak. Distal pancreatectomy is preferred if the leak is in the tail of the pancreas. Otherwise drainage into a Roux-en-Y limb of jejunum is effective. This approach is successful in at least 80% of patients who survive to undergo operation.

Bowel Obstruction

Intestinal obstruction secondary to chronic pancreatitis can occur in the duodenum, jejunum, or the colon. The pathogenesis can involve the direct spread of inflammation from the pancreas through the leaves of the mesentery to the affected intestine. Direct spread of the fibroinflammatory process in the pancreas or ischemia may also be responsible.

When the obstruction develops in association with an episode of acute inflammation of the pancreas, it may subside as the inflammation subsides. If it persists for 3–4 weeks, it is likely to require operative correction.

The diagnosis is made when a barium contrast examination reveals a discrete area of narrowing. In the duodenum the differential diagnosis is usually between ulcer disease and periampullary malignancy. In the colon, cancer is the main concern. Endoscopic examination reveals an intact mucosa when the stricture is secondary to pancreatitis.

Duodenal obstruction (usually involving the second or third portion) should be bypassed with a gastrojejunostomy. Colonic obstruction most commonly involves the transverse colon or the splenic flexure. Resection with end-to-end anastomosis is satisfactory in most cases.

Splenic Vein Thrombosis

Chronic pancreatitis is the most common etiology of splenic vein thrombosis. This creates a segmental form of portal hypertension which may result in gastric varices that can bleed. The incidence of the complication is probably higher than suspected, since varices may be overlooked and hemorrhage need not have occurred. Patients with chronic pancreatitis who have had upper gastrointestinal bleeding and/or in whom gastric varices are noted may be candidates for angiography to determine splenic vein patency. Although splenectomy is curative, the role of prophylactic splenectomy in patients who have not yet bled is unclear.

Hemorrhage

Hemorrhage in chronic pancreatitis usually occurs from pseudoaneurysms that involve the splenic, gastroduodenal, or pancreaticoduodenal arteries. They are commonly found in association with pseudocysts, and can rupture into the cyst or into the pancreatic duct. If the blood enters the gut and is manifest either as hematemesis or melena, endoscopy is a valuable diagnostic maneuver. Angiography is a great help because it provides precise localization of the bleeding source, and in poor-risk patients therapeutic embolization may be definitive. However, in some cases, the hemorrhage is too rapid for such diagnostic maneuvers. The preferred treatment is operation with either resection or suture ligation of the bleeding point.

Clinical Relevance of Cholestasis Syndrome in Chronic Pancreatitis – The Cape Town Experience*

P. C. Bornman, I. Kalvaria, A. H. Girdwood, and I. N. Marks[1]

Introduction

Common bile duct stenoses (CBDSs) are more frequently identified today with the increased use of modern imaging techniques in the diagnosis of chronic alcohol-induced pancreatitis (CAIP).

Despite numerous publications on this subject, uncertainty remains with regard to its natural history and in particular the risk of developing complications such as cholangitis and secondary biliary cirrhosis. The reported incidence of the latter complication varies from 0% to 16% [1, 2, 5–8, 10–14]. Most studies, however, are based on retrospective reviews of patients who required a biliary drainage operation while the few reports on the natural history have yielded conflicting results [1, 2, 5, 7, 8, 11, 12]. The discrepancies in these studies may in part be explained by differences in criteria used for patient selection, interpretation of liver histology, and factors such as continued alcohol abuse. This study was carried out to shed further light on the natural history of CBDS in chronic pancreatitis.

Material and Methods

Over a 7-year period (1979–1985) 60 patients with CAIP and CBDS were identified while undergoing endoscopic retrograde cholangiopancreatography (ERCP). This constituted 12% of 502 patients with CAIP investigated by ERCP over this period. There were 56 males and 4 females with a mean age of 44 years (range, 25–65 years). Most patients had a long-standing history of CAIP (mean of 8 years) and 90% had calcification at the time of the diagnosis.

Results

Three clinical groups have emerged from this study. There were ten asymptomatic or minimally symptomatic patients (group 1). In 21 patients, CBDSs were discovered during investigation for pain (group 2). The remaining 29 patients presented with

* Support from The South African Medical Research Council is acknowledged
[1] Surgical Gastroenterology and GIT Clinic, Groote Schuur Hospital and Departments of Surgery and Medicine, University of Cape Town, South Africa

Chronic Pancreatitis
Ed. by Beger, Büchler, Ditschuneit, and Malfertheiner
© Springer-Verlag Berlin Heidelberg 1990

jaundice of whom 3 had associated cholangitis and 4 had biliary calculi (group 3). These jaundiced patients had significantly more advanced disease (i. e., calcification, diabetes mellitus, and steatorrhea) than groups 1 and 2.

The mean alkaline phosphatase levels in the 31 nonjaundiced patients (groups 1, 2) were 290 IU ($N = $ < 115 IU). The majority of patients exhibited type I or III strictures [9] on ERCP. These strictures were equally distributed between the three groups. However, extrahepatic bile duct dilatation (CBD diameter of > 10 mm) with or without intrahepatic dilatation was significantly more common in the jaundiced group.

Twenty-nine patients underwent liver biopsy during the follow-up period. Histological evidence of extrahepatic biliary obstruction was present in almost half of the biopsies and was significantly more common in the jaundiced group (groups 1, 2: 4/14; group 3: 10/15; $p = $ < 0.05). Secondary biliary cirrhosis was not encountered in any of these biopsies.

Outcome

In the ten asymptomatic or minimally symptomatic patients nine remained well over a mean follow-up period of 46 months with no further deterioration of liver function tests.

Six of the 21 patients in group 2 came to surgery. Five underwent a biliary drainage operation and a pancreaticojejunostomy and one had biliary drainage with pancreatic cyst-jejunostomy. Of the remaining 15 patients treated nonoperatively, 6 of 10 in whom follow-up data were available remained well over a mean follow-up period of 29 months.

Seventeen of the 29 patients who presented with jaundice came to a biliary drainage procedure. The indications for surgery were jaundice alone in 13 patients and associated cholangitis in 3. In one patient an additional pancreatic duct drainage procedure was carried out for pain. The jaundice was transient in nature in the remaining 12 patients. Six of these patients remained well for a mean interval of 26 months. Among the other six nonoperated patients, two have subsequently died, one underwent a Whipple's resection for pain, and three were lost to follow-up.

The overall outcome of the 29 patients treated conservatively in the three groups was satisfactory in 72% of cases. No patient had clinical or biochemical evidence of deteriorating liver function.

The results of surgery were satisfactory in terms of the biliary systems in 20 of 21 patients (95%) in whom a follow-up was available, but 5 had ongoing pain.

Discussion

The results of the Cape Town experience confirm the benign nature of CBDS in CAIP and support a conservative management policy for the majority of patients.

None of the 29 nonjaundiced patients with markedly raised alkaline phosphatase levels who were treated conservatively have shown progressive biliary obstruction over a medium- to long-term follow-up period. Although liver histology was not obtained in all patients, none of these patients developed clinical or biochemical evidence of progressive liver damage. Secondary biliary cirrhosis was not encountered in this series and the incidence of cholangitis (three cases) and biliary calculi (four cases) was low.

The variability in the natural history of CBDS in CAIP makes it difficult to lay down clear guidelines for the indications and timing of surgical intervention. In some cases the obstruction may be reversible due to edema during acute flare-ups while in others it results from progressive fibrosis and calcification associated with end stage disease. Our experience validates a conservative approach in nonjaundiced patients with raised alkaline phosphatase levels and questions the risk of insidious progression to secondary biliary cirrhosis in such patients. However, a "prophylactic" biliary drainage operation in those patients with marked bile duct dilatation would be indicated when patients are undergoing a pancreatic drainage or resection for pain. In patients who present with obstructive jaundice, it seems reasonable to adopt a conservative policy of 2–3 weeks since jaundice was transient in half of our cases. However, if jaundice persists or recurs, or there are associated gallstones or cholangitis, early biliary decompression is indicated, particularly in the absence of recent alcohol ingestion.

The choice of biliary drainage lies between choldochoduodenostomy or a Roux-en-Y hepaticojejunostomy. The latter procedure is preferred when gross pancreatic enlargement separates the common bile duct from the duodenum. It can also be used when simultaneous drainage of the pancreatic duct is indicated [4]. It is now well accepted that cholecystojejunostomy does not provide adequate long-term biliary drainage and is often a source for recurrent attacks of cholangitis. Some cases with CBDS associated with gross disease in the head of the pancreas and intractable pain are probably best treated by a Whipple's resection.

Warshaw and Rattner [13] have warned against the pitfall of overlooking a fibrotic stenosis of the bile duct when the compression is allegedly due to a contiguous pancreatic cyst. In this situation, drainage of the cyst may not be sufficient and operative cholangiography is mandatory to exclude an associated fibrotic stricture.

Portal hypertension due to extrahepatic inflow obstruction from gross pancreatic fibrosis is a common problem in these patients and excessive bleeding may be encountered with routine cholecystectomy. In this situation we have found the technique of subtotal cholecystectomy [3] to be useful in minimizing blood loss. The operation entails leaving the posterior wall of the gallbladder attached to the liver with a piecemeal excision of the remaining gallbladder followed by a running suture to control excessive bleeding from the gallbladder wall. The cystic duct is closed with a pursestring suture from within the gallbladder, thus avoiding dissection in Calot's triangle.

There is growing evidence that CBDSs in CAIP run a relatively benign course in the majority of patients. Since no test at a given time can predict the outcome, an expectant policy with careful follow-up and monitoring of liver function tests would seem appropriate for the majority of cases.

References

1. Afroudakis A, Kaplowitz N (1981) Liver histopathology in chronic common bile duct stenosis due to chronic alcoholic pancreatitis. Hepatology 1:65–72
2. Aranha GV, Prinz RA, Freeark RJ, Greenlee HB (1984) The spectrum of biliary tract obstruction from chronic pancreatitis. Arch Surg 119:595–600
3. Bornman PC, Terblanche J (1985) Subtotal cholecystectomy for the difficult gallbladder in portal hypertension and cholecystitis. Surgery 98:1–6
4. Carter CD (1988) Pancreatitis and the biliary tree: the continuing problem. Am J Surg 155:10–17
5. Creaghe SB, Roseman DM, Saik RP (1981) Biliary obstruction in chronic pancreatitis: indications for surgical intervention. Am Surg 47:243–246
6. Gregg JA, Carr-Locke DL, Gallagher MM (1981) Importance of common bile duct stricture associated with chronic pancreatitis; diagnosis by ERCP. Am J Surg 141:199–203
7. Leger L, Lemaigre G, Roseau E, Lenriot JP (1972) Les lésions hépatiques des pancréatites chroniques, 50 observations. Nouv Presse Med 1:2159–2163
8. Petrozza JA, Dutta SK, Latham PS, Iber FL, Gadacz TR (1984) Prevalence and natural history of distal common bile duct stenosis in alcoholic pancreatitis. Dig Dis Sci 29:890–895
9. Sarles H, Sahel J (1978) Cholestasis and lesions of the biliary tract in chronic pancreatitis. Gut 19:851–857
10. Scott J, Summerfield JA, Elias E, Dick R, Sherlock S (1977) Chronic pancreatitis: a cause of cholestasis. Gut 18:196–201
11. Stabile BE, Calabria R, Wilson SE, Passaro E (1987) Stricture of the common bile duct from chronic pancreatitis. Surg Gynaecol Obstet 165:121–126
12. Stahl TJ, Allen M, Ansel HJ, Vennes JA (1988) Partial biliary obstruction caused by chronic pancreatitis: an appraisal of indications for surgical biliary drainage. Ann Surg 207:26–32
13. Warshaw AL, Rattner DW (1980) Facts and fallacies of common bile duct obstruction by pancreatic pseudocyst. Ann Surg 192:33–37
14. Warshaw AL, Schapiro RH, Ferrucci JT, Galdabini JJ (1976) Persistent obstructive jaundice, cholangitis and biliary cirrhosis due to common bile duct stenosis in chronic pancreatitis. Gastroenterology 70:562–567
15. Yadegar J, Williams R, Passaro E, Wilson SE (1980) Common duct stricture from chronic pancreatitis. Arch Surg 115:582–586

Pseudocysts in Chronic Pancreatitis:
Development and Clinical Implications

E. L. Bradley III[1]

Pancreatic pseudocysts are the most common complication of chronic pancreatitis, occurring at some time in the course of the disease in as many as 25% of patients [1]. Furthermore, even after satisfactory initial surgical drainage of pseudocysts, recurrence has been observed to develop in another 10% of cases during long-term follow-up [2]. The frequency of this complication, therefore, underscores the necessity for familiarity with the diagnosis and management of these patients.

Definitions

By definition, a pancreatic pseudocyst is a collection of pancreatic juice outside the normal boundaries of the ductal system, which is enclosed by a fibrous tissue membrane. The pseudocyst may be acute (< 3 weeks old) or chronic (> 3 weeks old). Since acute pseudocysts are rarely diagnosed in patients with chronic pancreatitis, unless there has been a documented recent history of an acute exacerbation of pancreatitis, patients with chronic pancreatitis should be considered to have chronic pseudocysts. The clinical distinction between acute and chronic pseudocysts is important, since behavior and appropriate treatment differ markedly [3]. In this chapter, we will only consider chronic pseudocysts arising in patients with chronic pancreatitis.

Pathology

Approximately three out of four chronic pseudocysts develop in patients with chronic alcoholic pancreatitis [4]. Chronic pseudocysts most commonly occur in males (1.5:1), and are usually seen in the 4th–6th decade of life [4]. Chronic pseudocysts occur more commonly in the body of the pancreas compared to the head or tail. They are most often single, but can present as multiple pseudocysts in approximately 10% of cases [5].

The distinction between pseudocysts and other cystic pancreatic diseases is established by biopsy of the pseudocyst wall. The demonstration of a fibrous lining, rather than the epithelial lining seen with neoplastic or true cysts, indicates the necessity for surgical drainage. In the absence of histologic information, neoplastic cysts have undergone internal drainage, rather than the required resection. Neoplastic cysts of

---

[1] Piedmont Professor of Surgery, Emory University, Atlanta, Georgia

Chronic Pancreatitis
Ed. by Beger, Büchler, Ditschuneit, and Malfertheiner
© Springer-Verlag Berlin Heidelberg 1990

the pancreas have been estimated to exist in as many as 20% of cases thought to represent pancreatic "pseudocysts" [6]. Since percutaneous or transendoscopic drainage techniques for "pseudocysts" do not obtain tissue for histology, inappropriate drainage of neoplastic cysts masquerading as "pseudocysts" is being seen with increasing frequency [7] (Fig. 1).

Diagnosis

Modern imaging techniques have greatly simplified the diagnosis of pancreatic pseudocysts. Ultrasonography, computed tomography, and endoscopic pancreatography may each play a role in the diagnosis and management of pseudocysts.

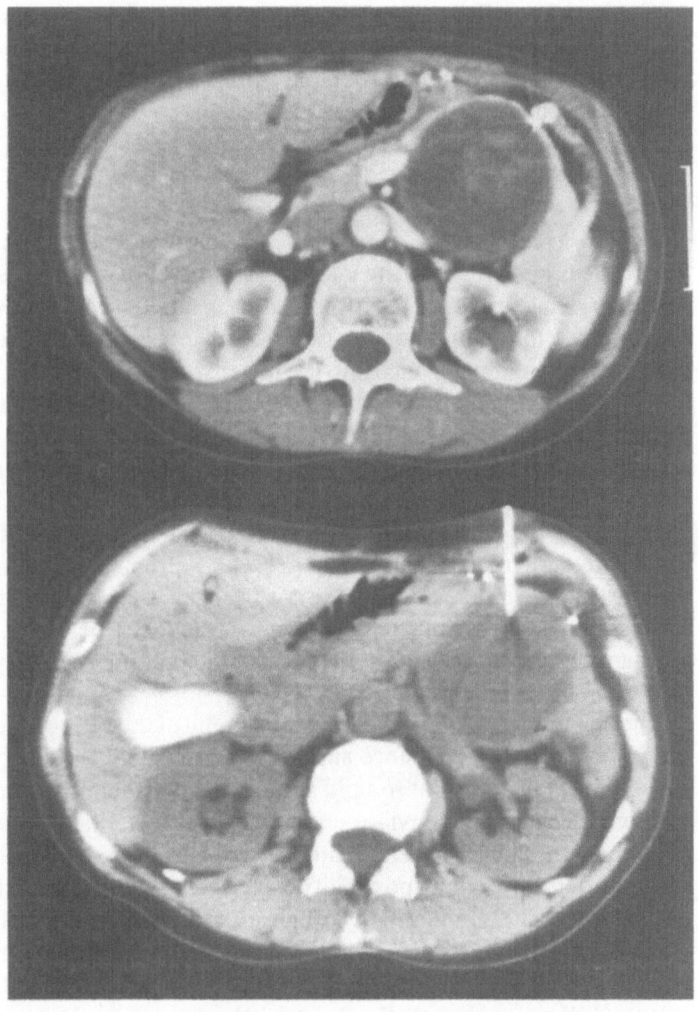

Fig. 1. Pancreatic "pseudocyst" *(top)*. CT-guided placement of drainage catheter *(bottom)*. Persistence of the "pseudocyst" led to referral and resection of a mucinous cystadenocarcinoma

However, computed tomography has emerged as the single most accurate method of diagnosing pancreatic pseudocysts [8]. In addition to accuracy rates exceeding 90%, CT is also capable of demonstrating the coexistence of an enlarged common duct or pancreatic duct, findings of particular relevance to the choice of an operative approach. In the presence of dilation of either or both of the common bile duct and pancreatic duct, pseudocyst drainage alone is rarely sufficient [9]. Sonography is best employed as a serial monitor of pseudocyst size in those patients in whom definitive drainage is delayed.

While some workers have advocated endoscopic pancreatography for all patients with pseudocysts [10, 11], the author has not found *routine* preoperative pancreatography desirable for the following reasons:

1. secondary infection of sterile pseudocysts occurs in 25% of patients [11];
2. 30%–50% of pancreatic pseudocysts fail to maintain a duct-pseudocyst connection and cannot be filled by contrast [12]; and
3. CT is safer, offers as much information, and is considerably less expensive. However, patients with recurrent pseudocysts should undergo endoscopic pancreatography as should patients with suspected concomitant common duct obstruction not demonstrated on CT.

Pathophysiology

Very little is known about the initial formation of pancreatic pseudocysts. Almost 90 years ago, Opie proposed that pseudocysts resulted from rupture of a pancreatic duct, activation of interstitial pancreatic juice, necrosis of the surrounding parenchyma, escape of the pancreatic juice into the lesser sac, and reaction of local mesothelial cells to wall off the collection by a fibrous membrane. Although plausible, even today this scenario remains conjectural.

Once initiated, however, the dynamics of pseudocyst formation are more clear. Because pancreatic ductal pressure is usually elevated in chronic obstructive pancreatitis [13], expansion of the embryonic pseudocyst continues until the surrounding tissue pressure equals pancreatic secretory pressure. Although not conclusively demonstrated, some evidence exists to suggest that the pancreatic juice contained within a pseudocyst can exchange with plasma (see below). If so, this may be one mechanism responsible for resorption of immature pseudocysts and spontaneous resolution of chronic pseudocysts.

Since it has long been known that thickening of the fibrous capsule of pseudocysts is time dependent [4], and since surgical internal drainage requires maturation of the pseudocyst wall sufficient to hold sutures, an optimum time exists for surgical intervention. Because the amylase contained in pseudocysts is degraded (deaminated) over time, and since the deaminated amylase from the pseudocyst can be detected in serum [14], the intriguing possibility exists that pseudocysts can be "dated" by a serum test. Unfortunately, the relative quantity of deaminated ("old") amylase has not as yet proved reliable in prospectively timing surgical intervention. For all practical purposes, however, surgical drainage may be undertaken in all patients with pseudocysts and chronic pancreatitis whenever the pseudocyst is diagnosed, *providing* there is no recent history of an acute episode of pancreatitis [15, 16].

Natural History

In contrast to acute pseudocysts, chronic pseudocysts infrequently undergo uncomplicated spontaneous resolution [4, 16]. This observation may be related to the duration of the pseudocyst, since wall thickness is known to increase with time. More specifically, large chronic pseudocysts (those > 6 cm) almost never resolve spontaneously without some type of complication [17, 18]. Small chronic pseudocysts (5 cm or less), on the other hand, may be safely observed as long as they do not increase in size, since complications are rare and spontaneous resolution more frequent [19].

The risk of complications in large chronic pseudocysts increases with the length of observation, and, after 7 weeks, the morbidity and mortality of persistent observation exceeds the risk of elective surgery [18]. It is clear that persistent conservative treatment of chronic pseudocysts, in the often vain hope of spontaneous resolution, exposes the patient to unwarranted risks. Overall, the risk of complications occurring in chronic pseudocysts during prolonged observation is approximately one-in-three, and for each patient experiencing a complication there is a similar risk for a fatal outcome [4].

Hemorrhage into a preexisting pseudocyst, with subsequent conversion into a pseudoaneurysm, is the most serious complication of chronic pseudocysts [20]. While hemorrhage has been estimated to occur in 5% of cases, it accounts for 40%–80% of all deaths from chronic pseudocysts [21]. Since bleeding most often occurs from a branch of the splenic artery, therapeutic embolization is often successful [22] (Fig. 2). Massive hemorrhage may also occur from gastric varices secondary to splenic vein obstruction, which, in turn, is usually due to perivenular fibrosis from the underlying chronic pancreatitis rather than pressure from the pseudocyst [23]. Because of the multiplicity of conditions and sites which may express bleeding in patients with chronic pseudocysts, angiography is mandatory in these patients.

Obstruction of the common bile duct is also common in patients with chronic pseudocysts. Untreated, common bile duct obstruction in chronic pancreatitis can lead to irreversible biliary cirrhosis. Again, the obstruction is usually due to entrapment of the common duct by chronic pancreatitis and fibrosis, rather than to pressure from the pseudocyst [24]. Failure to appreciate this admonition may lead to persistence of biliary obstruction after simple pseudocyst drainage. Operative cholangiography following pseudocyst drainage can prevent this error (Fig. 3). When intestinal obstruction results from compression of an adjacent segment of intestine by the pseudocyst, decompression of the pseudocyst provides relief.

Rupture of a pancreatic pseudocyst occurs more commonly than has been previously appreciated. While sudden massive intraperitoneal rupture may result in peritonitis, slow leaks occur more commonly, and result in pancreatic ascites. When the pseudocyst leaks into the pleural cavity, pancreatic hydrothorax results [25]. The majority of these internal fistulas will resolve with conservative treatment. Failure to control fistula output after 2 weeks of hyperalimentation is an indication for pancreatography in preparation for surgery. Rupture of a chronic pseudocyst may also occur directly into an adjacent segment of intestine, resulting in an autoenteric anastomosis [26]. Surgical intervention in these cases is limited to those few patients in whom autodrainage has not resulted in resolution, or for those with accompanying massive hemorrhage (Fig. 4).

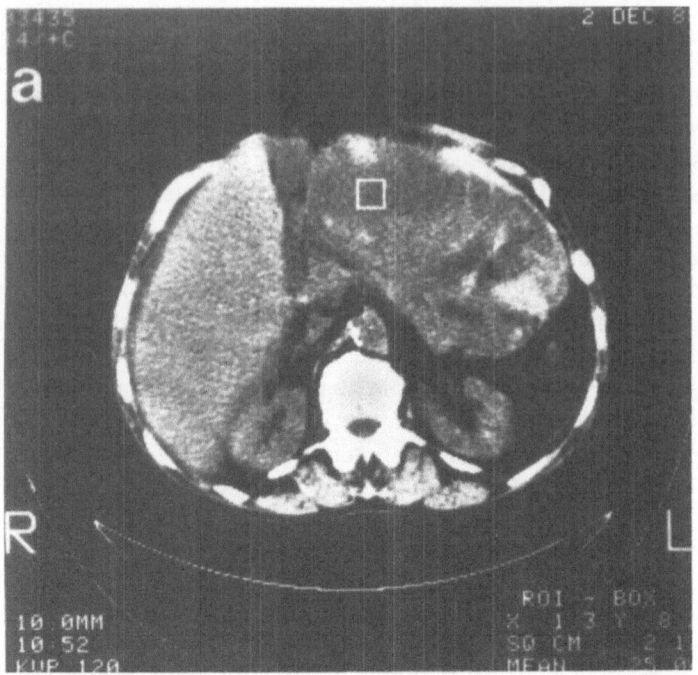

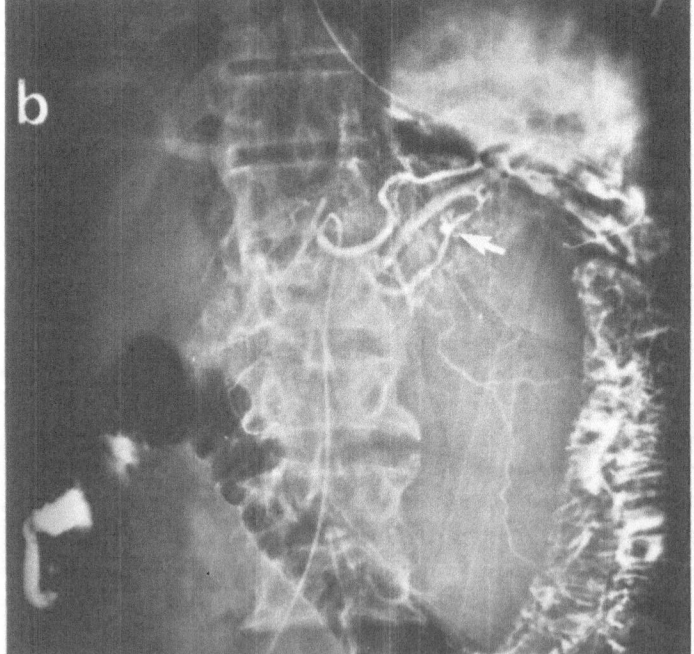

Fig. 2a, b. Pseudoaneurysm arising from a pancreatic pseudocyst. **a** CT scan in a patient with a known pseudocyst which underwent sudden painful enlargement. Note the mixture of densities within the large *left upper quadrant* mass. **b** Splenic arteriogram demonstrating leak from the pancreatic magna into the pseudocyst *(arrow)*

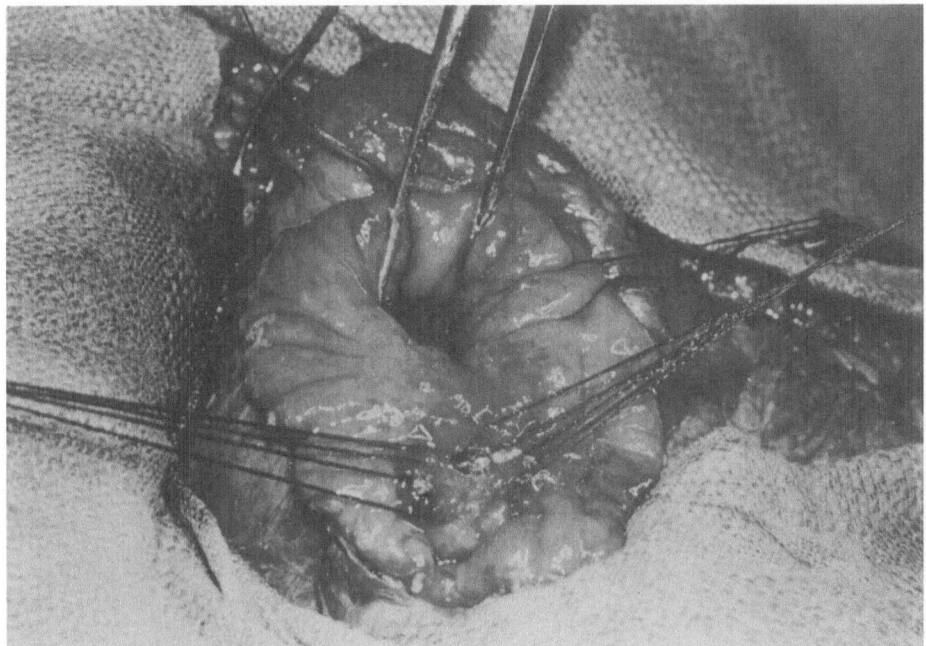

Fig. 3. Pseudocyst in head of pancreas thought to be obstructing the common duct. Tranduodenal cystoduodenostomy (forceps) did not relieve common duct obstruction on cholangiography. Sphincteroplasty for ampullary stenosis (note sutures and tip of Bake's dilator) resulted in free flow of contrast into duodenum [4]

Secondary infection can occur in chronic pseudocysts. However, bacteria may be present in pseudocyst fluid without evidence of invasive infection [27, 28]. More properly, this condition could be called bacterial contamination rather than infection. Contaminated pseudocysts can be safely drained into the intestinal tract without fear of anastomotic dehiscence [28]. On the other hand, if the fluid in a pseudocyst is purulent, or systemic sepsis has been present, it is safer to assume that an infected pseudocyst has progressed to a pancreatic abscess, and external drainage should be employed. If any doubt exists in a pancreatic pseudocyst, external drainage is always the wisest course.

Nonsurgical Drainage

Advances in medical technology have provided countless new therapeutic possibilities for the management of today's patients. As physicians first and surgeons second, our task is to critically evaluate the new proposals as they appear, comparing the risks and benefits of the new procedure with established treatments. Nonsurgical drainage of chronic pancreatic pseudocysts is a case in point. Essentially two nonsurgi-

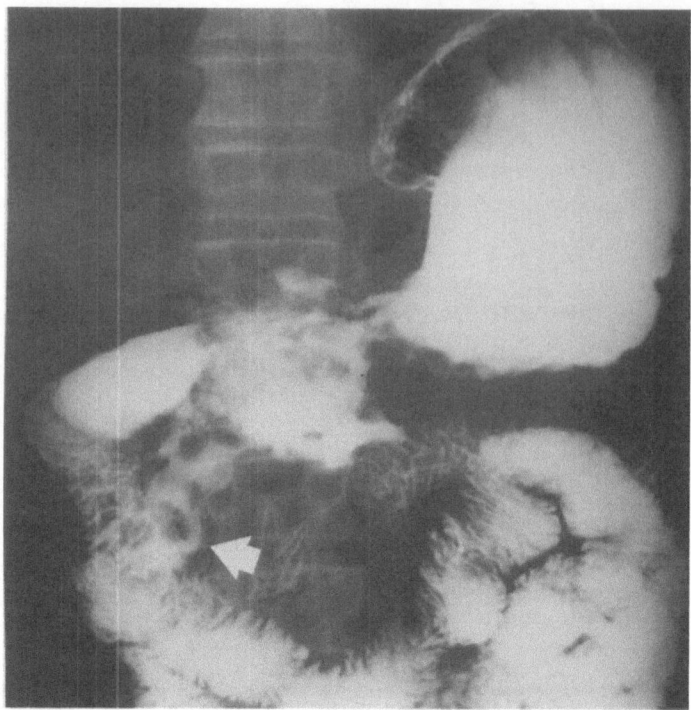

Fig. 4. Spontaneous rupture of a pancreatic pseudocyst into the third portion of the duodenum (arrow). A repeat GI series two weeks later demonstrated complete resolution

cal approaches to the management of chronic pseudocysts have been advocated; percutaneous aspiration [29] and transendoscopic drainage [30].

Percutaneous aspiration of pseudocysts by guided single puncture has been notoriously unsuccessful, with a worldwide recurrence rate approaching 70% [4]. Currently, single puncture aspiration cannot be recommended as definitive therapy, but can be helpful in preoperative preparation of patients with massive pseudocysts which result in marked diminution of pulmonary compliance. Prolonged percutaneous drainage by means of an indwelling catheter placed in the pseudocyst, on the other hand, has been much more successful. Resolution has occurred in as many as 70% of cases when drainage exceeds 1 week [31].

However, the risks of long-term transcutaneous intubation, secondary infection and hemorrhage, have not as yet been quantitated for comparison to known mortality and morbidity risks established for surgical drainage. Comparative studies are urgently needed. Furthermore, biopsy of the "pseudocyst" wall is not done with transcutaneous drainage, thereby providing the potential for inadvertent transcutaneous drainage of neoplastic cysts in as many as one case in seven of pancreatic „pseudocysts" [7].

Transenteric endoscopic drainage of pancreatic pseudocysts has been effected by direct puncture [30], electrocoagulation [32, 33], and various lasers [34]. As might be anticipated in procedures with limited exposure, both hemorrhage and intestinal perforation have occurred with fatal results. Most importantly, however, the principle of transendoscopic drainage *assumes adherence* between the pseudocyst and the adjacent segment of intestine [35]. Lacking such inflammatory adherence, the pseudocyst and enteric stoma may separate after the incisions are made. This would result in a high-risk, activated pancreaticoenteric fistula. In a personal operative series of 132 pancreatic pseudocysts, adherence to an adjacent segment of intestine was present in only 42% of cases. Transendoscopic drainage must therefore remain a potentially high risk procedure until such time as a nonoperative method for reliably determining adherence can be discovered. More traditional surgical methods of treatment of pancreatic pseudocysts are covered by Häring and Roscher in this volume.

References

1. Aranha GV, Prinz RA, Esguerra AC, Greenlee HB (1983) The nature and course of cystic pancreatic lesions diagnosed by ultrasound. Arch Surg 118:486–488
2. Sankaran S, Walt AJ (1975) The natural and unnatural history of pancreatic pseudocysts. Br J Surg 62:37–44
3. Bradley EL III, Gonzalez AC, Clements JL (1976) Acute pancreatic pseudocysts: incidence and implications. Ann Surg 184:734–737
4. Bradley EL III (ed) (1982) Pseudocysts In Complications of Pancreatitis. Saunders, Philadelphia, p 125
5. Bradley EL III, Austin H (1982) Multiple pancreatic pseudocysts: the principle of internal cystocystostomy in surgical management. Surgery 92:111–114
6. Warshaw AL, Rutledge PL (1987) Cystic tumors mistaken for pancreatic pseudocysts. Ann Surg 205:393–398
7. Lumsden A, Bradley EL III (1990) Differential diagnosis and initial management of cystic pancreatic lesions. Hepatogastroenterology 36:462–468
8. Williford ME, Foster WL, Halvorsen RA, Thompson WM (1983) Pancreatic pseudocyst: comparative evaluation by sonography and computed tomography. AJR 140:53–57
9. Munn JS, Aranha GV, Greenlee HB, Prinz RA (1987) Simultaneous treatment of chronic pancreatitis and pancreatic pseudocyst. Arch Surg 122:662–667
10. Sugawa C, Walt AJ (1979) Endoscopic retrograde pancreatography in the surgery of pancreatic pseudocysts. Surgery 86:639–647
11. O'Connor M, Kolars J, Ansel H, Silvis S, Vennes J (1986) Preoperative endoscopic retrograde cholangiopancreatography in the surgical management of pancreatic pseudocysts. Am J Surg 151:18–24
12. Laxson LC, Fromkes JJ, Cooperman M (1985) Endoscopic retrograde cholangiopancreatography in the management of pancreatic pseudocysts. Am J Surg 150:683–686
13. Bradley EL III (1982) Pancreatic duct pressure in chronic pancreatitis. Am J Surg 144:313–315
14. Warshaw AL, Lee K-H (1980) Aging changes of pancreatic isoamylases and the appearance of "old amylase" in the serum of patients with pancreatic pseudocysts. Gastroenterology 79:1246–1251
15. Ephgrave K, Hunt JL (1986) Presentation of pancreatic pseudocysts: implications for timing of surgical intervention. Am J Surg 151:749–753
16. Grace RR, Jordan PH (1976) Unresolved problems of pancreatic pseudocysts. Ann Surg 184:16–21
17. Imrie CW, Buist LJ, Shearer MG (1988) Importance of cause in the outcome of pancreatic pseudocysts. Am J Surg 156:159–162
18. Bradley EL III, Clements JL, Gonzalez AC (1979) The natural history of pancreatic pseudocysts: a unified concept of management. Am J Surg 137:135–141
19. Ashner AF, Collen MJ, Mackow RC, Chapman AB, Korenman JC, Ciarleglio CA, Benjamin SB, Rakowski TA (1987) Amylase, lipase, isoamylase and trypsin in patients with renal insufficiency and renal failure. Gastroenterology 92:1296

20. Wu TK, Zaman SN, Gullick HD, Powers SR (1977) Spontaneous hemorrhage due to pseudocysts of the pancreas. Am J Surg 134:408–410
21. Frey CF, Eckhauser F, Stanley JC (1982) Hemorrhage In Complications of Pancreatitis. Bradley EL III (ed) Saunders, Philadelphia, pp 96–119
22. Stabile BE, Wilson SE, Debas HT (1983) Reduced mortality from bleeding pseudocysts and pseudoaneurysms caused by pancreatitis. Arch Surg 118:45–51
23. Little AG, Moossa AR (1981) Gastrointestinal hemorrhage from left-side portal hypertension. Am J Surg 141:153–158
24. Skellenger ME, Patterson D, Foley NT, Jordan PH (1983) Cholestasis due to compression of the common bile duct by pancreatic pseudocysts. Am J Surg 145:343–348
25. Broe PJ, Cameron JL (1982) Pancreatic ascites and pancreatic pleural effusions in complications of pancreatitis. In: Bradley EL III (ed) Pseudocysts in complications of pancreatitis. Saunders, Philadelphia, pp 245–261
26. Bradley EL III, Clements JL (1976) Transenteric rupture of pancreatic pseudocysts: management of pseudocystenteric fistulas. Am Surg 42:827–837
27. Shatney CH, Lillehei RC (1979) Surgical treatment of pancreatic pseudocysts: analysis of 119 cases. Ann Surg 189:386–394
28. Mullins RJ, Malangoni MA, Bergamini TM, Casey JM, Richardson JD (1988) Controversies in the management of pancreatic pseudocysts. Am J Surg 155:165–172
29. Hancke S, Pedersen JF (1976) Percutaneous puncture of pancreatic cysts guided by ultrasound. Surg Gynecol Obstet 142:551–552
30. Rogers BHG, Cicurel NJ, Seed RW (1975) Transgastric needle aspiration of pancreatic cyst thru an endoscope. Gastrointest Endosc 21:133–134
31. Matzinger FR, Ho CS, Yee AC, Gray RR (1988) Pancreatic pseudocysts drained thru a percutaneous transgastric approach: further experience. Radiology 167:431–434
32. Sahel J, Bastid C, Pellat B, Schurgers P, Sarles H (1987) Endoscopic cystoduodenostomy of cysts of chronic calcifying pancreatitis: a report of 20 cases. Pancreas 2:447–453
33. Lamblin G, Joly JP, Delcenserie R, Delamarre J, Dupas JL (1989) Non surgical management of pseudocysts in acute and chronic pancreatitis. AGA Abstracts. Gastroenterology 96:285
34. Delmotte JS, Brunetaud JM, Desurmont P, Houcke P, Cortot A, Paris JC (1982) Treatment of pancreatic and biliary cysts by endoscopic argon laser. AGA Abstracts, Gastroenterology 82:1041
35. Bradley EL III (1985) Don't fix nothin' that ain't broke. Am J Surg 149:197

Pancreatic Ascites

J. P. NEOPTOLEMOS and M. C. WINSLET[1]

Introduction

Pancreatic ascites is defined as the persistent accumulation of "massive" amounts of intraperitoneal fluid during the course of chronic pancreatitis which is characterized by a high amylase level and a high protein content, usually over 3 g/l [14]. In most cases the ascites is serous in nature, but it may be serosanguinous, turbid or chylous.

Pancreatic ascites was first described by Bockus in 1946 [4], although he ascribed the ascites to compression of the portal vein by a large pseudocyst. It was not until 1951 that Davis and Kelsey [11] gave the classical description of the disease, referring to a young boy with chronic pancreatitis who suffered from gross ascites despite repeated paracentesis and drainage at laparotomy. The ascites of chronic pancreatitis is a different entity from the ascites of acute necrotizing pancreatitis [2]. In the latter situation the ascites is associated with a poor outcome [2, 24], and the colour and volume of fluid may be used as an accurate prognostic marker [25].

The incidence of ascites in chronic pancreatitis is difficult to estimate, but the prevalence is certainly under 1%. Although Leger et al. [22] reported five cases out of a total of 148 patients (3.4%) requiring surgery for chronic pancreatitis, this figure probably overestimates the general experience. The exact pathology varies considerably from patient to patient; unless patients are carefully investigated and treated, the mortality is 20%–30%. It is for this reason that ascites in chronic pancreatitis deserves special consideration.

Pathogenesis

The commonest underlying cause for pancreatic ascites is chronic pancreatitis secondary to alcohol abuse; in addition to trauma there is a growing list of unusual causes (Table 1). The concept that leakage of pancreatic juice into the peritoneal cavity was the primary mechanism of pancreatic ascites [6] gained steady recognition with the wider use of intra-operative pancreatography and subsequently pre-operative endoscopic retrograde cholangiopancreatography (ERCP) [7, 12, 32, 34, 37].

Persistent leakage of pancreatic juice into the peritoneal cavity may be either from the pancreatic duct itself or from a pseudocyst which is in communication with the duct (Fig. 1). Pancreatic ascites occurs in up to 15% of patients with a pseudocyst [32].

---

[1] University Department of Surgery, Dudley Road Hospital, Birmingham B18 7QH, UK

Chronic Pancreatitis
Ed. by Beger, Büchler, Ditschuneit, and Malfertheiner
© Springer-Verlag Berlin Heidelberg 1990

Table 1. Causes of pancreatic ascites in 247 cases from collected series [8, 9, 12–14, 17–20, 23, 26–31, 35, 36, 38–40, 42–46]

Cause	Number	Proportion
Alcohol	203	82.2%
Unknown	19	7.7%
Trauma	17	6.9%
Duplication cysts	2	
Carcinoma of pancreas	1	
Distal splenorenal shunt	1	
Stenosis of ampulla of Vater	1	3.2%
Pancreatic duct stones	1	
Carcinoid tumour[a]	1	
Hodgkin's lymphoma	1	

[a] Associated with trauma

On the other hand, around 60% of patients with ascites have pseudocysts, and these appear to be the commonest site for leakage [9, 14, 33]. In a series of 15 pancreatograms reported by Weaver et al. [45], it was suggested that leakage from a pseudocyst was responsible for ascites in 11 cases, in two there was leakage from the duct, and in two others a pseudocyst was present without any leakage demonstrated.

The exact pathophysiology responsible for duct or pseudocyst rupture is unknown. Localized pancreatic necrosis, perhaps with an element of increased duct pressure from downstream obstruction would seem a likely mechanism for duct rupture. Increased pressure within the pseudocyst, local erosion of the pseudocyst wall by autodigestion or ischaemia and increased abdominal pressure are possible factors contributing to pseudocyst leakage.

There are several reasons to suppose that pancreatic ascites is not due simply to leakage of pancreatic juice. Firstly, pancreatic enzyme levels in the ascites rarely reach those found in pancreatic juice. Secondly, the high levels of proteins found in the ascites, including albumin, cannot be entirely derived from either pancreatic juice itself or by transudation into the peritoneal cavity. In experimental circumstances direct leakage of pancreatic juice into the peritoneal cavity does not result in pancreatic ascites [15]. Although an exudative process is unquestionably present [1, 35], this does not appear to be due to pancreatic enzyme activity, which is absent in human pancreatic ascites [35]. Blockage of peripancreatic and peritoneal lymphatics [16] may be involved.

Clinical Presentation and Diagnosis

Pancreatic ascites affects men more than twice as often as women and usually occurs from the third to fifth decades [9, 14, 37, 45]; this would seem to be a reflection of alcohol drinking habits. Most patients present with increasing abdominal distention. Abdominal pain varies greatly in character but is often epigastric and bearable in intensity; pain may, however, be entirely absent. Nausea, intermittent vomiting, malaise, anorexia, weight loss and steatorrhoea occur with increasing length of

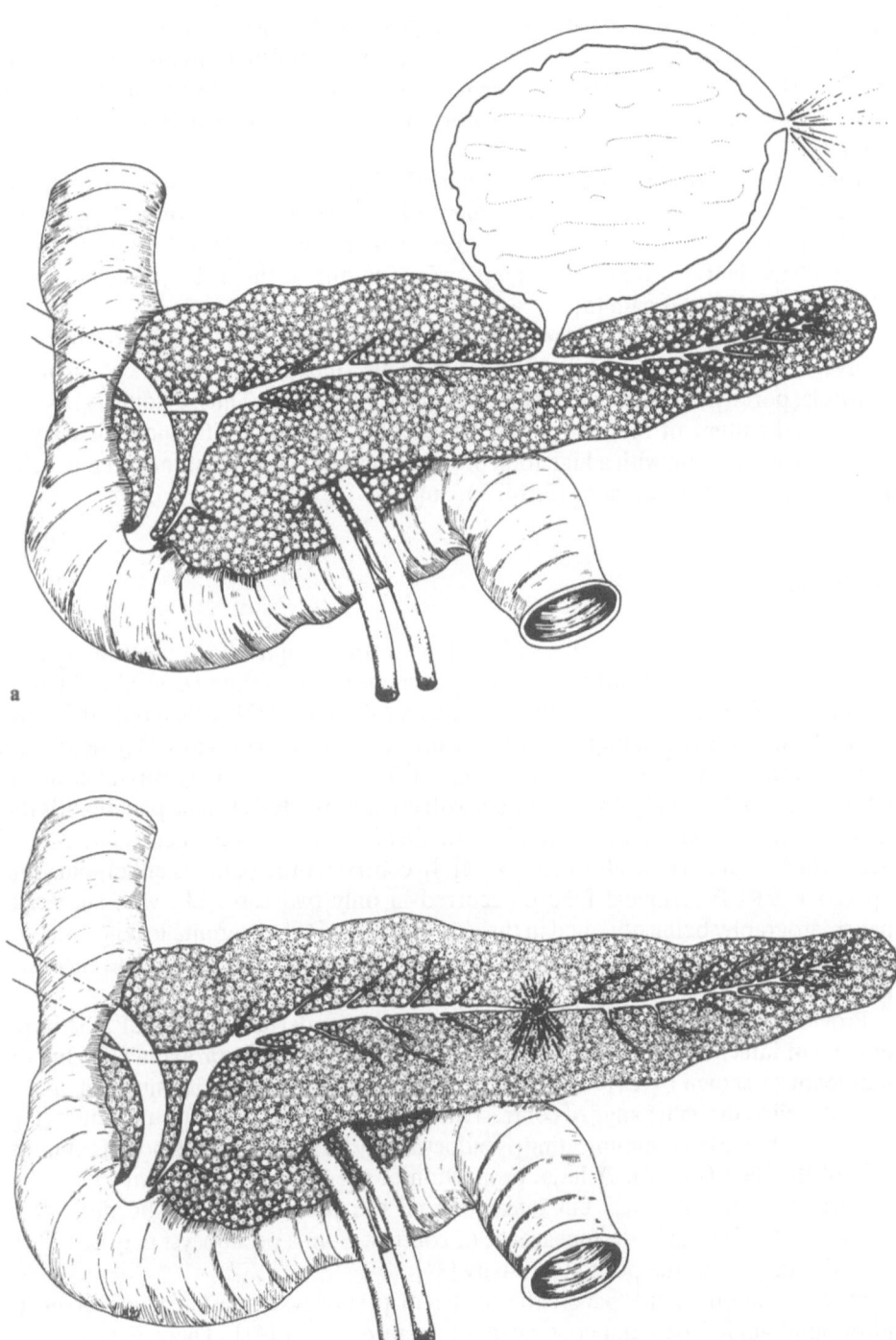

Fig. 1a, b. **a** Leakage from a pseudocyst which is in communication with the main pancreatic duct is considered to be the commonest cause of pancreatic ascites. **b** The only other mechanism reported is leakage from a main pancreatic duct

history. Up to two-thirds of patients may not give a recent history of an acute attack of pancreatitis [8, 9]. The ascites is readily apparent on clinical examination; cachexia may be striking. Erythematous subcutaneous nodules, usually on the limbs and representing fat necrosis are confirmatory of alcoholic pancreatitis but are rarely found.

There may be dyspnoea due to a sympathetic effusion or a pancreatico-pleural fistula; of 27 patients reported by Cameron [5], five also had a connecting pleural fistula. In the same series, another seven patients had a pleural effusion and a pancreatico-pleural fistula but without ascites; in one of these the presenting complaint was abdominal pain [5].

Diagnosis is achieved by undertaking an ascitic tap. This also helps to exclude other causes of ascites in a similar group of patients, including malignancy, alcoholic cirrhosis, portal or splenic vein thrombosis and tuberculosis. Thus, cytological examination and culture of the ascites may be relevant. Elevation of pancreatic enzyme levels in combination with a high total protein or albumin level is pathognomic, being found in at least 80% of cases [5, 14, 33, 36].

Investigations

Both ERCP and contrast-enhanced computed tomography (CT) are essential for management. Although intra-operative pancreatography might be used to identify the site of leakage, technical problems can be considerable [37]. This should therefore be used only if other techniques have been unsuccessful. In a series of 73 patients with pancreatic ascites prior to the introduction of ERCP, a site of leakage was identified in only 27 cases (40%) [14]. In 67 patients with ethanol-related chronic pancreatitis this limited information almost certainly contributed to an overall recurrence rate of ascites in 24% and a mortality of 34% [14]. In contrast, of 15 patients undergoing pre-operative ERCP technical failure occurred in only two cases but with successful pancreatography being obtained in these at operation [45]; a definite leakage site was identified in 13 (87%) of the cases which contributed to a zero recurrence and mortality.

Provided that careful but routine precautions are undertaken at ERCP, the introduction of infection into the pancreatico-biliary tree is rarely a problem [10]. Important features shown by ERCP include strictures and dilation of the main pancreatic duct as well as direct leakage of contrast into the peritoneal cavity from the duct (Fig. 2). A large but non-communicating pseudocyst may be revealed as a smooth compression of the duct (Fig. 2). A large proportion of pseudocysts are shown to be communicating with the duct, but leakage from the pseudocyst may be difficult to demonstrate. The rapid disappearance of contrast from a pseudocyst may be indicative of leakage into the peritoneal cavity [34].

Demonstration of the pancreatic duct and pseudocysts may be undertaken by ultrasound-guided percutaneous needle puncture (PCP) [41]. There is probably a greater risk of introducing infection by this route than by ERCP, and an internal fistula might be created following withdrawal of the needle; this is particularly so if there is a non-communicating pseudocyst, or if there is a pancreatic duct stricture.

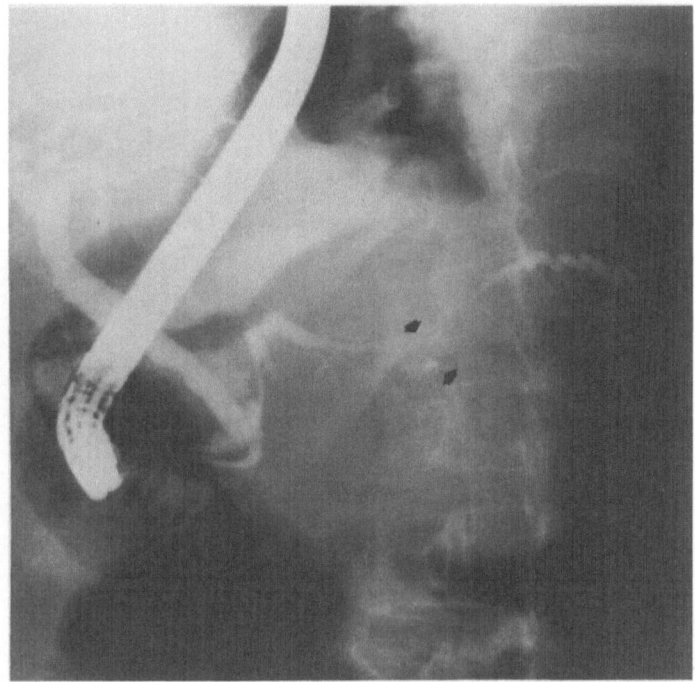

Fig. 2. ERCP showing leakage of contrast from the main pancreatic duct *(arrows)* directly into the peritoneal cavity

Nevertheless, PCP is the only pre-operative means by which to demonstrate a leak if ERCP has failed, or if there is a leaking but non-communicating pseudocyst.

A pancreatico-pleural fistula or communicating mediastinal pseudocyst might be revealed by ERCP but may require direct injection of contrast into the thorax [5, 40].

The detailed pathology of the pancreas in ascites due to chronic pancreatitis can be quite complex. This necessitates the use of CT in order to demonstrate the number and sites of any pseudocysts (Figs. 2–5). Contrast enhancement is important to identify any areas of pancreatic necrosis [3]. According to Cameron [5] a pancreatic duct leaking posteriorly is the cause of a pleural effusion, whereas a duct leaking anteriorly causes a pseudocyst. As illustrated in Figs. 2–5, large multiple non-communicating pseudocysts may be present in association with a pancreatic duct leaking into the peritoneal cavity via a retroperitoneal route.

Treatment

The majority of patients need to undergo surgery. A period of 2–3 weeks of medical treatment is warranted for three reasons:
1. Detailed investigations of the exact nature of the problem must be undertaken.
2. The nutritional status of the patient, which is often very poor, must be improved by intravenous nutrition.
3. Resolution of the ascites without surgery sometimes occurs.

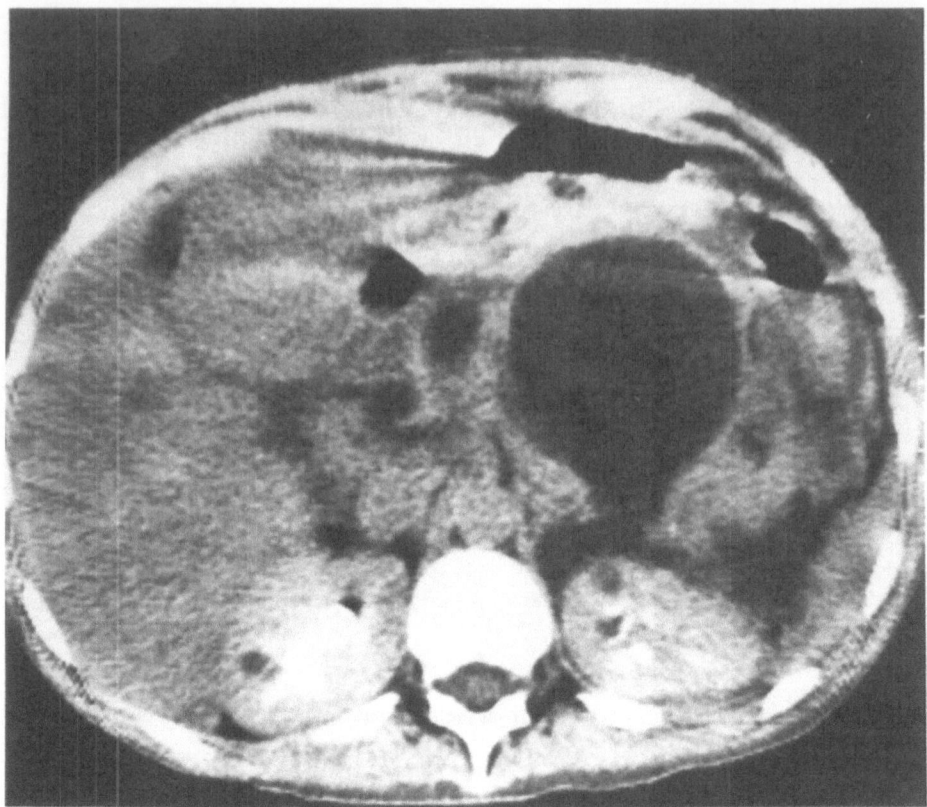

Fig. 3. Contrast-enhanced CT scan shows a large pseudocyst arising in the lesser sac in the same patient as in Fig. 2, confirming the ERCP findings

Fig. 5. Composite diagram of the radiological findings in Figs. 2–4 and confirmed at laparotomy. No communication was found at operation between the pancreatic duct and the lesser sac pseudocyst following i.v. injection of pancreozymin. The site of pancreatic duct rupture was identified only following mobilization of the left pancreas. At this point there was no pancreatic tissue remaining; pancreatic juice was flowing freely into the retroperitoneal space. More than 5 l dark brown (serosanguinous) fluid was removed from the peritoneal cavity. If the pseudocysts had been drained, this would not have prevented recurrent ascites. Both pseudocysts were resected along with the body and tail of the pancreas. An accompanying ascitic pleural effusion (high in amylase) also resolved following surgery. The patient, a young alcoholic who had presented with marked cachexia, made a rapid and uneventful recovery following surgery, which also included cholecystectomy for incidental gallstones

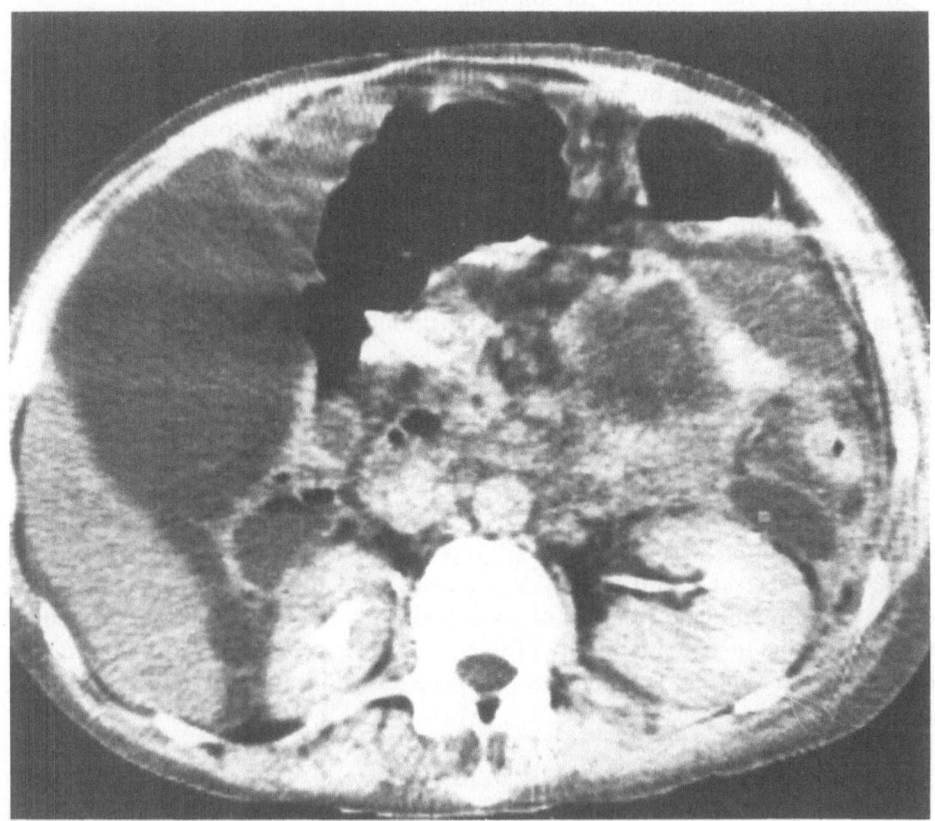

Fig. 4. CT scan at a higher level than that in Fig. 3, showing a completely separate and non-communicating pseudocyst which was shown to occupy the whole of the left diaphragmatic space

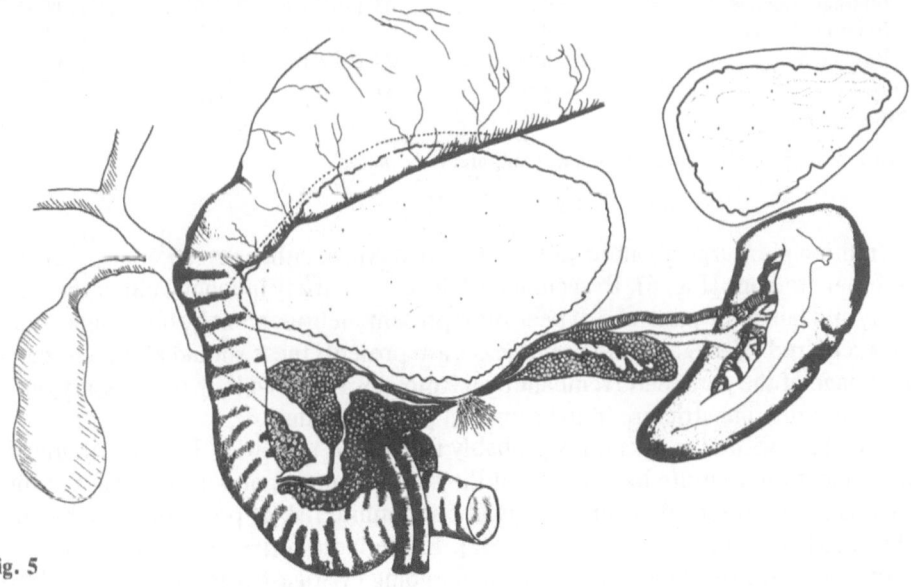

Fig. 5

Medical treatment includes the following:

1. Avoidance of food by mouth. Although some authors have also recommended a nasogastric tube, this seems necessary only if there is gastric outlet obstruction; allowing some water by mouth adds to the comfort of the patient.
2. Suppression of pancreatic secretion by agents such as somatostatin. Cameron [5] has used acetazolamide, and atropine and Satz et al. [35] have used calcitonin infusion with some success.
3. Repeated paracenteses to encourage sealing of the leakage site and to relieve pressure from the diaphragm in order to improve respiratory effort.
4. Intravenous nutrition to replace the high protein losses consequent on ascitic tapping as well as to improve the poor nutritional situation found at presentation.

Persistent or recurrent leakage after an initial period of conservative management necessitates operative intervention. Improved well-being of the patient after 2–3 weeks of medical treatment indicates successful preparation for surgery; it is not a reason for continued non-intervention. Failure to improve the overall clinical performance of the patient or deterioration without an apparent cause may require earlier intervention. Cameron et al. [8] reported on 17 patients treated for several weeks; this was successful in only seven cases, and four patients died whilst on conservative treatment. Analysis of published cases treated by prolonged medical therapy mirrors this high mortality (Table 2). Some success has been reported with external beam radiotherapy, but this is now largely of historical interest [11, 16, 21, 26, 28, 46].

Table 2. Results of surgical and non-surgical treatment in 189 cases of pancreatic ascites associated with excess alcohol intake from collected series [8, 9, 12–14, 18–20, 23, 26–30, 35, 36, 38–40, 44–46]

Treatment	Number	Successful	Recurrence	Mortality
Surgical				
Internal drainage	57	43 (76%)	3 (5%)	11 (19%)
External drainage	18	7 (39%)	7 (39%)	4 (22%)
Resection	29	23 (97%)	0	1 (3%)
Medical	57	31 (54%)	9 (16%)	17 (30%)
Other methods[a]	28	14 (50%)	10 (36%)	4 (14%)

[a] Includes laparotomy alone, LeVeen shunt, and radiotherapy

In principle, surgery can be divided into two types, either resection or permanent internal drainage (Fig. 6). Resection is of the distal variety involving either the tail or body and tail of the pancreas. If necrosis is present, débridement by blunt dissection is also required. If one or more pseudocysts are present, these should also be resected. Drainage of the pancreatic remnant by a Roux-en-Y jejunal loop is necessary only if there is a definite stricture in the proximal pancreatic duct.

Drainage without resection is probably inferior to resection. Internal drainage is dependent on accurate localization of the site of leakage, and a Roux-en-Y jejunal loop is again preferred. There is a small but definite risk of post-operative haemorrhage following internal drainage [8, 32]. In the large series by Weaver et al. [45], there were two deaths in 12 patients undergoing cystogastrostomy or cystojejunos-

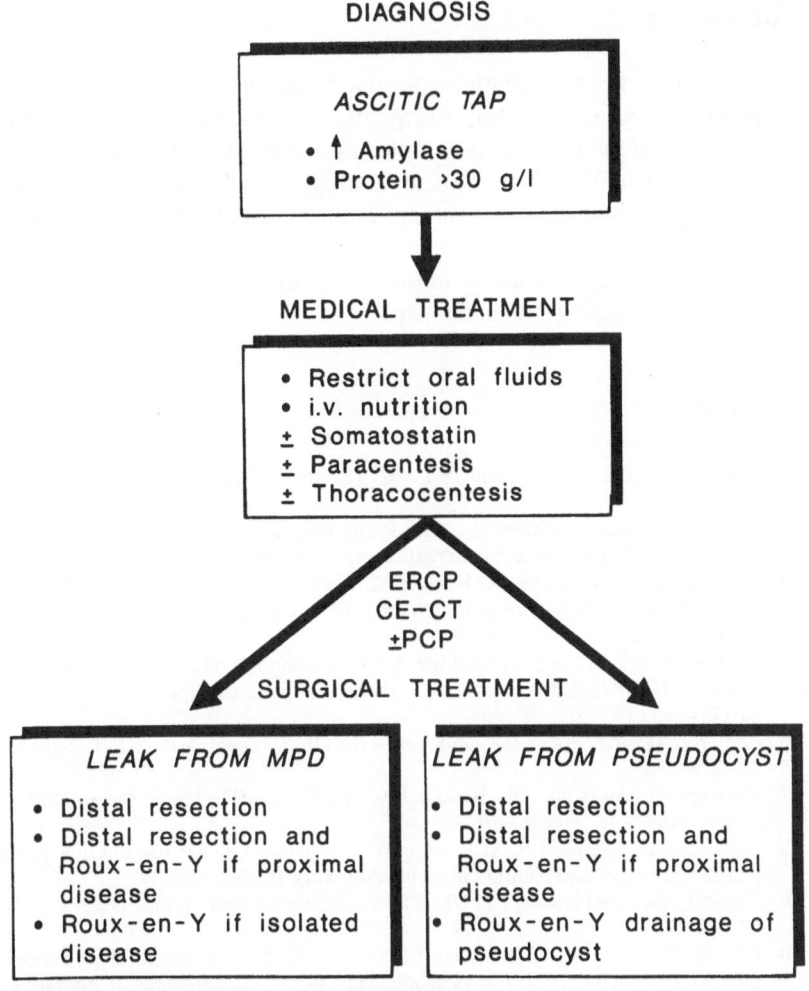

DIAGNOSIS

ASCITIC TAP

- ↑ Amylase
- Protein ›30 g/l

MEDICAL TREATMENT

- Restrict oral fluids
- i.v. nutrition
- ± Somatostatin
- ± Paracentesis
- ± Thoracocentesis

ERCP
CE–CT
±PCP

SURGICAL TREATMENT

LEAK FROM MPD

- Distal resection
- Distal resection and Roux‑en‑Y if proximal disease
- Roux‑en‑Y if isolated disease

LEAK FROM PSEUDOCYST

- Distal resection
- Distal resection and Roux‑en‑Y if proximal disease
- Roux‑en‑Y drainage of pseudocyst

Fig. 6. An algorithm for the management of pancreatic ascites

tomy and no deaths in 11 patients undergoing resection. Internal drainage is nevertheless to be preferred to resection if the pseudocyst is situated in the head of the gland.

Sometimes it is assumed that the presence of a pseudocyst is the cause of leakage, despite lack of radiological proof. Although drainage of such a pseudocyst may by chance be successful, failure to correctly identify the site of leakage partly accounts for the high recurrence and mortality associated with both internal and external drainage (Table 2). Even though resection is much more technically demanding, there is no reported recurrence following this procedure, and it is associated with a remarkably small mortality. A major pancreatico‑pleural fistula can also be dealt with entirely by the abdominal approach [5]; lesser pleural effusions always resolve if the abdominal pathology is correctly dealt with.

Conclusions

The mortality of patients with ascites due to chronic pancreatitis is remarkably high, standing at around 20%. Improvements in recent years have been possible by an appreciation of the potentially complex nature of the problem and the application of ERCP and CT to identify the exact pathology in each individual case. A combination of medical care and judicious surgery have contributed to an improving outcome.

Acknowledgements. We are grateful to Wendy Kemp for the artwork and to Dilys Thomas for preparing the manuscript.

References

1. Barua RL, Villa F, Steigmann F (1962) Massive ascites due to pancreatitis. Am J Dig Dis 7:900–906
2. Beger HG, Kunz R, Bittner R (1987) Prognostic criteria in necrotizing pancreatitis. In: Beger HG, Buchler M (eds) Acute pancreatitis. Springer, Berlin Heidelberg New York, pp 198–200
3. Block S, Maier W, Bittner R, Buchler M, Malfertheiner P, Beger HG (1986) Identification of pancreatic necrosis. Severe acute pancreatitis: imaging procedures versus clinical staging. Gut 27:1035–1042
4. Bockus HL (1946) Gastroenterology, Vol 3. Saunders, Philadelphia, p 840
5. Cameron JL (1978) Chronic pancreatic ascites and pancreatic pleural effusion. Gastroenterology 74:134–140
6. Cameron JL, Anderson RP, Zuidema GD (1967) Pancreatic ascites. Surg Gynecol Obstet 125:328–332
7. Cameron JL, Brawley RK, Bender HW, Zuidema GD (1969) The treatment of pancreatic ascites. Ann Surg 170:668–676
8. Cameron JL, Kieffer RS, Sanderson WJ, Zuidema GD (1976) Internal pancreatic fistulas: pancreatic ascites and pleural effusions. Ann Surg 184:588–593
9. Castle LAM, Terblanche J (1978) Pancreatic ascites and pleural effusions. Aust NZ J Surg 48:290–295
10. Classen DC, Jacobson JAB, Burke JP, Jacobson JT, Scott Evans R (1988) Serious pseudomonas infections associated with endoscopic retrograde cholangiopancreatography. Am J Med 84:590–596
11. Davis ML, Kelsey WM (1951) Chronic pancreatitis in childhood. Am J Dis Child 81:687–692
12. Davis RE, Graham DY (1975) Pancreatic ascites: the role of endoscopic pancreatography. Dig Dis 20:977–980
13. Devig PM, Cross GH, Mullen JT, Blanchard PB (1976) Pancreatic ascites. South Med J 69:1133–1135
14. Donowitz M, Herstein MD, Spiro HM (1974) Pancreatic ascites. Medicine (Baltimore) 53:183–195
15. Dragstedt LR, Haymond HE, Ellis JC (1934) Pathogenesis of acute pancreatitis. Arch Surg 28:233–291
16. Gambill EE, Walters W, Scanlon PW (1960) Chronic relapsing pancreatitis with extensive subacute peritonitis and chronic, recurrent massive "chylous" ascites. Am J Surg 28:668–670
17. Gekas MD, Nikoomanesh R, Smith GW (1979) Pancreatic ascites: a rare complication of distal splenorenal shunt. Am J Surg 138:710–712
18. Hotz J, Goebell M, Herforth G, Probst M (1977) Massive pancreatic ascites without carcinoma. Report of three cases. Digestion 15:200–216
19. Ingram DM, Sheiner HJ (1980) Massive pancreatic serous effusions. Aust NZ J Surg 50:137–140
20. Kalwinsky D, Fritelli G, Oski FA (1974) Pancreatitis presenting as unexplained ascites. Am J Dis Child 128:734–736

21. Kavin H, Sobel JD, Dembo AJ (1971) Pancreatic ascites treated by irradiation of pancreas. Br Med J 2:503–504
22. Leger L, Lenriot JP, Lemaigre G (1974) Five to twenty year follow-up after surgery for chronic pancreatitis in 148 patients. Ann Surg 180:185–191
23. Levine JB, Warshaw AL, Falchuk KR, Schapiro RH (1977) The value of endoscopic retrograde pancreatography in the management of pancreatic ascites. Surgery 81:360–362
24. McCarthy MC, Dickerman RM (1982) Surgical management of severe acute pancreatitis. Arch Surg 117:476–480
25. McMahon MJ, Playforth MJ, Pickford IR (1980) A comparative study of methods for the prediction of severity of attacks of acute pancreatitis. Br J Surg 67:22–25
26. Morton RE, Deluca R, Reisman TN, Radkin JB, Rogers AI (1976) Pancreatic ascites: successful treatment with pancreatic radiation. Dig Dis 21:333–336
27. Munoz JN, Bose S (1975) Pancreatic ascites: a case report and review of the literature. Am J Dig Dis 20:1178–1183
28. Ou Tim L, Sotomayor M, Segal I (1977) Pancreatic ascites. S Afr J Surg 15:201–204
29. Paloyan D, Skinner DB (1976) Clinical significance of pancreatic ascites. Am J Surg 132:114–117
30. Rawlings W, Bynum TE, Pasternak G (1977) Pancreatic ascites: diagnosis of leakage site by endoscopic pancreatography. Surgery 81:363–365
31. Roberts JC (1975) Traumatic pancreatitis and pleural effusion. Aust NZ J Surg 45:90–94
32. Sankaran S, Walt AJ (1975) The natural and unnatural history of pancreatic pseudocysts. Br J Surg 62:37–44
33. Sankaran J, Walt AW (1976) Pancreatic ascites, recognition and management. Arch Surg 111:430–434
34. Sankaran S, Sugawa C, Walt AJ (1979) Value of endoscopic retrograde pancreatography in pancreatic ascites. Surg Gynecol Obstet 148:185–192
35. Satz N, Uhlschmid G, Pei P, Streuli R, Ammann RW (1984) On the pathogenesis of pancreatic ascites. Eur Surg Res 16:170–174
36. Sileo AV, Chawla SK, Loprest PA (1975) Pancreatic ascites: diagnostic importance of ascitic lipase. Dig Dis 20:1110–1114
37. Smith RB, Warren WD, Rivard AA, Anderson JR (1973) Pancreatic ascites. Diagnosis and management with particular reference to surgical technics. Ann Surg 177:538–546
38. Sottomayor M, Nom Chong R, Dawson M (1978) Use of ERCP in the diagnosis of internal pancreatic fistula. Gut 19:244–246
39. Sparks FC, Levine JB, Henken EM (1979) Pancreatic ascites – management by caudal pancreatectomy and side-to-side pancreaticojejunostomy. Am J Surg 138:713–715
40. Tombroff M, Loisq A, de Koster JP, Englehom L, Govaerts J-P (1973) Pleural effusion with pancreaticopleural fistula. Br Med J 1:330–331
41. Van Sonnenberg E, Wittich GR, Casola G, Stauffer AE, Polansky AD, Coons HG, Cabrere OA, Gerver PS (1985) Complicated pancreatic inflammatory disease: diagnostic and therapeutic role of interventional radiology. Radiology 155:335–340
42. Varma JS (1985) Acute chylous ascites with carcinoid of the pancreas. Scott Med J 30:111
43. Verma GR, Sabharwal A, Rajvansh A, Kauskik SP (1983) Pancreatic ascites due to Hodgkin's lymphoma pancreas. Indian J Cancer 20:38–39
44. Ward PA, Raju S, Suzuki H (1977) Preoperative demonstration of the pancreatic fistula by endoscopic pancreatography in a patient with pancreatic ascites. Ann Surg 185:232–234
45. Weaver DW, Walt AJ, Sugawa C, Bouwan DL (1982) A continuing appraisal of pancreatic ascites. Surg Gynecol Obstet 154:845–848
46. Wilkinson AE, Richards AT (1972) Proceedings of surgical case conferences held at the Johannesburg Hospital. S Afr J Surg 10:235–237

Diagnosis

Role of Serum Enzymes in Chronic Pancreatitis

G. Del Favero, C. Fabris, D. Basso, T. Meggiato, P. Fogar, and R. Naccarato[1]

A large number of enzymes of different classes (e. g., proteolytic, lipolytic, nucleolytic) are synthesized by the acinar cells of the exocrine pancreas and secreted into the pancreatic ducts [1]. Although the secretory pathway of the acinar cells leads to the discharge of enzymes through the secretory pole of the cell, small amounts may be released into the bloodstream, as occurs in endocrine secretion. Therefore small quantities of pancreatic enzymes may be detected in the circulation of healthy humans.

When the pancreatic gland has acute damage, large amounts of pancreatic enzymes are released into the serum [2–6]. This phenomenon has been widely studied and utilized for diagnostic purposes in acute pancreatitis. Extremely high levels of amylase, lipase, and trypsin are almost invariably a component of the clinical picture of this disease [2, 4].

Chronic pancreatitis is a heterogeneous disease and its pathogenesis is not yet well understood. The features of the inflammatory process, leading to acinar cell destruction and gland scarring, can vary; this depends on the different etiological factors and on their duration of action. In fact, chronic pancreatitis may either resemble acute pancreatitis or have an insidious and subclinical course. Clinical relapses are usually frequent in the early phases of the disease, while the progressive substitution of the exocrine parenchyma by fibrous tissue accompanies remission of pain and the onset of exocrine and endocrine insufficiency in the later stages [7].

Variations that may be observed in serum pancreatic enzymes reflect the different phases of chronic pancreatitis [2], although they have particular properties which account for differences in their behavior patterns. All the exocrine pancreatic enzymes are low molecular weight proteins, the mol. wt. ranging from about 15000 to 50000. Because of this, they are ultrafiltrable in the kidney and this explains the high rate of disappearance of amylase and lipase from the circulation after an acute attack of pancreatitis [3, 5]. The behavior and biochemical properties of proteolytic enzymes are different from those of amylase. Both trypsin and elastase 1 are present in the circulation as free and inhibitor-bound forms [8, 9]. Their routes of disappearance from the circulation are different, since free enzymes are excreted via the kidney, while the bound forms are probably taken up by the reticuloendothelial system. A great part of immunoreactive trypsin is present in the circulation in the form of free enzyme, whereas elastase 1 is mainly accounted for by alpha-1-antitrypsin-bound

---

[1] Istituto di Medicina Interna, Cattedra di Malattie Apparato Digerente, Università degli Studi di Padova, Padua, Italy

Chronic Pancreatitis
Ed. by Beger, Büchler, Ditschuneit, and Malfertheiner
© Springer-Verlag Berlin Heidelberg 1990

forms [8, 9]. This probably explains why elastase 1 levels continue to be high after an acute pancreatitis attack, the period being longer then that of other enzymes which are rapidly cleared by the kidney [3].

In chronic pancreatitis, serum pancreatic enzymes levels are usually within the normal range [4, 10, 11]. However high levels may be found in some patients with clinical signs of relapse [2]. The increase may involve all the different pancreatic enzymes or some of them, the remaining values being normal. Rarely is it three- to fourfold the upper normal range; it may be transient, or, if the pancreatic relapse does not subside, persistent. The presence of pseudocysts seems to be associated with a high frequency of abnormal values; other complications, such as pancreatic calcifications, do not seem to be linked to high serum enzyme levels.

In chronic pancreatitis low serum values for all pancreatic enzymes may be observed [2, 4]. This finding, however, is significant only for trypsin, an enzyme of exclusively pancreatic origin [12, 13]. Patients with an important exocrine insufficiency may have decreased immunoreactive trypsin values, and this finding is observed only in pancreatic diseases. Therefore, low-level immunoreactive trypsin has a low sensitivity but a high specificity for pancreatic exocrine insufficiency. The behavior of elastase 1 seems to be similar to trypsin, but with a less evident diagnostic utility [14].

All these observations indicate that the determination of serum pancreatic enzymes plays a limited role in the diagnosis of chronic pancreatitis and in the detection of its complications. However, it may be of physiopathological interest to consider their variations in chronic pancreatic diseases.

Starting from the concept that pancreatic enzymes are ultrafiltrable, their urinary excretions have been investigated in pancreatic diseases [8, 9, 15, 16]. It is well known that increased amylasuria mirrors amylasemia, since the former reflects a passive phenomenon. It has been observed, however, that in the course of pancreatic inflammation, the renal handling of amylase, expressed by its fractional clearance, is frequently altered [17]: irrespective of the serum amylase level a higher percentage of ultrafiltered enzyme is excreted by the kidney into the urine. It has been suggested that various factors play a role in enhancing amylase urinary clearance. Among them a diminished tubular reabsorption of this enzyme may play a predominant role. In fact, usually only small amounts of the ultrafiltered amylase can be detected in urine, because most of the ultrafiltered amylase is reabsorbed by the tubular cells. In acute, as well as in chronic, pancreatitis factors of unknown origin can alter renal tubular cells and enhance fractional amylase clearance [18].

The renal clearance of other pancreatic enzymes, such as trypsin and elastase 1, has been investigated [8, 9]. It has been reported that the renal clearance of both these proteases is different from that of amylase [8, 9]. The amounts of both enzymes bound to inhibitors decrease in the presence of pancreatic inflammation and this fact interferes with their urinary clearance [8–10, 15]. Furthermore, free proteases possess a lower mol. wt. and their biochemical properties (e.g., the isoelectric point) are different from those of amylase. All these factors may determine variations in the ultrafiltration and tubular reabsorption between amylase and proteases. In effect, the amount of protease excretion is far lower than that of amylase, for a given serum level.

In chronic pancreatitis the urinary clearances of both trypsin and elastase 1 increases in a number of patients, as is observed for amylase [9, 17, 19]. The presence of pancreatic inflammation increases the percentage of free proteases in the circulation, leading to an increased ultrafiltered load. However, this aspect seems to play a minor role in explaining the altered clearances of both proteases in chronic pancreatitis. The presence of tubular damage, on the other hand, as already suggested for amylase, plays a major role in increasing the plasma-urine transfer of trypsin and elastase 1 [18].

Urinary proteases might be expected to be almost exclusively accounted for by free, unbound enzymes. However, chromatographic studies have demonstrated that both free and inhibitor-bound trypsin forms can be detected in the urine of patients with chronic pancreatitis [15]. The origin of these bound forms, in particular if derived from the circulation or form in urine, is unknown.

We may conclude that even if the evaluation of serum pancreatic enzymes is not of great utility to the clinician in any attempt to promptly and reliably diagnose chronic pancreatitis, it is, on the contrary, of constant value in biochemical and pathophysiological studies.

References

1. Rinderknecht H (1986) Pancreatic secretory enzymes. In: Go VLW, Gardner JD, Brooks FP, Lebenthal E, DiMagno EP, Scheele GA (eds) The exocrine pancreas. Raven, New York, pp 163–183
2. Fahrenkrug J, Magid E (1980) Concentration of immunoreactive trypsin and activity of pancreatic isoamylase in serum compared in pancreatic diseases. Clin Chem 26:1573–1576
3. Murata A, Ogawa M, Fujimoto K, Kitahara T, Kosaki G (1982) Changes in serum immunoreactive elastase 1 in acute pancreatitis. Hepatogastroenterology 29:278–280
4. Ventrucci M, Gullo L, Daniele C, Bartolucci C, Priori P, Platé L, Bonora G, Labò G (1983) Comparative study of serum pancreatic isoamylase, lipase, and trypsin-like immunoreactivity in pancreatic disease. Digestion 28:114–121
5. Flamion B, Delhaye M, Horanyi Z, Delange A, Demanet H, Quenon M, van Melsen A, Cremer M, Delcourt A (1987) Comparison of elastase 1 with amylase, lipase, and trypsin-like immunoreactivity in the diagnosis of acute pancreatitis. Am J Gastroenterol 82:532–535
6. Buamah PK, Cornell C, Cassells-Smith AJ, Skillen AW (1987) Serum human pancreatic elastase I levels in pancreatic disease. Clin Chim Acta 166:57–60
7. DiMagno EP, Clain JE (1986) Chronic pancreatitis. In: Go VLW, Gardner JD, Brooks FP, Lebenthal, DiMagno EP, Scheele GA (eds) The exocrine pancreas. Raven, New York, pp 541–575
8. Fabris C, Benini L, del Favero G, Cavallini G, Basso D, Vantini I, Bonvicini P, Brocco G, Piccoli A, Tonon M, Naccarato R, Scuro LA (1987) Molecular size distribution of immunoreactive trypsin and renal tubular dysfunction: role in trypsin plasma-urine transfer. Enzyme 37:174–181
9. Fabris C, Basso D, Benini L, Meggiato T, del Favero G, Cavallini G, Panozzo MP, Fogar P, Angonese C, Vantini I, Piccoli A, Plebani M, Naccarato R (1989) Urinary elastase 1 in chronic pancreatic disease. Enzyme 42:80–86
10. Fabris C, del Favero G, Panucci A, Plebani M, di Mario F, Piccoli A, Basso D, Burlina A, Naccarato R (1986) Serum elastase 1 and immunoreactive trypsin in chronic pancreatic disease: is there any relationship with trypsin inhibitors? Enzyme 35:82–86
11. Lesi C, Melzi d'Eril GV, Pavesi F, Scandellari A, Faccenda F, Casertano MG, Savoia M, Zoni L, Peppi M (1985) Clinical significance of serum pancreatic enzymes in the quiescent phase of chronic pancreatitis. Clin Biochem 18:235–238
12. Steinberg WM, Anderson KK (1984) Serum trypsinogen in diagnosis of chronic pancreatitis. Dig Dis Sci 29:988–993
13. Steinberg WM, Goldstein SS, Davis ND, Anderson KK, Shamma'a JM (1985) Predictive value of a low serum trypsinogen. Dig Dis Sci 30:547–551

14. Malfertheiner P, Buchler M, Stanescu A, Uhl W, Ditschuneit H (1987) Serum elastase 1 in inflammatory pancreatic and gastrointestinal diseases and in renal insufficiency. A comparison with other serum pancreatic enzymes. Int J Pancreatol 2:159–170
15. Fabris C, Benini L, Basso D, del Favero G, Vantini I, Piccoli A, Cavallini G, Scuro LA, Naccarato R (1988) Renal factors in serum trypsinogen 1 metabolism and excretion in chronic pancreatic disease. Pancreas 3:25–29
16. Junge W, Malyusz M, Ehrens HJ (1985) The role of the kidney in the elimination of pancreatic lipase and amylase from blood. J Clin Chem Clin Biochem 23:387–392
17. Grosberg SJ, Wapnick S, Purow E, Purow JR (1979) Specificity of serum amylase and amylase creatinine clearance ratio in the diagnosis of acute and chronic pancreatitis. Am J Gastroenterol 72:41–45
18. Fabris C, Basso D, del Favero G, Piccoli A, Angonese C, di Mario F, Plebani M, Bonvicini P, Burlina A, Naccarato R (1989) Renal tubular dysfunction in pancreatic cancer and chronic pancreatitis. Nephron 51:56–60
19. Farini R, Fabris C, del Favero G, Bonvicini P, de Besi T, Piccoli A, Baccaglini U, Plebani M, Pedrazzoli S, Kind R, Ceriotti G, Naccarato R (1981) Role of trypsin/creatinine clearance ratio in the differential diagnosis of chronic pancreatic disease. Gastroenterology 81:242–246

Value and Clinical Role of Intubation Tests in Chronic Pancreatitis

L. Gullo[1]

In recent years, the diagnosis of pancreatic diseases has been greatly facilitated by the introduction of several functional and imaging techniques into the clinic. Duodenal intubation, a test which is more than 50 years old, is being performed less and less frequently, mainly because of its complexity. The topic I will address in this communication is: does duodenal intubation still have a valid role in the diagnosis of chronic pancreatitis?

In an attempt to answer this question, I will present some data from our laboratory obtained in a large series of patients with chronic pancreatitis.

In our clinic, duodenal intubation is one of the investigations usually carried out on patients suspected of having chronic pancreatitis, and our data indicate that in a significant number of patients, mainly in those with mild disease, this test is very useful for the diagnosis. We use a Sarles tube for gastric and duodenal juice aspiration and, to stimulate the pancreas, we use a prolonged intravenous infusion (90 min) of secretin (1 clinical unit/kg per hour) plus cerulein (100 ng/kg per hour) [1]. Using this type of pancreatic stimulation, we have shown that, in patients with chronic pancreatitis, pancreatic secretion of enzymes tends to decrease with prolonged stimulation, whereas in normal subjects it remains constant or increases (Fig. 1). This behavior allows a better and more complete discrimination between normal subjects and chronic pancreatitis patients, if we consider the outputs of enzymes during the last 30 min of pancreatic stimulation [1, 2].

Table 1 summarizes the sensitivity and the specificity of the secretin-cerulein test in the diagnosis of pancreatic insufficiency. These data are based on tests performed in

Table 1. Diagnostic value of the secretin-cerulein test in chronic pancreatitis

	%
Sensitivity	97.1
($n = 140$)	
Specificity	97.9
($n = 96$)	
+ Pred. value	98.5 (70)*
− Pred. value	95.9 (99.8)*

* corrected for a prevalence of chronic pancreatitis of 0.05

[1] Institute of Medicine and Gastroenterology, University of Bologna, St. Orsola Hospital, Bologna, Italy

Chronic Pancreatitis
Ed. by Beger, Büchler, Ditschuneit, and Malfertheiner
© Springer-Verlag Berlin Heidelberg 1990

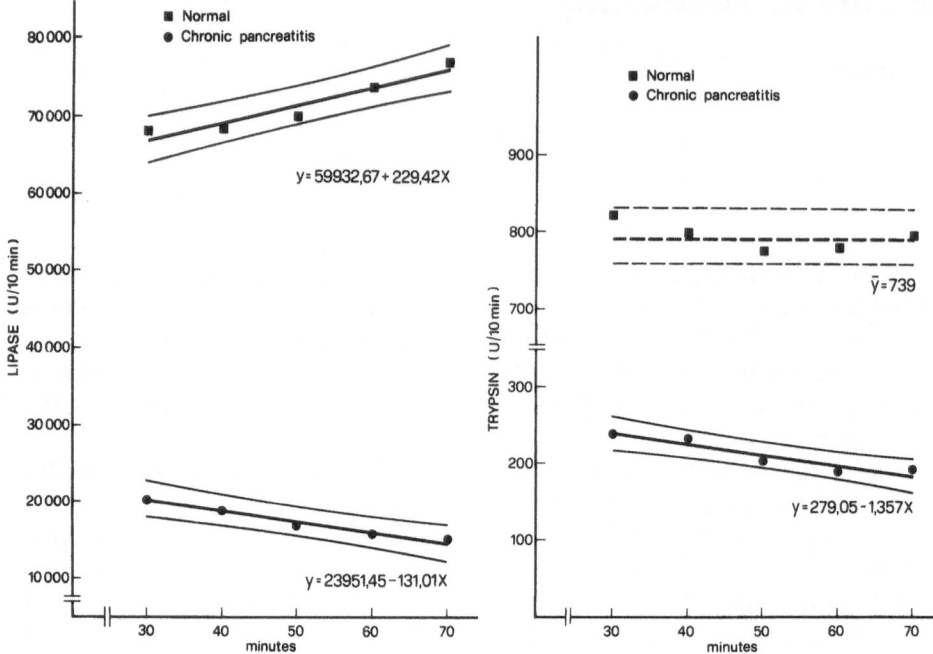

Fig. 1. Behavior of pancreatic enzyme secretion during 90-min pancreatic stimulation with secretin (1 clinical unit/kg per hour) and cerulein (100 ng/kg per hour) in 32 patients with chronic pancreatitis and in 30 healthy normal subjects (analysis of variance)

140 patients with chronic pancreatitis and in 96 controls (normal subjects and patients suffering from various nonpancreatic digestive diseases) [3]. The diagnosis of chronic pancreatitis was based on clinical history (recurrent attacks of upper abdominal pain with raised serum levels of pancreatic enzymes) and was confirmed by at least two of the following criteria: rx-evidence of pancreatic calcification, typical ductal changes at endoscopic retrograde cholangiopancreatography, morphologic changes at ultrasonography, and pancreatic exocrine insufficiency. The sensitivity of the secretin-cerulein test was 97% and the specificity 98%. In the vast majority of patients (about 80%) ultrasound and endoscopic retrograde pancreatography were also carried out, and the sensitivity of these two techniques was lower, i.e., about 70% and 90%, respectively. Our experience with computed tomography has so far involved fewer patients; however, the results obtained indicate that its sensitivity in chronic pancreatitis is similar to that of ultrasound. It is interesting to note that if we consider only those patients with earlier forms of chronic pancreatitis, i.e., no pancreatic calcification, steatorrhea, or diabetes (about 40% of the total), the sensitivity of duodenal intubation always remains above 90%, whereas that of ultrasound and endoscopic retrograde pancreatography (but above all ultrasound) further decrease. Thus, these data clearly indicate that the diagnostic value of the secretin-cerulein test is greater than that of the modern imaging techniques in patients with chronic pancreatitis, even in earlier forms of the disease which are, as is well known, the most difficult to diagnose.

Table 2. Relationship between the duration of clinical history[a] and exocrine pancreatic insufficiency in chronic pancreatitis. Percentage of pathological results with the secretin-cerulein test

	Bicarbonate %	Lipase %	Chymotrypsin %
≤ 1 year (n = 27)	74	96	81
2–3 years (n = 34)	94	97	97
4–5 years (n = 17)	94	94	94
6–10 years (n = 33)	94	94	94
> 10 years (n = 17)	94	100	88
Total (n = 128)	90	96	91

[a] Patients were divided into five groups according to the time elapsed between the first typical attack of abdominal pain and the study

Table 2 shows the relationship between exocrine pancreatic insufficiency and the clinical duration of chronic pancreatitis in 128 of the above-mentioned 140 patients. The patients were divided into five groups according to the duration of clinical history: those studied within 1 year of the clinical onset of pancreatitis (first attack of abdominal pain), those studied within 2–3 years, within 4–5 years, 6–10 years, and those studied more than 10 years from the clinical onset. As regards patients studied more than 1 year after the clinical onset of pancreatitis, there are no important differences in the percentages of pathologic results. The vast majority of them (more than 90%) had pancreatic insufficiency involving both bicarbonate and enzymes. However, as regards the 27 patients studied within 1 year of the clinical onset of pancreatitis (i.e., very early in the clinical course of the disease), 7 (25%) had normal bicarbonate output, 5 (19%) had normal chymotrypsin output, but only 1 (4%) had normal lipase output. These data indicate: first, that pancreatic insufficiency occurs early in the clinical course of chronic pancreatitis, and, second, that enzyme secretion, mainly that of lipase, is impaired first in this disease. The fact that an isolated deficiency of lipase secretion is an early sign of pancreatic insufficiency in chronic pancreatitis has been confirmed by sequential studies of pancreatic function carried out in our laboratory [4] in which we have seen the development of global pancreatic insufficiency (bicarbonate and enzymes) during the follow-up in patients with isolated lipase insufficiency at the first evaluation.

In a recent study [5] in which we compared the results of the secretin-cerulein test with those of ultrasound in 42 patients with chronic pancreatitis, we have shown that most of the patients with mild impairment of enzyme secretion, including patients with isolated lipase deficiency, had a normal ultrasonographic pattern. These results further confirm the superiority of the secretin-cerulein test over ultrasound in the diagnosis of chronic pancreatitis, and indicate that patients found to have mild enzyme impairment, or isolated lipase deficiency at the secretin-cerulein test, indeed, have mild or early pancreatic lesions.

Unfortunately, duodenal intubation is unpleasant for the patient and time consuming, so several efforts have been made in recent years to develop more simple, tubeless pancreatic function tests. Several tubeless tests are currently available, but their sensitivity in detecting pancreatic insufficiency is significantly lower than that of duodenal intubation, especially in patients with mild to moderate insufficiency [6–8]. For this reason, the clinical usefulness of these tests is rather limited.

So, on the basis of my own experience with patients with chronic pancreatitis, and with pancreatic function tests, I believe that, as far as the clinical role of the intubation tests is concerned, it is reasonable to conclude as follows: basically, we see three types of patients with chronic pancreatitis: those with early or mild disease, those with moderate disease, and those with severe and advanced disease. Those with advanced disease and, generally, most of those with moderate disease, do not present any diagnostic difficulties. The clinical history by itself is usually sufficient to diagnose the disease, and ultrasonography and/or endoscopic retrograde pancreatography plus some tubeless function test are sufficient to confirm the diagnosis. In these patients duodenal intubation is not usually necessary. However, for patients with early or mild disease, the confirmation of clinical diagnosis is often difficult since most of the other tests available, including ultrasonography, computed tomography, and endoscopic retrograde pancreatography, are not able to demonstrate pathology at this stage. In these patients, duodenal intubation is the only test capable of reliably confirming the clinical suspicion of chronic pancreatitis in the vast majority of cases.

References

1. Gullo L, Costa PL, Fontana G, Labò G (1976) Investigation of exocrine pancreatic function by continuous infusion of caerulein and secretin in normal subjects and in chronic pancreatitis. Digestion 14:97–107
2. Gullo L, Costa PL, Labò G (1978) A comparison between injection and infusion of pancreatic stimulants in the diagnosis of exocrine pancreatic insufficiency. Digestion 18:64–69
3. Gullo L (1986) Direct pancreatic function test (duodenal intubation) in the diagnosis of chronic pancreatitis. Gastroenterology 90:799–800
4. Gullo L, Barbara L, Labò G (1988) Effect of cessation of alcohol use on the course of pancreatic dysfunction in alcoholic pancreatitis. Gastroenterology 95:1003–1008
5. Bolondi L, Priori P, Gullo L, Santi V, Li Bassi S, Barbara L, Labò G (1987) Relationship between morphological changes detected by ultrasonography and pancreatic exocrine function in chronic pancreatitis. Pancreas 2:222–229
6. Ventrucci M, Gullo L, Daniele C, Priori P, Labò G (1983) Pancreolauryl test for pancreatic exocrine insufficiency. Am J Gastroenterol 78:806–809
7. Ventrucci M, Gullo L, Daniele C, Priori P, Bartolucci C, Canali S, Agostini D, Labò G (1985) Evaluation of BT PABA test in the diagnosis of pancreatic exocrine insufficiency. Ital J Gastroenterol 17:1–4
8. Gullo L (1986) Pancreatic function test by means of duodenal intubation. In: Malfertheiner P, Ditschuneit H (eds) Diagnostic procedures in pancreatic diseases. Springer, Berlin Heidelberg New York, pp 201–207

Value of Indirect Pancreatic Function Tests

P. G. LANKISCH[1]

Introduction

Two principally different procedures are available for investigating exocrine pancreatic function (Table 1):
1. Direct pancreatic function tests, measuring the contents of pancreatic secretion (bicarbonate and enzymes)
2. Indirect pancreatic function tests, whereby diminished digestive capability signifies exocrine pancreatic insufficiency.

Table 1. Applicability of pancreatic function tests

1. Suspected chronic pancreatitis in
– Relapsing abdominal complaints
– Diarrhea
– Steatorrhea
– Calcifications in the pancreas region on X-ray examination
2. Follow-up investigations in verified chronic pancreatitis
3. Clarification of the diagnosis after an attack of acute pancreatitis

Since direct pancreatic function tests, such as the secretin-pancreozymin test (SPT) and the Lundh test, are invasive, time-consuming, and expensive, they are usually performed only in specialized laboratories. The indirect pancreatic function tests consist in measuring an enzyme output (e.g., fecal chymotrypsin and trypsin, pancreatic isoamylase, or immunoreactive trypsin in serum), or in determining the enzyme effect (NBT-PABA test, pancreolauryl test).

This survey aims to describe these pancreatic function tests, how they are performed, their practicability, as well as their reliability in confirming or excluding exocrine pancreatic insufficiency resulting from chronic pancreatitis or other diseases. The chapter by Del Vavero deals specifically with measurements of pancreatic serum isoamylase and immunoreactive trypsin outputs.

---

[1] Department of Internal Medicine, Municipal Hospital of Lüneburg, Bögelstrasse 1,
D-2120 Lüneburg, FRG

Chronic Pancreatitis
Ed. by Beger, Büchler, Ditschuneit, and Malfertheiner
© Springer-Verlag Berlin Heidelberg 1990

Table 2. Measurement of fecal chymotrypsin

False-normal results can be obtained
– In mild to moderate exocrine pancreatic insufficiency
– When enzyme replacement therapy was not stopped in time
False-pathological results can be obtained
– In diarrhea
– In protein deficiency condition (lack of endogenic stimulation)
– In celiac disease
– In cachexia (because of chronic inflammatory diseases; tumors)
– In anorexia nervosa
– After Billroth II resection of the stomach
– In obstructive jaundice

Performance of Indirect Pancreatic Function Tests

Measuring Fecal Chymotrypsin and Trypsin

Fecal chymotrypsin and trypsin (Table 2) amount to only 5‰ of total enzymes excreted by the pancreas [1]. Nonetheless, fecal measurements can be useful in drawing conclusions about pancreatic secretion. Because of the poor correlation in earlier studies between fecal trypsin levels and clinical signs, this test has been abandoned [1]. The titrimetric method for measuring chymotrypsin is not very popular because of the odor involved, but it can be replaced by the new photometric procedures [10, 29].

NBT-PABA Test

In the NBT-PABA test (PFT Roche, Hoffmann-La Roche AG, Diagnostika, CH-7889 Grenzach-Wyhlen) the patient ingests with the test meal the pancreas stimulant N-benzoyl-L-tyrosyl-para-aminobenzoic acid. The *para*-aminobenzoic acid (PABA) is released in the duodenum by the esterolytic activity of pancreas-specific chymotrypsin. The PABA is absorbed in the gut, conjugated in the liver, and excreted in the urine. The concentration levels in the urine indicate whether the exocrine pancreatic function is normal or insufficient.

The NBT-PABA test may lead to false-abnormal results when absorption in the gut, conjugation in the liver, or renal function are disturbed. Repetition of the test with only the split-off product (pure PABA) may improve specificity [27]. With radioactive-marked PABA, this control test can be performed together with the usual NBT-PABA test on the same day [3, 28, 32]. In order to avoid possible interference in the test results, all medication, except for digitalis preparations, should be stopped 2 days prior to the test. Specifically, sulfonamides, sulfonyl carbamide, laxatives, diuretics, vitamins, and preparations containing pancreatic enzymes are to be discontinued. Forty-eight hours prior to and during the test, no benzoic acid preserved food should be allowed because benzoic acid could also interfere with the test. False-abnormal test results are also possible, given bacterial overgrowths in the gut containing special intestinal bacteria that are capable of splitting off the NBT-PABA peptide [12].

Pancreolauryl Test

In the second oral pancreatic function test, the pancreolauryl test (PLT; Temmler-Werke, 3550 Marburg, FRG), the patient ingests with the test meal fluorescein dilaurate, which is split by the pancreas-specific cholesterol esterase. The fluorescein component is absorbed and excreted in the urine. The test is repeated 2 days later with only fluorescein in order to exclude possible disturbances in absorption in the gut, conjugation in the liver, or renal function. The T/C ratio is calculated on the basis of the results on the test day (T) and the control day (C).

Vitamin B2 and salazosulfopyridine preparations as well as pancreatic enzymes interfere with test results and, therefore, have to be discontinued 5 days prior to the test. False-abnormal test results have been obtained from patients after Billroth II resection of the stomach (postcibal asynchrony?), with biliary diseases (insufficient hydrolysis of the ester?) and chronic inflammatory bowel disease [11, 14, 24].

Serum NBT-PABA Test and PLT Test

The difficulties of urine collection from elderly or severely ill patients or outpatients, and the need for shortening the duration of the test, have inspired efforts to use measurements of PABA or fluorescein in serum for evaluating exocrine pancreatic function [2, 4, 6, 15, 20].

However, modifications of the serum test have already been developed using metoclopramide and secretin to stimulate pancreatic secretion [25, 26].

Quantitative Fecal Fat Analysis

In cases of proven exocrine pancreatic insufficiency, both fecal weight and fat [33] should be measured over a period of at least 72 h to find out whether the exocrine pancreatic insufficiency requires enzyme replacement therapy. Quantitative fecal fat analysis may be used as an indirect pancreatic function test when performed prior to and after pancreatic enzyme replacement. This older method of fecal fat analysis yields results as good as a new method using "nuclear magnetic resonance" (NMR). The latter, however, is not yet widely used [30].

Measuring Plasma Amino Acids Following Stimulation with Secretin and Pancreozymin

A new interesting exocrine pancreatic function test measures amino acid levels in plasma following stimulation of the exocrine pancreas with secretin and pancreozymin. All patients with normal exocrine pancreatic function showed a minimum 12% decrease in amino acids; in patients with moderate to severe pancreatic insufficiency, this decrease was less than 12% [8, 13]. Results from further current investigations, especially in patients with mild exocrine pancreatic insufficiency, will be of great interest.

Breath Analysis Tests

Repeated efforts to use breath analysis as a substitute for direct pancreatic function tests have been unsuccessful [17]. A recently developed breath analysis test seems to be diagnostically valuable only in cases of severe exocrine pancreatic insufficiency [5]. Here again, further attempts to use breath analysis tests for detecting mild exocrine pancreatic insufficiency would be of great interest.

Value of Indirect Pancreatic Function Tests to Confirm or to Exclude Exocrine Pancreatic Insufficiency

The most commonly used indirect pancreatic function tests (fecal chymotrypsin measurements, NBT-PABA test, pancreolauryl test, and fecal fat analysis prior to and after pancreatic enzyme substitution) are now standardized, and have the advantage of no risks or side effects for the patient. With the exception of the quantitative fecal fat analysis, all indirect pancreatic function tests are easily performed. The results of the individual test depend more on competent laboratory performance than on the experience of the investigator, in contrast to morphological procedures, such as ultrasound, computed tomography, and endoscopic retrograde cholangiopancreatography (ERCP), which require an experienced investigator.

The results of indirect pancreatic function tests depend to a large extent on:
1. Selection of the patients:
   When patients are selected on the basis of exact case histories, a higher prevalence of chronic pancreatitis is to be expected, thus biasing the predictive value of the function test [11].
2. Instructions given to the patients:
   When, for example, in the NBT-PABA or pancreolauryl test, the patient takes the test pills before or after breakfast, instead of in the middle of the test meal, this can often lead to a false test result because of postcibal asynchrony.
3. Severity of exocrine pancreatic insufficiency:
   In cases of mild exocrine insufficiency, all indirect pancreatic function tests may yield false-normal results.

Sensitivity of fecal chymotrypsin test results is high, especially in patients with severe exocrine pancreatic insufficiency [1, 9, 18, 19, 31]. False-normal and false-abnormal test results are, nonetheless, possible (Table 2).

All previous studies have shown that the pancreolauryl and the NBT-PABA tests are very reliable detectors of severe exocrine pancreatic insufficiency, but not so in cases of mild or moderate insufficiency where false-normal test results have been

Table 3. Correlation of different indirect pancreatic function tests with the secretin-pancreozymin test and fecal fat analysis [19]

Exocrine pancreatic insufficiency	Pancreolauryl test Abnormal ($n = 53$)	NBT-PABA test Abnormal ($n = 52$)	Fecal chymotrypsin Abnormal ($n = 47$)
Mild	67%	73%	25%
Moderate	88%	88%	60%
Severe	100%	97%	92%

registered [19, 24, 31]. In comparative investigations in patients with pancreatogenic steatorrhea, the sensitivity of all three tests lay between 92% and 100%. In patients with mild to moderate exocrine pancreatic insufficiency, tubeless pancreatic function tests proved to be more reliable than fecal chymotrypsin measurements [19] (Table 3).

At a symposium in Ulm [23], all surveys existing at that time on sensitivity and specificity of indirect pancreatic function tests were summarized (Tables 4, 5). An explanation for the wide range of specificity and sensitivity in the survey probably lies in the above-mentioned dependent variables, namely selection of and instructions to the patients and severity of exocrine pancreatic insufficiency.

Table 4. Specificity of indirect pancreatic function tests [23]

Test	Studies	Patients	Specificity (%)
Fecal chymotrypsin	4	256	84 (73– 89)
NBT-PABA test[a]	2	384	87 (87– 88)
Pancreolauryl test	11	604	82 (39–100)

[a] One gram NBT-PABA + 6-h collection period

Table 5. Sensitivity of indirect pancreatic function tests [23]

Test	Studies	Patients	Specificity (%)
Fecal chymotrypsin	10	361	78 (50–100)
NBT-PABA test[a]	3	255	87 (85– 94)
Pancreolauryl test	11	371	90 (55–100)

[a] One gram NBT-PABA + 6-h collection period

Our serum tests have yielded the same sensitivity and specificity as our urine tests [20]. Other investigators have had more reliable results from serum tests [25, 26]. In our study, the optimal cutoff point for separating normal from abnormal pancreatic function was 210 min in the pancreolauryl test, and 150 min in the NBT-PABA test. The latter test was slightly less sensitive and specific than the pancreolauryl test (Figs. 1, 2) [20].

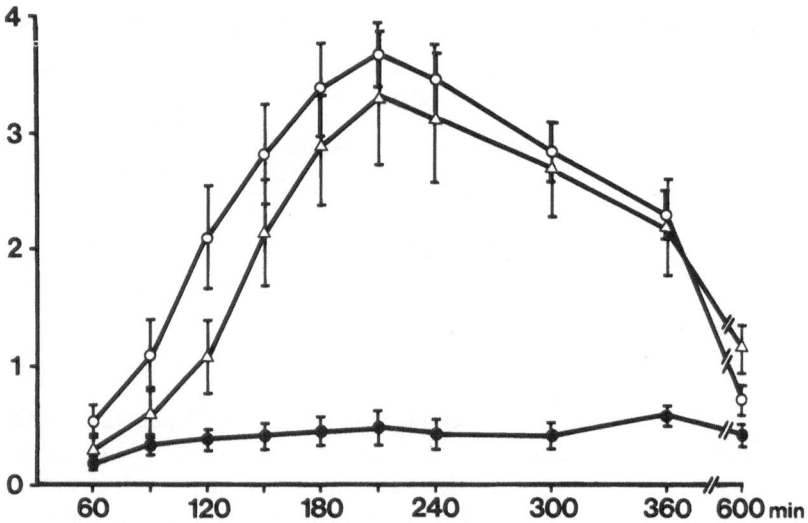

Fig. 1. Fluorescein concentration in the serum (micrograms per milliliter; mean ± SEM) on the test day in 22 healthy controls (○), 17 patients with nonpancreatic diseases and normal pancreatic function (△), and 31 patients with exocrine pancreatic insufficiency (●) [20]

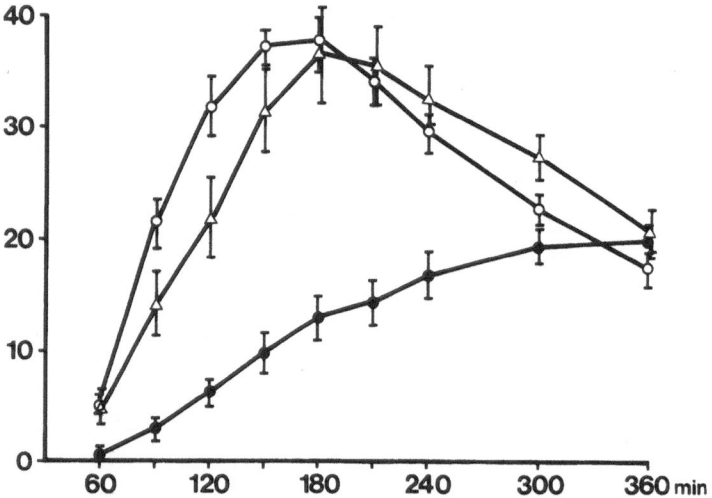

Fig. 2. p-Aminobenzoic acid concentration in the serum (nanomoles per milliliter; mean ± SEM) in 22 healthy controls (○), 17 patients with nonpancreatic diseases and normal pancreatic function (△), and 31 patients with exocrine pancreatic insufficiency (●) [20]

The fact that normal stool contains a certain amount of fat (< 7 g/day) renders quantitative fecal fat analyses obsolete [16]. Whether the simple fecal weight measurement could replace the more complicated fecal fat analysis has also been discussed. Comparing fecal weight and fat analyses in 1269 investigations, Lembcke [22] found no correlation in 26.3% of the cases: 12.8% of the patients had steatorrhea in spite of

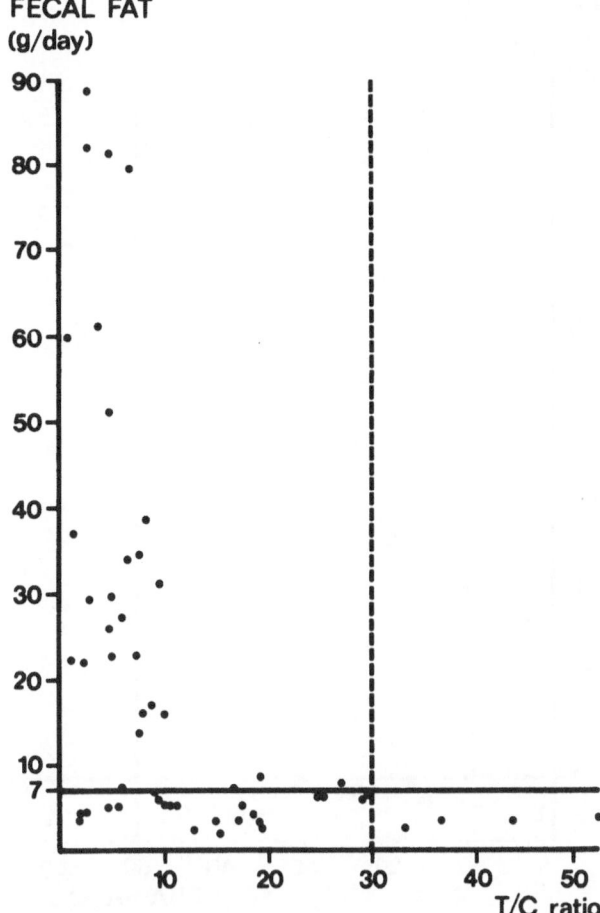

Fig. 3. Comparison of daily fecal fat excretion with the results of the urine pancreolauryl test in 54 patients with exocrine pancreatic insufficiency proven by the secretin-pancreozymin test

normal fecal weight, and 13.5% had normal fecal fat content along with increased fecal weight. Therefore, steatorrhea cannot be reliably diagnosed by means of fecal weight measurements.

Indirect and direct pancreatic function tests are useful for determining whether exocrine pancreatic insufficiency (steatorrhea) requires pancreatic enzyme replacement therapy. DiMagno et al. [7] found steatorrhea only when the stimulated lipase secretion fell below 10% of the normal mean. We recently showed that the pancreolauryl test yields a similar correlation (Fig. 3), but not the NBT-PABA test [21]. The T/C ratio was higher than 10 in 21 patients; only 3 of these patients had borderline steatorrhea (7–8.5 g/day). With a T/C ratio of 10 adopted as the cutoff figure, lower levels were indicative of pancreatic steatorrhea, with a sensitivity of 89.3%. Such a useful cutoff limit indicating steatorrhea did not occur in the NBT-PABA test (Fig. 4) [21].

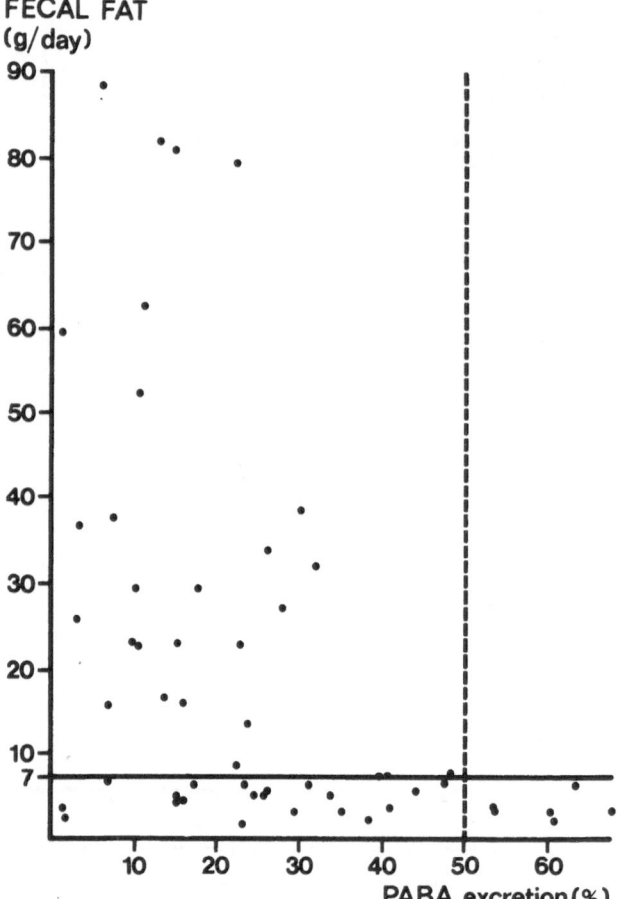

Fig. 4. Comparison of daily fecal fat excretion with the results of the urine NBT-PABA test in 54 patients with pancreatic insufficiency proven by the secretin-pancreozymin test

Value of Indirect Pancreatic Function Tests for the Diagnosis of Chronic Pancreatitis

The major symptom should guide diagnostic procedures for chronic pancreatitis: If epigastric complaints dominate, ERCP should be performed prior to indirect pancreatic function tests. If weight loss, diarrhea, and/or steatorrhea dominate, indirect pancreatic function tests should be performed prior to ERCP (Fig. 5). However, if chronic pancreatitis is still suspected despite normal ERCP findings and normal indirect pancreatic function test results, a direct function test should be performed to confirm or refute the tentative diagnosis, for chronic pancreatitis may involve in its early stages only the small pancreatic ducts, which cannot always be detected by ERCP, and indirect pancreatic function tests may yield false-normal test results in cases of mild to moderate exocrine pancreatic insufficiency.

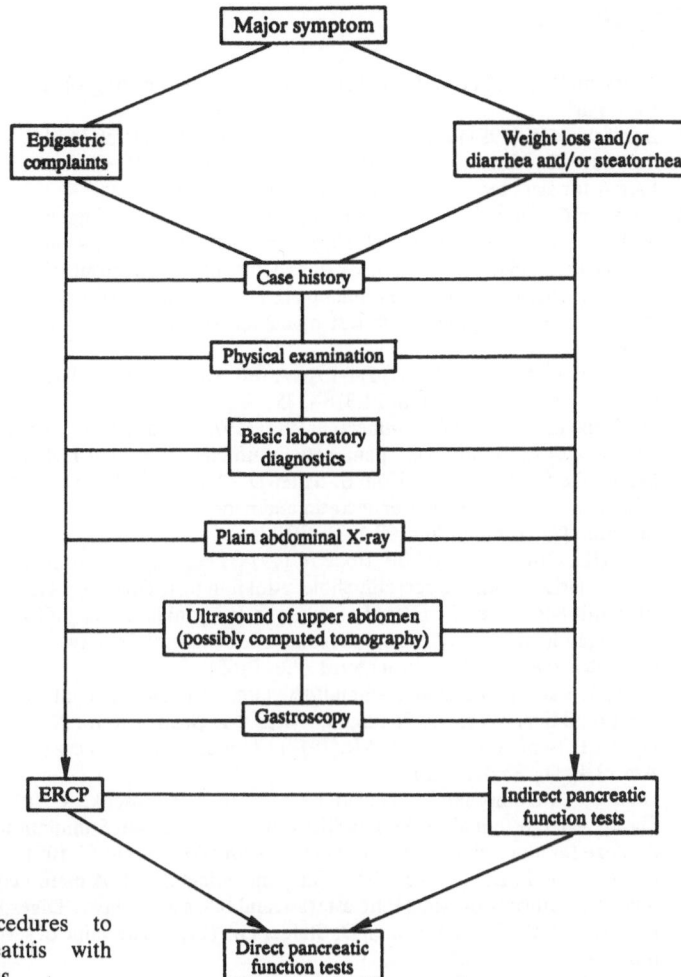

Fig. 5. Diagnostic procedures to prove chronic pancreatitis with different major symptoms

Conclusions

Indirect pancreatic function tests are a practicable alternative to direct pancreatic function tests for diagnosing exocrine pancreatic insufficiency. Indirect pancreatic function tests allow staging of the disease and thereby facilitate comparison of different studies. They are also useful in some cases for determining whether pancreatic enzyme replacement therapy is necessary or not. In contrast to morphological procedures, they involve neither side effects or risks for the patient, nor complications for patients, investigators, and laboratory staff alike. The procedures being standardized, the test results depend to a lesser extent on the experience of the investigator, and more on the selection of and the instructions to the patient, and to some extent on the severity of the exocrine pancreatic insufficiency.

Like all pancreatic function tests, the indirect tests do not give a clue to etiology, nor do they help investigators differentiate between pancreatic insufficiency due to chronic pancreatitis and that due to pancreatic cancer.

References

1. Ammann R (1967) Fortschritte in der Pankreasfunktionsdiagnostik. Springer, Berlin Heidelberg New York
2. Bornschein W (1981) Der PABA-Peptid-Serum Test. Dtsch Med Wochenschr 106:1676–1677
3. Braganza JM, Kay GH, Tetlow VA, Herman KJ (1983) Observations on the BT/PABA/^{14}C-PABA tubeless test of pancreatic function. Clin Chim Acta 130:339–347
4. Cavallini G, Piubello W, Brocco G, Micciolo R, Chech G, Angelini G, Benini L, Riela A, dalle Molle L, Vantini I, Scuro LA (1985) Serum PABA and fluorescein in the course of Bz-Ty-PABA and pancreolauryl test as an index of exocrine pancreatic insufficiency. Dig Dis Sci 30:655–663
5. Cole SG, Rossi S, Stern A, Hofmann AF (1987) Cholesteryl octanoate breath test. Preliminary studies on a new noninvasive test of human pancreatic exocrine function. Gastroenterology 93:1372–1380
6. Delchier JC, Soule JC (1983) BT-PABA test with plasma PABA measurements: evaluation of sensitivity and specifity. Gut 24:318–325
7. DiMagno EP, Go VLW, Summerskill WHJ (1973) Relations between pancreatic enzyme outputs and malabsorption in severe pancreatic insufficiency. N Engl J Med 288:813–815
8. Domschke S, Heptner G, Kolb S, Sailer D, Schneider MU, Domschke W (1986) Decrease in plasma amino acid level after secretin and pancreozymin as an indicator of exocrine pancreatic function. Gastroenterology 90:1031–1038
9. Dürr HK, Otte M, Forell MM, Bode JC (1978) Fecal chymotrypsin: a study on its diagnostic value by comparison with the secretin-cholecystokinin test. Digestion 17:404–409
10. Ehrhardt-Schmelzer S, Otto J, Schlaeger R, Lankisch PG (1984) Faecal chymotrypsin for investigation of exocrine pancreatic function: a comparison of two newly developed tests with the titrimetric method. Z Gastroenterol 22:647–651
11. Freise J, Ranft U, Fricke K, Schmidt FW (1984) Chronische Pankreatitis: Sensitivität, Spezifität und prädiktiver Wert des Pankreolauryltests. Z Gastroenterol 22:705–712
12. Gyr K, Felsenfeld O, Imondi AR (1978) Chymotrypsin-like activity of some intestinal bacteria. Am J Dig Dis 23:413–416
13. Heptner G, Domschke S, Schneider MU, Kolb S, Domschke W (1987) Aminosäurespiegel im Plasma – dargestellt als α-Amino-Stickstoff – reagieren auf Stimulation des exokrinen Pankreas: Ansätze für einen Pankreasfunktionstest. Klin Wochenschr 65:1054–1061
14. Kay G, Hine P, Braganza J (1982) The pancreolauryl test. A method of assessing the combined functional efficacy of pancreatic esterase and bile salts in vivo? Digestion 24:241–245
15. Lang C, Gyr K, Tonko I, Conen D, Stalder GA (1984) The value of serum PABA as a pancreatic function test. Gut 25:508–512
16. Lankisch PG (1982) Progress report: exocrine pancreatic function tests. Gut 23:777–798
17. Lankisch PG, Lembcke B (1984) Indirect pancreatic function tests: chemical and radioisotope methods. Clin Gastroenterol 13:717–737
18. Lankisch PG, Ehrhardt-Schmelzer S, Koop H, Caspary WF (1980) Der NBT-PABA-Test in der Diagnostik der exokrinen Pankreasinsuffizienz. Dtsch Med Wochenschr 105:1418–1423
19. Lankisch PG, Schreiber A, Otto J (1983) Pancreolauryl test. Evaluation of a tubeless pancreatic function test in comparison with other indirect and direct tests for exocrine pancreatic function. Dig Dis Sci 28:490–493
20. Lankisch PG, Brauneis J, Otto J, Göke B (1986) Pancreolauryl and NBT-PABA tests. Are serum tests more practicable alternatives to urine tests in the diagnosis of exocrine pancreatic insufficiency? Gastroenterology 90:350–354
21. Lankisch PG, Otto J, Brauneis J, Hilgers R, Lembcke B (1988) Detection of pancreatic steatorrhea by oral pancreatic function tests. Dig Dis Sci 33:1233–1236
22. Lembcke B (1984) Malassimilationsdiagnostik. In: Caspary WF (ed) Maldigestion, Malabsorption. Klinik, Differentialdiagnose, Therapie. Kali-Chemie Pharma, Hannover, pp 47–86 (Gastroenterologische Reihe, vol 21)
23. Malfertheiner P, Ditschuneit H (1985) Diagnostic procedures in pancreatic disease. Springer, Berlin Heidelberg New York
24. Malfertheiner P, Peter M, Junge U, Ditschuneit H (1983) Der orale Pankreasfunktionstest mit FDL in der Diagnose der chronischen Pankreatitis. Klin Wochenschr 61:193–198

25. Malfertheiner P, Büchler M, Müller A, Ditschuneit H (1987) Fluorescein dilaurate serum test: a rapid tubeless pancreatic function test. Pancreas 2:53–60
26. Malfertheiner P, Büchler M, Müller A, Ditschuneit H (1987) Fluoresceindilaurat-Serumtest nach Metoclopramid- und Sekretinstimulation zur Pankreasfunktionsprüfung. Beitrag zur Diagnose der chronischen Pankreatitis. Z Gastroenterol 25:225–232
27. Mitchell CJ, Humphrey CS, Bullen AW, Kelleher J, Losowsky MS (1979) Improved diagnostic accuracy of a modified oral pancreatic function test. Scand J Gastroenterol 14:737–741
28. Mitchell CJ, Field HP, Simpson FG, Parkin A, Kelleher J, Losowsky MS (1981) Preliminary evaluation of a single-day tubeless test of pancreatic function. Br Med J 282:1751–1753
29. Münch R, Bühler H, Ammann R (1983) Chymotrypsinaktivität im Stuhl: Vergleich eines neuen photometrischen Verfahrens mit der titrimetrischen Standardmethode. Schweiz Med Wochenschr 113:1794–1797
30. Schneider MU, Demling L, Jones SA, Barker PJ, Domschke S, Heptner G, Domschke W (1987) NMR spectrometry. A new method for total stool fat quantification in chronic pancreatitis. Dig Dis Sci 32:494–499
31. Stock K-P, Schenk J, Schmack B, Domschke W (1981) Funktions-"Screening" des exokrinen Pankreas. FDL-, N-BT-PABA-Test, Stuhl-Chymotrypsinbestimmung im Vergleich mit dem Sekretin-Pankreozymin-Test. Dtsch Med Wochenschr 106:983–987
32. Tanner AR, Fisher D, Ward C, Smith CL (1984) An evaluation of the one-day NBT-PABA/^{14}C-PABA in the assessment of pancreatic exocrine insufficiency. Digestion 29:42–46
33. Van de Kamer JH, ten Bokkel Huinink H, Weijers HA (1949) Rapid method for the determination of fat in feces. J Biol Chem 177:347–355

How to Position Exocrine and Endocrine Function Tests in the Diagnostic Approach to Chronic Pancreatitis

P. P. Toskes[1]

Patients with chronic impairment of pancreatic exocrine function usually present with abdominal pain or with diarrhea, steatorrhea, and weight loss. Those patients who have abdominal pain as their chief complaint may develop diarrhea, steatorrhea, and weight loss or may always have abdominal pain as their major symptom and never evolve to frank exocrine insufficiency. Approximately 15% of patients with chronic pancreatitis never manifest abdominal pain and present initially with diarrhea, steatorrhea, and weight loss.

In adults, the usual causes of pancreatic exocrine impairment are alcohol-induced chronic pancreatitis, pancreatic resection, pancreatic cancer, and idiopathic chronic pancreatitis. In children the usual cause is cystic fibrosis.

The diagnosis of chronic pancreatitis in general is difficult to make and is often done by exclusion. This is especially true in those patients whose main manifestation is pain, since they often have only mild to moderate impairment of exocrine function while those with steatorrhea have severe impairment of exocrine function. Often the diagnosis of chronic pancreatitis has necessitated the use of invasive tests that are uncomfortable for the patient, time consuming for both patient and physician, and expensive; consequently, the diagnosis is often not made. Now, however, a group of pancreatic function tests (bentiromide, trypsinlike immunoreactivity) have emerged that are simple to perform and provide the clinician with good sensitivity and specificity, especially in those patients with pancreatic steatorrhea. These tests of pancreatic function are characterized by their ease of performance and excellent acceptance by patients. They are noninvasive and inexpensive and can be performed in an office or clinic setting. For patients with mild to moderate impairment of exocrine function, i.e., those with chronic abdominal pain and no steatorrhea, direct tube tests, such as the secretin or secretin-cholecystokinin (CCK) test and endoscopic retrograde cholangiopancreatography (ERCP), remain the most consistent way to make the diagnosis of chronic pancreatitis.

Table 1 lists 14 diagnostic tests that are used with varying degrees of frequency to diagnose and classify patients suspected of having chronic pancreatitis. The direct tube tests with analysis of pancreatic secretion following stimulation of the pancreas with secretin, CCK, etc. are the most sensitive and specific tests and have served as the gold standard for evaluation of pancreatic exocrine function. Yet these tests are not widely used in the United States, precipitating the search for simple, noninvasive tests.

---

[1] Division of Gastroenterology, Hepatology and Nutrition, University of Florida College of Medicine, Gainesville, FL 32610, USA

Chronic Pancreatitis
Ed. by Beger, Büchler, Ditschuneit, and Malfertheiner
© Springer-Verlag Berlin Heidelberg 1990

Table 1. Tests for chronic pancreatitis

1. Direct tube tests: secretin, cholecystokinin, secretin-cholecystokinin, secretin-bombesin
2. Indirect tube tests: Lundh test, small-bowel perfusion
3. Stool fat before and after pancreatic enzymes
4. Fecal chymotrypsin
5. Cobalamin (vitamin B_{12}) urinary excretion test
6. D-xylose urinary excretion test
7. Bentiromide test
8. Pancreaolauryl test
9. Serum trypsinlike immunoreactivity
10. Isoamylase determination
11. Serum pancreatic polypeptide
12. Lactoferrin content of duodenal secretions
13. Plain film of abdomen
14. Endoscopic retrograde cholangiopancreatography

The only tubeless tests of exocrine function which are commercially available in the United States and have been extensively evaluated are bentiromide and serum trypsinlike immunoreactivity. Analysis of feces for fat or proteases has fallen out of favor. Isoamylase determinations are no longer commercially available unless one performs electrophoresis, which is cumbersome. Although the urinary xylose excretion is not, strictly speaking, a test of pancreatic function, it is used to separate pancreatic steatorrhea from small-bowel steatorrhea since it is normal in most patients with pancreatic steatorrhea.

Plain film of the abdomen and ERCP are not function tests but are frequently used to diagnose patients with chronic pancreatitis. Although it is generally appreciated that diffuse calcification of the pancreas on plain film examination signifies significant exocrine impairment, the meaning of focal calcification or calcification detected only by CT examination is still being defined.

The bentiromide test and serum trypsinlike immunoreactivity are good tests for documenting severe pancreatic exocrine insufficiency. Both tests lack appropriate sensitivity for detecting those patients with mild to moderate impairment of exocrine function, for example, abdominal pain with normal fat absorption. Figure 1 demonstrates 6-h cumulative urinary arylamie excretion following oral administration of 500 mg bentiromide in 120 subjects (chronic pancreatitis and controls). No normal subject had a value below 50%. Overlap between normals and patients with chronic pancreatitis occurred only in those pancreatic patients with normal fat absorption [1]. Although we have found no specificity problems with the bentiromide test in patients with biopsy-proven small-bowel or liver disease [2], other investigators have reported abnormal bentiromide tests in patients with small-bowel or liver disease. This may be due to the fact that in these latter studies a large dose of bentiromide (2 g) was used. Nevertheless, as Fig. 2 demonstrates, a depressed serum trypsin level is virtually specific for pancreatic steatorrhea and can thus complement the bentiromide test [3].

Thus, there is great need for a simple, noninvasive test that detects mild to moderate impairment of exocrine function – a tubeless secretin-CCK test!

To that end we have demonstrated that plasma pancreatic polypeptide (PP) response following intramuscularly administered ceruletide (800 ng/kg) clearly sepa-

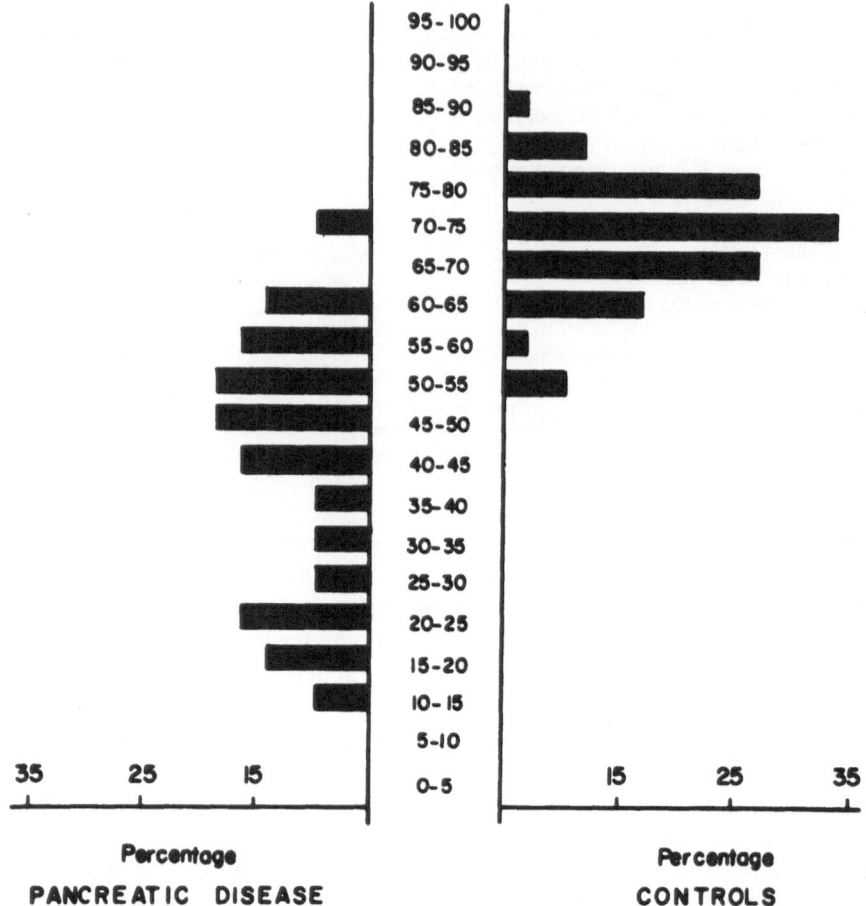

Fig. 1. Cumulative 6-h urinary arylamine excretion following oral administration of 500 mg bentiromide. (From [1])

rated normal control subjects from patients with mild to moderate impairment of pancreatic exocrine function, as well as those with pancreatic steatorrhea [4]. Table 2 demonstrates the integrated and single time point analysis of PP in 53 subjects. At 30 min, the integrated PP response was significantly different between control subjects (mean ± SEM), 11.1 ± 2.4 ng min^{-1} ml^{-1}, those with mild to moderate chronic pancreatitis, 2.6 ± 0.9 ng min^{-1} ml^{-1} ($p < 0.01$), and those with pancreatic steatorrhea, 2.9 ± 1.6 ng min^{-1} ml^{-1} ($p < 0.01$). The integrated PP response of patients with small-bowel steatorrhea or those with nonpancreatic abdominal pain did not differ from controls. In the same patients, peak and integrated plasma CCK levels following intravenously administered CCK 8 (40 ng/kg bolus over 2 min followed by 20 ng/kg over 30 min) were 45% and 32%, respectively, of values achieved following intramuscular ceruletide administration. Near-maximal PP stimulation may be required to detect patients with chronic pancreatitis of mild to moderate severity.

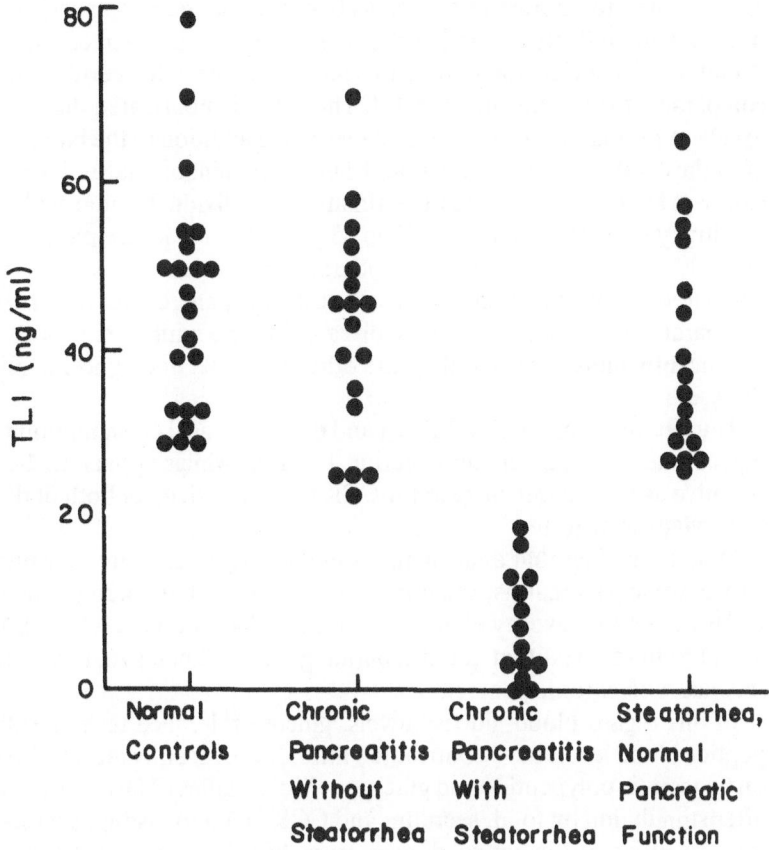

Fig. 2. Serum trypsinlike immunoreactivity in chronic pancreatitis patients and control subjects. (From [3])

Table 2. Sensitivity, specificity and efficiency of pancreatic polypeptide response (percentages)

	30 min I PPR	45 min I PPR	15 min single sample	30 min single sample	45 min single sample
Sensitivity	76	67	62	48	71
Specificity	87	93	86	93	87
Efficiency	81	78	71	66	78

Sensitivity, probability of a positive result in pancreatitis patients with and without steatorrhea; specificity, probability of a negative test in normal controls; efficiency, the proportion of correct results

The amino acid consumption test is a new tubeless pancreatic function test. As originally reported by Domschke and associates, patients with chronic pancreatitis demonstrated less of a decrement in plasma amino acid concentration than control subjects following intravenous administration of secretin and CCK [5]. Another report from this laboratory demonstrated that only the amino acid consumption test as contrasted to indirect tests such as bentiromide, pancreolauryl, and fecal chymo-trypsin, truly reflected exocrine pancreatic function in gastrectomized patients [6].

Gullo and associates simplified this test and showed that cerulein alone gave results comparable to secretin and CCK [7]. They also demonstrated that they could achieve excellent results with just one blood sample, in addition to the basal sample, at 60 min after the cerulein infusion, and that the measurement of total amino acids photometri-cally was as discriminatory as the estimation of individual amino acids. They found the sensitivity of this test to be 91.4% in 35 patients with severe pancreatic insufficiency and 80% in those with mild to moderate impairment of exocrine function. When compared to the fecal chymotrypsin test and pancreolauryl, all three tests were comparable for diagnosing severe disease, but the amino acid consumption test was significantly more sensitive than the other two tests in diagnosing mild to moderate disease.

Thus, both the ceruletide-PP test and the amino acid consumption test are interest-ing new tests of pancreatic exocrine function which appear to be about 80% as sensitive as the secretin or secretin-CCK test. Specificity of both of these tests has yet to be vigorously tested.

Despite the fact that abnormalities in endocrine function are common in patients with chronic pancreatitis, the hope that some test of endocrine function might accu-rately reflect the severity of exocrine function has not been fulfilled. It would also be useful to have a test that could separate genetic diabetes mellitus from the diabetes secondary to chronic pancreatitis.

In this regard blood glucose levels, glucose tolerance tests, insulin levels and C peptide blood levels have contributed little. More recently attention has been focused on pancreatic polypeptide and glucagon. Most studies of fasting PP levels or PP levels after stimulation by food, secretin, and CCK failed to distinguish those patients with mild to moderate exocrine disease from healthy control subjects. Integrated PP response following intramuscularly administered ceruletide as described above seems to be a potential worthwhile contribution in diagnosing mild to moderate exocrine damage.

In regard to separating genetic diabetes from secondary diabetes, Keller and coworkers recently demonstrated that pancreatic blood glucagon levels failed to increase during arginine infusion in patients with diabetes secondary to chronic pancreatitis [8]. Those with genetic diabetes demonstrated the same degree of gluca-gon release as did control subjects. The unique contribution of these investigators was the employment of a pancreatic glucagon-specific antibody in their radio-immunoassay.

Figure 3 is a schematic depiction of when commonly employed diagnostic tests become abnormal in a typical patient with alcohol-induced chronic pancreatitis. An abnormal hormone stimulation test or subtle abnormalities on ERCP may occur at 60%–70% damage to the exocrine gland. More typical pancreatic ductal changes occur somewhat later. Calcification of the pancreas by CT or sonography may be as sensitive as a hormone stimulation test, but more evaluation of this observation must be carried out. Diffuse pancreatic calcification on plain film of the abdomen and an abnormal bentiromide test are noted at about 80% damage, abnormal endocrine function at 85% damage, and decreased serum trypsin levels and increased fecal fat at greater than 90% damage.

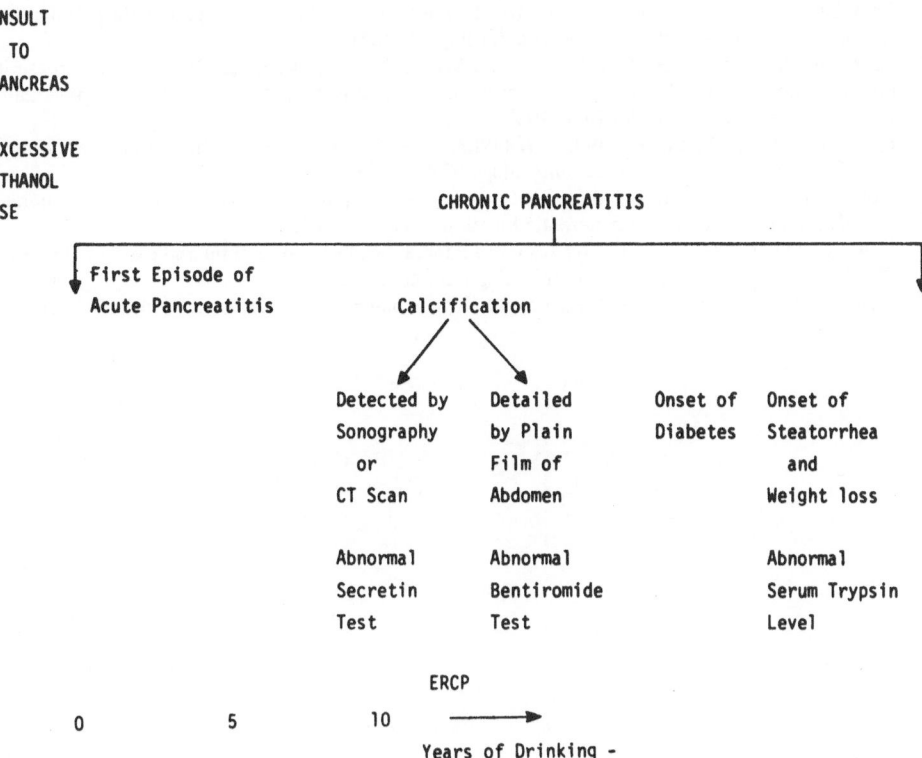

Fig. 3. Development of abnormal function tests in chronic pancreatitis. (From [9])

In summary, the detection of severe pancreatic exocrine dysfunction has become quite reliable with the use of a number of simple, tubeless tests. To date no consistently reliable simple test of pancreatic function has been established to replace direct tube-hormone stimulation tests. The recent introduction of the integrated PP response following administration of large doses of intramuscular ceruletide and the amino acid consumption test appear promising. The challenge remains to firmly establish a reliable, simple, tubeless test of pancreatic exocrine function which can detect mild to moderate damage.

References

1. Toskes P (1983) Bentiromide as a test of exocrine pancreatic function in adult patients with pancreatic exocrine insufficiency: determination of appropriate dose and urinary collection period. Gastroenterology 85:565–569
2. Meyer B, Campbell D, Curington C, Toskes P (1987) The bentiromide test is not affected in patients with small bowel disease of liver disease. Pancreas 2:44–47
3. Jacobson D, Curington C, Connery K, Toskes P (1984) Trypsin-like immunoreactivity as a test for pancreatic insufficiency. N Engl J Med 310:1307–1309

4. Campbell D, Slaff J, McGuigan J, DesJardin L, Toskes P (1985) Integrated pancreatic polypeptide response in pancreatic diseases. Gastroenterology 88:1341
5. Domschke S, Heptner G, Kolb S, Sailer D, Schneider MU, Domschke W (1986) Decrease in plasma amino acid level after secretin and pancreozymin as an indicator of exocrine pancreatic function. Gastroenterology 90:1031–1038
6. Heptner G, Domschke S, Domschke W (1989) Exocrine pancreatic function after gastrectomy. Specificity of indirect tests. Gastroenterology 97:147–153
7. Gullo L, Pezzilli R, Ventrucci M (1989) Cerulein-induced plasma amino acid decrease: a simple, sensitive, and specific test of pancreatic function. Pancreas 4:619
8. Keller U, Szollosy E, Varga L, Gyr K (1984) Pancreatic glucagon secretin and exocrine function (BT-PABA test) in chronic pancreatitis. Dig Dis Sci 29:853–857
9. Toskes P, Greenberger N (1983) Acute and chronic pancreatitis. Disease-a-Month 29:1–81

Magnetic Resonance Imaging and Computed Tomography in Chronic Pancreatitis

W. Maier[1]

As a result of recent advances in sectional imaging, modern imaging techniques have become the standard diagnostic tests after the patient's complaints indicate that pancreatic disease may be the underlying problem. Ultrasound is the preferred initial procedure, but in most cases it does not provide the breadth of information that is drawn from a comprehensive computed tomographic (CT) study. The results of magnetic resonance imaging (MRI) in pancreatic diseases are increasingly comparable to those obtained from CT, but at present the method cannot supplant CT or ultrasound as an initial procedure in patients with suspected pancreatic disease. Because of the high sensitivity of CT in the evaluation of pancreatic disease the greatest part of this chapter is devoted to CT.

Magnetic Resonance Imaging in Chronic Pancreatitis

The normal pancreas is easily demonstrated as a structure of moderate intensity lying anterior to the splenic and portal veins (Fig. 1). Its intensity is similar to that of the liver, as also shown by spin echo and inversion recovery techniques. Calculated T_1 and T_2 relaxation times correspond to those of the normal pancreas and liver.

In chronic pancreatitis most MRI findings are similar to the findings observed with CT scanning (discussed in more detail below). MRI is able to demonstrate diffuse or focal enlargement of the gland (Fig. 2) but is unable to distinguish an inflammatory mass from a neoplasm [2]. Fibrosis of peripancreatic fat planes is of similar intensity as the normal pancreas and is apparent only when pancreatic margins are obscured [2]. Because of motion and volume averaging, small pancreatic calcifications cannot be seen on MRI. Only larger ones (more than 1 cm in diameter) can be detected, as ill-defined low intensity areas [1]. Detection of pancreatic pseudocysts on MRI is restricted to those larger than 1.5–2 cm in diameter. However, some cysts are not as well delineated as in CT (Fig. 3). Dilatation of the duct of Wirsung is also not reliably demonstrated on MRI.

---

[1] Radiological Clinic of the University of Ulm, Steinhövelstrasse 2, 7900 Ulm, FRG

Chronic Pancreatitis
Ed. by Beger, Büchler, Ditschuneit, and Malfertheiner
© Springer-Verlag Berlin Heidelberg 1990

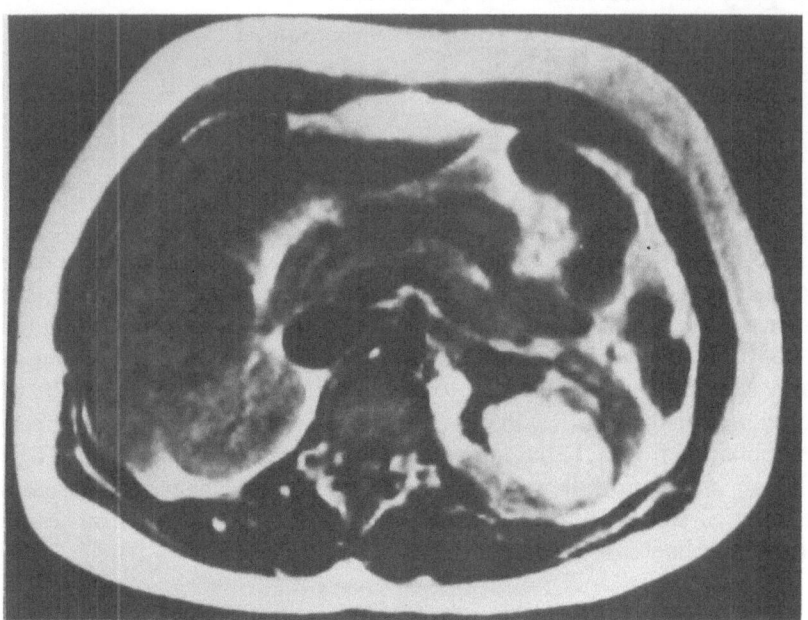

Fig. 1. MRI. Normal pancreas

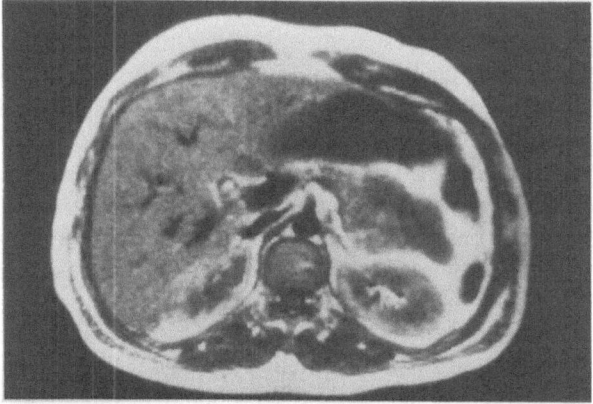

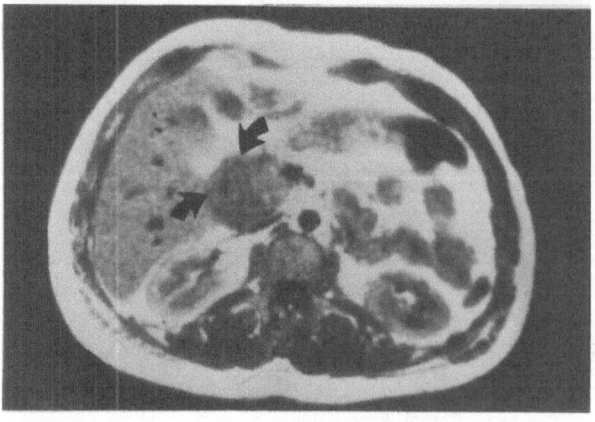

Fig. 2. MRI. Focal enlargement of the pancreatic head due to chronic pancreatitis

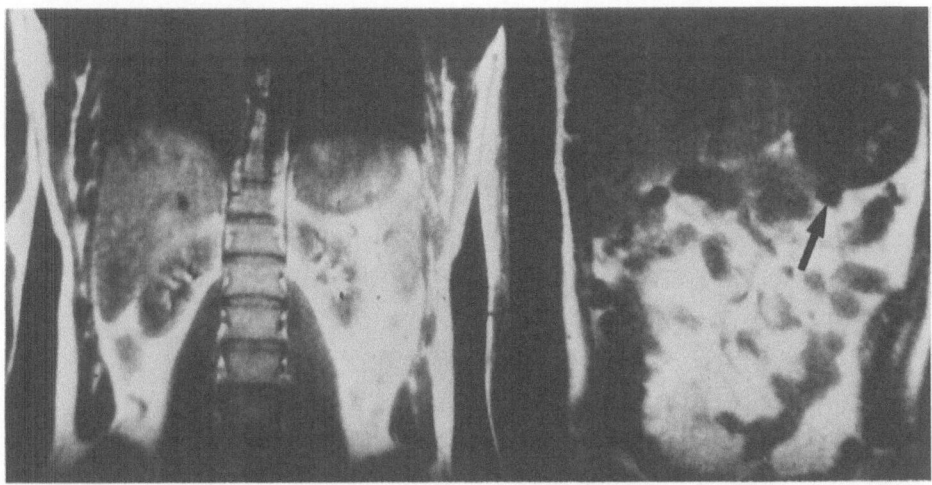

Fig. 3. MRI. Small pseudocyst of the tail of the pancreas in chronic pancreatitis

Computed Tomography in Chronic Pancreatitis

With the aid of modern, fast CT scanners numerous pathoanatomic features of chronic pancreatitis can be visualized which alone or in combination allow a safe diagnosis. This section discusses the value of CT findings for diagnosis and differential diagnosis of chronic pancreatitis.

Pancreatic Size

In the early stage of chronic pancreatitis the pancreas may be normal in size and CT density. In the absence of other signs, such as ductal dilatation or calcifications, a specific diagnosis of (mild) chronic pancreatitis cannot be made on CT. According to Ferrucci and coworkers a normally sized pancreas is encountered in 15%–20% of patients suffering from chronic pancreatitis [3].

Atrophy of the gland with or without fatty replacement is encountered in advanced cases. Atrophy is a nonspecific sign of chronic pancreatitis and can also be due to chronic ductal obstruction in pancreatic cancer (Fig. 4). Especially atrophy limited to the body and tail of the pancreas can be an indicator of an underlying neoplasm. Because atrophy can be part of the aging process, in any evaluation of pancreatic size the patient's age must be taken to account (Fig. 5).

Enlargement of the gland in chronic pancreatitis can be diffuse (Fig. 6) or focal. In about one-third of cases with chronic pancreatitis the gland is enlarged [1]. Since pancreatic enlargement may also be caused by pancreatic neoplasm, differentiation of an inflammatory mass from a carcinoma is a major problem when there are no other CT signs of chronic pancreatitis (see below). In our experience, pancreatic enlargement combined with a normal contrast enhancement pattern is due to an inflammatory pseudotumor in most cases, whereas in pancreatic carcinoma a characteristic ill-

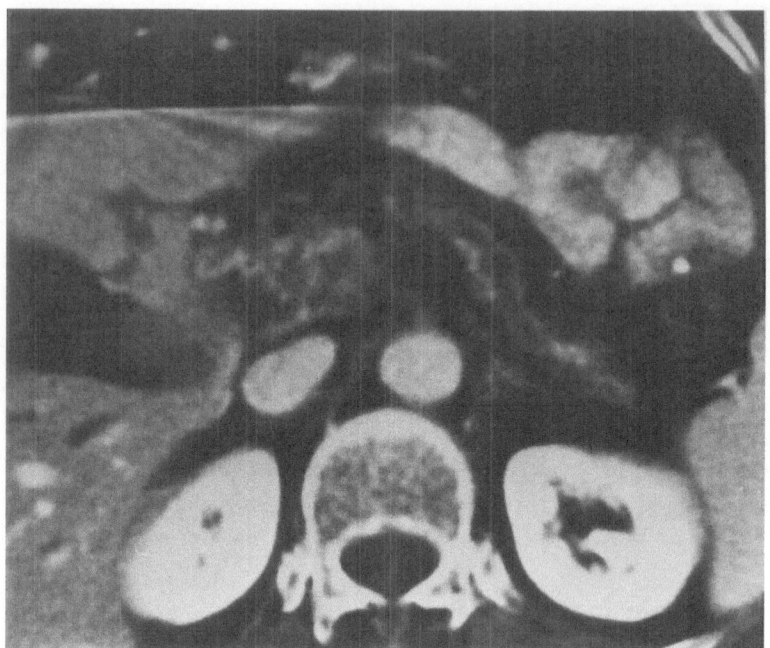

Fig. 4. Glandular atrophy due to chronic ductal obstruction in pancreatic carcinoma

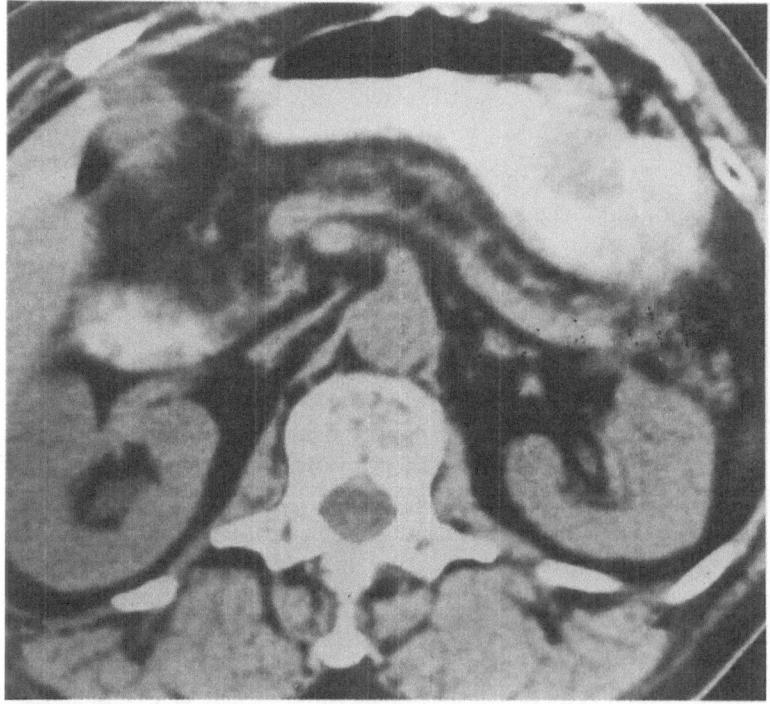

Fig. 5. Pancreatic atrophy in the elderly

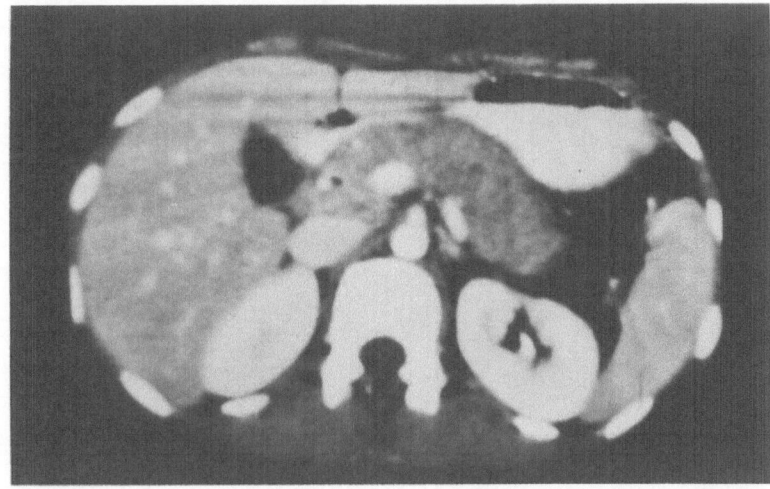

Fig. 6. Diffuse enlargement of the pancreas in chronic sclerosing pancreatitis (microscopy confirmed)

defined enhancement defect can be found (Fig. 7). Pancreatic enlargement due to acute pancreatitis can easily be appreciated by recognizing other CT signs of the disease such as peripancreatic infiltration or necrosis and characteristic clinical symptoms.

Calcifications

Deposition of calcium carbonate and calcium phosphate is the hallmark of chronic pancreatitis. Pancreatic calcifications can be parenchymal or ductal in location (Fig. 8). Appreciation of ductal involvement is important because some surgeons are of the opinion that managing pancreatic duct obstruction may be beneficial to the patient. Pancreatic calcification can vary in location and amount, but they generally occur first in the head. Occasionally, splenic artery calcifications mimic pancreatic calculi, but thin collimation and the use of intravenous contrast material in general obviates this mistake. Whereas MRI is not able to demonstrate small calculi, CT is the most sensitive of all radiographic methods for diagnosis and localization of pancreatic calcifications.

Ductal Dilatation

The normal duct or Wirsung can be visualized in a large proportion of cases using current-generation CT scanners [4] and appropriate flow-controlled contrast medium application [5–7]. If adequate technique is used, the dilated pancreatic duct may be visualized in 80%–90% of cases.

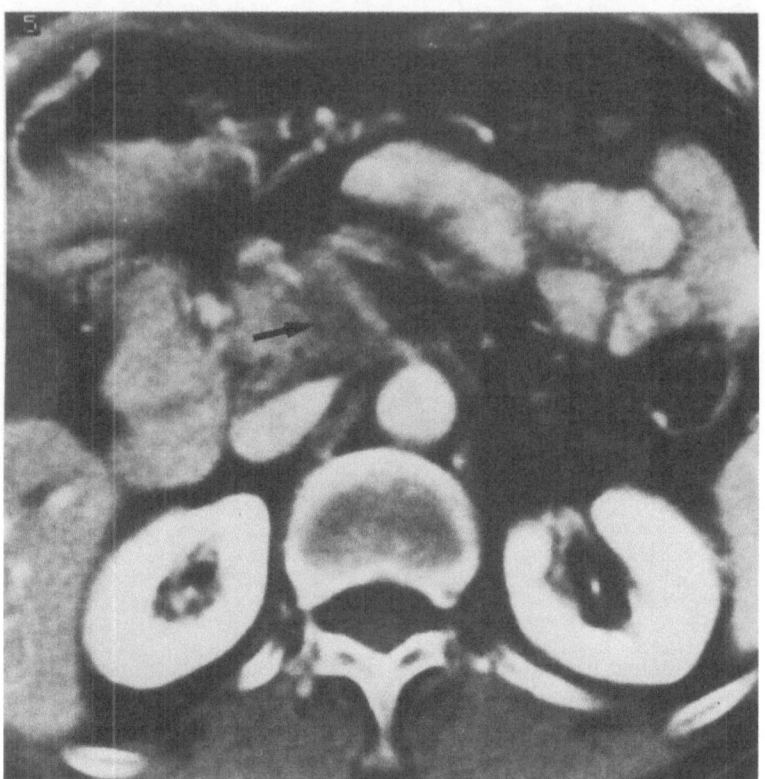

Fig. 7. Mass lesion with enhancement defect in pancreatic carcinoma

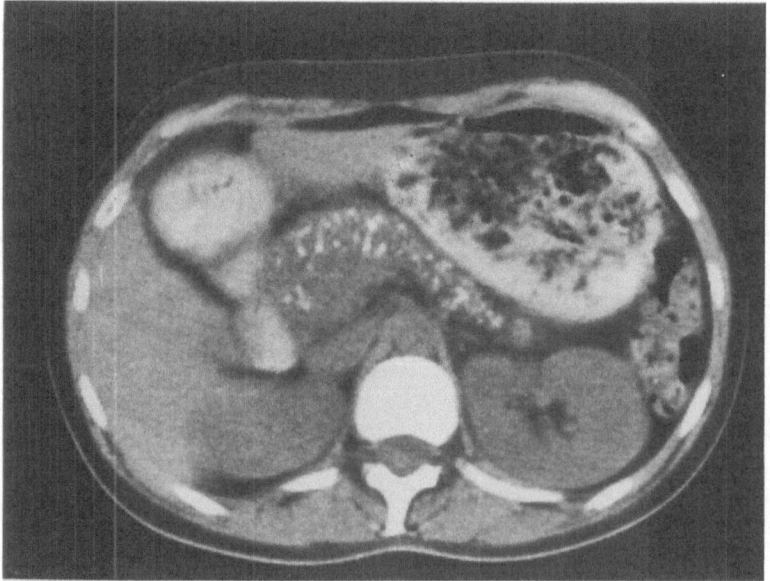

Fig. 8. Pancreatic calcification in chronic pancreatitis

Dilatation of the duct of Wirsung occurs in acute and chronic pancreatitis as well as in pancreatic cancer [8–9]. Whereas ductal dilatation as a sign of acute pancreatitis can easily be appreciated considering secondary CT signs and the clinical setting, differentiation between chronic pancreatitis and pancreatic cancer on the basis of an enlarged duct may be difficult or impossible. However, the morphology of the dilated duct aids to some degree in differential diagnosis. Out of 49 cases of pancreatic carcinoma we found a ductal dilatation in 24, in which the dilatation was smooth in 62% and beaded in 37.5%; worthy of note is that an irregular dilatation was not found in this series. On the other hand, out of 33 cases of chronic pancreatitis we found a dilated duct of Wirsung in 21, in which dilatation was irregular in 71% and beaded in 29%. While there is a statistical difference in ductal morphology in chronic pancreatitis and pancreatic cancer, there is clearly an overlap of the CT pattern of the dilated duct in the two entities.

The ratio of duct width to total gland width yields characteristic values for chronic pancreatitis and pancreatic carcinoma [10]. In our own series we found a mean value of 0.50 (confidence interval between 0.45 and 0.55) for pancreatic cancer and a mean value of 0.26 (confidence interval between 0.19 and 0.33) for chronic pancreatitis.

In rare cases an impacted calculus gives rise to ductal obstruction and subsequent (smooth) dilatation.

Fluid Collections

Pancreatic fluid collections can occur in acute and chronic pancreatitis and in pancreatic cancer. Pseudocysts are most commonly found in chronic pancreatitis (Fig. 9).

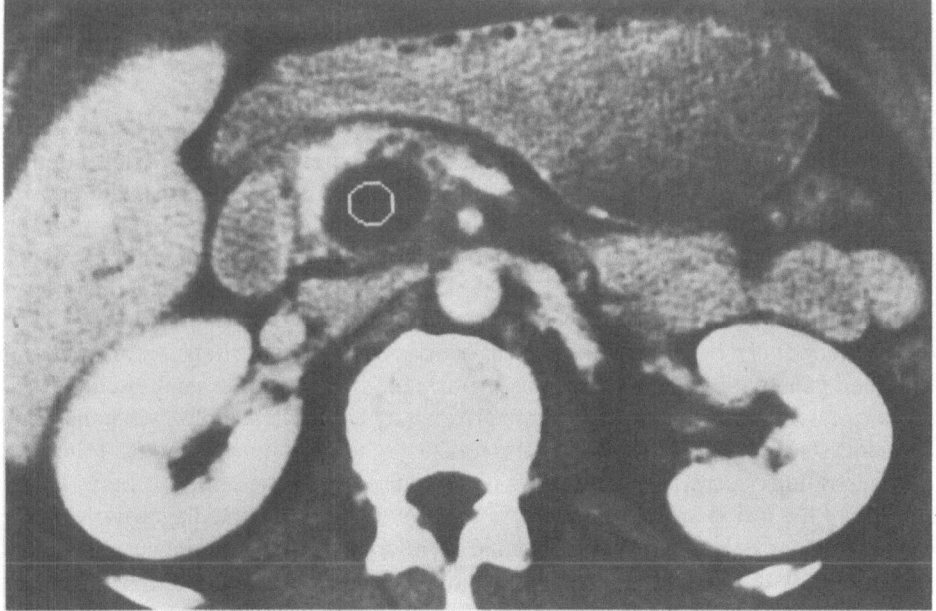

Fig. 9. Pancreatic pseudocyst in chronic pancreatitis

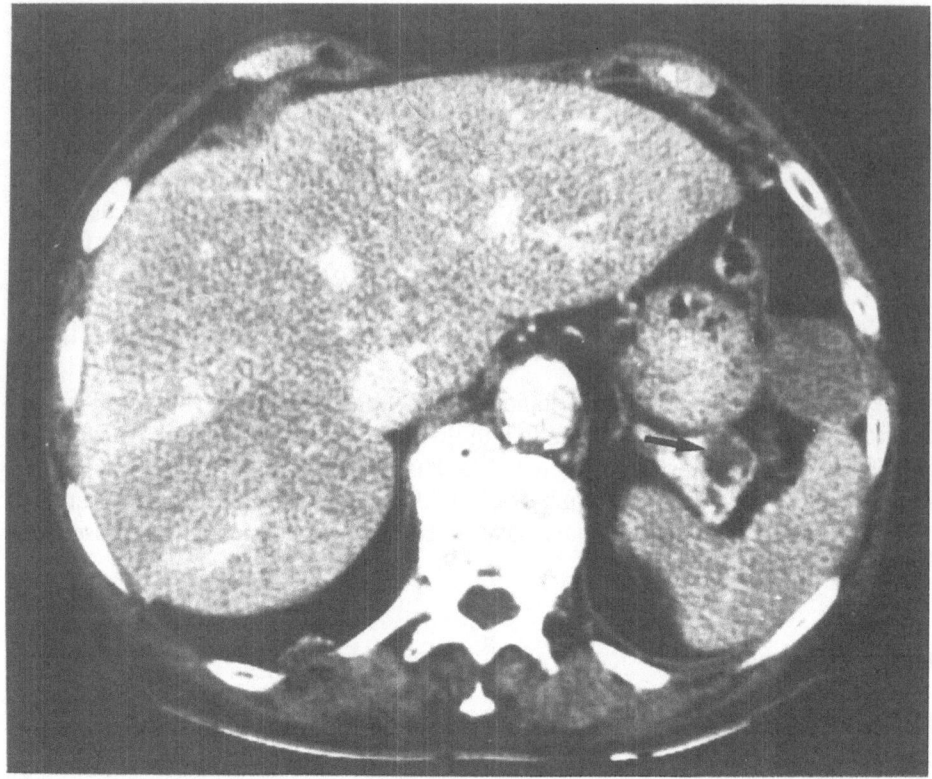

Fig. 10. False aneurysm of the splenic artery mimicking a pseudocyst

They are either located within the pancreas or are extrapancreatic. In the latter case they can be seen contiguous to the gland or at remote sites such as the mediastinum or the pelvis. On CT pseudocysts are readily appreciated as mass lesions with central density values equivalent to that of water. However there is some variation in the attenuation values of pseudocysts depending on the content of protein and cellular debris. High attenuation values suggest the presence of pseudocyst infection or hemorrhage.

Pseudocysts can be confused with a variety of pancreatic disorders. A tortuous and enlarged pancreatic duct may be indistinguishable from multiple small pseudocysts. True or false aneurysms of the splenic artery may closely resemble extrapancreatic pseudocysts (Fig. 10). However, characteristically they (in part) enhance following administration of contrast medium. On nonenhanced scans the similarity between the density of the lesion and the density of blood gives a hint for the diagnosis.

Necrotic or cystic tumors may resemble pseudocysts. However, they usually occur in patients without a history of pancreatitis, alcohol, or trauma. Cystic tumors commonly exhibit thick, irregular walls that only rarely calcify, as opposed to the smooth and occasionally calcified capsule of a pseudocyst.

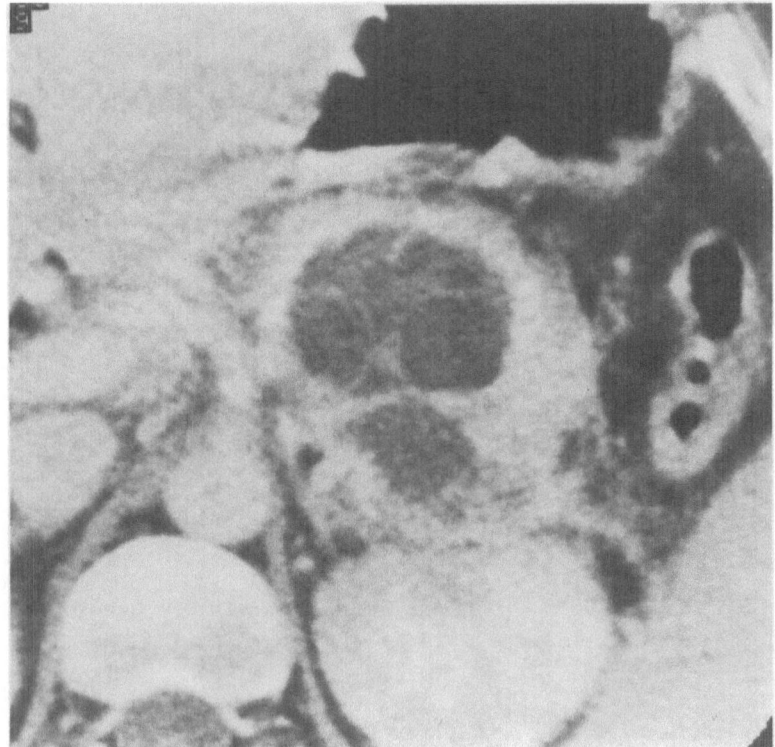

Fig. 11. Benign cystadenoma of the pancreas mimicking a pseudocyst

Rarely, a pseudocyst may be septated and thus be indistinguishable from a benign cystadenoma (Fig. 11).

Extrapancreatic Fibrosis

Diffuse extrapancreatic fibrosis (Fig. 12) may sometimes be encountered in chronic pancreatitis. Thickening of the renal fascia is frequently associated with chronic pancreatitis. They all reflect spread of the inflammatory process into the peripancreatic space and may occasionally be indistinguishable from extrapancreatic inflammation in acute pancreatitis, lymphomatous involvement of the retroperitoneum, inflammatory renal disease or edema secondary to congestive heart failure [11].

Vascular Complications

Thrombosis of the splenic vein, splenic artery aneurysm, or pseudoaneurysm are sometimes found in chronic pancreatitis. Like other signs already mentioned, they are nonspecific and can be encountered in pancreatic cancer as well as in chronic or acute pancreatitis [11].

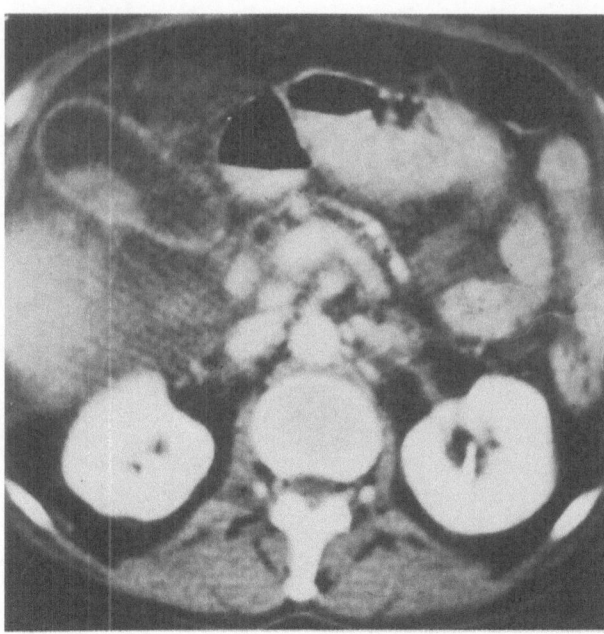

Fig. 12. Extrapancreatic fibrosis in chronic pancreatitis (autopsy confirmed)

References

1. Margulis AR, Higgins CB, Kaufmann L, Crooks LE (1983) Clinical magnetic resonance imaging. Radiologie Research and Education Foundation, San Francisco
2. Kerman J, Haaga JR (1989) Magnetic resonance imaging of the abdomen and pelvis. In: Taveras MJ, Ferrucci JT (eds) Radiology. Lippincott, Philadelphia
3. Ferrucci JF, Kirkpatrick RH, Hall DH (1979) Computed body tomography in chronic pancreatitis. Radiology 130:175–182
4. Berland LL et al. (1981) Computed tomography of the normal and abnormal pancreatic duct: correlation with pancreatic ductography. Radiology 141:715–724
5. Maier W (1987) Early objective diagnosis and staging of acute pancreatitis by contrast-enhanced computed tomography. In: Beger HG, Buechler M (eds) Acute pancreatitis. Springer, Berlin Heidelberg New York, pp 132–140
6. Maier W (1986) Experimentelle und Klinische Untersuchungen zur Rolle der Computertomographie in der Stadieneinteilung der Akuten Pancreatitis. University of Ulm
7. Maier W (1988) Frühdiagnose und Staging der Akuten Pankreatitis durch Computertomographie. Fortschr Röntgenstr 148:251–254
8. Fishman A et al. (1979) Significance of dilated pancreatic duct on CT examination. AJR 132:251–254
9. Gold RR, Seaman WB (1981) Computed tomography and the dilated pancreatic duct: an ominous sign. Gastrointest Radiol 6:35–38
10. Itaiy et al. (1982) Computed tomographic appearance of resectable pancreatic carcinoma. Radiology 143:719–726
11. Freeny PC, Lawson TL (1982) Radiology of the pancreas. Springer, New York Heidelberg Berlin

Role of ERCP in Chronic Pancreatitis

T. Rösch and M. Classen[1]

The diagnosis of chronic pancreatitis is made by tests of pancreatic function as well as by demonstration of morphological changes. Endoscopic retrograde cholangiopancreatography (ERCP) has been established as the standard procedure for defining pathologic findings in the ductal system [1, 2]. The main features of chronic pancreatitis in ERCP have been described in numerous studies and several grading systems have been proposed.

Pathomorphology of Chronic Pancreatitis

The normal limits of the main pancreatic duct have been described [3]. The most important morphological features of chronic pancreatitis [4] are inflammatory changes and irregular sclerosis and scarring within the pancreatic parenchyma with consecutive ductal changes (irregularities with stenoses and dilatation) and, finally, a gradual loss of glandular tissue. These changes can be diffusely distributed or they can be focal as in pancreas divisum or "groove pancreatitis"; in a series of 77 cases with focal pancreatitis, half were located in the pancreatic tail [5].

Using a histological workup of 359 patients with chronic pancreatitis, Sahel and Sarles [6] discerned two distinct forms of inflammatory changes: chronic calcifying pancreatitis, often correlated to alcoholism, and chronic obstructive pancreatitis due to obstruction of the pancreatic duct (Table 1); the main differences between these

Table 1. Histomorphological differences of the two main forms of chronic pancreatitis. [6]

	Chronic calcifying pancreatitis ($n = 313$)	Chronic obstructive pancreatitis ($n = 46$)
Dilatation		
Intralobular ducts	68%	38%
Interlobular ducts	89%	70%
Plugs	55%	15%
Calcified stones	31%	–
Epithelial atrophy	40%	4%
Connective tissue fibrosis	92%	80%

[1] Department of Internal Medicine II, Technical University of Munich, Ismaninger Str. 22, D-8000 München 80, FRG

Chronic Pancreatitis
Ed. by Beger, Büchler, Ditschuneit, and Malfertheiner
© Springer-Verlag Berlin Heidelberg 1990

two forms were found to be plugs and calcified concrements predominantly found in the first form of the disease.

Morphology of Chronic Pancreatitis with ERCP

The ductal changes of chronic pancreatitis can be visualized by ERCP with a high degree of accuracy. For correct interpretation of the pancreatic duct system and to achieve comparability between different centers performing ERCP, a high standard of imaging quality should be maintained, for which several prerequisites should be kept in mind:
1. Optimal radiological equipment.
2. Pre-ERCP control (plain) film to detect pre-filling changes of parenchyma.
3. Thorough filling of main duct and side branches; parenchymography should be avoided in order to prevent post-ERCP pancreatitis.
4. Films should be taken during the filling and emptying phase, i.e., because intraductal concrements can be overlooked due to overfilling of the duct. Furthermore, a prolonged emptying period points toward a morphological or functional obstruction
5. Movements, blurring, or artifacts due to injection of air bubbles should be avoided.

The main ERCP features of chronic pancreatitis are:
1. Pancreatic calcifications on the pre-filling plain film.
2. Ductal changes in endoscopic retrograde pancreatography (ERP), as irregularities due to stenoses and dilatation, which are found in the main pancreatic duct as well as in the side branches. Furthermore, intraductal plugs–calcified or not–can be demonstrated by accurate ductal filling; in some cases, larger intraductal stones can lead to a complete ductal obstruction (Fig. 1, 2).
3. Endoscopic retrograde cholangiography (ERC): The biliary system can be involved in chronic inflammation of the pancreatic head which leads to a smoothly tapered distal common bile duct stenoses with prestenotic dilatation in advanced cases (Fig. 3).

Grading Systems for Chronic Pancreatitis

In order to classify the ERCP findings of chronic pancreatitis according to their severity, several grading systems have been proposed. The most widely used are the classification of Kasugai et al. [7] and the so-called Cambridge classification (Table 2) [8]. None of these has emerged to be without shortcomings and so no uniform classification has been used in studies of chronic pancreatitis. Recently, Cremer et al. [9] have proposed a morphological classification which does not grade severity, but defines different types of chronic pancreatitis with respect to localization of the disease and the presence of obstructive changes (Fig. 4). Since the gold standard to control ERCP findings of chronic pancreatitis is the histological workup of the resected pancreas, it is not exactly known if morphological deterioration of ERP

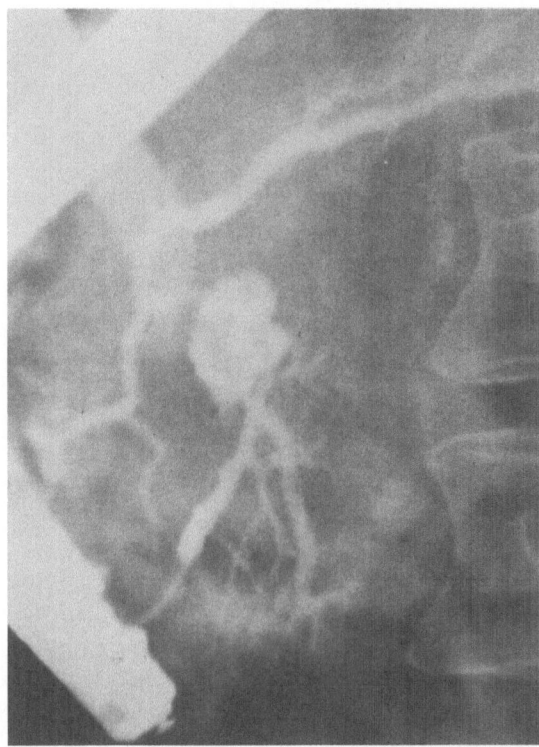

Fig. 1. Chronic pancreatitis in ERP with irregularities of the main pancreatic duct and side branches and cystic changes

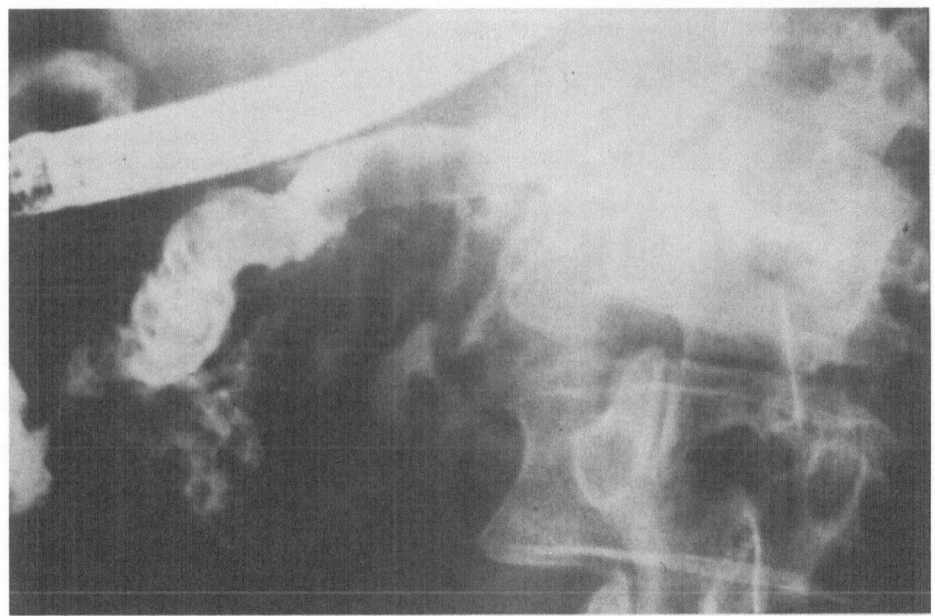

Fig. 2. Chronic pancreatitis in ERP with massive dilatation of the main pancreatic duct and multiple large intraductal concrements

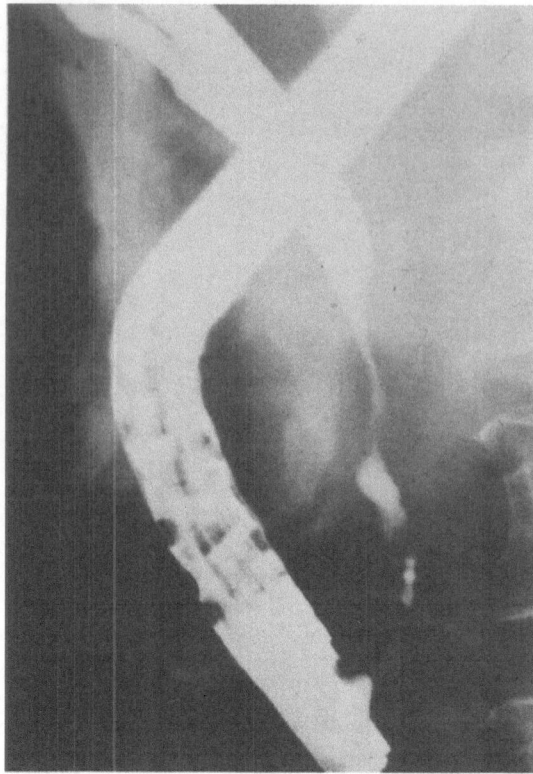

Fig. 3. Common bile duct in chronic pancreatitis: smoothly tapered distal stenosis due to inflammation of the pancreatic head

Table 2. Cambridge classification of chronic pancreatitis. [8]

	Main duct	Side branches
Normal	Normal	Normal
Equivocal	Normal	<3 abnormal
Mild changes	Normal	>3 abnormal
Moderate changes	Abnormal	>3 abnormal
Marked changes	Abnormal	>3 abnormal
	+ one or more of:	
	Large cavity	
	Obstruction	
	Filling defects	
	Severe dilatation/irregularity	

findings really represents histological progression of the disease; however, it does not necessarily mean functional deterioration (see below).

Accuracy of ERCP in Diagnosing Chronic Pancreatitis

The accuracy of ERCP in the diagnosis of chronic pancreatitis has been evaluated in a number of studies. Sensitivity rates of 72%–92% are reported (Table 3). However,

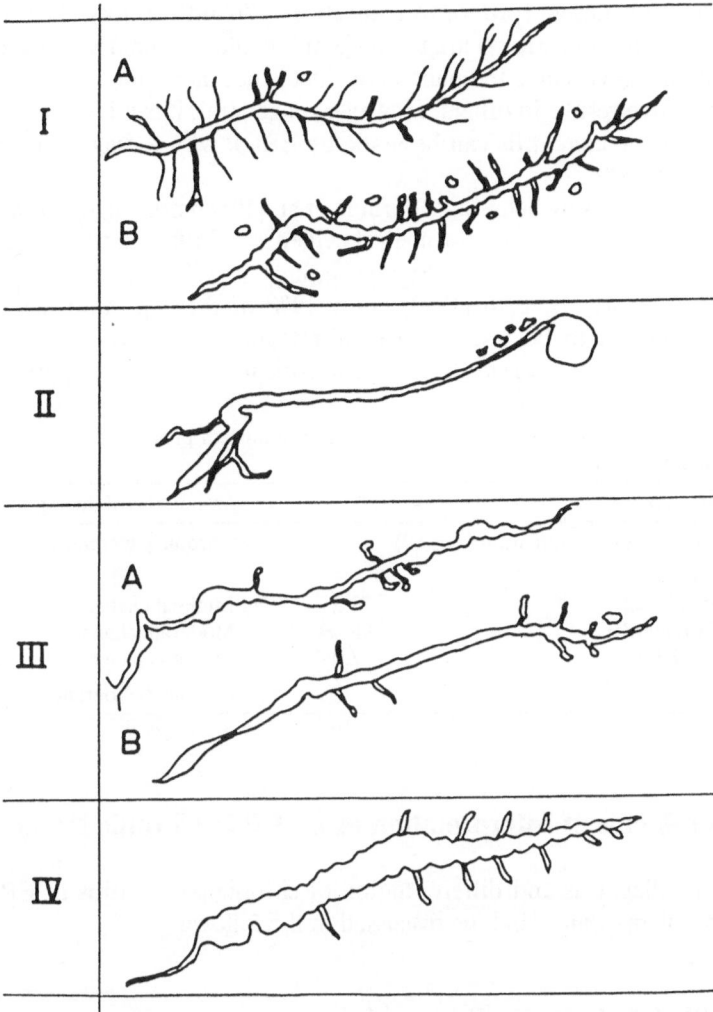

Fig. 4. Endoscopic retrograde cholangiopancreatography classification of ductal changes in chronic pancreatitis by Cremer et al. [9]

Table 3. Diagnostic accuracy of ERCP in chronic pancreatitis

Authors	Patients (n)	Correct diagnosis	False negative	Failure
Classen et al. [36]	25	68%	32%	–
Rolny et al. [16]	30	70%	30%	–
Valentini et al. [15]	65	80%	14%	6%
Branganza et al. [12]	45	82%	18%	–
Anacker et al. [37]	269	83%	3%	14%
Malfertheiner et al. [13]	74	89%	11%	–
Belohlavek [38]	193	92%	8%	–

the study design (pro- or retrospectively, "blind" or not), the selection of cases, and the evaluation criteria are too different to allow comparison. In some of these studies failure to visualize the pancreatic duct is not mentioned or it is mixed up with false-negative results in others. However, in general, it can be stated that the diagnosis of chronic pancreatitis can be made by ERCP with a diagnostic accuracy of approximately 90%.

In a series by Schmitz-Moorman et al. [10] comprising 69 postmortem ductograms of pancreata without histological evidence of inflammation, chronic pancreatitis was diagnosed out of the ductogram findings in 37% (minimal), 33% (moderate), and 11% (marked), respectively; only 19% of these postmortem filling studies were considered to be normal. The histologic work-up of these pancreata, however, showed only different degrees of fibrosis in 72%–88% of patients (Table 4).

Table 4. Correlation between changes in postmortem pancreatic ductograms and histopathologic findings. [10]

Histology		Evaluation of ductogram	
No signs of inflammation ($n = 69$)		Chronic pancreatitis	
Fibrosis			
Periductal	72.5%	Minimal changes	37.2%
Intralobular	88.4%	Moderate changes	33.3%
Perilobular	87.0%	Marked changes	10.4%
		Normal ductogram	19.1%

Problems of Interpretation of ERCP in Chronic Pancreatitis

The diagnosis and differentiation of chronic pancreatitis in ERCP still pose some problems which shall be discussed in the following:

Which Gold Standard?

There are two possible methods of controlling the accuracy of ERCP in the diagnosis of chronic pancreatitis: function testing and histological workup.

Pancreatic exocrine function is markedly reduced in far advanced disease; in earlier stages of chronic pancreatitis only some of the secretory parameters might be decreased [11]. Quite a few studies show a good correlation between advanced stages of ductal changes in ERP and a marked hyposecretion in the secretin-pancreozymin test [12–16] or the Lundh test meal [17]. In the early phase of the disease, however, the correlation between functional and ductal changes is usually weak [12, 13] (Table 5). One potential explanation for this discrepancy has been given by the study of Di Magno et al. [18], who showed a correlation between the degree of exocrine hyposecretion and the length of opacified duct in ERP: An exocrine secretory insufficiency was detectable only when more than 90% of the duct length is obstructed. This might be especially valid for the obstructive form of chronic pancreatitis.

Table 5. Correlation between morphological changes in ERP and function testing (secretin-pancreozymin test) in chronic pancreatitis. [13]

SP test: Grading of hyposecretion	Correlation with ERCP grading (according to Kasugai)
I	44%
II	32%
III	75%

$n = 74$

The correlation of ERCP findings and histological workup also seems to be weak, although only limited data are available. Heji et al. [19] investigated 18 patients with surgical resection of their pancreas because of chronic pancreatitis. The preoperative ERP grading (due to Kasugai's classification) correlated only weakly with the degree of several histological findings (Table 6).

Table 6. Severity of chronic pancreatitis: correlation between ERP grading and histopathological findings. [19]

ERP grading (Kasugai)	Correlation with histological grading, regarding		
	Atrophy	Dilatation	
		Main duct	Side ducts
I	1/ 1	0	0
II	1/ 5	1/ 3	0
III	4/12	4/11	2/17

$n = 18$ (surgical resection)

Differentiation from Changes Following Acute Pancreatitis and from Pancreatic Carcinoma

The scarring of the pancreas following acute pancreatitis may involve the ductal system and thus mimic the morphologic pattern of chronic disease. In up to 10% of cases a conclusive differential diagnosis between chronic pancreatitis and pancreatic carcinoma cannot be made out of the ERCP findings, although high sensitivity rates of ERCP for both conditions are reported in the literature [1]. An Italian study of 130

Table 7. Diagnostic yield of ERCP in patients with upper abdominal symptoms. [20]

ERCP findings: chronic pancreatitis with	Final Diagnoses		
	Chronic pancreatitis	St. p. acute pancreatitis	Pancreatic carcinoma
Moderate changes	76.6%	7.8%	15.7%
Marked changes	72.2%	3.8%	24.0%

$n = 130$

patients [20] with ERCP features suggestive of chronic pancreatitis showed that up to 8% and 24% of patients ended up with the final diagnoses "status post acute pancreatitis" and "pancreatic carcinoma," respectively (Table 7).

Pancreatic Duct Changes with Aging ("Presbypancreas")

Ductal changes of the pancreas may occur with aging and can mimic chronic pancreatitis. In a series by Kreel and Sandin [21], including 120 necropsy cases without inflammatory features of the pancreas, an inflammatory-like ductal pattern was observed in the postmortem ductogram in up to three-fourths of cases and occurred significantly more often in persons over 60 years of age (Table 8). This corresponds to a decreasing pancreatic function with age [22], although this has been doubted [23].

Table 8. Diagnostic yield of ERCP in patients with upper abdominal symptoms. [31]

| | Normal | ERP findings | |
		Chronic pancreatitis	Pancreatic carcinoma
Suspected pancreatic disease (history, clinical data) $n = 26$	57%	34.6%	7.7%
No suspicion of pancreatic disease $n = 49$	83%	8.2%	8.2%

Circumscript Forms

The circumscript froms of chronic pancreatitis may pose difficulties in diagnosis and differentiation to the clinician in the assessment of ERP. In up to 10% of patients with chronic inflammatory changes of the pancreas this segmental form can be found [5]; in 50% it is located in the region of the body and tail of the organ; in 14% a correlation with pancreas divisum can be found. The so-called groove pancreatitis affects the pancreatic head and the inflammatory and fibrotic process is localized in the groove between the head of the organ and the duodenum [2]. It is thought to arise as a sequela of a localized acute necrotizing pancreatitis limited to the head of the organ. In ERP the main pancreatic duct is normal but can be displaced by the fibrotic process [24] and thus may mimic a pancreatic head tumor. Furthermore, inflammatory changes of small ducts in the respective region are observed in segmental pancreatitis.

Follow-up of Patients with Chronic Pancreatitis

Since chronic pancreatitis runs a rather variable course depending on the cause of the disease and several other features [25], the pathology of the parenchyma and the ductal system may also change during the long-term course of the disease. From studies of abdominal plain films it is known that pancreatic calcifications decrease in about one-third of cases during a mean follow-up period of 10–12 years [26]. There is only one series from Japan in which the authors followed 79 patients with chronic pancreatitis by serial ERCP over a mean period of 2.3 years [27]: Morphological deterioration was observed in 80% of patients with alcoholic and 19% of patients with non-alcoholic chronic pancreatitis. Of cases with suspected chronic pancreatitis, 22% developed more marked signs of inflammation, while 19% of normal controls (with various other diseases) turned out to have chronic pancreatitis during the follow-up period. Similar results have recently been reported [28].

Clinical Role of ERCP in Chronic Pancreatitis

The primary diagnosis of chronic pancreatitis is achieved by ERCP in a high percentage (usually about 90%) of cases; ERCP thus serves as standard method for detecting morphological changes of this disease. Although there is a high reproducibility of ERP findings by histopathologic workup of resection specimens [29], the detection and classification of mild inflammatory changes is still difficult in the clinical setting and sometimes needs a follow-up and/or a complementary function testing. Several conditions (status post acute pancreatitis, carcinoma, changes with aging) have to be considered in the differential diagnosis of chronic pancreatitis demonstrated in ERCP.

Endoscopic retrograde cholangiopancreatography has been used in the evaluation of patients with upper abdominal pain, although there are only a few reports of the diagnostic yield of ERCP in this clinical setting. Ruddell et al. investigated 140 patients with unexplained abdominal pain of more than 3 month's duration; ERCP was performed after numerous other investigative procedures. In five patients previously unrecognized gallstones were detected and pancreatography was abnormal in 18% with one carcinoma [30]. Another clinical study from Italy [31] revealed a considerably higher incidence of chronic pancreatitis or pancreatic carcinoma in patients with but also without suspicion of pancreatic disease examined by ERCP (Table 8); however, the selection criteria are somewhat unclear in this series.

Endoscopic retrograde cholangiopancreatography is also very useful in patients with previously diagnosed chronic pancreatitis and abdominal pain. Winstanley et al. [32] investigated 115 patients with confirmed chronic pancreatitis and sustained abdominal pain; ERCP revealed surgically treatable findings (e.g., strictures, cysts, or focal pancreatitis) in 46% of cases. With the increasing role of endoscopic therapy of chronic pancreatitis – dilatation or stenting of strictures, stone extraction after extracorporal shock wave lithotripsy, endoscopic cystostomy [9, 33] – ERCP may become increasingly important in selecting patients who benefit from endoscopic (or surgical) therapy.

In conclusion, ERCP is essential for establishing the diagnosis of chronic pancreatitis and for planning of therapy in these patients. With the advent of endoscopic ultrasound [34, 35] and eventually endosonographically guided target biopsy as well as of endoscopy of pancreatic ducts, the clinical value of endoscopy in chronic pancreatitis will be considerably extended.

References

1. Niederau C, Grendell JH (1985) Diagnosis of chronic pancreatitis. Gastroenterology 88:1973–1975
2. Rösch W (1987) ERCP in acute and chronic pancreatitis. In: Sivak MV (ed) Gastroenterologic endoscopy. Saunders, Philadelphia, pp 780–793
3. Classen M, Hellwig H, Rösch W (1973) Anatomy of the pancreatic duct. Endoscopy 5:14–18
4. Heitz PU, Klöppel G (1984) Pathomorphology of pancreatitis. In: Gyr KE, Singer MV, Sarles H (eds) Pancreatitis, concepts and classification. Excerpta Medica, Amsterdam, pp 83–85
5. Rösch W (1983) Die segmentäre Pankreatitis. Leber Magen Darm 13:49–54
6. Sahel J, Sarles H (1984) Chronic calcifying pancreatitis and obstructive pancreatitis – two entities. In: Gyr KE, Singer MV, Sarles H (eds) Pancreatitis, concepts and classification. Excerpta Medica, Amsterdam, pp 47–49
7. Kasugai T, Kuno N, Kizu M, et al. (1972) Endoscopic pancreatocholangiography. II. The pathological endoscopic pancreatocholangiogramm. Gastroenterology 63:227–234
8. Axon ATR, Classen M, Cotton PB, et al. (1984) Pancreatography in chronic pancreatitis: international definitions. Gut 25:1107–1112
9. Cremer M, Deviere J, Engelholm L (1989) Endoscopic management of cysts and pseudocysts in chronic pancreatitis: long-term follow-up after 7 years of experience. Gastrointest Endosc 35:1–9
10. Schmitz-Moormann P, Himmelmann GW, Brandes JW, et al. (1985) Comparative radiological and morphological study of human pancreas. Pancreatitis-like changes in postmortem ductograms and their morphological pattern. Possible implication for ERCP. Gut 26:406–414
11. Gullo L, Costa PL, Fontana G, Labo G (1976) Investigation of exocrine pancreatic function by continuous infusion of cerulein and secretin in normal subjects and in chronic pancreatitis. Digestion 14:97–107
12. Braganza JM, Hunt LP, Warwick F (1982) Relationship between pancreatic exocrine function and ductal morphology in chronic pancreatitis. Gastroenterology 82:1341–1347
13. Malfertheiner P, Büchler M, Stanescu A, Ditschuneit H (1986) Exocrine pancreatic function in correlation to ductal and parenchymal morphology in chronic pancreatitis. Hepatogastroenterology 33:110–114
14. Nakano S, Horiguchi Y, Takeda T, et al. (1974) Comparative diagnostic value of endoscopic pancreatography and pancreatic function tests. Scand J Gastroenterol 9:383–390
15. Valentini M, Cavallini G, Vantini I, et al. (1981) A comparative evaluation of endoscopic retrograde cholangiopancreatography and the secretin-cholecystokinin test in the diagnosis of chronic pancreatitis: a multicenter study in 124 patients. Endoscopy 13:64–67
16. Rolny P, Lukes JP, Gamklou R, et al. (1978) A comparative evaluation of endoscopic retrograde pancreatography and secretin-CCK test in the diagnosis of pancreatic disease. Scand J Gastroenterol 13:777–781
17. Ashton MG, Axon ATR, Lintott DJ (1978) Lundh test and ERCP in pancreatic disease. Gut 19:910–915
18. DiMagno EP, Malagelada JR, Go VLW (1979) The relationship between pancreatic ductal obstruction and pancreatic secretion in man. Mayo Clin Proc 54:157–162
19. Heji HA, Obertrop H, van Blankenstein M, et al. (1987) Comparison of endoscopic retrograde pancreatography with functional and histologic changes in chronic pancreatitis. Acta Radiol 28:289–293
20. Cavallini G, Riela A, Angelini GP, et al. (1986) Limitations in the interpretation of endoscopic retrograde pancreatography findings in chronic pancreatitis. In: Malfertheiner P, Ditschuneit H (eds) Diagnostic procedures in pancreatic disease. Springer, Berlin Heidelberg New York, pp 175–184
21. Kreel L, Sandin B (1973) Changes in pancreatic morphology associated with aging. Gut 14:962–970
22. Laugier R, Baez-Santana C, Dupuy P, Sarles H (1989) Human pancreatic exocrine secretion decreases with age. Gastroenterology 96:A289
23. Gullo L, Priori P, Daniele C, et al. (1983) Exocrine pancreatic function in the elderly. Gerontology 29:407–411

24. Stolte W, Weiss W, Volkholz H, Rösch W (1982) A special form of segmental pancreatitis: "groove pancreatitis". Hepatogastroenterology 29:198–208
25. Ammann RW, Akovbiantz A, Largiader F, Schueler G (1984) Course and outcome of chronic pancreatitis. Gastroenterology 86:820–828
26. Ammann RW, Muench R, Otto R, et al. (1988) Evolution and regression of pancreatic calcification in chronic pancreatitis. Gastroenterology 95:1018–1028
27. Nagata A, Homma T, Tamai K, et al. (1981) A study of chronic pancreatitis by serial endoscopic pancreatography. Gastroenterology 81:884–891
28. Miyake H, Harada H, Kinichika K, et al. (1987) Clinical course and prognosis of chronic pancreatitis. Pancreas 2:378–385
29. Stolte M, Schaffner O, Trommsdrof L, et al. (1981) Diagnostischer Wert der Pankreatographie. Inn Med 8:150–155
30. Ruddell WSJ, Lintott DJ, Axon ATR (1983) The diagnostic yield of ERCP in the investigation of unexplained abdominal pain. Br J Surg 70:74–75
31. Angelini G, Antolini G, Bovo P, et al. (1987) Frequency of pancreatographic changes in subjects with upper abdominal symptoms and its relationship to alcohol intake. Int J Pancreatol 2:305–310
32. Winstanley PA, Manning AP, Lintott DJ, Axon ATR (1986) Endoscopic retrograde cholangio-pancreatography in pancreatitis with persistent or recurrent pain. Int J Pancreatol 1:407–412
33. Soehendra N, Grimm H, Schreiber W (1986) Endoskopische transpapilläre Drainage des Ductus Wirsungianus bei der chronischen Pankreatitis. Dtsch Med Wochenschr 111:727–731
34. Lees WR (1986) Endoscopic ultrasonography of chronic pancreatitis and pancreatic pseudocysts. Scand J Gastroenterol [Suppl 123], 21:123–129
35. Rösch T, Dancygier H, Lorenz R, et al. (1989) The role of endoscopic ultrasonography in chronic pancreatitis. In: Dancygier H, Classen M (eds) 5th International Symposium on Endoscopic Ultrasonography. Z Gastroenterol [Suppl] Demeter-Verlag S. 26–28
36. Classen M, Koch H, Demling L (1972) Diagnostische Bedeutung der endoskopischen Kontrast-darstellung des Pankreasgangsystems. Leber Magen Darm 2:79–83
37. Anacker H, Weiss HD, Kramann B, Gmelin E (1981) Die Treffsicheheit der endoskopischen retrograden Pankreatiko-Cholangiographie in der Diagnostik der Pankreaskrankheiten. Dtsch Med Wochenschr 106:230–233
38. Belohlavek D (1977) Diagnostische Möglichkeiten der endoskopisch retrograden Cholangiopan-kreatikographie. *Habilitationsschrift*, University of Ulm

Imaging of Chronic Pancreatitis: A Synopsis

P. C. Freeny[1]

Radiologic imaging has become essential in the diagnosis and evaluation of patients with chronic pancreatitis. The primary techniques include the cross-sectional modalities of ultrasonography (US), computed tomography (CT), and magnetic resonance (MR), as well as endoscopic retrograde cholangiopancreatography (ERCP), and angiography.

Role of Imaging

Radiologic imaging has four primary roles in the evaluation of patients with chronic pancreatitis:
1. diagnosis,
2. staging the severity of the disease,
3. detection of complications, and
4. assistance in choosing treatment alternatives.

Diagnosis

Diagnosis of chronic pancreatitis is based upon *clinical* findings, assessment of endocrine and exocrine pancreatic *function,* and *morphologic* changes in the gland as depicted by imaging studies. Evaluation of all three parameters is essential, since many patients with chronic pancreatitis will have abnormalities of only one or two.

Ultrasonography

The use of high-resolution real-time scanners, as well as the techniques of endoscopic and intraoperative sonography, have made US a major imaging procedure in the evaluation of patients with suspected chronic pancreatitis. The findings of chronic pancreatitis include alterations in size, shape, and echotexture of the gland, pancreatic and bile duct dilatation, calculi, fluid collections, and portal venous obstruction (Fig. 1). The frequency of these findings varies and is dependent upon the severity and

[1] Clinical Professor of Radiology, University of Washington, Virginia Mason Clinic, PO Box 900, Seattle, WA 98111, USA

Chronic Pancreatitis
Ed. by Beger, Büchler, Ditschuneit, and Malfertheiner
© Springer-Verlag Berlin Heidelberg 1990

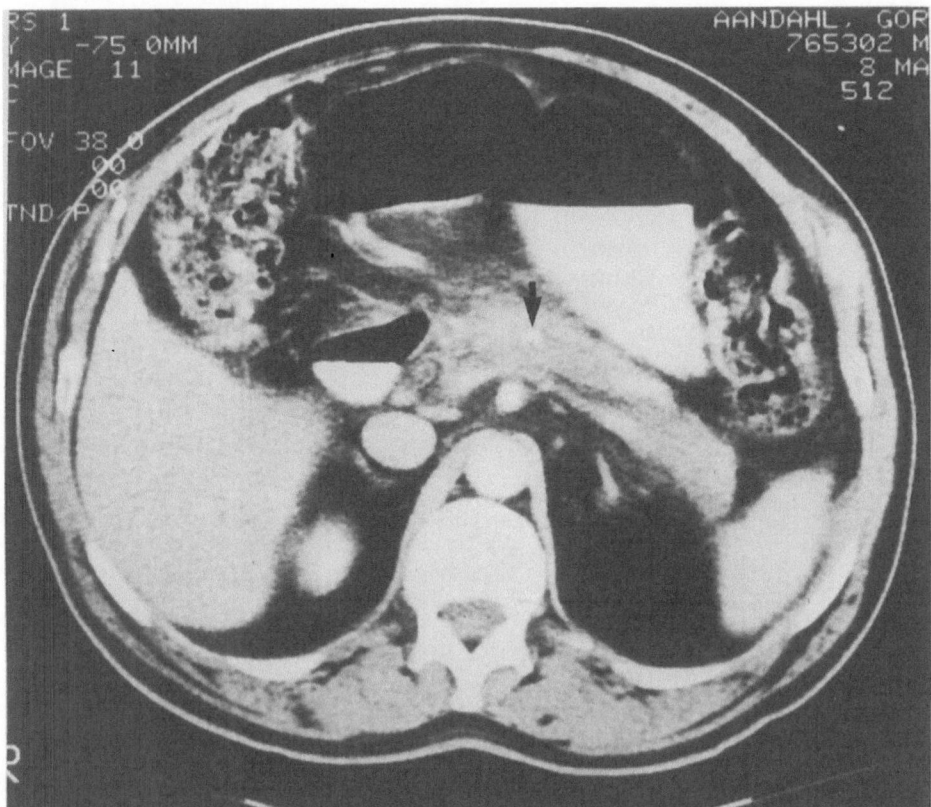

Fig. 1A

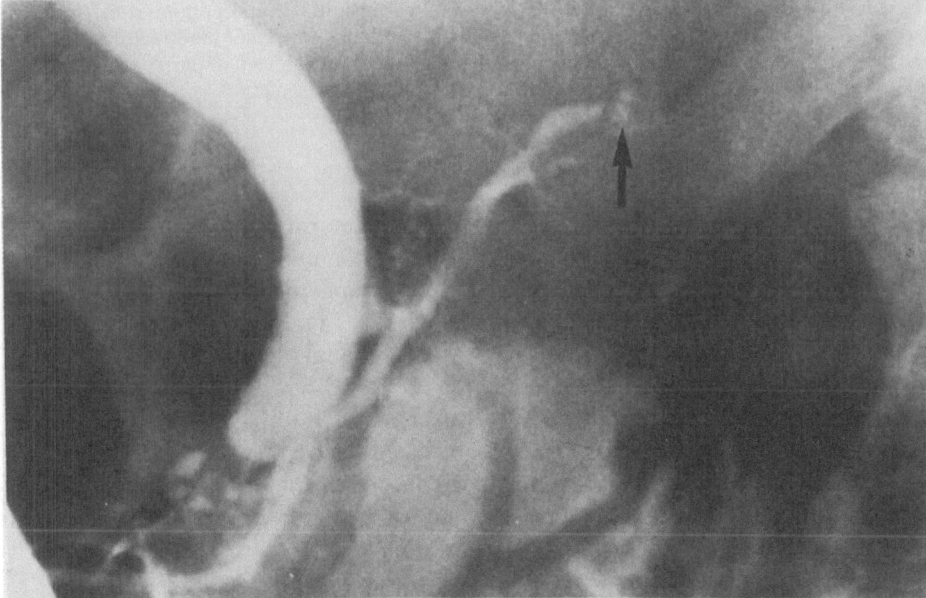

Fig. 1B

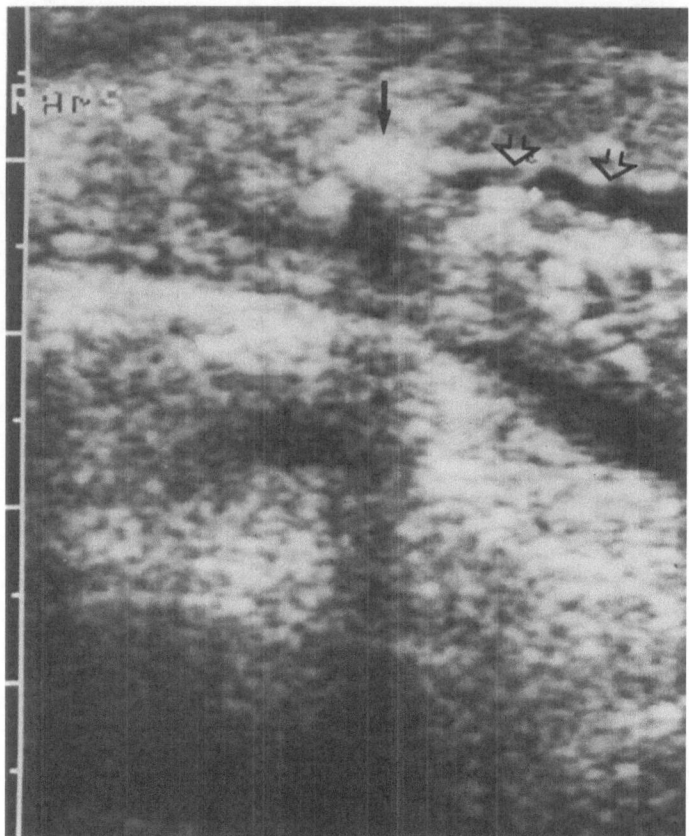

Fig. 1A–C. Chronic pancreatitis. **A** CT shows small calculus in the mid-portion of the pancreas *(arrow)*. Pancreatic duct is not seen. **B** ERCP shows obstruction of pancreatic duct by calculus *(arrow)* and nonfilling of the upstream duct. **C** Intraoperative US shows ductal calculus *(arrow)* and dilatation of upstream duct *(open arrows)*. Patient underwent a Whipple's resection

duration of the disease [1]. In particular, US may be normal in patients with early or mild disease. The use of secretin stimulation and simultaneous US imaging of the main pancreatic duct can uncover changes which may aid in diagnosis, such as absent or decreased (< 50%) pancreatic duct caliber change or persistent duct dilatation (> 100%) at 15 min [1]. Bolondi et al. [1] have reported that the sensitivity of this test in diagnosis of chronic pancreatitis is 87%.

The sensitivity of US in diagnosis of chronic pancreatitis ranges from 48% to 96%, with an average of about 60% – 70% [1]. The false-negative rate is about 25%, and the percentage of unsatisfactory US examinations due to inability to adequately image the pancreas is about 20% [1]. Despite these limitations, the low cost of US makes it an excellent screening examination.

Computed Tomography

The CT findings of chronic pancreatitis are similar to those of US: alterations in size and shape of the gland, changes in parenchymal attenuation, calculi, pancreatic and bile duct dilatation, fluid collections, and vascular involvement (portal venous obstruction, arterial pseudoaneurysms) (Fig. 1). As with US, the frequency of abnormal findings is dependent upon the severity of the disease.

There is considerable variation in the reported sensitivity of CT in diagnosis of chronic pancreatitis, ranging from 50% to 90%. However, most of the studies appeared prior to the introduction of current generation scanners and the use of 5-mm collimated scans and dynamic incremental bolus contrast enhancement technique [2, 3]. A current paper by Luetmer et al. [4], utilizing state-of-the-art CT, reports a false-negative rate of only 7% (4 of 56 patients) in CT detection of chronic pancreatitis. However, the clinical/functional severity of the disease in their patients was not reported.

Although CT is more expensive than US and requires administration of intravenous contrast, it has some significant advantages: high detail depiction of both pancreatic and peripancreatic anatomy, including vascular structures and the surrounding gastrointestinal tract, virtual absence of technically unsatisfactory examinations, and high contrast sensitivity for pancreatic calcifications (Figs. 1, 2). The main limitations of CT are partial volume effect and slice misregistration, both of which can inhibit detection of mild-moderate degrees of pancreatic duct dilatation (see Fig. 1).

Endoscopic Retrograde Cholangiopancreatography

Endoscopic retrograde cholangiopancreatography has been widely used as a primary modality for diagnosis of chronic pancreatitis and the findings are well known. They include caliber changes of the main pancreatic duct, lateral side branches, and the common bile duct, intraductal filling defects or calculi, and cysts or fluid collections which communicate with the pancreatic duct (Fig. 1).

Endoscopic retrograde cholangiopancreatography is abnormal in about 80%–85% of patients with chronic pancreatitis [5]. If one excludes cases in which there is a failure to cannulate the pancreatic duct, a correct ERCP diagnosis is possible in about 90% of patients [6]. Because subtle changes of the main pancreatic duct and lateral side branches can be detected by ERCP, it continues to be the "gold standard" for diagnosis of chronic pancreatitis and is essential for planning operative strategy.

Magnetic Resonance

Magnetic resonance has had minimal use in evaluation of patients with chronic pancreatitis. MR is significantly inferior to CT in identifying the margins of the gland, depicting the pancreatic duct, and imaging the surrounding gastrointestinal tract. In addition, calculi which are smaller than 5 mm in diameter are rarely seen using current MR techniques. At the present time, MR has no significant role in diagnosis of chronic pancreatitis.

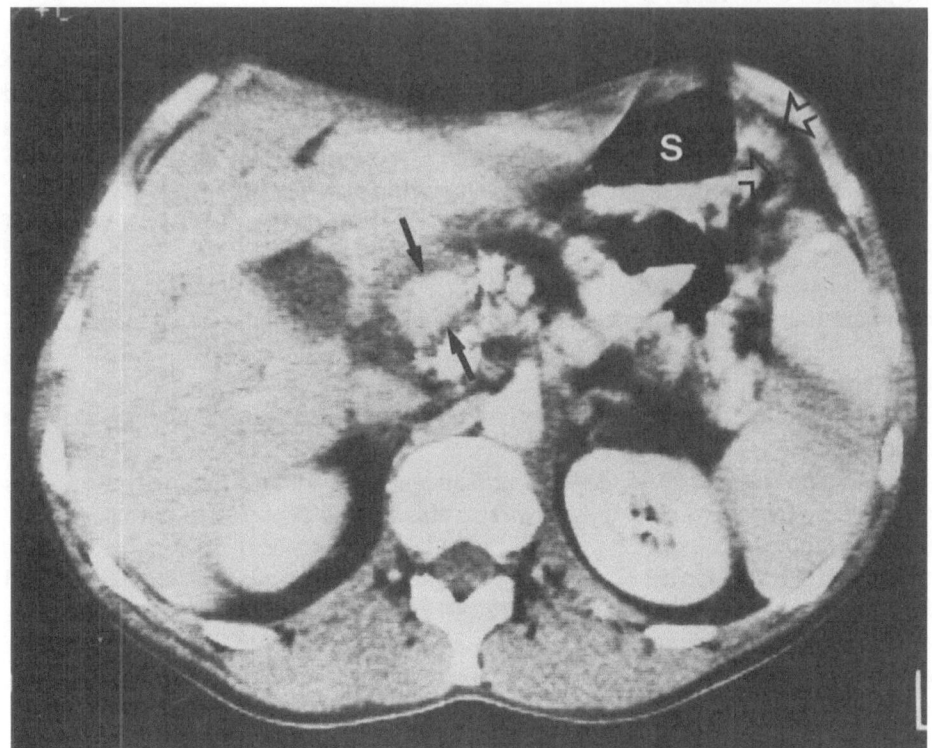

Fig. 2A

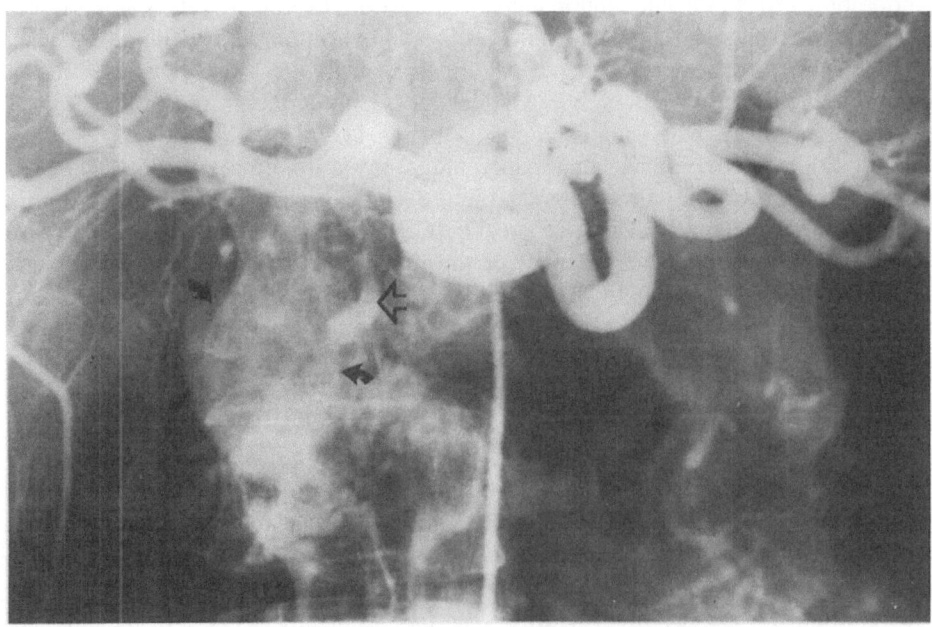

Fig. 2B

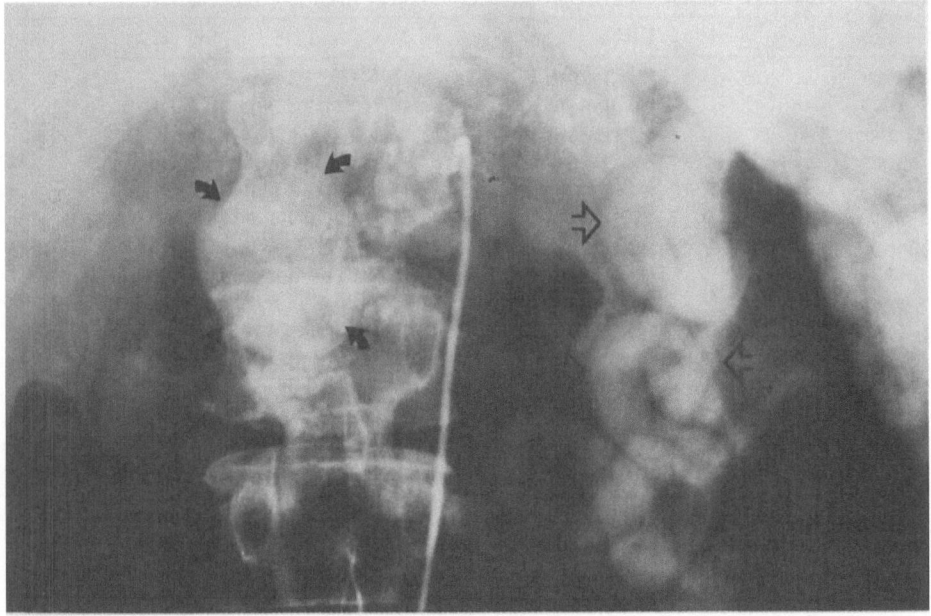

Fig. 2A–C. Chronic pancreatitis. **A** CT shows a pseudoaneurysm *(arrows)* in the head of the pancreas, multiple pancreatic duct calculi, and a large varix *(open arrows)* around the stomach *(S)*. **B** Preoperative arteriogram shows early filling of the pseudoaneurysm *(arrows)* from the gastroduodenal artery *(open arrow)*. **C** Venous phase shows the pseudoaneurysm *(arrows)* and the large perigastric varices *(open arrows)*

Morphologic Staging of Chronic Pancreatitis

The severity of chronic pancreatitis can be staged on the basis of clinical symptoms, usually pain, diminished exocrine and/or endocrine function, and morphologic changes in or around the gland, as depicted by imaging studies.

The 1983 Cambridge meeting introduced a new morphologic grading system for chronic pancreatitis based on US, CT, and ERCP [7] (Table 1). This system generally has been accepted as the international standard for classifying the severity of the morphologic changes of chronic pancreatitis. However, no reports have as yet appeared comparing the Cambridge classification of morphologic severity to the severity of the clinical/functional changes in patients with chronic pancreatitis.

A variety of reports have appeared over the last decade comparing morphologic changes of chronic pancreatitis depicted by US, CT, and ERCP with clinical symptoms (pain) and functional changes (measured by various pancreatic function tests) [8–16]. In general, there has been good correlation between the severity of clinical symptoms and functional impairment and the severity of morphologic changes in patients with advanced chronic pancreatitis. However, in patients with mild or moderate symptoms and functional impairment, correlation with morphologic changes has been poor. For example, Lankisch et al. [11] showed that 50% of patients with chronic

Table 1. Cambridge classification of pancreatic morphology in chronic pancreatitis

Changes	ERCP	CT and US
Normal	MPD normal No abnormal LSBs	MPD ≤ 2 mm Normal gland size, shape
Equivocal	MPD normal < 3 abnormal LSBs	Homogeneous parenchyma Only one of the following signs: MPD 2–4 mm Gland enlarged (< 2× normal) Heterogeneous parenchyma
Mild	MPD normal > 3 abnormal LSBs	Two or more signs for diagnosis: MPD 2–4 mm Slight gland enlargement Heterogeneous parenchyma
Moderate	MPD changes + LSB changes	Small cysts < 10 mm MPD irregularity Focal acute pancreatitis Increased echogenicity of MPD walls MPD walls Gland contour irregularity

Severe
Any of the above changes plus one or more of the following:
                  Cyst > 10 mm
                  Intraductal filling defects
                  Calculi
                  MPD obstruction, stricture
                  Severe MPD irregularity
                  Contiguous organ invasion

MPD, main pancreatic duct; LSB, lateral side branch ducts
Focal change: less than one-third of gland involved

pancreatitis and ductal calcifications (Cambridge classification: severe morphologic changes) had only slight or moderate functional impairment. Malfertheiner et al. [16] also showed that in patients with severe clinical/functional changes morphologic abnormalities depicted by CT or ERCP were mild in 14% and 20% of patients, respectively. Virtually all investigators have concluded that in general the severity of clinical/functional impairment cannot be predicted by the degree of morphologic changes, and vice versa [8–16].

Complications of Chronic Pancreatitis

The primary complications of chronic pancreatitis include formation of fluid collections (pseudocyst, abscess), spread of the inflammatory reaction to involve the gastrointestinal tract, bile ducts, and vascular system, and pancreatic ascites. A major role of imaging is detection and precise definition of these complications. In addition, imaging studies can be used to guide interventional techniques, such as endoscopic or percutaneous catheter drainage of fluid collections, transhepatic or endoscopic biliary decompression, transcatheter embolization for control of hemorrhage, and endoscopic pancreatic duct stent placement (Fig. 3).

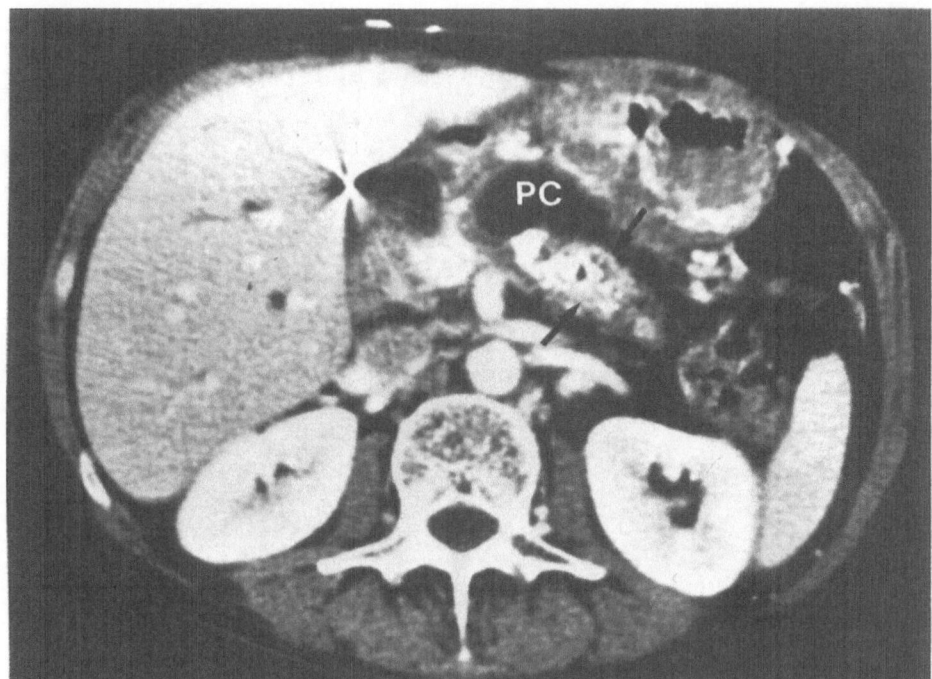

Fig. 3A

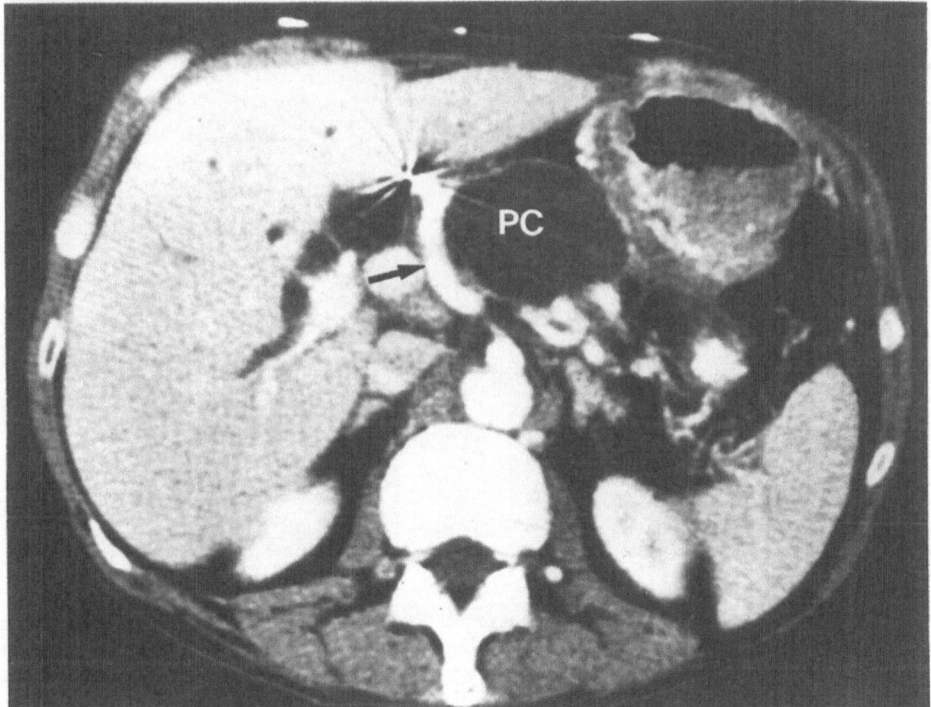

Fig. 3B

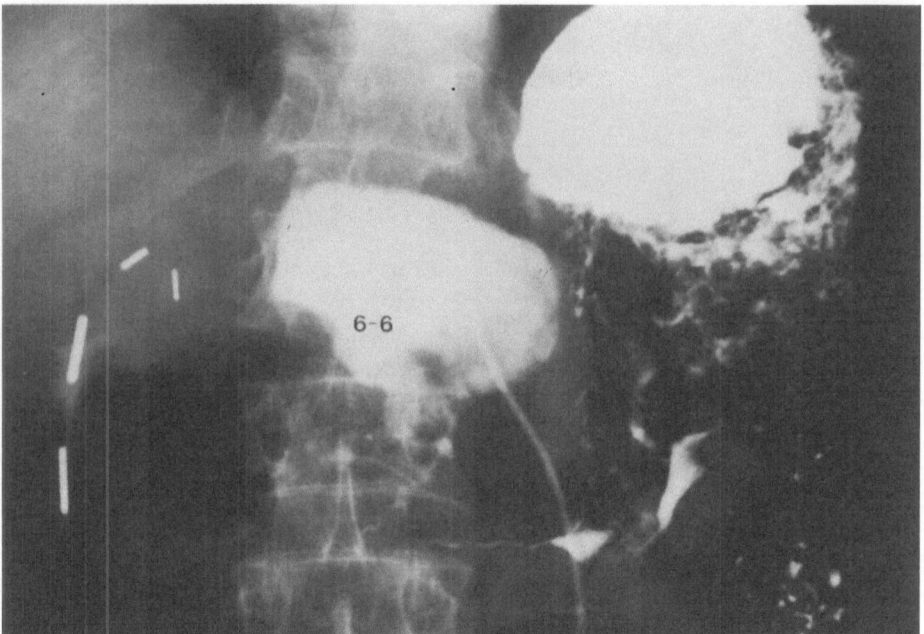

Fig. 3C

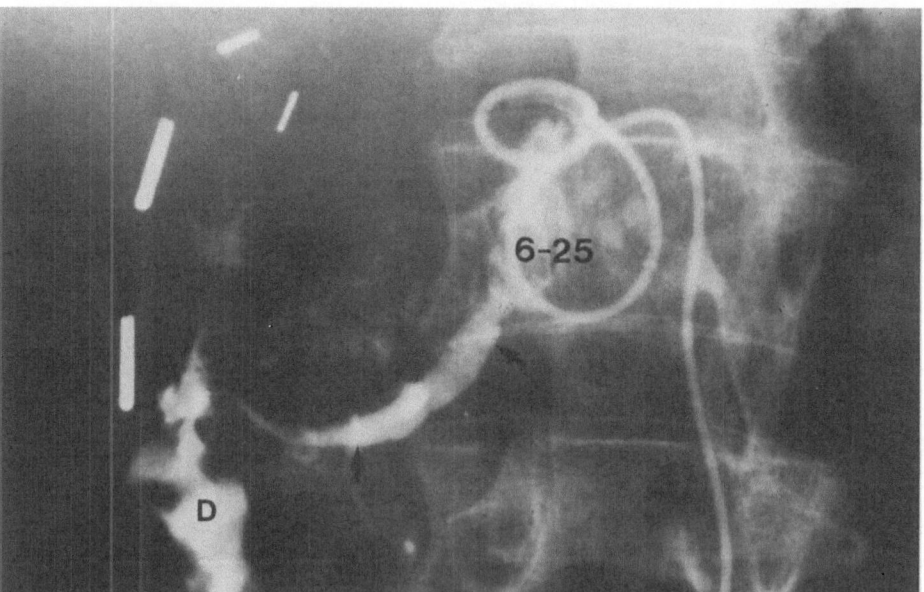

Fig. 3D

Fig. 3A–D. Percutaneous pseudocyst drainage. **A** CT shows a pseudocyst *(PC)* anterior to the heavily calcified tail of the pancreas *(arrows)*. **B** Scan caudal to **A** shows the cyst *(PC)* and an adjacent large varix *(arrow)*. **C** Percutaneous catheter drainage *(6–6)* shows contrast within pseudocyst. **D** Contrast study 18 days later *(6–25)* shows resolution of cyst and communication with downstream pancreatic duct *(arrows)*, with drainage into duodenum *(D)*. Catheter was removed and cyst did not recur

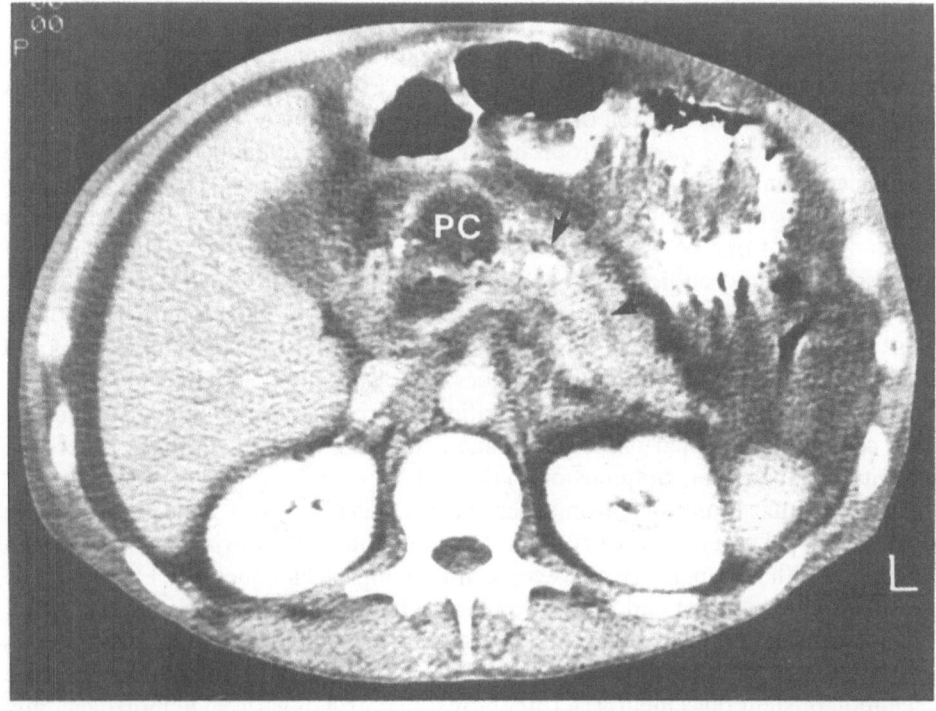

A

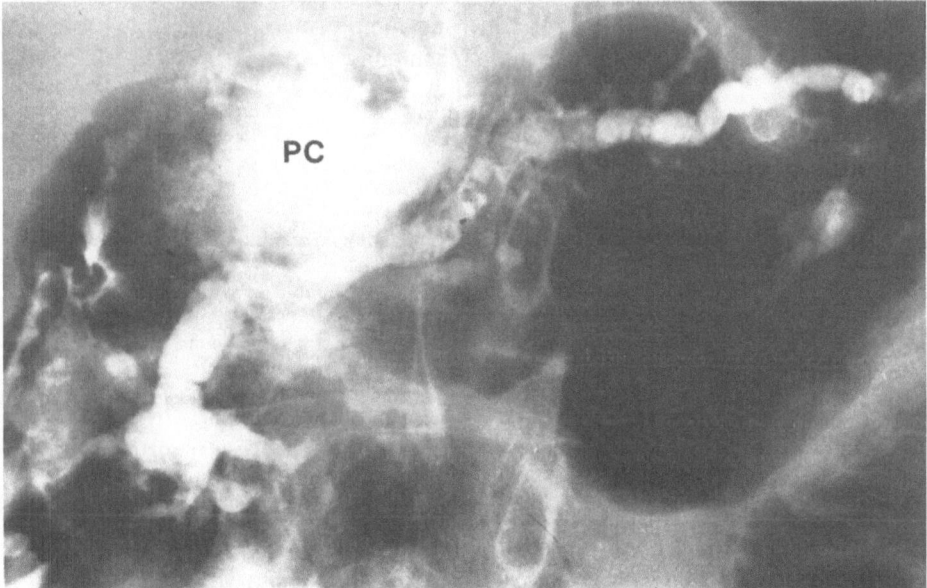

B

Fig. 4A, B. Chronic pancreatitis. **A** CT shows a pseudocyst *(PC)* in the head of the pancreas with upstream pancreatic duct dilatation and calculi *(arrows)*. **B** Preoperative ERCP shows communication of the dilated pancreatic duct and the pseudocyst *(PC)*. The cyst was unroofed and a longitudinal pancreaticojejunostomy was performed

Treatment Alternatives

Patients with chronic pancreatitis can be treated with conservative medical therapy, surgery, or interventional endoscopic or radiologic techniques. Imaging procedures play a crucial role in selection of the appropriate therapeutic approach.

Medical therapy is most appropriate for management of endocrine and exocrine insufficiency and for control of pain during acute exacerbations [17, 18]. Chronic, unremitting pain, usually requiring increasing levels of narcotics for control, or development of one of the complications of pancreatitis, are indications for more aggressive therapy, surgical, endoscopic, or radiologic.

The primary indications for surgery are persistent pain and treatment of complications of chronic pancreatitis [19]. Imaging studies are used to detect complications and possible causes for pain, such as a pseudocyst or obstruction of the pancreatic or bile duct, and to select the appropriate operation for treatment of a complication or for pain control, such as partial or total pancreatectomy versus a drainage procedure (longitudinal pancreaticojejunostomy) (Fig. 4).

Some complications of chronic pancreatitis, such as fluid collections, biliary obstruction, pancreatic duct calculi and strictures, and acute arterial hemorrhage, can be treated with nonoperative endoscopic or radiologic techniques (see Fig. 3). These include percutaneous or endoscopic drainage of fluid collections, endoscopic removal of pancreatic duct calculi, endoscopic or transhepatic dilatation of bile duct strictures and placement of stents for decompression, endoscopic pancreatic duct stricture dilatation or stent placement, sclerotherapy for control of variceal hemorrhage, and transcatheter embolotherapy for control of arterial hemorrhage or pseudoaneurysm formation [20–24]. Radiologic guidance and monitoring are crucial for safe and efficacious performance of most of these techniques.

References

1. Bolondi L, Bassi SL, Gaiani S, et al. (1989) Sonography of chronic pancreatitis. Radiol Clin North Am 27:815–833
2. Ferrucci JT Jr, Wittenberg J, Black EB, et al. (1981) Computed body tomography in chronic pancreatitis. Radiology 130:175–182
3. Savarino V (1980) Computed tomography in the diagnosis of pancreatic disease. Ital J Gastroenterol 12:265–269
4. Luetmer PH, Stephens DH, Ward EM (1989) Chronic pancreatitis: reassessment with current CT. Radiology 171:353–357
5. Caletti G, Brocchi E, Agostini D, et al. (1982) Sensitivity of endoscopic retrograde pancreatography in chronic pancreatitis. Br J Surg 69:507–509
6. Swobodnik W, Meyer W, Brecht-Kraus D, et al. (1983) Ultrasound, computed tomography and endoscopic retrograde cholangiopancreatography in the morphologic diagnosis of pancreatic disease. Klin Wochenschr 61:291–296
7. Freeny PC (1989) Classification of pancreatitis. Radiol Clin North Am 27:1–3
8. Elsborg L, Bruusgaard L, Strandgaard L, et al. (1981) Endoscopic retrograde pancreatography and the exocrine pancreatic function in chronic alcoholism. Scand J Gastroenterol 16:941–944
9. Jensen R, Matzen p, Malchow-Moller A, Christofferson I, et al. (1984) Pattern of pain, duct morphology, and pancreatic function in chronic pancreatitis. Scand J Gastroenterol 19:334–338
10. Girdwood AH, Hatfield ARW, Bornman PC, et al. (1984) Structure and function in noncalcific pancreatitis. Dig Dis Sci 8:721–726

11. Lankisch PG, Otto J, Erkelenz I, et al. (1986) Pancreatic calcifications: no indicator of severe exocrine pancreatic insufficiency. Gastroenterology 90:617–621
12. Valentini M, Cavallini G, Vantini I, et al. (1981) A comparative evaluation of endoscopic retrograde cholangiopancreatography and the secretin-cholecystokinin test in the diagnosis of chronic pancreatitis: a multicentre study in 124 patients. Endoscopy 13:64–67
13. Braganza JM, Hunt LP, Warwick F (1982) Relationship between pancreatic exocrine function and ductal morphology in chronic pancreatitis. Gastroenterology 82:1341–1347
14. Bornman PC, Marks IN, Girdwood AH, et al. (1980) Is pancreatic duct obstruction or stricture a major cause of pain in calcific pancreatitis? Br J Surg 67:425–428
15. Bolondi L, Priori P, Gullo L, et al. (1987) Relationship between morphological changes detected by ultrasonography and pancreatic exocrine function in chronic pancreatitis. Pancreas 2:222–229
16. Malfertheiner P, Buchler M, Stanescu A, et al. (1986) Exocrine pancreatic function in correlation to ductal and parenchymal morphology in chronic pancreatitis. Hepatogastroenterology 33:110–114
17. Worning H (1984) Chronic pancreatitis: pathogenesis, natural history and conservative therapy. Clin Gastroenterol 13:871–894
18. Lankisch PG, Creutzfeldt W (1984) Therapy of exocrine and endocrine pancreatic insufficiency. Clin Gastroenterol 13:985–999
19. Frey CF, Bodai BI (1984) Surgery in chronic pancreatitis. Clin Gastroenterol 13:913–940
20. Freeny PC, Lewis GP, Traverso LW, et al. (1988) Infected pancreatic fluid collections: percutaneous catheter drainage. Radiology 167:435–442
21. Classen M, Phillip J (1984) Endoscopic retrograde cholangiopancreatography (ERCP) and endoscopic therapy in pancreatic disease. Clin Gastroenterol 13:819–842
22. Huibregtse K, Schneider B, Vrji AA, et al. (1988) Endoscopic pancreatic drainage in chronic pancreatitis. Gastrointest Endosc 34:9–15
23. Cremer M, Deviere J, Engelholm L (1989) Endoscopic management of cysts and pseudocysts in chronic pancreatitis: longterm follow-up after 7 years of experience. Gastrointest Endosc 35:1–9
24. Vujic I (1989) Vascular complications of pancreatitis. Radiol Clin North Am 27:81–91

Conservative Treatment

The Role of Analgesic Treatment in Chronic Pancreatitis

W. Domschke[1]

According to the pattern of clinical symptoms in chronic pancreatitis (CP), medical therapy aims at
a) pain relief,
b) compensation of exocrine pancreatic insufficiency, and
c) management of diabetes mellitus.
This review deals particularly with the first point.

Natural History of Pain

In almost all patients with CP pain is the chief symptom, occurring either intermittently or chronically, and it has the greatest impact on life-style in terms of repeated hospitalization, loss of time at work, use of and addiction to analgesics and alcohol. The magnitude of the problem is illustrated by the fact that about 20% of patients even require frequent doses of narcotics for pain relief [30]. Principally, the frequency of pain and, consequently, the role of analgesic treatment differ in alcohol-induced and non-alcohol-induced (idiopathic) CP in that in the former group the incidence of primary painless disease was reported to be as low as 4.9%, while it is high (53.7%) in idiopathic CP [3]. Usually CP progresses to calcification and exocrine/endocrine insufficiency, which is said to be closely associated with the onset of pain relief [2]. From their longitudinal study in alcohol-induced CP, Ammann et al. (Fig. 1) con-

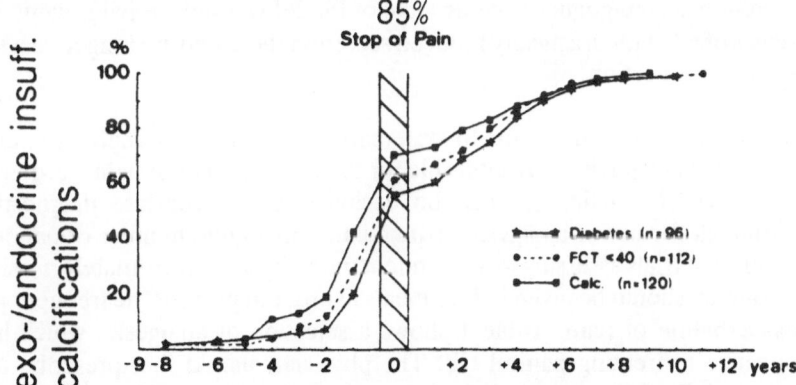

Fig. 1. Natural history of chronic pancreatitis. Increase in calcifications (■——■) and dysfunction (*——* diabetes; ●---● exocrine insufficiency) and pain relief over years. (From [2])

---

[1] Department of Medicine, University of Erlangen-Nürnberg, D-8520 Erlangen, FRG

Chronic Pancreatitis
Ed. by Beger, Büchler, Ditschuneit, and Malfertheiner
© Springer-Verlag Berlin Heidelberg 1990

cluded that 85% of patients obtain lasting relief from pain at a median of 4.5 years from onset of the disease. However, in some cases the concerted development of calcification, pancreatic insufficiency, and pain alleviation may take no less than 18 years, which is clearly a burden to the patience of patients and their physicians. The concept of pain relief due to increasing destruction of pancreatic glandular tissue has not been unanimously accepted [18, 24]. At least in idiopathic CP, pain relief may occur despite normal pancreatic exocrine function [3]. In any case, during periods of severe pain patients must be offered an appropriate analgesic treatment.

Analgesic Treatment Modalities

This review concentrates on medical treatment modalities that have been advocated for pain relief in CP. Surgical procedures – drainage, resection, denervation – are presented separately here.

Abstinence from Alcohol. Considerable time should be spent with the patient to convince him/her of the paramount importance of total abstinence. Accordingly, it is advisable to refer the patient to specific psychotherapy and guidance within a local Alcoholics Anonymous group. Efforts along these lines seem urgently indicated, as pancreatic deterioration does appear to occur more rapidly when alcoholics continue to drink than when they reform and abstain; the same holds true for the development of pain relief, the rate of which is usually higher in abstinent patients [12, 14, 20, 23]. In three studies, however, no correlation between changes in abdominal pain and abstinence from alcohol was observed [22, 24, 27]. This discrepancy may be due, at least in part, to the fact that not all reports differentiated systematically between alcohol-induced and idiopathic CP. Furthermore, the incidence of pain in response to alcohol drinking should be separately evaluated in early- and late-stage CP. It may well be, namely, that in the early stage of the disease with relatively normal exocrine secretion secretagogues such as alcohol [5, 26] can induce pain, while in advanced stages of CP with drastically reduced secretion there may no longer be a substrate for such alcohol action.

Analgesics. Naturally, prior to systematic treatment with analgesics, any anatomic reasons which might be responsible for the development of pain – e.g., pseudocysts, bile duct obstruction – must be excluded by appropriate diagnostic work-up. Although the use of analgesics is mandatory in a great number of patients with CP, controlled trials assessing this treatment modality are unfortunately missing. Usually, analgesics should be given before meals in order to prevent the frequent postprandial exacerbation of pain. Table 1 shows a selection of analgesics which have proven effective in treating painful CP. The physician should first prescribe nonnarcotic, peripherally acting agents, i.e., spasmolytics/analgesics. However, in many severe cases opiate analgesics are urgently required, and they should not be withheld because of the risk of inducing narcotic addiction, which generally seems to be overestimated. Nevertheless, the use of simpler drugs, such as salicylates or paracetamol, should be maximized by increasing dose strength or frequency before switching to stronger or narcotic alternatives. Adjuvant analgesic drugs – antidepressants, anxiolytics – are

Table 1. Analgesic and adjuvant analgesic drugs in chronic pancreatitis

First step:	*Second step:*
Spasmoanalgesics	Opioid analgesics
– Salicylates and NSAIDs	– Codeine
– Paracetamol	– Tilidine
– Pyrazolones	– Pentazocine
Antidepressants	– Pethidine
Anxiolytics	– Buprenorphine
	– Tramadol

often helpful, and their use may mean that analgesics are not required or can be given at a lower dose. Drug doses should be determined individually and should be the lowest compatible with controlling pain. Analgesics should always be prescribed on a time-contingent basis, as round-the-clock medication is clinically more effective and, additionally, can decrease the total amount of drug required over a 24-h period.

Diet. Avoidance of alcohol in any form or quantity is of paramount importance. Otherwise, there are no prospectively controlled trials which have demonstrated a relevant relationship between dietary measures and the occurrence of pain. Conventionally, patients are recommended to eat frequent, small meals (6 meals per day) of a bland diet with fats being restricted to 25% of the calorie intake, i. e., about 80–110 g fat per day [25]. Thus, it is hoped that postprandial pancreatic secretion does not exceed moderate magnitude, and that pain is consequently largely prevented.

Enzyme Therapy. Large oral doses of pancreatic extracts have been reported to induce pain relief in a number of patients with CP [17, 28]. This effect was interpreted to be due, at least in part, to a negative feedback control on the endogenous production of pancreatic enzymes by the orally administered exogenous enzymes [8]. However, other authors were unable to find significant pain reduction following pancreatic enzyme supplementation or found pain relief to be related to reduction of steatorrhea leading to decreased colonic motility [1, 13]. This controversial issue is discussed fully in another chapter of this volume.

Endoscopic-Sonographic Stenting. In selected cases, particularly in the obstructive type of CP, interventional endoscopy and/or sonography may alleviate pain. After endoscopic pancreatic sphincterotomy, therapeutic measures include aspiration of protein plugs or extraction of calculi from the main pancreatic duct, intraductal insertion of endoprostheses [10, 16, 29], and sonographically guided placement of stents into pseudocysts for external or internal drainage [6, 15]. Long-term follow-up and success rates of such new technologies await further investigation.

Acupuncture. In two prospective trials with a crossover design, the pain-relieving effect of electroacupuncture or transcutaneous electric nerve stimulation was studied; neither modality was effective [4].

Celiac Plexus Block. Another treatment to control pain is celiac plexus block by percutaneous, radiologically or sonographically guided injection of absolute ethanol. This procedure has been used in smaller uncontrolled series of patients for years, with contradictory results. The occasional benefits almost never last for more than a few months [19], and repeated treatment may not be as effective and exposes the patient to the well-documented dangers of the procedure [11]. In a comparative study of celiac plexus block and pancreaticogastrostomy, pain was relieved most effectively by surgery [21].

Epidural Anesthesia. In patients with severely painful CP who are unwilling to undergo or are unsuitable for surgery, as the last nonsurgical treatment resort epidural administration of opiates may be considered. Via an epidural catheter connected to a pump or port system, intermittent injections or continuous infusion of narcotics can be performed, providing superior pain control while preserving to an appreciable extent the patient's quality of life.

If all medical measures fail to relieve pain, most clinicians will opt – although this indication is still controversial [7] – for an appropriate surgical intervention [9], particularly in case of debilitating pain with its deteriorating effects on the patient's life-style and social and personal relationships.

References

1. Adler G (1988) Enzymsubstitution zur Behandlung der Schmerzen bei chronischer Pankreatitis. Dtsch Med Wochenschr 113:1075–1079
2. Ammann RW, Akovbiantz A, Largiader F, Schueler G (1984) Course and outcome of chronic pancreatitis. Longitudinal study of a mixed medical-surgical series of 245 patients. Gastroenterology 86:820–828
3. Ammann RW, Buehler H, Muench R, Freiburghaus AW, Siegenthaler W (1987) Differences in the natural history of idiopathic (nonalcoholic) and alcoholic chronic pancreatitis. A comparative long-term study of 287 patients. Pancreas 2:368–377
4. Ballegaard S, Christophersen SJ, Gamwell Dawids S, Hesse J, Vestergaard Olsen N (1985) Acupuncture and transcutaneous electric nerve stimulation in the treatment of pain associated with chronic pancreatitis. Scand J Gastroenterol 20:1249–1254
5. Clain JE, Barbezat GO, Marks IN (1981) Exocrine pancreatic enzyme and calcium secretion in health and pancreatitis. Gut 22:355–358
6. Classen M, Phillip J (1984) Endoscopic retrograde cholangio-pancreatography and endoscopic therapy in pancreatic disease. Clin Gastroenterol 13:819–842
7. Creutzfeldt W (1987) Chirurgische Therapie der chronischen Pankreatitis – Advocatus diaboli-Kommentar. Langenbecks Arch Chir 372:373–378
8. Dlugosz J, Fölsch UR, Czajkowski A, Gabryelewicz A (1988) Feedback regulation of stimulated pancreatic enzyme secretion during intraduodenal perfusion of trypsin in man. Eur J Clin Invest 18:267-272
9. Domschke W, Encke A (1988) Schmerztherapie bei chronischer Pankreatitis – Kontroverse Standpunkte. Z Gastroenterol 23:136–142
10. Fuji T, Amano H, Ohmura R, Akiyama T, Aibe T, Takemoto T (1989) Endoscopic pancreatic sphincterotomy – technique and evaluation. Endoscopy 21:27–30
11. Greiner L (1985) Punktionssonographische Alkoholneurolyse der Coeliakalganglien. Dtsch Med Wochenschr 110:833–836
12. Gullo L, Barbara L, Labò G (1988) Effect of cessation of alcohol use on the course of pancreatic dysfunction in alcoholic pancreatitis. Gastroenterology 95:1063–1068

13. Halgreen H, Pedersen NT, Worning H (1986) Symptomatic effect of pancreatic enzyme therapy in patients with chronic pancreatitis. Scand J Gastroenterol 21:104–108
14. Hayakawa T, Kondo T, Shibata T, Sugimoto Y, Kitagawa M (1989) Chronic alcoholism and evolution of pain and prognosis in chronic pancreatitis. Dig Dis Sci 34:33–38
15. Heyder N, Flügel H, Domschke W (1988) Catheter drainage of pancreatic pseudocysts into the stomach. Endoscopy 20:75–77
16. Huibregtse K, Schnider B, Vrij AA, Tytgat GNJ (1988) Endoscopic pancreatic drainage in chronic pancreatitis. Gastrointest Endosc 34:9–15
17. Isaksson G, Ihse I (1983) Pain reduction by an oral pancreatic enzyme preparation in chronic pancreatitis. Dig Dis Sci 28:97–102
18. Kondo T, Hayakawa T, Noda H, et al. (1981) Follow-up study of chronic pancreatitis. Gastroenterol Jpn 16:46–53
19. Leung JWC, Aveling W, Bowen-Wright M, Shorvon PJ, Cotton PB (1982) Coeliac plexus block for pain control in pancreatic cancer and chronic pancreatitis. Gut 23:A451
20. Little JM (1987) Alcohol abuse and chronic pancreatitis. Surgery 101:357–360
21. Madsen, P, Hansen E (1985) Coeliac plexus block versus pancreaticogastrostomy for pain in chronic pancreatitis. Scand J Gastroenterol 20:1217–1220
22. Marks IN, Girdwood AH, Bank S, Louw JH (1980) The prognosis of alcohol-induced calcific pancreatitis. S Afr Med J 57:640–646
23. Miyake H, Harada H, Kunichika K, Ochi K, Kimura I (1987) Clinical course and prognosis of chronic pancreatitis. Pancreas 2:378–385
24. Pedersen NT, Andersen BN, Pedersen G, Worning H (1982) Chronic pancreatitis in Copenhagen. Scand J Gastroenterol 17:925–931
25. Sarles H (1986) Latest developments in the pathophysiology and treatment of chronic pancreatitis. In: Dobrilla G (ed) Problems and controversies in gastroenterology. Raven, New York, pp 231–238
26. Sarles H, Devaux MA, Noel-Jorand MC (1984) Action of ethanol on the pancreas. In: Gyr KE, Singer MV, Sarles H (eds) Pancreatitis, concepts and classification. Elsevier, Amsterdam, pp 183–187
27. Sarles JC, Nacchiero M, Garani F, Salase B (1982) Surgical treatment of chronic pancreatitis. Am J Surg 144:317–322
28. Slaff J, Jacobson D, Tillman R, Curington C, Toskes P (1984) Protease-specific suppression of pancreatic exocrine secretion. Gastroenterology 87:44–52
29. Soehendra N, Grimm H, Schreiber HW (1986) Endoskopisch-transpapilläre Drainage des Ductus Wirsungianus bei der chronischen Pankreatitis. Dtsch Med Wochenschr 111:727–731
30. The Copenhagen Pancreatitis Study Group (1981) An interim report from a prospective epidemiological multicenter study. Scand J Gastroenterol 16:305–312

Modern Treatment of Exocrine Pancreatic Insufficiency

M. Otte and A. Heufelder[1]

The clinical manifestation of exocrine pancreatic insufficiency is a late symptom of chronic pancreatitis. Steatorrhea due to maldigestion of dietary fats does not occur until the pancreatic secretory capacity is less than 10% of normal [1]. Quantification of steatorrhea requires the analysis of stool fats, a method most laboratories feel thrilled with. This commonly makes pancreatic insufficiency only a clinical diagnosis, when patients with known chronic pancreatitis present with weight loss despite adequate nutritional intake.

However, as the decision to establish supplementary treatment means life-long therapy causing daily costs of approximately U.S. $ 4-$ 5, a diagnosis of severe pancreatic insufficiency should be confirmed. Adequate proof seems to come from tubeless tests of pancreatic exocrine function. Only recently, Lankisch et al. [7] could demonstrate a high probability of steatorrhea when the pancreolauryl test resulted in a T/C ratio below 10.

Treatment of pancreatogenic steatorrhea requires preparations containing high doses of lipase and sufficient amounts of colipase. Based on normal pancreatic secretion following almost maximal stimulation by caerulein and secretin (according to the method approved by the European Pancreatic Club), a secretory capacity of 10% corresponds to approximately 100000 Fédération International Pharmaceutique (FIP) units, regardless of whether the mean or the median acts as the value of reference (Fig. 1).

Of all pancreatic extracts currently available, the preparation richest in lipase releases 36000 FIP units of lipase. By calculation, three capsules per meal should guarantee proper treatment. In contrast, several commercially available pancreatin preparations contain considerably lesser amounts of lipase. Among those available in the Federal Republic of Germany there is a range of 2000–36000 FIP units of lipase, most preparations are declared as containing 10000 FIP units or more [9]. Of the popular preparations used in therapeutic trials in the United States, Pancrease contains approximately 4900 FIP units, Cotazym about 8800 and Viokase about 3500.

The main therapeutic problem in using pancreatic extracts is their degradation by gastric acid [4]. Pancreatic enzymes, especially lipase, are irreversibly denatured by pH values below 4. With chronic pancreatitis, gastric pH values usually fall below this figure. Even within the duodenal bulb, pH values demonstrate considerable acidity [11]. Only the more distal regions of the duodenum constantly exhibit pH values above 5. This is why conventional enzyme supplementation without acid protection

---

[1] Klinik für Innere Medizin, Medizinische Universität Lübeck, D-2400 Lübeck 1, FRG

Chronic Pancreatitis
Ed. by Beger, Büchler, Ditschuneit, and Malfertheiner

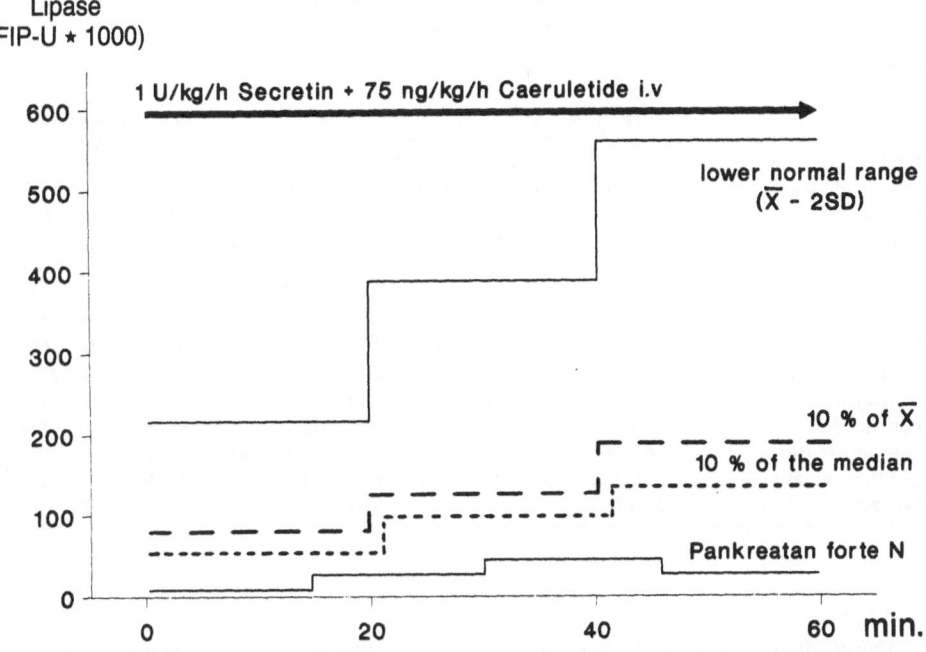

Fig. 1. In vitro release of lipase from Pankreatan forte N in comparison to submaximally stimulated pancreatic secretion in man. Lipase levels within 10% of the median and the mean of normal secretory capacity are presented

results in low lipase activities, with only 3.5%–15% of the orally administered amounts reaching the duodenum [2, 5].

There have been reports of improved success rates with simultaneous application of antacids or a H_2 receptor blocking agent [3, 12], underscoring the clinical relevance of acid inactivation. Therefore, acid-protected preparations have been designed that release their enzyme content only with pH values above 5.5.

In order to allow the mixing of food with enzymes in the stomach, thus solving the problems with slow break-up of protected tablets, several manufacturers now offer pancreatin preparations as pellets or microtablets with acid-proof coating. Application with gelatine capsules permits prompt dissolution on contact with gastric juice.

Still another important point of relevance for a good pancreatic enzyme preparation has been largely disregarded so far. With weakly acid or alkaline pH values, it usually takes considerable time until enzyme release is achieved, and enzymes are fully available for digestion. This time factor is of importance for the treatment of exocrine pancreatic insufficiency.

In vitro testing of several preparations has been used successfully to demonstrate marked differences of enzyme release [9]. With the best preparations, full lipase availability could be demonstrated within 15 min. In contrast, there was only partial release of lipase from other preparations even after 120 min (Table 1).

Table 1. Lipase content of various preparations during incubation over 120 min at pH 6.6, compared to total content as declared by the respective manufacturer

Preparation	Lipase content (FIP units)	Time (min)							
		15	30	45	60	75	90	105	120
Pankreatan forte N	36000	3008	26600	35950	32370	29500	26900	25500	24000
Panzytrat 20000	20000	18530	19470	18550	17700	16800	15450	14770	14210
Kreon	10000	11500	13900	12500	11600	10500	9800	9900	8400
Fermento duodenal	15000	7500	12150	14400	16200	13900	13050	12150	11250
Combizym forte	30000	600	7800	13500	22200	24900	27600	27000	26700
Gillazym	10500	3675	5985	7770	7980	9975	9030	8920	8610
Enzym gallo sanol	15000	2700	3450	4650	6150	6000	4950	4500	4050
Ozym	12000	2280	5400	5520	5880	5280	5400	5760	6120
Panpur (1985)	28000	0	0	5040	6720	7000	12880	25200	26320
Nutrizym	12500	1250	2375	3250	3375	4375	7125	9500	8000
Pancholtruw	15750	0	1440	2500	4320	6120	6480	7200	7560
Panzynorm forte	6000	0	1560	1980	3360	4020	4440	5160	6820
Cholspasminase	8000	0	560	800	2400	4800	4560	4560	4600
Lipazym	13000	0	0	780	1170	910	780	780	650

The clinical relevance of rapid intestinal availability of pancreatic enzymes becomes clear with respect to the duodenal-cecal transit time. This passage takes 67–160 min, depending on whether liquid or solid food has been consumed [6, 8]. It is only this time span that digestion and absorption have at their disposal.

This theoretical background and the in vitro studies mentioned earlier demonstrate three main criteria that every good pancreatic extract must meet: high enzyme content, rapid-release kinetics, and acid stability.

Treatment using such potent preparations promises adequate therapeutic success; with 100000 FIP units of lipase per day, stool fat excretion can be reduced by 50%, with 200000 FIP units by even 70% [10]. However, complete restoration to normal seems rare. This would probably require even higher doses of lipase, such as 100000 FIP units with each meal.

However, most patients do fairly well with a clear reduction of stool fat excretion. Changes in body weight allow for a reliable parameter of what treatment has achieved. There are only very few patients with inadequate weight gain despite high-dose lipase supplementation with an excellent preparation. This form of treatment failure may ensue when the break-up of the acid-resistant coating occurs too late or fails to occur at all due to very low pH values in the duodenum and upper jejunum. In this situation, the trial of a H_2 receptor blocking agent may be worthwhile. Another form of treatment would be the use of fungal lipases, which have been shown to function effectively even in an acid milieu.

References

1. DiMagno EP, Go VLW, Summerskill WHJ (1973) Relation between pancreatic enzyme outputs and malabsorption in severe pancreatic insufficiency. N Engl J Med 288:813–815

2. DiMagno EP, Malagelada JR, Go VLW, Moertel CG (1977) Fate of orally ingested enzymes in pancreatic insufficiency. Comparison of two dosage schedules. N Engl J Med 296:1318–1322
3. Graham DY (1982) Pancreatic enzyme replacement. The effect of antacids or cimetidine. Dig Dis Sci 27:485–490
4. Heizer WD, Cleaveland CR, Iber FL (1965) Gastric inactivation of pancreatic enzyme supplements. Bull Johns Hopkins Hosp 116:261–270
5. Ihse I, Lilja P, Lundquist I (1980) Intestinal concentrations of pancreatic enzymes following pancreatic replacement therapy. Scand J Gastroenterol 15:137–144
6. Kellow JE, Borody TJ, Phillips SF, Haddad AC, Brown ML (1986) Sulfapyridine appearance in plasma after salicylazosulfapyridine. Gastroenterology 91:396–400
7. Lankisch P, Otto J, Brauneis J, Hilgers R, Lembcke B (1988) Detection of pancreatic steatorrhea by oral pancreatic function tests. Dig Dis Sci 33:1233–1236
8. Malagelada JR, Robertson JS, Brown ML, Remington M, Duenes JA, Thomforde M, Carryer PW (1984) Intestinal transit of solid and liquid components of a meal in health. Gastroenterology 87:1255–1263
9. Otte M, Ridder P, Dageförde J (1987) In-vitro-Untersuchungen zur Pankreasenzymsubstitution. Dtsch Med Wochenschr 112:1498–1502
10. Otte M, Ridder P, Gutowski HD (1989) Substitutionsbehandlung der Pankreasinsuffizienz mit Pankreatin-Fertigarzneien. Intern Prax 29:185–189
11. Ovesen L, Brendtsen F, Tage-Jensen U, Pedersen NT, Gram BR, Rune SJ (1986) Intraluminal pH in the stomach, duodenum, and proximal jejunum in normal subjects and patients with exocrine pancreatic insufficiency. Gastroenterology 90:958–962
12. Regan PT, Malagelada JR, DiMagno EP, Glanzman SL, Go VLW (1977) Comparative effects of antacids, cimetidine and enteric coating on the therapeutic response to oral enzymes in severe pancreatic insufficiency. N Engl J Med 297:854–858

Enzyme Supplementation for Pain in Chronic Pancreatitis

I. Ihse and J. Permerth[1]

Pain is the dominant clinical problem in chronic pancreatitis. However, its cause or causes are still poorly understood. The idea that increased intraductal pressure is associated with pain has lately gained support from several studies. In 1982 Bradley [7] reported significantly increased ductal pressure in 19 patients with chronic pancreatitis as measured during operation for pain. A drawback with this study was that the control values were obtained endoscopically (patients without any signs of pancreatic disease). The findings were repeated however, by Sato et al. [27], who in an intraoperative study found elevation of both ductal perfusion and residual pressure in patients with chronic pancreatitis compared to controls who had surgery for gastric cancer. Also, Madsen and Winkler [22] reported high ductal pressure as measured intraoperatively in patients with chronic pancreatitis. In an endoscopic study Okazaki et al. [23] made similar findings, and they could even demonstrate a statistically significant increase of the ductal pressure in chronic pancreatitis patients with pain by comparison with a group of patients with painless disease. Interestingly, Ebbehöj et al. [9] were able to record pancreatic tissue pressure during surgery and measured higher values in chronic pancreatitis than in controls, and after ductal drainage a significant drop in tissue pressure was found.

Opponents of the ductal hypertension theory often point out the frequent lack of correlation between pancreatographic changes and the presence of pain. They further emphasize the failure rate of about 30% reported after duct drainage procedures [14, 15, 18]. However, it is possible that obstruction and hypertension not only of the main duct but also of separate secondary or tertiary branches or of pseudocysts may contribute to pancreatic pain. Also, the ductal hypertension theory is consistent with the observed correlation between disappearance of pain in some patients with severely disturbed exocrine pancreatic function [4]. Other suggested causes of pain are recurrent autodigestive tissue necrosis and a possible increase in size and number of nerves, as recently suggested by Bockman et al. [5]. Unfortunately, similar histological changes are also present in patients with painless pancreatitis [20]. Thus, a critical review of the current literature suggests that the origin of pain in chronic pancreatitis is multifactorial, and that increased intraductal pressure is a strong candidate as one of the causes, as long as there is preserved exocrine secretory capacity of the gland. It is therefore not surprising that pain treatment in chronic pancreatitis has largely been directed against duct decompression either surgically [15, 18] or endoscopically [31].

---

[1] Department of Surgery, University Hospital, 58185 Linköping, Sweden

Chronic Pancreatitis
Ed. by Beger, Büchler, Ditschuneit, and Malfertheiner
© Springer-Verlag Berlin Heidelberg 1990

A theoretical alternative of pharmacological duct decompression presented itself when the protease-specific feed-back regulation of pancreatic secretion was suggested in man in 1977 [16]. It is now legitimate to ratify its existence in man since several different groups have come to the same result [1–3, 6, 8, 12, 21, 24, 25, 29, 33]. Still, however, it is not settled whether cholecystokinin (CCK) is the only mediator, or whether other factors are operating in addition [3, 32]. As to the possible association between the feedback mechanism and pain relief the hypothesis was [16] that the low intraduodenal protease activity in chronic pancreatitis would trigger the release of stimulatory factors (CCK, secretin, and/or cholinergic factors?) leading to augmented secretion, which in the presence of ductal obstructions and/or stones would cause intraductal hypertension and pain. Consequently, addition of pancreatic enzyme supplements capable of increasing intraduodenal protease levels [17] could be expected to diminish pain.

In a double-blind crossover study we [19] found pain relief in 15 out of 19 patients with chronic pancreatitis. In the whole group there was a decrease in pain intensity of 30% whereas it was 70% in the ten "good responders." Furthermore, there was a statistically significant reduction in the number of pain attacks in patients on active enzymes. Slaff et al. [29] studied 20 patients with chronic pancreatitis and pain in a double-blind crossover study using a preparation which, like the one that we used, was known to increase intraduodenal protease activities in the dose regimen used. Among nine patients with mild to moderate pancreatic insufficiency 8 experienced pain reduction whereas only 2 of 11 with severe insufficiency found the treatment helpful. Recently, Rämö et al. [26] reported statistically significant pain relief after self-administration (ad libitum) of an enzyme preparation as compared to administration of the regular dose in ten patients with persistent abdominal pain due to chronic pancreatitis. Like Slaff et al. [29] they also recorded a statistically significant reduction in the need of analgetics during the study period. Self-administration led to an increase in the intake of enzyme preparations by more than 100%. Halgreen et al. [11] used the same preparation as Rämö and co-workers [26] and in the regular dose as recommended by the manufacturer. Although there was a tendency to reduction in pain and analgetic consumption in the patients with steatorrhea when treated with active pancreatic enzymes, statistical significance was not reached [11]. However, in ancillary experiments the authors were unable to confirm any increase in intraduodenal protease activity by the dose and preparation used. One may speculate that self-administration of the preparation leading to more than doubling of the amount of capsules per day resulted in increase of intraduodenal protease activities as an explanation of the observed pain relief in the study by Rämö et al. [26]. Grouped together, the three double-blind studies demonstrating good results by enzyme treatment [19, 26, 29] comprise 49 patients, of whom 36 (73%) experienced more or less pronounced pain relief. Further studies are, however, mandatory to definitely settle the role of the treatment. Similarly, the mechanism behind a possible pain-relieving effect of pancreatic enzyme medication in chronic pancreatitis needs elucidation: Is it an exclusive effect of the feedback mechanism? Is it an effect via reduction in the number of bowel movements? Indirectly the above-mentioned four studies lend support to the feedback mechanism. It would, in this context, be of interest to investigate whether any of the new, specific, and potent CCK antagonists cause pain reduction in chronic pancreatitis. In fact, elevated serum levels of CCK in chronic pancreatitis have been demonstrated by some authors [10, 13, 28, 30], again supporting the existence of the feedback mechanism in man.

Available data on the value of enzyme treatment for pancreatic pain and the absence of true side effects allow us to make the following recommendations provided that the preparation used is known to increase duodenal protease levels. We suggest that in patients with pancreatic pain an efficient pancreatic enzyme preparation should be attempted in an adequate dose for 1–2 months. If no effect is apparent after this time interval, the patients should be recommended self-administration for another 1–2 months. If still no effects are discernible, the treatment should be stopped if pain relief is the only reason for the medication.

References

1. Adler G, Mullenhoff A, Bozkurt T, Göke B, Koop J, Arnold R (1988) Comparison of the effect of single and repeated administration of a protease inhibitor (camostate) on pancreatic secretion in man. Scand J Gastroenterol 23:158–162
2. Adler G, Mullenhoff A, Koop J, Bozkurt T, Göke B, Beglinger C, Arnold R (1988) Stimulation of pancreatic secretion in man by a protease inhibitor (camostate). Eur J Clin Invest 18:98–104
3. Adler G, Reinshagen M, Koop J, Göke B, Schafmayer A, Rovati LC, Arnold R (1989) Differential effects of atropine and a cholecystokinin receptor antagonist on pancreatic secretion. Gastroenterology 96:1158–1164
4. Amman RW, Buehler H, Bruehlmann W, Kehl O, Muench R, Stamm R (1986) Acute (non-progressive) alcoholic pancreatitis: prospective longitudinel study of 144 patients with recurrent alcoholic pancreatitis. Pancreas 1:195–203
5. Bockman DF, Buchler M, Malfertheiner P, Beger HG (1988) Analysis of nerves in chronic pancreatitis. Gastroenterology 94:1459–1469
6. Boyd EJS, Cumming JGR, Cushieri A, Wormsley KG (1985) Aspects of feed-back control of pancreatic secretion in man. Ital J Gastroenterol 17:18–22
7. Bradley EL (1982) Pancreatic duct pressure in chronic pancreatitis. Am J Surg 144:313–316
8. Calan J, Bojarski JC, Spriner CJ (1987) Raw soya-bean flour increases cholecystokinin release in man. Br J Nutr 58:175–179
9. Ebbehöj N, Svendsen LB, Madsen P (1984) Pancreatic tissue pressure: techniques and patho-physiological aspects. Scand J Gastroenterol 19:1066–1068
10. Fumakoshi A, Nakano J, Shinozaki H, Tateishi K, Hamaoka T, Ibayashi H (1986) High plasma cholecystokinin levels in patients with chronic pancreatitis having abdominal pain. Am J Gastroenterol 81:1174–1178
11. Halgreen H, Thorsgaard Pedersen N, Worning H (1986) Symptomatic effect of pancreatic enzyme therapy in patients with chronic pancreatitis. Scand J Gastroenterol 21:104–108
12. Hanssen L, Osnes M, Myren J (1978) Pancreatic secretion obtained by endoscopic cannulation of the main pancreatic duct and secretin release after duodenal acidification in man. Scand J Gastroenterol 13:325–330
13. Harvey R, Rey JF, Howard JM, Read AE, Elderle A, Vantini J, Groarke JF, Fitzgerald JF (1977) Bioassay and radioimmunoassay of serum cholecystokinin in patients with pancreatic disease. Rend Gastroenterol 9:15–16
14. Holmberg JT, Isaksson G, Ihse I (1985) Long-term results of pancreaticojejunostomy in chronic pancreatitis. Surg Gynecol Obstet 160:339–346
15. Ihse I, Lankisch PG (1988) Treatment of chronic pancreatitis. Acta Chir Scand 154:553–558
16. Ihse I, Lilja P, Lundquist I (1977) Feed-back regulation of pancreatic enzyme secretion by intestinal trypsin in man. Digestion 15:303–308
17. Ihse I, Lilja P, Lundquist I (1980) Intestinal concentrations of pancreatic enzymes following pancreatic replacement therapy. Scand J Gastroenterol 15:137–144
18. Ihse I, Borch K, Larsson J (1988) Chronic pancreatitis – results of operations for relief of pain. World J Surg 12:866–870

19. Isaksson G, Ihse I (1983) Pain reduction by an oral pancreatic enzyme preparation in chronic pancreatitis. Dig Dis Sci 28:97–102
20. Klöppel G (1989) Pathology of chronic pancreatitis and pancreatic pain. Acta Chir Scand (in press)
21. Liener JE, Goodale RL, Deshmukh A, Satterberg TL, Ward G, DiPietro C, Bankey PE, Bormer JW (1988) Effect of a trypsin inhibitor from soya-beans (Bowman-Birk) on the secretory activity of the human pancreas. Gastroenterology 94:419–427
22. Madsen P, Winkler K (1982) The intraductal pancreatic pressure in chronic obstructive pancreatitis. Scand J Gastroenterol 17:553–554
23. Okazaki K, Yamamoto Y, Kagiyama S, Tamura S, Sakamoto Y, Nakazama Y, Morita M, Yamamoto Y (1988) Pressure of papillary zone and pancreatic main duct in patients with chronic pancreatitis in the early state. Scand. J Gastroenterol 23:501–506
24. Owyang C, Louie D, Tatum D (1986) Feed-back regulation of pancreatic enzyme secretion. J Clin Invest 77:2042–2047
25. Owyang C, May D, Louie D (1986) Trypsin suppression of pancreatic enzyme secretion. Gastroenterology 91:637–643
26. Rämö OJ, Puolakkainen PA, Seppälö K, Schröder TM (1989) Self-administration of enzyme substitution in the treatment of exocrine pancreatic insufficiency. Scand J Gastroenterol 24:688–692
27. Sato T, Miyashita E, Yamauchi H, Matsumu S (1986) The role of surgical treatment for chronic pancreatitis. Ann Surg 203:266–271
28. Schafmayer A, Becker HD, Werner M, Fölsch UR, Creutzfeldt W (1985) Plasma cholecystokinin levels in patients with chronic pancreatitis. Digestion 32:136–139
29. Slaff J, Jacobson D, Tillman CR, Curlington C, Toskes P (1984) Protease-specific suppression of pancreatic exocrine secretion. Gastroenterology 87:44–52
30. Slaff J, Wolfe M, Toskes P (1985) Elevated fasting cholecystokinin levels in pancreatic exocrine impairment: evidence to support feedback regulation. J Lab Clin Med 105:282–285
31. Soehendra N, Grimm H, Schreiber H (1986) Endoscopic transpapillary drainage of the pancreatic duct in chronic pancreatitis. Dtsch Med Wochenschr 111:727–731
32. Sum G, Lee KY, Chang TM, Chey WY (1989) Effect of pancreatic juice diversion on secretin release in rats. Gastroenterology 96:1173–1179
33. Yasui A, Nimura Y, Hayakawa N, Hayakawa T, Shibata T, Kondo T, Naruse S, Shionoya S (1988) Feed-back regulation of basal pancreatic secretion in humans. Pancreas 6:681–687

Diabetes Mellitus in Chronic Pancreatitis

B. GLASBRENNER, P. MALFERTHEINER, and H. DITSCHUNEIT[1]

Introduction

The endocrine compartment in the pancreas is small, accounting for 1%–2% of the total gland, but is essential for the regulation of glucose homeostasis [1, 2]. In order to understand the pathological changes in the endocrine pancreas in the course of chronic pancreatitis better, the basic anatomy and function of endocrine cells in the pancreas are briefly reviewed.

The Endocrine Compartment

No capsule or basement membrane surrounds the islets and therefore endocrine and exocrine pancreatic tissue compartments are in close contact. Both cell-to-cell contacts between exocrine and endocrine cells and direct connections between capillaries of islets and acini have been shown in careful anatomical studies [3–5]. These morphological findings explain the intimate regulatory connections between islet hormones and exocrine pancreatic secretion. Glucagon [6, 7], somatostatin [8–10], and pancreatic polypeptide (PP) [11–13] have been shown to inhibit pancreatic exocrine secretion in various animals and humans, at least in pharmacological doses, whereas insulin potentiates the stimulatory effect of cholecystokinin (CCK) on pancreatic exocrine secretion and regulates the synthesis of amylase [14–17]. The role of insulin was shown to be specific, since insulin receptors on acinar cells were detected [18, 19].

The release of insulin is controlled by several metabolic (glycemia), hormonal, and neural factors and is enhanced by an "incretin" factor from the gut mucosa [20, 21]. The gut hormone gastric inhibitory polypeptide (GIP) is one of the incretin candidates [22, 23], but other factors originating from the gut may participate to increase the insulin response.

Morphology and Function of the Endocrine Pancreatic Compartment in Chronic Pancreatitis

In morphological studies of the endocrine pancreas in chronic pancreatitis, distinct qualitative and quantitative changes have been discerned. The qualitative changes are

---

[1] Department of Internal Medicine II, Gastroenterology, Robert-Koch-Str. 8, D-7900 Ulm, FRG

Chronic Pancreatitis
Ed. by Beger, Büchler, Ditschuneit, and Malfertheiner
© Springer-Verlag Berlin Heidelberg 1990

characterized by focal accumulation of islets in the slcerotic tissue, occasional neoformation of islets through ductuloinsular proliferation (nesidioblastosis), and perisinusoidal fibrosis of the sclerotic islets [24]. Perisinusoidal fibers often split the islets into separate lobules. The proportion of beta cells is reduced to about 60% of control values [24].

Fasting insulin levels in chronic pancreatitis were found to be normal or slightly increased [25, 26], whereas insulin release following intravenous glucose stimulation was found to be reduced [27], showing a depletion of insulin reserve in chronic pancreatitis. Following partial pancreatectomy, the diabetic state depends on the amount and portion of the gland removed [28]. These observations show that a decrease in the number of beta cells and a disturbed responsiveness to stimulation may account for the development of diabetes in chronic pancreatitis. A possible local factor is the sclerosis that affects islet integrity by impairing local circulation and glucose diffusion [29].

The alpha cells appear to be more resistant to pancreatic sclerosis than beta cells, and morphological studies in chronic pancreatitis revealed a relative increase in the number of alpha cells in the islets [24], resulting in a shift in the alpha:beta ratio from 1:3–1:3.5 in controls to 1:0.4–1:1.7 in patients with chronic pancreatitis [24]. This explains the observed rise in glucagon plasma concentration after an oral glucose load in chronic pancreatitis that contrasts with the decrease in glucagon release in healthy controls [30]. Since hyperglycemia has no suppressive effect on glucagon release in the absence of insulin [30], the relative hyperglucagonemia and alpha cell hyperplasia observed in chronic pancreatitis are likely to be secondary to insulin deficiency. The opposite has, however, also been found to be true, i. e., decreased glucagon secretion after stimulation with arginine in patients with chronic pancreatitis [32–34]. These conflicting data on glucagon release in chronic pancreatitis confirm the heterogeneity of the populations studied.

The number of PP cells appears to be increased in chronic pancreatitis [24] and therefore a functional defect of PP cells must be assumed, since the impaired release of PP in response to hormonal and nutritional stimulation is a well established factor in chronic pancreatitis [35–37]. Some authors have reported that the impairment of the PP response corresponds to the degree of exocrine deficiency [38], but other investigators have not confirmed this strong correlation [39]. Nevertheless, a deficiency in pancreatic enzyme secretion into the duodenum seems to result in diminished PP secretion, and perfusion of the duodenum with pancreaticobiliary juice may stimulate PP release in patients with chronic pancreatitis [40].

Morphological studies have not demonstrated abnormalities in the number of D cells in chronic pancreatitis [24]. The absence of morphological changes does not exclude the possibility of functional abnormalities in somatostatin release, but data on somatostatin in chronic pancreatitis are lacking.

Table 1 summarizes the main morphological changes found in the endocrine islets in chronic pancreatitis compared with healthy subjects.

Table 1. Quantitative changes in the islet cells in chronic pancreatitis compared to healthy subjects (according to [24])

Type of islet cell studied	Quantitative change observed
beta cells	decreased to 60% of control values
alpha cells	increased in number
alpha : beta ratio	1:0.4–1:1.7
	(controls 1:3.0–1:3.5)
PP cells	increased in number
D-cells	normal number

The Relationship Between Chronic Pancreatitis and Pancreatic Diabetes

The overall incidence of impaired glucose tolerance and frank diabetes mellitus secondary to chronic pancreatitis varies between 40% and 90%. Seventy per cent of the patients with noncalcified and 90% of the patients with calcified chronic pancreatitis have impaired glucose tolerance during the follow-up; 10%–30% develop diabetes at some time [41, 42]. The mean duration between the diagnosis of chronic pancreatitis and the onset of pancreatic diabetes was reported to be between 7 and 15 years [43–45].

From the clinical point of view, diabetes induced by pancreatitis has more similarities with the juvenile type I diabetes than with type II diabetes (Table 2). Patients with diabetes and chronic pancreatitis are often young and have a rather low body weight. Serum cholesterol and -lipids are generally low [42]. In this context, it is to note that a number of studies have shown abnormal pancreatic responses to secretin and CCK in type I diabetes [46–49]. Pancreatic dysfunction with decreased secretion of amylase, trypsin, lipase, and bicarbonate is often found in type I diabetes, and the degree of dysfunction correlates with the duration of the disease [48]. Morphologically, the pancreas in type I diabetic patients is frequently atrophic and infiltrated with fat [50], so that the decreased mass of exocrine tissue might account for the exocrine functional damage. The pathophysiology and clinical relevance of these findings are under debate. Possibly, these abnormalities are related to the lack of the stimulatory action of insulin on pancreatic acini [51], but increased glucagon plasma levels with their inhibitory effects upon the exocrine pancreas [52, 53] and visceral neuropathy [54] might also be contributing factors.

Table 2. Differences between diabetes in chronic pancreatitis (dm/cp) and diabetes mellitus type II (dm type II)

	dm/cp	dm type II
age of onset	< 50 years	> 50 years
body weight	low	high
insulin sensitivity	high	low
risk of hypoglycemia	high	low
serum lipids	normal	increased
serum insulin	low	high
therapy	diet, insulin	diet, sulfonylurea

Insulin Treatment

In every patient with chronic pancreatitis, glucose tolerance should be tested regularly, so that the onset of pancreatic diabetes can be recognized early. For clinical practice, diabetes in chronic pancreatitis should be regarded as an insulinopenic diabetes, since treatment with sulfonylurea is generally not successful. Insulin sensitivity is generally not disturbed in chronic pancreatitis and treatment with insulin must be started cautiously and under clinical control especially because of the risk of hypoglycemia, which is the main clinical problem in these patients. A number of factors may account for hypoglycemia. Glucagon release is known to be an important homeostatic response to hypoglycemia in humans, and a disturbed glucagon release in chronic pancreatitis (as discussed above) or coexisting liver disease may result in prolonged hypoglycemia [55–57]. Further risk factors are prolonged alcoholism, dietary irregularities, and food/insulin asynchrony due to bad compliance and/or steatorrhea.

An interesting finding is the relative infrequency of ketosis; if diabetic coma occurs, it is rather of the hyperosmolar-non-ketotic type [55]. Vasculopathy (vascular disease, retinopathy, nephropathy) is also less frequent in pancreatic diabetes than in congenital diabetes patients when age and duration are taken into account [58, 59]. Concerning neuropathy, only few data are available [41].

Due to the complexity of pancreatic diabetes and different stages and courses of chronic pancreatitis, there is a wide variation of insulin requirements not only in different patients, but also in a single patient in the course of the disease. The necessity of beginning the therapy cautiously has already been mentioned, a general dose recommendation cannot be given. To achieve a stable metabolic situation, it is essential for there to be a good compliance with regular diet, food/insulin synchrony and no alcoholism.

Enzyme Replacement Therapy

In the case of pancreatic exocrine function, there is no doubt that steatorrhea must be treated with enzyme replacement therapy to get a better and more constant assimilation of dietary components. To investigate whether patients with diabetes in chronic pancreatitis benefit from enzyme replacement therapy even in the early stages of the disease, we performed a study in ten patients with diabetes and chronic pancreatitis (Table 3). Only two of the ten patients (Nos. 6 and 7) suffered from steatorrhea, the others had only mild to moderate exocrine insufficiency [60]. All patients were treated in a randomized double-blinded crossover trial for about 5 days with either placebo or pancreatin (6×2 capsules, 6×300 mg/d). During these days 1–4, blood glucose levels were determined seven times every day and night. On day 5, seven of the ten patients were attached to a glucose sensor and blood glucose was adjusted to 120 ng/dl until 8.00 A.M. At. 8.30 A.M., the patients received a test meal with two capsules of either placebo or pancreatin. Blood glucose was monitored continuously. Blood samples were taken ten times in the following 4 h in order to determine the levels of C peptide [61], glucagon [62], and PP [63].

Table 3. Data of patients with diabetes mellitus induced by chronic pancreatitis

| | Patient no. | | | | | | | | | |
	1	2	3	4	5	6	7	8	9	10
age at onset (y)	54	47	57	51	46	35	54	43	40	52
time from onset of chronic pancreatitis (y)	1/2	2	4	4	6	8	12	14	15	16
time from onset of diabetes mellitus (y)	1/4	2	4	1	0.5	2	4	4	13	9
total dose of insulin (U)										
mo	48	30	16	36	16	16	36	14	6	28
ev	34	16	6	24	8	8	20	10	4	26
maximal fluorescein serum levels in PLT serum test (ng/ml)	4.02	1.80	2.66	4.36	4.34	0.34	0.92	3.26	3.18	3.82
Broca index	0.90	1.05	0.95	0.73	0.78	0.78	0.82	0.88	1.08	1.04

y, years; U, units; mo, morning; ev, evening; PLT, pancreolauryl test; (see reference [60])

Figures 1–5 summarize the findings of this study. Some of the patients (Nos. 1–4, No. 7) benefited from enzyme replacement in that they responded with lower blood glucose values and others did not; the effect was therefore not statistically significant (Fig. 1). Similar curves were also found after the test meal on day 5 with continuous blood glucose monitoring (Fig. 2).

The main reason for the unaltered blood glucose levels was that an increased endogenous insulin release could not be achieved by pancreatin medication, as

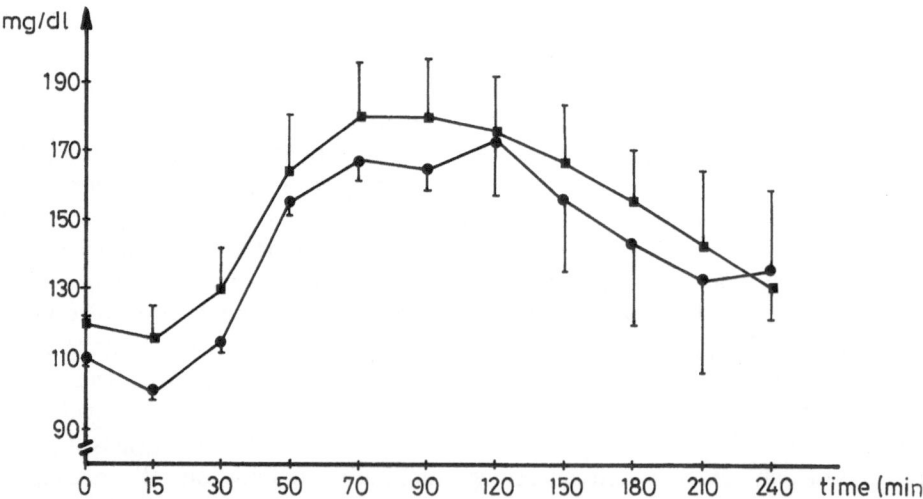

Fig. 2. Blood glucose levels means ± standard errors of the means) in seven patients with chronic pancreatitis and diabetes before and after a test meal with placebo *(squares)* or pancreatin *(circles)* medication

assessed by measuring C peptide levels (Fig. 3). We had assumed that pancreatin might be insulinotropic due to an increased incretin release. Creutzfeld and coworkers have found an increase of plasma GIP concentrations in patients with chronic pancreatitis induced by pancreatin [64]. The effect of pancreatin upon CCK plasma levels seems to be dose-dependent and is under debate; both a decrease [65] and an

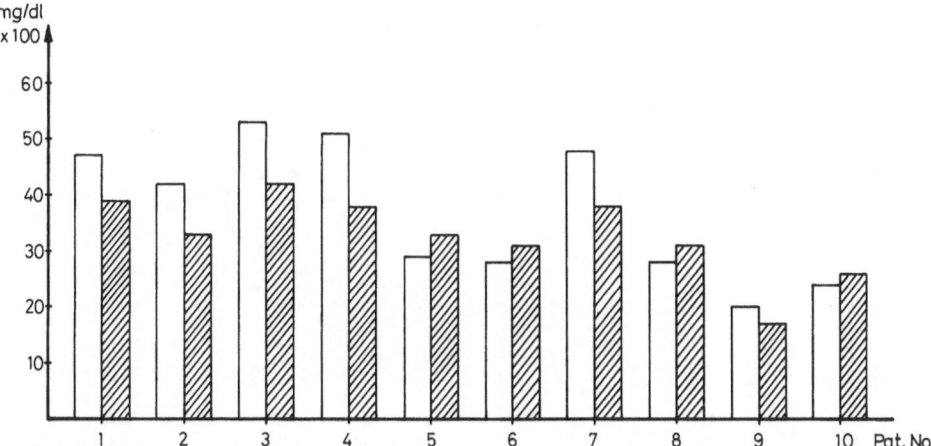

Fig. 1. Influence of 6 × 2 capsules (6 × 300 mg) pancreatin upon blood glucose levels in patients Nos. 1–10, shown as sum the of all blood glucose measurements over about 3 days (7×3 = 21 measurements). Each column n = 10; *open columns*, patients under placebo; *hatched columns*, patients under pancreatin treatment

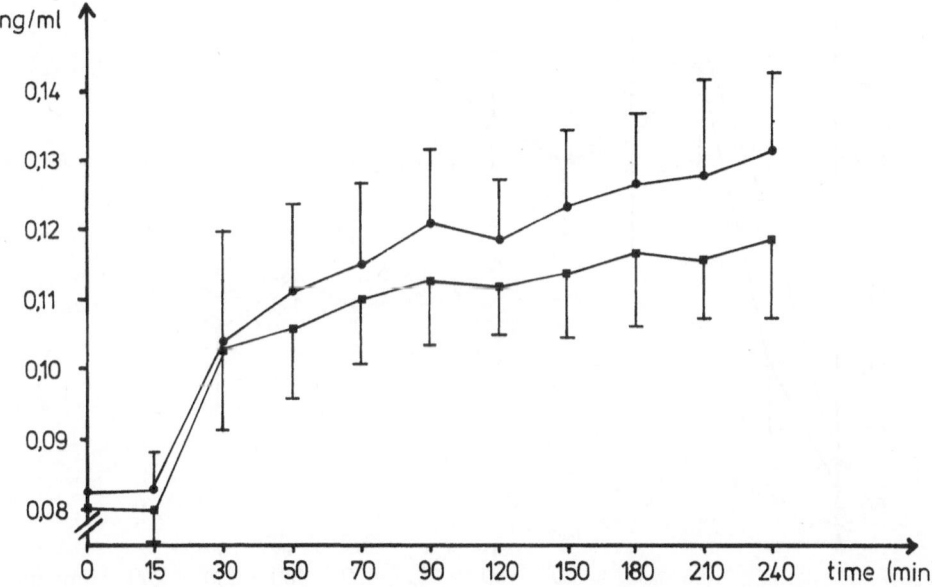

Fig. 3. Plasma C peptide levels (means ± standard errors of the means) in seven patients with chronic pancreatitis and diabetes before and after a test meal with placebo *(squares)* or pancreatin *(circles)* medication

increase [67] of CCK after the administation of pancreatin medication in chronic pancreatitis have been described. Nevertheless, if an incretin is released by enzyme replacement, it is doubtful whether this incretin can exert its insulinotropic activity in patients with pancreatic diabetes.

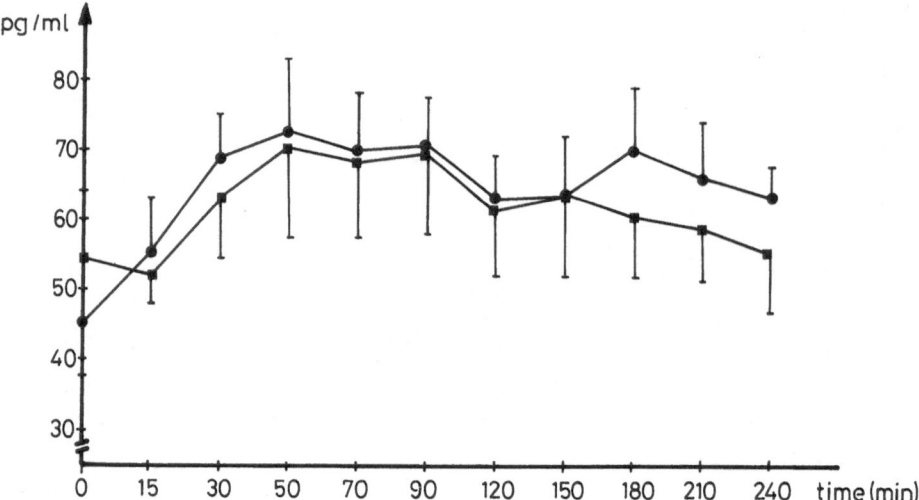

Fig. 4. Plasma glucagon levels (means ± standard errors of the means) in seven patients with chronic pancreatitis and diabetes before and after a test meal with placebo *(squares)* or pancreatin *(circles)* medication

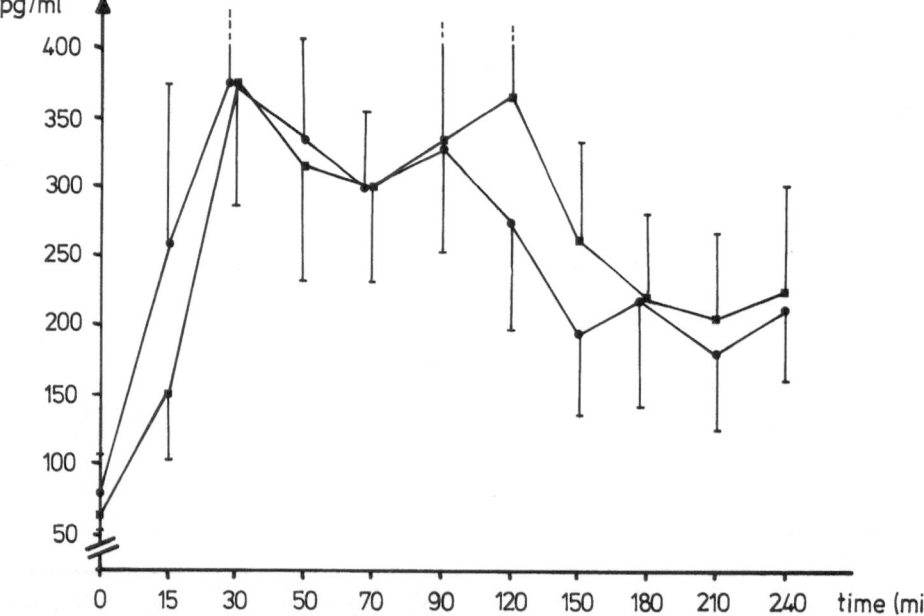

Fig. 5. Plasma PP levels (means ± standard errors of the means) in seven patients with chronic pancreatitis and diabetes before and after a test meal with placebo *(squares)* or pancreatin *(circles)* medication

Normal basal values and a moderate postprandial increase in glucagon and PP plasma levels were found in this study. There was no difference in the amounts released of either of these two hormones whether or not there was enzyme supplementation (Figs. 4, 5). A correlation between the postprandial PP response and exocrine impairment (as assessed using an indirect exocrine function test) was not found in these ten patients.

Using statistical analysis, we could not find any parameter correlating with the effect of pancreatin on blood glucose or on plasma hormones in these few patients. From the present state of knowledge, enzyme replacement continues to be strictly recommended only in those patients with clinical signs of steatorrhea. Avoidance of alcoholic beverages, dietary discipline, food/insulin synchrony, and the treatment of steatorrhea with enzyme replacement remain the four cornerstones in the management of pancreatic diabetes until new therapeutic efforts result from a better understanding of the pathophysiology of diabetes in chronic pancreatitis.

References

1. Williams JA, Goldfine ID (1986) The insulin-acinar relationship. The exocrine pancreas: biology, pathobiology, and diseases, Raven, New York, pp 347–360
2. Orci L (1982) Macro- and micro-domains in the endocrine pancreas. Diabetes 31:538–565
3. Wharton GK (1932) The blood supply of the pancreas, with special reference to that of the islands of Langerhans. Anat Rec 53:55–81
4. Ando S (1959) A study of the vascular supply in the pancreas Fukuoka Acta Med 50:4247–4274
5. Lifson N, Kramlinger KG, Mayrand RR, Lender EJ (1980) Blood flow to the rabbit pancreas with special reference to the islets of Langerhans. Gastroenterology 79:466–473
6. Dyck WP, Texter EC, Lasater JM, Higetower NC (1970) Influence of glucagon on pancreatic exocrine secretion in man. Gastroenterology 58:532–539
7. Fontana G, Costa PL, Tassari R, Labo G (1975) Effect of glucagon on pure human exocrine pancreatic secretion. Am J Gastroenterol 63:490–494
8. Creutzfeld W, Lankisch PG, Fölsch UR (1975) Hemmung der sekretin- und cholecystokinin-pankreozymininduzierten Saft- und Enzymsekretion des Pankreas und der Gallenblasenkontraktion beim Menschen durch Somatostatin. Dtsch Med Wochenschr 100:1135
9. Domschke S, Domschke W, Rösch W, et al. (1977) Inhibition by somatostatin of secretin-stimulated pancreatic secretion in man: A study with pure pancreatic juice. Scand J Gastroenterol 12:59
10. Miller TA, Tepperman FS, Fang WF, et al. (1979) Effect of somatostatin on pancreatic protein secretion induced by cholecystokinin. J Surg Res 26:488–493
11. Taylor IL, Solomon TE, Walsh JH, Grossman MI (1979) Pancreatic polypeptide: metabolism and effect on pancreatic secretion in dogs. Gastroenterology 76:524–528
12. Greenberg GR, McCloy RF, Chadwick VS, Adrian TE, Baron JH, Bloom SR (1979) Effect of bovine pancreatic polypeptide on basal pancreatic and biliary outputs in man. Am J Dig Dis 24:11–14
13. Beglinger C, Taylor IL, Grossman MI, Solomon TE (1984) Pancreatic polypeptide inhibits exocrine pancreatic responses to six stimulants. Am J Physiol 246:286–291
14. Söling HD, Unger KO (1972) The role of insulin in the regulation of alpha-amylase synthesis in the rat pancreas. Eur J Clin Invest 2:199
15. Adler G, Kern HF (1975) Regulation of exocrine pancreatic secretory process by insulin in vivo. Horm Metab Res 7:296
16. Kanno T, Saito A (1976) The potentiating influence of insulin on pancreozymin-induced hyperpolarization and amylase release in the pancreatic acinar cell. J Physiol (Lond) 261:505–521
17. Goldfine ID, Williams JA (1984) Actions of cholecystokinin and insulin on the acinar pancreas. In: Cantin M (ed) Cell biology of the secretory process. Karger, Basel, pp 389–422

18. Korc M, Sankaran H, Wong KY, Williams JA, Goldfine ID (1978) Insulin receptors in isolated mouse pancreatic acini. Biochem Biophys Res Commun 84:293–299
19. Sjödin L, Holmberg K, Lyden A (1984) Insulin receptors on pancreatic acinar cells in guinea pigs. Endocrinology 115:1102–1109
20. Zenz E, LaBarre J (1929) Contribution à l'étude des variations physiologiques de la sécrétion interne du pancréas: Relations entre les sécrétions externe et interne du pancréas. Arch Int Physiol Biochim 31:20–44
21. Creutzfeldt W (1979) The incretin concept today. Diabetologia 16:75–85
22. Brown JC, Dryburgh JR, Ross SA, Dupre J (1975) Identification and actions of gastric inhibitory polypeptide. Recent Prog Horm Res 31:487–532
23. Elahi D, Andersen DK, Brown JC, Debas H, Herhcopf RJ, Raizes GS, Tobin JD, Andres R (1979) Pancreatic alpha and beta-cell responses to GIP infusion in normal man. Am J Physiol 237:E185–E191
24. Klöppel G, Bommer G, Commandeur G, Heitz PU (1978) The endocrine pancreas in chronic pancreatitis: Immunocytochemical and ultrastructural studies. Virchows Arch [A] 377:157–174
25. Keller P, Bank S, Marks IN, O'Reilly IG (1965) Plasma insulin levels in pancreatic diabetes. Lancet 2:1211–1214.
26. Peters N, Dick AP, Hales CN, Orrell DH, Sarner M (1966) Exocrine and endocrine pancreatic function in diabetes mellitus and chronic pancreatitis. Gut 7:277–281
27. Joffe BJ, Bank S, Jackson WPU, Keller P, O'Reilly IG, Vinik AI (1968) Insulin reserve in patients with chronic pancreatitis. Lancet 2:890–892
28. Nieschlag E, Gilfrich BJ, Nagel M (1971) Insulinsekretion nach Pankreasresektion. Dtsch Med Wochenschr 96:859–862
29. Bommer G, Heitz PU, Klöppel G (1976) Immunohistologische und ultrastrukturelle Untersuchungen des endokrinen Pankreas bei chronischer Pankreatitis. Verh Dtsch Ges Pathol 60:485
30. Muller WA, Faloona GF, Unger R (1971) The effect of experimental insulin deficiency of glucagon secretion. J Clin Invest 50:1992–1999
31. Unger RH, Orci L (1977) Role of glucagon in diabetes. Arch Intern Med 137:482–491
32. Kalk WJ, Vinik AI, Bank S, et al. (1974) Glucagon responses to arginine in chronic pancreatitis. Possible pathogenic significance in diabetes. Diabetes 23:257–263
33. Kannan V, Nabarro JDN, Cotton PB (1979) Glucagon secretion in chronic pancreatitis. Horm Res 11:203–212
34. Keller U, Szöllösy E, Varga L, Gyr K (1984) Pancreatic glucagon secretion and exocrine function (BT-PABA test) in chronic pancreatitis. Dig Dis Sci 29:853–857
35. Adrian TE, Besterman HS, Mallinson CN, et al. (1979) Impaired pancreatic polypeptide release in chronic pancreatitis with steatorrhoea. Gut 20:98–101
36. Stern AI, Hansky J, Korman MG (1980) Pancreatic polypeptide after secretion: a new test for chronic pancreatitis. Gastroenterology 78:270
37. Glaser B, Vinik AI, Sive AA, et al. (1980) Plasma human pancreatic polypeptide response to administered secretin: Effects of vagotomy, cholinergic blockade and chronic pancreatitis. Clin Endocrinol Metab 50:1094–1099
38. Owyang C, Scarpello JH, Vinik AI (1982) Correlation between pancreatic enzyme secretion and plasma concentration of human pancreatic polypeptide in health and in chronic pancreatitis. Gastroenterology 83:55–62
39. Malfertheiner P, Feurle GE, Büchler M, Kemmer T, Ditschuneit H (1984) Chronische Pankreatitis: diagnostische Bedeutung des pankreatischen Polypeptids. Münch Med Wochenschr 126 [41] 1183–1185
40. Owyang C, Thueson C, Scarpello JH, Vinik AI (1981) Modulation of pancreatic polypeptide release by pancreatico-biliary secretion in health and in chronic pancreatitis. Gastroenterology 80:1246
41. Bank S, Marks IN, Vinik AI (1975) Clinical and hormonal aspects of pancreatic diabetes. Am J Gastroenterol 64:13–22
42. Bank S (1986) Chronic pancreatitis: clinical features and medical management. Am J Gastroenterol 153–166
43. Bour M (1971) Pancreatites chroniques, diabete sucré et microangiopathie specifique. Sem Hop Paris 47, 2403–2409
44. Dettwyler W (1964) Le diabéte des pancréatopathies. Semin Hôp Paris 40:1676–1682

45. Martin NM (1963) New trends in diabetes detection. Am J Nurs 63:101–103
46. Vacca J, Henke WJ, Knight WA (1964) The exocrine pancreas in diabetes mellitus. Ann Intern Med 61:242–247
47. Domschke W, Tympner F, Domschke S, Demling L (1975) Exocrine pancreatic function in juvenile diabetics. Dig Dis Sci 20:309–312
48. Frier BM, Saunders JHB, Wormsley KG, Bouchier IAD (1976) Exocrine pancreatic function in juvenile-onset diabetes mellitus. Gut 17:685–691
49. Lankisch PG, Manthey G, Otto J, Koop H, Talaulicar M, Willms B, Creutzfeldt W (1982) Exocrine pancreatic function in insulin-dependent diabetes mellitus. Digestion 25:211–216
50. Gepts W (1965) Pathologic anatomy of the pancreas in juvenile diabetes mellitus. Diabetes 14:619–633
51. Henderson JR, Daniel PM, Fraser PA (1981) The pancreas as a single organ: the influence of the endocrine upon the exocrine part of the gland. Gut 22:158–167
52. Sato M, Yamamoto K, Mayama H, Yamashiro Y (1984) Exocrine pancreatic function in diabetic children. J Pediatr Gastroenterol Nutr 3:415–420
53. Unger RH, Dobbs RE, Orci L (1978) Insulin, glucagon, and somatostatin secretion in the regulation of metabolism. Ann Rev Physiol 40:307–343
54. El-Newihi H, Staples J, Dooley CP, Suad C, Zeidler A, Valenzuela JE (1984) Exocrine pancreatic function in patients with diabetic diarrhea. Dig Dis Sci 29:A-8
55. Bank S (1981) Acute and chronic pancreatitis. In: Dent TL (ed) Pancreatic disease diagnosis and therapy. Grune and Stratton, New York, pp 167–188
56. Pitchumoni CS (1984) Special problems of tropical pancreatitis. Clin Gastroenterol 13 (3):941–959
57. Marks IN, Bank S (1976) Chronic pancreatitis, relapsing pancreatitis, pancreatic lithiasis and calcification of the pancreas. Part 2. Clinical aspects. In: Bockus III (ed) Gastroenterology. 3rd edn. vol III. Saunders, Philadelphia, pp 1052–1069
58. Horiuchi N, Kitamura T, Nakagawa F (1971) Clinical pattern of diabetes complicated by pancreatic cancer and lithiasis. Jap J Clin Med 29:2146–2151
59. Tiengo A, Segato T, Briani G, Setti A, Del Prato S, Devidé A, Padovan D, Virgili F, Crepaldi G (1983) The presence of retinopathie in patients with secondary diabetes following pancreatectomy or chronic pancreatitis. Diabetes Care 6:570–579
60. Malfertheiner P, Büchler M, Müller A, Ditschuneit H (1987) Fluorescein dilaurate serum test: a rapid tubeless pancreatic function test. Pancreas 2:53–60
61. Beyer J, Krause U, Cordes U (1979) C-peptide: its biogenesis, structure, determination and clinical significance. Giornale Italiano Chimica Clinica 4: [Suppl 1]:9–22
62. Unger RH, Eisentraut AM, Melall MS, Keller S, Lanz HC, Madison LL (1959) Glucagon antibodies and their use for immunoassay of glucagon. Proc Soc Exp Biol Med 102:621–623
63. Taylor IL (1987) RIA of the pancreatic polypeptide family. J Clin Immunoassay 10:43–49
64. Creutzfeldt W, Ebert R (1986) The enteroinsular axis. The exocrine pancreas: biology, pathobiology, and diseases. Raven, New York, pp 333–346
65. Slaff J, Wolfe MM, Toskes PP (1984) Pancreatic extract inhibition of plasma CCK levels. Dig Dis Sci 29:A-31
66. Mössner J, Back T, Regner U, Fischbach W (1989) Plasma-Cholezystokininspiegel bei chronischer Pankreatitis. Z Gastroenterol 27:401–405
67. Maschee AAM, Jansen JBMJ, Cossteus FHM, Lamers CBHW (1989) Reversible gallbladder dysfunction in severe pancreatic insufficiency. Gut 30:866–872

Interventional Treatment

Direct Cholangiopancreatoscopy and Use of Pancreatic Duct Stents and Drains in the Treatment of Pancreatitis

R. A. Kozarek[1]

Miniscopes

Background

Small-caliber endoscopes that could be passed through prototype duodenoscopes to visualize the pancreatic and bile ducts were first developed by the Japanese in the early 1970s [1]. Subsequent reports from Europe and Japan were published documenting the feasibility of this technology [2, 3], but widespread application was never realized. Instrument costs and fragility and the development and utilization of computed tomography and ultrasound imaging precluding the need for more invasive endoscopic procedures were all reasons why subsequent miniscope development languished [4].

Recently there has been renewed interest in the utilization of instruments which can directly visualize the pancraticobiliary tree. This is based upon the developing realization that other diagnostic studies including ERCP, ultrasound, magnetic resonance imaging, computed tomography, and angiography remain imperfect for diagnosis. Thus, the diagnosis of early pancreatic malignancy remains elusive. Miniscopes have the potential to define precancerous or dysplastic ductal changes, particularly if cytology brushes and biopsy forceps can be further miniaturized. In addition to diagnosis, the potential to apply directed therapy within the pancreatic or bile duct may be expanded with direct visualization capabilities [5, 6]. A case in point is the development of tunable dye and q-switched Nd-YAG lasers that can effect biliary or pancreatic duct stone fracture via energy transmitted down a 250-μm quartz fiber [7, 8]. Similar fibers could be utilized to transmit laser energy to treat cholangiocarcinomas or obstructing pancreatic duct neoplasms. Moreover, directional instruments have the potential to be utilized to pass quidewires through tight stenoses or even into the gallbladder. Balloon dilation, insertion of nasoduct or gallbladder drains, and stent placement could thereby be facilitated.

Because of the above, I have evaluated 13 prototype miniscopes over the past 4 years (Fig. 1) [5, 9]. Instruments could be divided into visual probes which utilize single quartz fibers for illumination and visulization and miniaturizations of conventional endoscopes in which glass fibers are arranged in parallel. Whereas the former are relatively cheap to produce, acute angulation can result in fiber fracture and complete optical blackout.

---

[1] Chief of Gastroenterology, Virginia Mason Clinic, PO Box 900, Seattle, WA 98111, USA

Chronic Pancreatitis
Ed. by Beger, Büchler, Ditschuneit, and Malfertheiner
© Springer-Verlag Berlin Heidelberg 1990

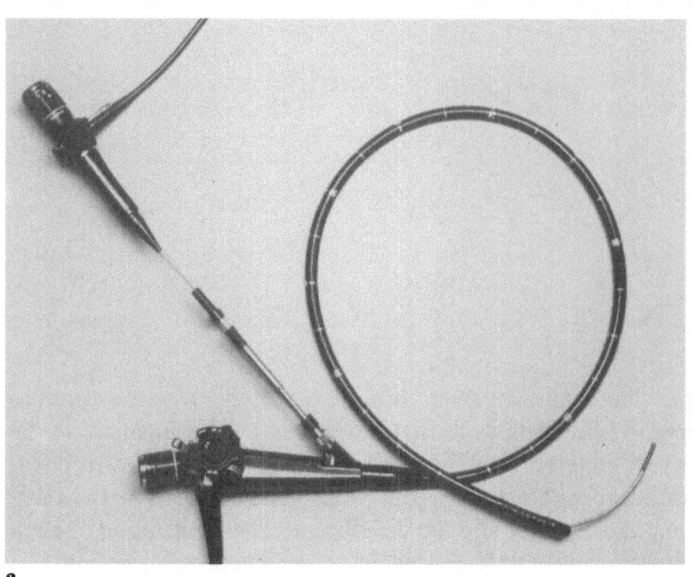

a

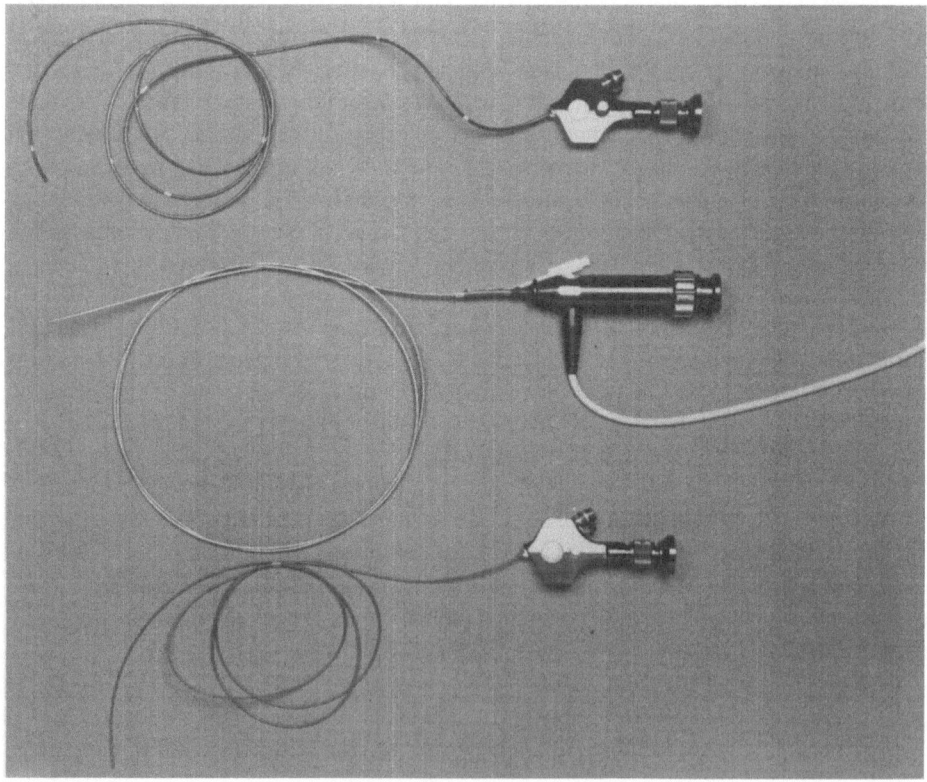

b

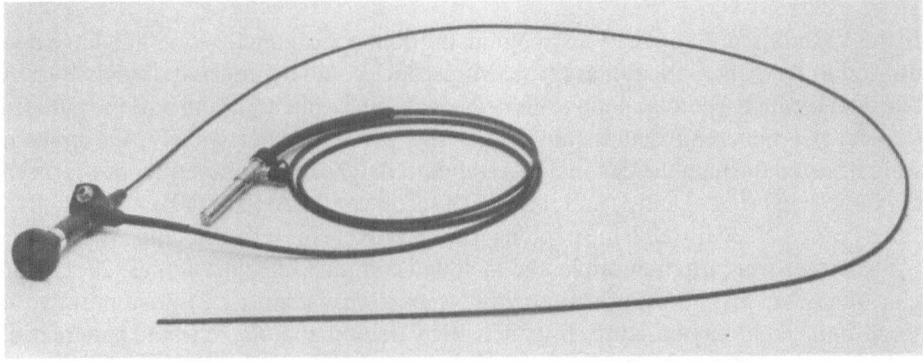

Fig. 1a–d. Miniscopes. **a** an 11-F Olympus Ultra-thin passed through 4.2-mm channel therapeutic duodenoscope. **b** 7-F Reichert *(top)*, 6-F Microvasive *(middle)*, and 5-F Reichert *(bottom)* miniscopes. Microvasive instrument is visual probe and has a fixed eyepiece with disposable shafts. **c** 180-cm, 7-F Pentax miniscope with 3-F instrument channel. **d** 6-F visual probe, American Edwards

Types

Instruments were produced by Schott Fiberoptics (formerly Reichert), Pentax, Microvasive, American-Edwards, and Olympus and ranged in diameter from 1 to 14.1 F and in length from 15–200 cm. Only the larger Olympus instruments had two-way tip deflection, and the 14.1 F Olympus Ultrathin was also the only one to include automatic suction and air-water capacities. Instruments smaller than 5 mm had no working channel.

Indications

In the 100 miniscope applications at our institution, approximately one-half have been utilized in the pancreaticobiliary tree. Miniscopes could be inserted directly into the bile duct through a percutaneous biliary drainage or T-tube tract and into the pancreatic duct if a pancreaticocutaneous fistula was present. Alternatively, the majority were inserted through the channel of a standard diagnostic, therapeutic, or prototype duodenoscope (Fig. 2 and 3) and required a second endoscopist's presence. Finally, a subset were passed through the papilla intraoperatively prior to scheduled septotomy.

Diagnoses were often multiple and included common bile duct stones, 20; cholangiocarcinoma, 5; sclerosing cholangitis, 4; papillary stenosis, 6; postoperative or stone-induced biliary stricture, 6; pancreatic carcinoma, 5; and chronic pancreatitis, 8. Eight attempts were unsuccessful, and visualization was judged to be suboptimal in fully one-third of the successful cases. Despite this, we were able to visualize biliary calculi missed at time of sphincterotomy, clarify the etiology of biliary strictures, and obtain tissue diagnoses of pancreatic carcinoma [10]. Of particular note are the ductal ectasia, calculi, proteinaceous debris, and ductal irregularity noted in the setting of chronic pancreatitis.

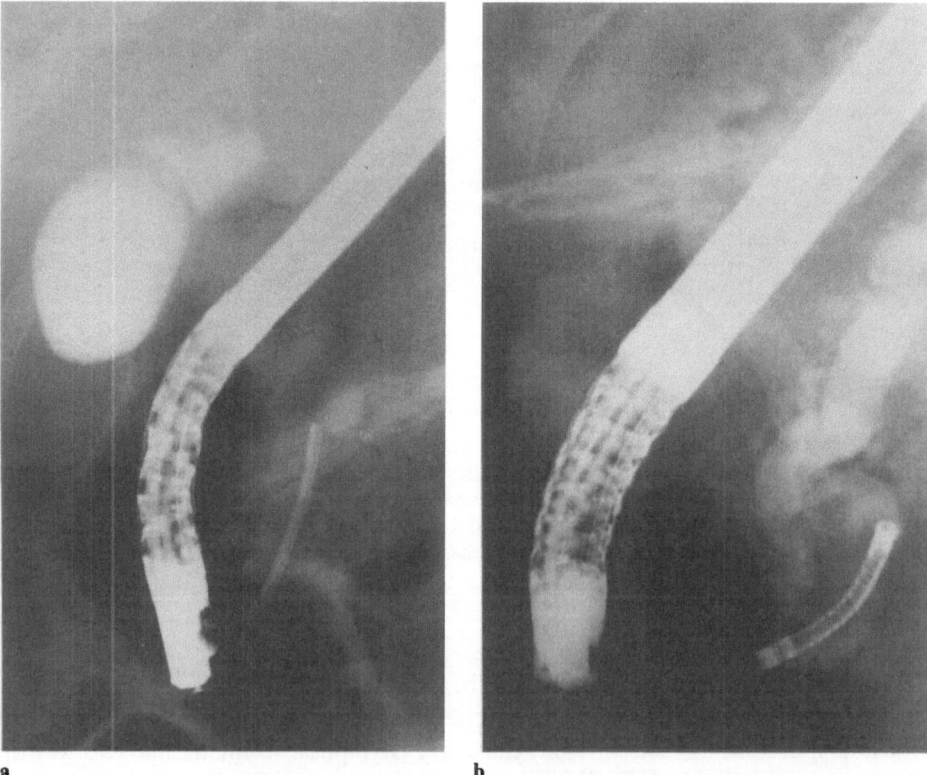

a   b

Fig. 2a, b. Patient with chronic pancreatitis. **a** 7-F miniscope passed to level of genu. **b** 11-F miniscope in proximal pancreatic duct in setting of chronic pancreatitis. Sphincterotomy done

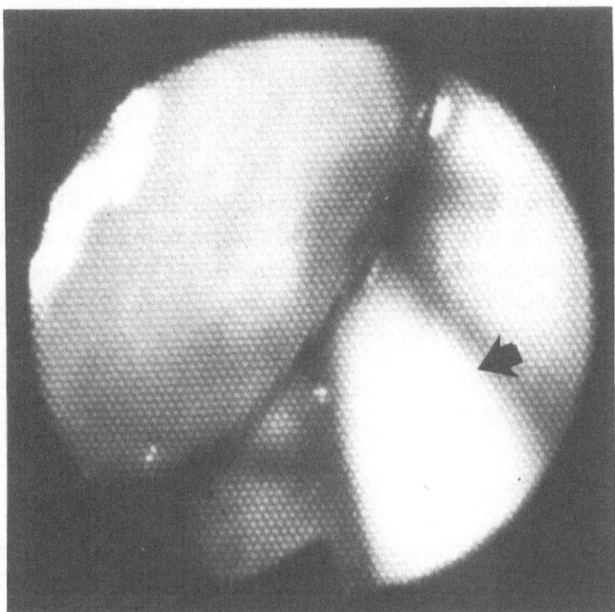

Fig. 3. Nasobiliary drain
(arrow). Note calculus 1–8
o'clock position

In addition to the improved diagnostic capabilities alluded to above and also confirmed in several recent publications [11–14], miniscopes have also been utilized therapeutically. Thus, we have fractured a pancreatic duct calculus using energy from a coumarin green tunable dye laser transmitted through a miniscope, used them to selectively cannulate pancreatic ductal stenoses, and in conjunction with other investigators at Duke and Harvard successfully fractured 13 of 14 large common bile duct calculi [6, 7, 15].

Limitations

Despite the above, all but the larger instruments were exceedingly fragile, and instruments larger than 7 F could not be passed into a normal-caliber pancreatic duct or bile duct without initial sphincterotomy. In particular, fused bundle systems had a tendency to fracture acutely, leading to visual blackout when angulated over the duodenoscope elevator. The use of finer fibers and more durable sheath material and passage over guidewires or through protective sheaths may enhance durability. Because visual probes can be produced for approximately one-tenth the cost of parallel fiber bundles, another approach that has been developed includes the use of a permanent eyepiece in conjunction with a disposable shaft of variable length and diameter, depending upon the indications for which the instrument is utilized.

Whereas the largest Olympus instrument had two-way tip deflection and automatic air-water insufflation, none of the other miniscopes was so equipped. This required passage over a guidewire for most and air or saline introduction through the working channel. The former could be problematic and occasionally led to piecemeal visualization of the duct. The latter was essential in the setting of bile or viscous pancreatic juice.

Future

Despite the list of technical limitations delineated above, further instrument refinements to include dependable directionality and the miniaturization of accessory equipment should ensure the miniscope's resurgence. Such instruments will likely play a limited but definable role in the future of diagnostic and therapeutic pancreaticobiliary endoscopy.

Pancreatic Drains and Stents

Overview

In contrast to the investigational character of miniscopes, endoscopically placed biliary drains and stents have received widespread application for benign and malignant strictures, biliary fistulas, and occasionally choledocholithiasis [16–19]. Temporary pancreatic drains and semipermanent stents have also been placed, but little data are available regarding insertion technique, usage patterns, clinical results, or side effects.

To date, two major papers have appeared in the literature. McCarthy et al. [20] were successful in placing 19 stents through the minor sphincter and into the dorsal pancreatic duct in 22 patients with chronic abdominal pain and pancreas divisum. Seventeen were felt to have a significant improvement in their pain, and stents were exchanged at 4–6 month intervals. In a second group of 15 patients with recurrent or chronic pancreatitis and a dominant stricture, approximately one-half improved following stent placement.

Huibregtse et al. [21] in turn, utilized pancreatic drains and stents in 32 patients with a variety of problems including patients with pancreatic duct stones, dominant strictures, ductal disruptions, or pseudocysts. Those patients with chronic pain as their main problem fared significantly less well than those with bouts of relapsing pancreatitis. Complications in the latter series included two episodes of pancreatitis, development of a pancreatic abscess secondary to an occluded stent in two patients, stent-induced ulceration on the contralateral duodenal wall in two patients, and a single mortality related to duodenal perforation following a pancreatic sphincterotomy. McCarthy et al. [20] in turn, had two episodes of pain exacerbation and two instances of stent migration into the pancreas.

Indications

Over the past 2 years, we have placed drains and stents into the pancreatic duct in a heterogenous patient group with both ongoing or recurrent, acute as well as chronic pancreatitis (Figs. 4–7). Thirty-five patients had six nasopancreatic drains and 38

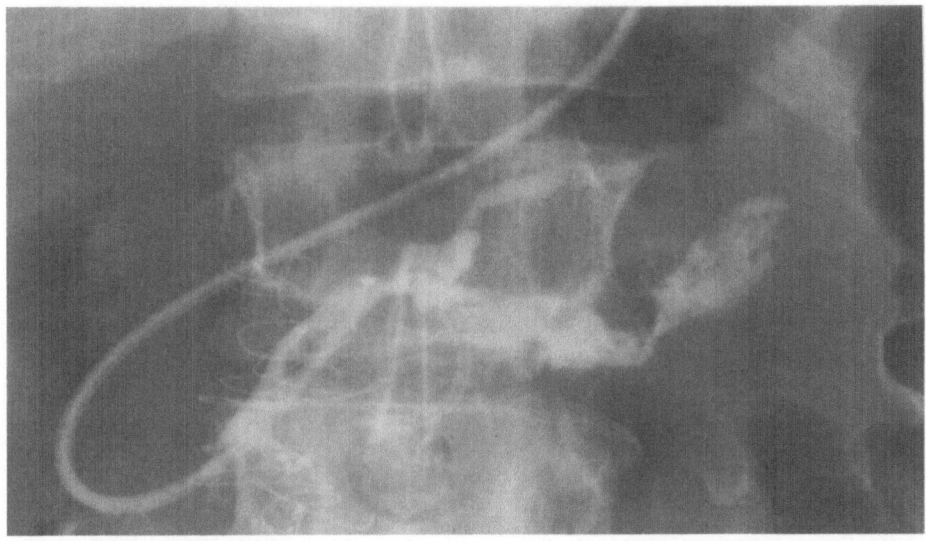

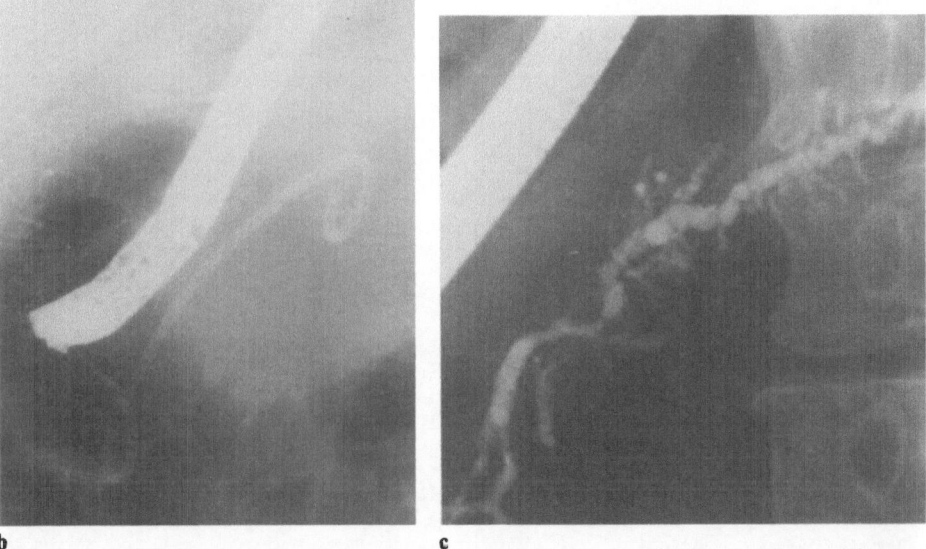

Fig. 4a–c. Patient with ductal disruption with pseudocyst in chronic pancreatitis. **a** Pigtail of 7-F stent into cyst cavity. **b** Double pigtail stent placed after 4 days of nasocyst drainage. **c** Pancreatogram obtained immediately after stent removal, stent in place for 6 weeks. Changes of chronic pancreatitis

internal pancreatic stents placed through the papilla. Indications have included a symptomatic disrupted duct/pseudocyst, 11; hypertensive pancreatic sphincter with recurrent pancreatitis, 5, or chronic pancreatic type pain without hyperamylasemia, 6; dominant ductal stricture, 7; pancreas divisum with relapsing pancreatitis attacks, 5; and villous adenoma of the papilla, 1.

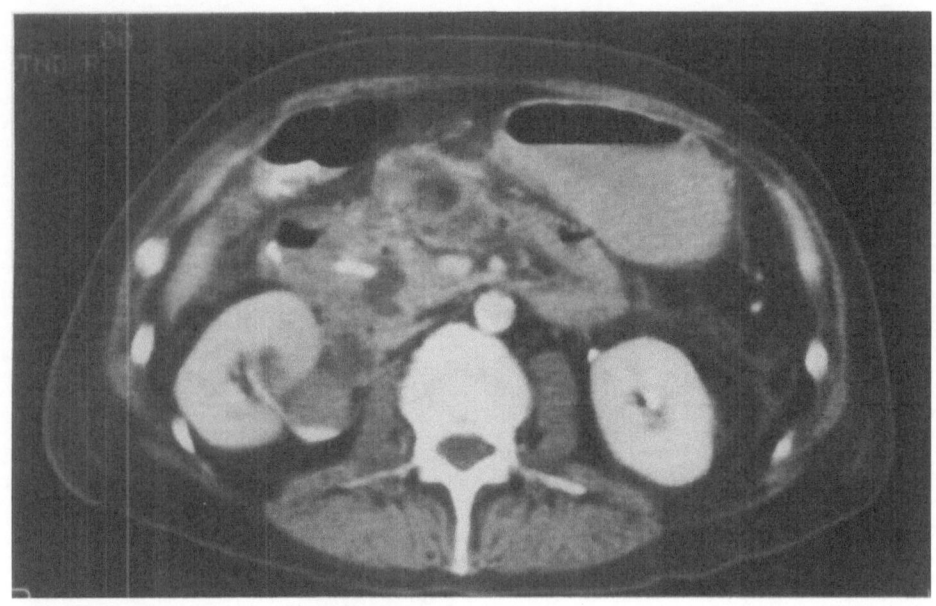

a

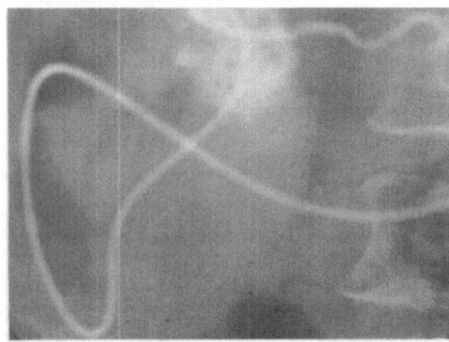

b

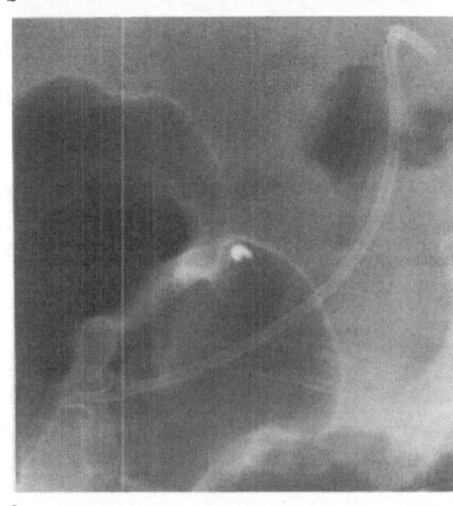

d

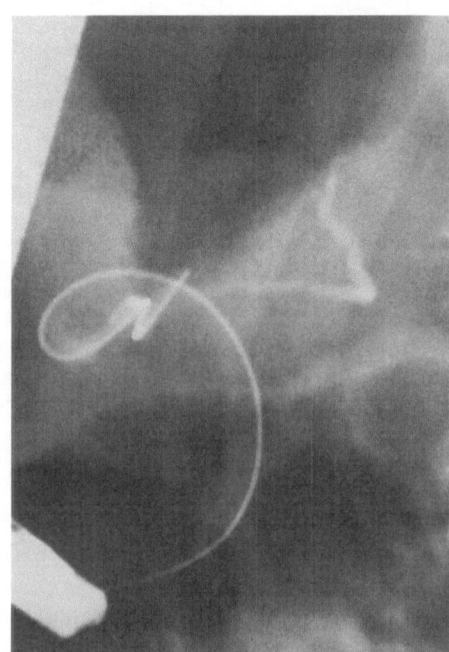

c

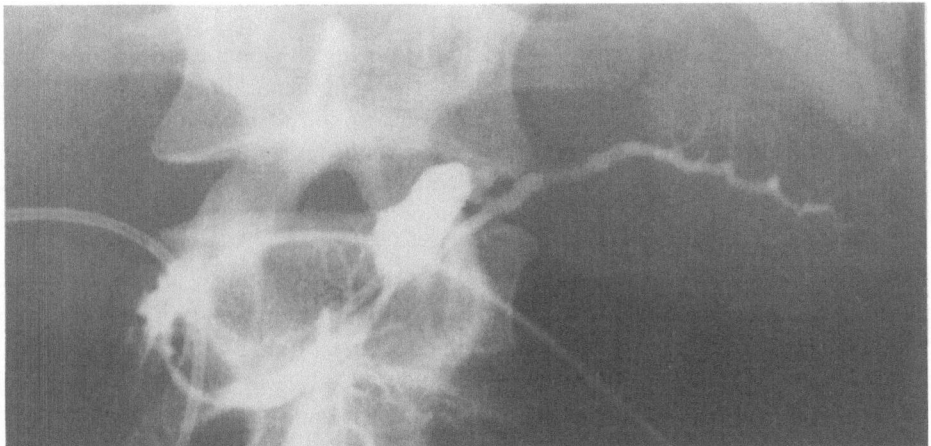

Fig. 6. Nasopancreatic drain at site of disrupted duct/traumatic pseudocyst. Note percutaneous biliary tube *(right)* placed for hemobilia

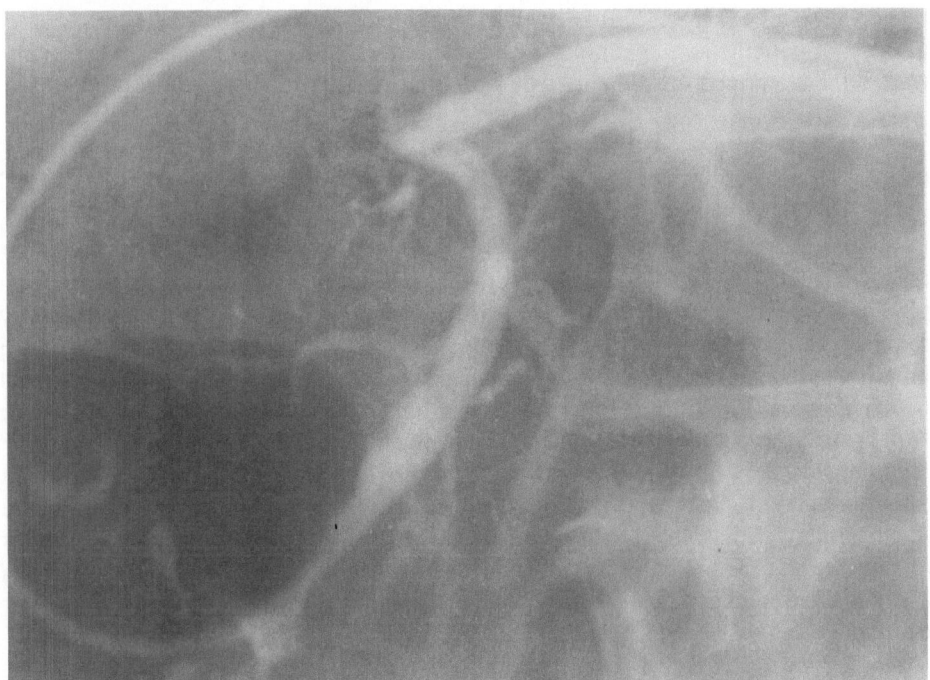

Fig. 7. Nasopancreatic drain in patient who underwent endoscopic resection of papilla of Vater. Drain pulled at 24 h

Fig. 5a–d. Patient with ongoing pancreatic phlegmon. **a** CT scan 6 weeks after development of post-ERCP pancreatitis at another institution. **b** Nasopancreatic drain at genu and site of ongoing ductal disruption. **c** Guidewire beyond genu. Drain was pulled at 6 days and replaced by stent **(d)** to occlude disrupted duct. **d** 5-F pancreatic duct stent. Clinical response was dramatic, and patient discharged 2 days post-stent on solid food. Stent retrieved at 6 weeks

Technique

Technically, patients had conventional ERCP utilizing an Olympus JF 1-T or JF 4.2-mm channel duodenoscope after premedication with meperidine and/or diazepam and cefotetan antibiotic precoverage. Ductal disruption with pseudocyst formation was treated with free cannulation through the papilla and guidewire passage directly into the cyst. Alternatively, the guidewire could be passed beyond the ductal disruption and into the distal duct if the cyst was small (< 2 cm). Larger collections were initially drained using a 350 cm long 6- or 7- F drain (Wilson-Cook Medical, Winston-Salem NC, USA) directly into the cyst, followed by scope removal and drain transposition to the nose. Drainage was continued until cyst drainage was negligible, and follow-up contrast cystogram confirmed reduction in size to 1–2 cm. Thereafter, a 5 to 7-F polyethylene stent with additional barbs and side holes was placed across the level of disruption and left in place for an additional 6–8 weeks prior to removal.

In patients who had previously undergone surgical sphincteroplasty or spincterotomy but had a residual hypertensive pancreatic duct sphincter mechanism as determined by pancreaticobiliary manometry, plus relapsing pancreatitis or chronic pancreatic-type pain, 5-F stents were placed beyond the genu using an ERCP catheter as a pushing tube. These stents as well as those placed into the dorsal pancreatic duct in divisum patients and beyond a dominant stenosis in chronic pancreatitis patients were either removed or exchanged at 4-month intervals.

Clinical Results

Published as a smaller series in 1989 [22] the results of pancreatic drain and stent placement have been encouraging. Ten of the original 11 pseudocysts were completely drained and pancreatic reconstituted ducts. Four of these subsequently required surgery, however: one residual pseudocyst, one recurrent pseudocyst at 6 months, one ongoing pancreatic-type pain, and one liver abscess. Of the 11 patients with hypertensive sphincter, four of the six with relapsing pancreatitis have improved, and three of these have had septotomy. In contrast, none of the patients with chronic pain improved. Four of the five patients with divisum improved, and one has had a minor sphincteroplasty which has stenosed and is again being stented. Five of the seven patients with isolated strictures have had decreased pain and recurrent episodes of pancreatitis. The single patient who had resection of his papilla for a villous adenoma had an uneventful course with the nasopancreatic drain placed to assure that edema did not occlude his pancreatic duct.

Complications. There were two minor flares of pancreatitis and four stents passed spontaneously at a mean of 1 month (range, 7 days–3 months). Nine of the stents occluded, leading to definable ductal changes in six: four diffuse dilations, one formation of a pseudocyst in the pancreatic tail, and one enlargement and infection of an existing pseudocyst. Both pseudocyst complications and three of the cases of ductal dilation resolved with stent exchange or removal. In addition to the above, an additional three patients, all of whom had normal-appearing proximal pancreatic ducts prior to stenting, developed areas of stenosis and side branch ectasia, probably secondary to side branch occlusion by the stent. Endoscopically resembling chronic pancreatitis, two of three ERCPs have normalized by 6 months, and the third has been left with some degree of residual but improving stenosis.

This series confirms that both stents and drains can be utilized in the pancreatic duct for a variety of pancreatic inflammatory conditions. Such conduits proved most useful in draining small pseudocysts and treating disrupted ducts. Because of their small diameter, as well as the complications noted in both this and the Amsterdam series, I would not at this time recommend their use in large or complex pseudocysts. Stents also proved useful as a diagnostic tool in the setting of hypertensive pancreatic duct sphincter mechanism and acute relapsing pancreatitis associated with pancreas divisum. We have subsequently sent a number of these patients to surgery, although recent reports suggest that periodic stent exchange for 1 year in the latter group is associated with markedly fewer pancreatitis episodes for up to 1 year following stent removal [23]. Finally, stents seemed to be useful in the setting of chronic pancreatitis and a dominant stricture. We have used this information to recommend surgery in several patients and to periodically exchange stents in several other high-risk individuals.

Future

While therapeutically dramatic in a significant number of patients, the side effects related to stent placement could also be dramatic. To this end, trade-out prior to occlusion seems desirable. Moreover, further work is needed to define the etiology of the frightening but apparently reversible duct stenoses and ectasias noted in 9% of patients in this series, all of whom had a patent stent at retrieval [24]. Additional side holes, softer material, shorter stents, stents of small diameter, and shorter placement periods may all factor in their prevention.

Further data are needed prior to widespread application of this technique.

References

1. Takekoshi T, Mariyama M, Sugiyama N, et al. (1975) Retrograde cholangiopancreatoscopy (in Japanese). Gastroenterol Endosc 17:678–683
2. Rösch W, Koch H, Demling L (1976) Peroral cholangioscopy. Endoscopy 8:172–173
3. Nakajima M, Akasaka Y, Yamaguchi K (1978) Direct endoscopic visualization of the bile and pancreatic duct systems by peroral cholangiopancreatoscopy (PCPS). Gastrointest Endosc 24:141–145
4. Kozarek RA (1989) Direct cholangiopancreatoscopy. In: Jacobs I (ed) ERCP. Diagnostic and therapeutic applications. Elsevier, New York, pp 251–262
5. Kozarek RA (1988) Miniscopes – a technology in search of an application. J Clin Gastroenterol 10:475–478
6. Kozarek RA, Ball TJ, Lowe DE (1988) Therapeutic uses of miniscopes (Abstr). Gastrointest Endosc 34:205
7. Ell CH, Lux G, Hochberger J, et al. (1988) Laser lithotripsy of common bile duct stones. Gut 29:746–751
8. Kozarek RA, Low DE, Ball TJ (1988) Tunable dye laser lithotripsy: in vitro studies and in vivo treatment of choledocholithiasis. Gastrointest Endosc 34:418–420

9. Kozarek RA (1990) Miniscopes: technology that bridges subspecialties. Ann Otol Rhinol Laryngol (in press)
10. Kozarek RA (1988) Direct cholangioscopy and pancreatoscopy at time of endoscopic retrograde cholangiopancreatography. Am J Gastroenterol 83:55–57
11. Bar-Meir S, Rotmensch S (1987) A comparison between peroral choledochoscopy and endoscopic retrograde cholangiopancreatography. Gastrointest Endosc 33:13–14
12. Bar-Meir S, Rotmensch S (1984) Investigation of obstructive jaundice by an ultra-thin caliber endoscope: a new technique for potential use in pregnancy. Annu J Obstet Gynecol 150:1003–1004
13. Ponchon T, Chavaillon A, Ayela P, et al. (1988) Retrograde biliary endoscopy for biopsy of stenoses and for lithotripsy (Abstr). Gastrointest Endosc 34:191
14. Riemann JF, Kohler B, Harloff M, Weber J (1988) Peroral cholangioscopy – an improved method in the diagnoses of common bile duct diseases (Abstr). Gastroenterology 99:37
15. Cotton PB, Putnam WS, Weinreth J, Kozarek R, et al. (1989) Endoscopic laser lithotripsy of large bile duct stones (Abstr). Gastrointest Endosc 35:163
16. Siegel JH, Snady H (1986) The significance of endoscopically placed prostheses in the management of biliary obstruction due to carcinoma of the pancreas: results of nonoperative decompression in 277 patients. Am J Gastroenterol 81:634–641
17. Huibregtse K, Katon RM, Coene PP, Tytgat GNJ (1986) Endoscopic palliative treatment in pancreatic cancer. Gastrointest Endosc 32:334–338
18. Brandabur JJ, Kozarek RA, Ball TJ, et al. (1988) Nonoperative versus operative treatment of obstructive jaundice in pancreatic cancer – cost and survival analysis. Am J Gastroenterol 83:1132–1139
19. Cotton PB, Forbes A, Leung JWC, Dineen L (1987) Endoscopic stenting for long-term treatment of large bile duct stones: 2–5 year follow-up. Gastrointest Endosc 33:411–412
20. McCarthy J, Geenen JE, Hogan WJ (1988) Preliminary experience with endoscopic stent placement in benign pancreatic diseases. Gastrointest Endosc 34:16–18
21. Huibregtse K, Schneider B, Vrij AA, Tytgat GNJ (1988) Endoscopic pancreatic drainage in chronic pancreatitis. Gastrointest Endosc 34:9–15
22. Kozarek RA, Patterson DJ, Ball TJ, Traverso LW (1989) Endoscopic placement of pancreatic stents and drains in the management of pancreatitis. Ann Surg 209:261–266
23. Prabhu M, Geenen JE, Hogan WJ, et al. (1989) Role of endoscopic stent placement in the treatment of acute recurrent pancreatitis associated with pancreas divisum (Abstr). Gastrointest Endosc 35:165
24. Kozarek RA (1989) Pancreatic stents can induce ductal changes consistent with chronic pancreatitis (Abstr). Gastrointest Endosc 35:191

Nonoperative Management of Pancreatic Pseudocysts: Selective Expectant Management

M. G. Sarr and G. J. Vitas[1]

Introduction

The development of a persistent pancreatic pseudocyst is generally considered to be a complication which requires operative intervention. Such current surgical "dictum" has arisen from retrospective reviews of patients who have been treated surgically, often under emergent conditions, for pancreatic pseudocysts [2, 6, 8, 9]. Because these series involve patients treated operatively, they entail an obvious bias, making it difficult or impossible to ascertain the natural history of pancreatic pseudocyst disease from the published literature. The one prospective study conducted by Bradley et al. [5] followed a population consisting largely of inner city alcoholics who developed an ultrasound-documented pancreatic pseudocyst. As with other studies of patients with acute pancreatitis [1, 3, 4], about 40% of the "pseudocysts" resolved within 6 weeks; thereafter, however, few resolved and a large percentage of patients (17 of 30) developed a significant complication related to the pseudocyst. Because this seemed to be at variance with our experience, we reviewed our results with the management of pancreatic pseudocysts at the Mayo Clinic in an attempt to better define the natural history of pancreatic pseudocysts in a more representative patient population.

Methods

The medical records of all consecutive patients seen at the Mayo Clinic with a diagnosis of pancreatic pseudocyst from 1980 through 1985 were reviewed retrospectively. Multiple clinical and laboratory parameters were abstracted, including etiology, underlying or previous pancreatic disease, clinical presentation, hospital course, and development of complications. Follow-up was conducted by telephone interview with the patient, the next of kin (if deceased), and, when necessary, with the home physician concerning the development of related complications, the need for surgery, or resolution of the pseudocyst. Attempts were made to obtain radiographic documentation of pseudocyst size on follow-up whenever possible. However, because our practice is primarily on a referral basis, radiographic surveillance of patients discharged with pancreatic pseudocysts was incomplete and was conducted at the discretion of the home physician.

---

[1] Department of Surgery, Mayo Clinic and Mayo Foundation, 200 First Street S.W., Rochester, MN 55905, USA

Chronic Pancreatitis
Ed. by Beger, Büchler, Ditschuneit, and Malfertheiner
© Springer-Verlag Berlin Heidelberg 1990

Results

From 1980 through 1985, we treated 114 patients with pancreatic pseudocysts documented by an objective imaging test (ultrasound, computerized tomography, endoscopic retrograde pancreatography). Patients were seen either in an outpatient setting or during hospitalization. Because of clinically significant symptoms related to the pancreatic pseudocyst, 46 patients underwent *primary* operative therapy. The remaining patients were treated expectantly at initial presentation either because of the lack of significant symptoms, or because the pseudocyst was related to coexistent acute pancreatitis, and the treating physicians elected to observe the patient for potential resolution. Patients with asymptomatic or minimally symptomatic pseudocysts were generally managed expectantly without operative, percutaneous, or endoscopic invasive intervention.

Characteristics of Pseudocysts

Sixty-eight patients over this 5-year interval were managed expectantly, including 48 men and 20 women with a mean age of 46 years (range, 8–81 years). The presumed etiology of the pseudocyst was related to alcoholic pancreatitis in 37%, gallstones in 18%, trauma in 6%, familial pancreatitis in 3%, and was of unknown cause in 35%. Of these 68 patients, 35% were hospitalized for acute pancreatitis, during which the pseudocyst was first recognized. The mean size of the pseudocysts was 5 cm (range, 2–30 cm); 10% (seven patients) had pseudocysts greater than 10 cm. The pseudocysts appeared as single collections in 66% and as multiple, separate collections in the remaining 34%; 33% were multiloculated and 23% contained "debris," i.e., were filled with a nonhomogeneous fluid-density and particulate matter on CT or ultrasound. At the time of pseudocyst recognition, the best estimate of cyst age (time from a documented event such as acute pancreatitis, trauma, etc.) was less than 2 weeks in 12%, 2–6 weeks in 16%, 6–12 weeks in 12%, greater than 12 weeks in 29%, and unknown or indeterminant in 26%. The pseudocysts(s) involved the anatomic head/neck of the gland in 60%, the body in 32%, and the tail of the gland in 46%.

At the time of presentation, the majority of patients (87%) had an element of abdominal pain; however, this was judged to be severe only in those patients with coexistent acute pancreatitis. A minority had some complaints of nausea and vomiting, early satiety, or weight loss. Hyperamylasemia was present in 53%. On physical examination, fever was present in 13%, a mass in 22%, and in those patients without acute pancreatitis, the physical examination was essentially normal.

Outcome of Expectant Management – Early and Late Complications

With a mean follow-up of 46 months, 44 of these 68 patients (65%) have been managed successfully with a nonoperative, noninterventional approach. One patient admitted with severe acute pancreatitis died of multiple organ system failure related to the pancreatitis. Of the remaining 23 patients who eventually underwent operation, not all were operated on for complications related to the pancreatic pseudocyst.

Indeed, catastrophic complications related directly to the pseudocyst occurred in only six of 68 patients (9%), including intracystic hemorrhage in two, perforation in three, and sepsis/pseudocyst infection in one. Five of these six patients required operation, and all recovered; one patient with hemorrhage was successfully treated by angiographic embolization of a bleeding site in the wall of the pseudocyst. Thus, the incidence of significant, catastrophic complications related to the expectant management of these 68 selected patients with documented pancreatic pseudocysts was only 9%.

Overall, other complications related to either the pseudocyst, the associated acute pancreatitis, or progression of underlying chronic pancreatitis developed in another 13 patients (19%), ten of whom eventually underwent operative therapy for these problems (Table 1). In addition, 13 other patients underwent operation because of development of pain believed related to the pseudocyst, allegedly increased size of the pseudocyst on follow-up radiographic surveillance (without new symptoms), or to rule out malignancy. The remaining 44 patients have remained well without further therapy.

Table 1. Indications for surgical intervention in 23 of 68 patients with pancreatic pseudocysts managed expectantly

Surgical Indication	Number of Patients
Perforation	3*
Infected cyst	1*
Intracystic hemorrhage	1*
Increased size on follow-up	6
Pain	6
Obstruction	
Gastric	2
Biliary	1
Exclude malignancy	1
Chronic GI bleed	1
Elective	1

* emergency operations

We examined the clinical presentations of the six patients who developed catastrophic complications in an attempt to identify possible risk factors for the development of serious complications related directly to the pseudocyst. Three of these six patients presented with severe acute pancreatitis and developed their complication within the ensuing 8 weeks. Only one of 18 patients with concomitant chronic pancreatitis and a pseudocyst developed a serious complication. Of the 24 patients who had a pancreatic pseudocyst of unknown etiology, two developed complications.

Characteristics of the pancreatic pseudocysts that appeared to be associated with a greater risk of serious complications included multiloculated or debris-filled cavities. Of the 13 multiloculated pseudocysts, three (23%) developed a complication; similarly, three of the nine patients with debris-filled pseudocysts (33%) went on to develop a serious complication. Although a greater percentage of the patients with the larger pseudocysts (over 10 cm) tended eventually to undergo some type of operative treatment, about one-half were successfully managed expectantly.

Radiologic Surveillance of Pseudocyst

Complete surveillance of pseudocyst size by follow-up CT or ultrasonography was obtained in 24 of the 44 patients successfully managed expectantly. The pseudocyst resolved in 13 patients (54%) at a mean time of 19 months; five of these resolved at greater than 6 months after their time of origin. Two increased in size (without symptoms), two decreased, and seven remained stable in size. Six other patients underwent elective surgical drainage of the pseudocyst because of increased size on follow-up examination despite the lack of any new symptoms.

Discussion

Our study suggests that all pancreatic pseudocysts that persist for greater than 6 weeks do not necessarily require operative, percutaneous, or endoscopic interventional drainage. An expectant approach to the management of asymptomatic pseudocysts or those with clinically insignificant symptoms may be safely undertaken with a small risk (approximately 10%) of serious acute complications. While we acknowledge that catastrophic complications do occur with pancreatic pseudocysts, they do not appear to be as frequent as has been implied in previous retrospective reviews of surgical series.

Our findings are somewhat at variance with the only good, prospective series of the natural history of pancreatic pseudocysts. Bradley et al. [5] prospectively followed 54 patients with pancreatic pseudocysts documented objectively with ultrasonography. A large percentage of these patients were inner city alcoholics who presented with acute pancreatitis. These investigators found that if resolution of the acute pseudocyst was to occur, it did so within 6 weeks; thereafter, the incidence of pseudocyst-related complications increased markedly, leading this group to advocate surgical drainage for pseudocysts that persisted for greater than 6 weeks. Obviously, our experience differs from their study, possibly for several reasons. First, our patient population was more diverse and had a minority of indigent inner city alcoholics with acute pancreatitis. Secondly, at least 26% presented with pseudocysts of indeterminant age, many of which have been present for a long time and thus may have represented a preselected group.

When we examined the risk of development of acute catastrophic complications related directly to the pseudocyst, we found that the etiology of the pseudocyst was of little significant or predictive importance. This risk was about 13% (3 of 23) with acute pancreatitis, 6% (1 of 18) with chronic pancreatitis, and 8% (2 of 24) with pancreatic pseudocysts of clinically indeterminant etiology. Many past studies have reported experience with the management of catastrophic complications related to pancreatic pseudocysts such as hemorrhage, perforation, or sepsis [2, 8]. However, these reviews consist of series of patients treated operatively and thus are preselected; more difficult to differentiate or quantitate are those patients with pancreatic pseudocysts who have minimal or no symptoms and are treated expectantly. Pollak et al. [7] described their experience with 54 patients, 32 of whom underwent operation. Of the remaining 19 patients, only three required rehospitalization for development of a complication. Similarly, Wade [10] followed 19 selected patients with pseudocysts, with only one patient developing a complication. Thus, there is a precedent for expectant management of selected patients. We believe that our experience with 68 patients supports this approach.

We acknowledge that acute, catastrophic complications do occur with pancreatic pseudocysts. During the time interval of this study, we treated 46 patients with *primary* operative therapy, six of whom required emergency surgery for cholangitis (two), hemorrhage (two), infected pseudocyst (one), or variceal hemorrhage (one). Also, six of the 68 patients treated expectantly went on to develop a catastrophic complication. Of these latter six patients, five developed their complication within the 8 weeks following diagnosis. In addition, this subgroup had a greater incidence of multiloculated or debris-filled pseudocysts, suggesting an element of pancreatic or peripancreatic necrosis. Thus, such patients may be at increased risk for expectant management; however, about two-thirds of the patients with a similar presentation were managed successfully with a noninterventional approach.

We acknowledge that not all of the 62 patients who did not develop an acute, catastrophic complication avoided operation. About one-third eventually underwent elective operation for development of pain, gastrointestinal obstruction, asymptomatic enlargement of the cyst, on for other miscellaneous reasons. Many of these operations were not for problems directly attributable to the pancreatic pseudocyst but rather to effects of the underlying acute or chronic pancreatitis. Nevertheless, 46 of the 68 patients avoided operative intervention.

In summary, expectant management of asymptomatic or minimally symptomatic pancreatic pseudocysts can be employed successfully with a risk of acute, catastrophic complications of about 10%. Another 20% may eventually require elective operative treatment for the development of symptoms or nonacute complications related to either the pseudocyst or the underlying pancreatic disease. However, about two-thirds of patients treated expectantly will avoid operation. Patients with multiloculated or debris-filled "pseudocysts," especially in the setting of severe acute pancreatitis may be at increased risk of developing an acute, catastrophic complication.

References

1. Agha FP (1984) Spontaneous resolution of acute pancreatic pseudocysts. Surg Gynecol Obstet 158:22–26
2. Aranha GV, Prinz RA, Freeark RJ, Kruss DM, Greenlee HB (1982) Evaluation of therapeutic options for pancreatic pseudocysts. Arch Surg 117:717–721
3. Aranha GV, Prinz RA, Esguerra AC, Greenlee HB (1983) The nature and course of cystic pancreatic lesions diagnosed by ultrasound. Arch Surg 118:486–488
4. Bourliere M, Sarles H (1989) Pancreatic cysts and pseudocysts associated with acute and chronic pancreatitis. Dig Dis Sci 34:343–348
5. Bradley EL III, Clements JL Jr, Gonzales AC (1979) The natural history of pancreatic pseudocysts: a unified concept of management. Am J Surg 137:135–141
6. Crass RA, Way LW (1981) Acute and chronic pancreatic pseudocysts are different. Am J Surg 142:660–663

7. Pollak EW, Michas CA, Wolfman EF Jr (1978) Pancreatic pseudocyst: management in fifty four patients. Am J Surg 135:199–201
8. Sankaran S, Walt AJ (1975) The natural and unnatural history of pancreatic pseudocysts. Br J Surg 62:37–44
9. Shatney CH, Lillehei RC (1981) The timing of surgical treatment of pancreatic pseudocysts. Surg Gynecol Obstet 152:809–812
10. Wade JW (1985) Twenty-five year experience with pancreatic pseudocysts: are we making progress. Am J Surg 149:705–708

Nonoperative Management of Chronic Pancreatic Pseudocysts

F. W. Henriksen and S. Hancke[1]

It is generally agreed that patients with chronic pancreatic pseudocysts run a high risk of developing complications such as rupture, hemorrhage, and obstruction of the common bile duct and duodenum. Whereas cysts occurring after acute pancreatitis often resolve spontaneously, this rarely happens in chronic pancreatitis, and therefore operative treatment is widely recommended [1–5]. Operative treatment usually consists of an internal drainage procedure (cystogastrostomy, cystoduodenostomy or Roux-en-Y cystojejunostomy) or resection of the affected part of the pancreas with the cyst. The use of external surgical drainage is not recommended, as it results in complication rates between 37% and 50% [8–10] and a lethality rate up to 28% [8]. Internal surgical drainage shows much more favorable results, with a complication rate between 6.4% and 29% and lethalities from 0% to 8.6% [8–10].

The appearance of new technical facilities such as ultrasound scanning, CT scanning and endoscopy with flexible endoscopes has led to new, nonoperative therapeutic methods as alternatives to surgical treatment. Repeated ultrasound-guided, percutaneous punctures was the first nonoperative therapy to be attempted [6, 7]. However the cysts often recur after simple aspiration. Percutaneous external drainage also has been shown to be inferior to internal drainage as regards complication rates (40% versus 15%) [9]. Transgastric, external drainage was attempted by Kuligowska and Olsen [11] in six patients. In only one patient, who had the catheter in situ for 7 days, was the treatment successful.

Many authors have used endoscopy to perform an internal drainage procedure of pancreatic pseudocysts. As early as 1975 Rogers et al. [12] published a case in which they punctured a pseudocyst contiguous to the stomach, via a gastroscope. In 1984 Hershfield [13] reported on a case of succesful drainage of a pseudocyst, adhering to the posterior wall of the duodenum, by repeated aspiration during ERCP. During endoscopy Kozarek et al. [14] found pseudocysts bulging into the posterior wall of the stomach or duodenum in four patients, and via the duodonoscope they made an incision into the cysts by electrocautery, thus creating an endoscopic cystogastrostomy/-duodenostomy. One patient had a significant bleeding episode, and two patients were cured by the method. A fourth patient died from liver failure. Using the same technique, but leaving a transnasal drain for several days, Cremer and Deviere [15] in 1986 presented a preliminary report on 18 patients treated in this way. At present (1989) their series includes 33 patients [16], 22 with cystoduodenostomy and

[1] Department of Surgical Gastroenterology D and the Ultrasonic Laboratory, Gentofte University Hospital, Copenhagen, Denmark

Chronic Pancreatitis
Ed. by Beger, Büchler, Ditschuneit, and Malfertheiner
© Springer-Verlag Berlin Heidelberg 1990

11 with cystogastrostomy; the success rate has been 96% in the former group and 100% in the latter. In the cystoduodenostomy one patient had a retroperitoneal infection (4.5%); in the cystogastrostomy group one patient developed an absces in the cyst, and one patient had a significant arterial bleeding (18.2% complication rate). Twenty patients had pain relief (61%). The authors emphasize that the method requires that the cyst be endoscopically seen bulging into the stomach or duodenum. If so, they recommend that this method should be first choice, before surgery. Using the same method as the Brussels group [16], Sahel et al. [17] have treated 20 patients with an endoscopic cystoduodenostomy. They obtained almost the same results, except for a higher complication rate (28%) from bleeding and perforation. Also, these authors stress the importance of visible compression into the duodenal wall. Buchi et al. [18] in 1986 published one case in which they employed the same technique, but used a Nd:YAG laser instead of electrocautery for making the cystogastrostomy. No bleeding occurred.

The above-mentioned methods are based exclusively on endoscopic techniques and are therefore dependent on what can be seen in the endoscope. Bernardino and Amerson [19] in 1984 presented one case in which the internal drainage was made under CT guidance without endoscopic assistance. They introduced a double Malecot biliary stent transcutaneously, through the stomach into the retrogastric cyst, so that the distal winged section of the catheter was placed in the cyst, and the proximal in the gastric lumen. The cyst disappeared completely within 8 weeks, and the catheter was removed endoscopically. This technique does not seem to have been used since.

Based on simultaneous use of ultrasonography and endoscopy we developed during the years 1982–1984 a method in which a polyethylene double-pigtail catheter was placed between the cyst and the stomach [20]. The catheter (8.5 F) was mounted on a puncture needle and introduced percutaneously and transgastrically into the cyst, so that the inner curl of the pigtail was placed in the cyst and the outer in the stomach. This was performed during external ultrasound scanning, with gastroscopy at the same time to control the placement of the catheter. In a preliminary report [21] on 31 patients the catheter was succesfully placed in 30 (97%). Complications occurred in five patients (17%). In two patients the entire catheter slipped into the cyst. One patient, with a cyst adjacent to the common bile duct, immediately developed biliary leak, and two patients who eventually exhibited a pancreatic cancer, developed abscesses in the cyst cavity. One patient died 4 days after the procedure from a myocardial infarction.

The new methods for nonoperative treatment of pancreatic pseudocysts are not yet fully developed. The methods in which only endoscopy is used present the problem that only when a bulging of the cyst into the stomach or duodenum is seen endoscopically can the technique be used. This problem might be overcome if endoscopy is used together with ultrasonography or CT scanning to localize the cyst. The problem of bleeding, when cutting is made in the gastric or duodenal wall, could possibly be solved by using laser cutting instead of electrocautery.

The main problem with the method using pigtail catheters for internal drainage is infection in the cystic cavity after placing of the catheter. This probably depends on obstruction of the catheter by detritus or necrotic material. This problem may be solved by use of catheters with a larger lumen, and by a careful selection of patients without solid material in the cyst. The fact that the entire pigtail catheter in few cases, at the initial phase of the series, slipped into the cyst is considered a beginner's problem.

At present the new nonoperative methods for internal drainage of pancreatic pseudocysts have the same or lower complication rate as compared with operative treatment and a definitively lower lethality. Also, they are less traumatizing for the patients, for whom the hospital stay may be shortened. With further refinement of these methods they can be expected to be the first choice of treatment, instead of surgery, in a large but selected group of patients with chronic pancreatic pseudocysts.

References

1. Crass RA, Way LW (1981) Acute and chronic pancreatic pseudocysts are different. Am J Surg 142:660–663
2. Bradley EL, Clements JL, Gonzales AC (1979) The natural history of pancreatic pseudocysts: a unified concept of management. Am J Surg 137:135–141
3. Sankaran S, Walt AJ (1975) The natural and unnatural history of pancreatic pseudocysts. Br J Surg 62:37–44
4. Maule WF, Reber HA (1986) Diagnosis and management of pancreatic pseudocysts, pancreatic ascites and pancreatic fistulas. In: Go VLW et al. The Exocrine Pancreas. Raven, New York, pp 601–610
5. Grace RR, Jordan PH (1976) Unresolved problems of pancreatic pseudocysts. Ann Surg 184:16–21
6. Hancke S, Pedersen JF (1976) Percutaneous puncture of pancreatic cysts guided by ultrasound. Surg Gynec Obst 142:551–552
7. Hancke S, Holm HH, Koch F (1985) Ultrasonically guided puncture of pancreatic mass lesions. In: Holm HH, Kristensen JK (eds) Interventional ultrasound. Copenhagen, Munksgaard
8. Shatney CH, Lillehei RC (1979) Surgical treatment of pancreatic pseudocysts. Ann Surg 189:386–394
9. Andrén-Sandberg A, Evander A, Isaksson G, Ihse I (1983) Management of pancreatic pseudocysts. Acta Chir Scand 149:203–206
10. Warshaw AL, Rattner DW (1985) Timing of surgical drainage for pancreatic pseudocysts. Ann Surg 202:720–724
11. Kuligowska E, Olsen WL (1985) Pancreatic pseudocysts drained through a percutaneous transgastric approach. Radiology 154:79–82
12. Rogers BHG, Cicurel NJ, Seed RW (1975) Transgastric needle aspiration of pancreatic pseudocyst through an endoscope. Gastrointest Endosc 21:133–134
13. Hershfield NB (1984) Drainage of a pancreatic pseudocyst at ERCP. Gastrointest Endosc 30:269–270
14. Kozarek RA, Brayko CM, Harlan J et al. (1985) Endoscopic drainage of pancreatic pseudocysts. Gastrointest Endosc 31:322–328
15. Cremer M, Deviere J (1986) Endoscopic management of pancreatic cysts and psuedocysts. Gastrointest Endosc 32:367–368
16. Cremer M, Deviere J, Engelholm L (1989) Endoscopic management of cysts and pseudocysts in chronic pancreatitis: long-term follow-up after 7 years of experience. Gastrointest Endosc 35:1–9
17. Sahel J, Bastid C, Pellat B, et al. (1987) Endoscopic cystoduodenostomy of cysts of chronic calcifying pancreatitis: a report of 20 cases. Pancreas 2:447–453
18. Buchi KN, Bowers JH, Dixon JA (1986) Endoscopic pancreatic cystogastrostomy using the Nd:YAG laser. Gastrointest Endosc 32:112–114
19. Bernardino ME, Amerson JR (1984) Percutaneous gastrocystostomy: a new approach to pancreatic pseudocyst drainage. Am J Radiol 143:1096–1097
20. Hancke S, Henriksen FW (1985) Percutaneous pancreatic cystogastrostomy guided by ultrasound scanning and gastroscopy. Br J Surg 72:916–917
21. Henriksen FW, Hancke S (1987) Ultrasound-guided percutaneous pancreatic cystogastrostomy. Digestion 38:24 (Abstr)

Surgical Treatment: Indication

Indications for Surgical Treatment in Chronic Pancreatitis

A. L. WARSHAW[1]

In any discussion of surgery for chronic pancreatitis, the first question must be, "Can chronic pancreatitis be treated?" Current evidence suggests that chronic pancreatitis is a disease which, once it begins, never stops. Removing the underlying cause of the disease, such as alcohol, may slow the process of deterioration, but generally deterioration continues nonetheless [1, 2]. Therefore, progression of the disease with ultimate destruction of the gland is to be expected, and recovery of function is exceptional. In this setting, surgical treatment may reduce symptoms or deal with specific complications, but there is no evidence that it will halt the progression of the disease or improve function.

It has been argued that the role of surgery is further limited by the fact that the natural history of the disease leads ultimately to autodestruction of the pancreas and, as that occurs, to relief of pain spontaneously. Since pain is, numerically speaking, the principal indication for surgical treatment, some would argue that patients should be encouraged to wait for spontaneous relief of pain rather than embarking on a surgical misadventure. Studies of the natural history of chronic pancreatitis show that the average time for spontaneous pain relief is in excess of 5 years, with a range up to 18 years and with only 80% of patients followed for that length of time achieving pain relief [3]. In addition, the pattern of pain is important in ascertaining the prognosis. Patients with intermittent pain or recurrent attacks of pain are more likely to achieve pain relief. Patients with constant severe pain are less likely to be relieved. The same comments appear to apply to nonsurgical treatment with pancreatic enzymes, which are least likely to work in patients who have severe persistent pain.

The principal indications for operation in chronic pancreatitis are the following:

Intractable pain	Pancreatic ascites
Large pseudocyst (> 5 cm)	Pleural effusion
Biliary obstruction	Splenic vein occlusion with variceal bleeding
Duodenal obtruction	Inability to exclude carcinoma

Of these, the most common indication is pain [1]. If the symptoms caused by pseudocysts are included, pain is the principal reason for operation in over 95% of patients. Biliary obstruction in association with pain is the next most common indication, occurring in up to one-third of all patients coming to operation for chronic pancreatitis [1]. Painless biliary obstruction is rare.

---

[1] Harvard Medical School and Massachusetts General Hospital, 15 Parkman St., Boston, MA 02114, USA

Chronic Pancreatitis
Ed. by Beger, Büchler, Ditschuneit, and Malfertheiner
© Springer-Verlag Berlin Heidelberg 1990

When considering the indications for operation in patients with chronic pancreatitis, one must also take into account circumstances which are either not indications for surgery or are contraindications. For example, even the most impressive pancreatic duct dilation, calcifications, or intraductal stones do not require surgery in a patient who is not symptomatic, or whose symptoms are manageable without surgery. Similarly, the natural history of small pseudocysts would appear to be harmless enough in the absence of symptoms that these lesions can be observed expectantly. The hopes that pancreatic duct drainage would improve pancreatic function by returning enzymes to the intestinal tract for digestion or might stabilize pancreatic function and prevent further deterioration by eliminating the obstructive injury have not thus far been borne out. What evidence exists suggests that pancreatic deterioration continues in spite of successful decompression, although there is one short-term study that suggests that pancreatic function may not deteriorate as rapidly after pancreatojejunostomy [4]. Certainly resection of the gland accelerates functional loss. Occlusion of the portal vein is increasingly being recognized as a complication of chronic pancreatitis [5], much as splenic vein occlusion has been noted for some years. However, portal vein occlusion creates such irremediable difficulties with varices around the head of the pancreas and bile duct that surgical procedures are made much more difficult and difficult and resection of the pancreatic head is probably not possible. We have seen superior mesenteric and portal vein obstruction in between 5% and 10% of late chronic pancreatitis.

The next major consideration in surgery for this disease is the nature of the duct abnormality. For reasons that are not known, approximately 40%–50% of patients develop a dilated pancreatic duct, with or without obstruction in the head of the gland and other partial obstructions along the length of the duct. The remainder develop a scarred contracted duct which has been compared to a leafless tree in winter. The opportunities provided by these two different duct patterns are quite different. The big-duct pattern, when the duct is greater than 7 mm in diameter, allows for long side-to-side pancreatojejunostomy, usually of the modified Puestow type, using a Roux-en-Y loop of jejunum. This operation is desirable because it is simple, safe and does not compromise pancreatic function by resection. However, when the duct pattern is of the small-caliber type, drainage procedures are ineffective and not an option. In these circumstances resection of the gland is the only option. This is less desirable because of the ablation of pancreatic tissue, and also because the operations become more complex, including resection of the pancreatic head and duodenum (Whipple-type operation) or duodenum-sparing resection of the pancreatic head (Beger-type operation) [6].

Consideration of surgery for pain relief from chronic pancreatitis must consider the mechanism of that pain. When the duct is dilated, it is assumed that there is pancreatic duct obstruction and pancreatic duct hypertension, but the evidence for this is relatively limited. Against this concept is the fact that there are usually relatively easy cannulation of the duct for pancreatography and relatively ready emptying of the duct. Two studies have measured duct pressures and found them elevated nonetheless [7, 8]. Other theoretical possibilities for the cause of pain include blockage of small side ducts by stones, protein plugs, or scar. Relief of major duct obstruction should not affect this. In addition, there has been considerable interest recently in abnormalities of sensory nerves in chronic pancreatitis, including increased numbers and size of sensory afferents [9].

The current state of the art for the modified Puestow pancreatojejunostomy can be summarized by stating that it is a safe and effective operation. Its morbidity should be less than 5%, mortality less than 2%, and effective pain relief on the order of 80% [1, 2]. Our own studies have shown that this successful relief of pain is unrelated to the development of either exocrine or endocrine insufficiency [1], in contradistinction to the assertions that pain relief comes only when pancreatic function has deteriorated to a terminal stage of the burned out pancreas. We have noted that pain relief after pancreatojejunostomy is immediate and irrespective of pancreatic function. Pancreatic function does continue to deteriorate irrespective of pain relief also.

The natural history of this disease often includes stenosis of other structures associated with the pancreas, in particular the common bile duct in its intrapancreatic portion and the duodenum as it passes around the head of the pancreas. Obstruction of either of these structures can in and of itself be an indication for surgical correction. Obstruction of the bile duct occurs in up to one-third of patients with advanced chronic pancreatitis and is characterized by a long, tapered stricture within the pancreatic head. The earliest biochemical manifestation is the elevation of alkaline phosphatase and later the presence of jaundice which is fixed and does not fluctuate or disappear. In such patients there is a risk of cholangitis and a small risk in the long term of secondary biliary cirrhosis [10]. The onset of functionally significant biliary stricture may not be coincident with the presentation with pain but may occur years after successful surgical treatment of a pain syndrome and be manifested as a reccurrence of symptoms [1, 10].

Similarly obstruction of the duodenum my occur asynchronously or synchronously with the presentation with pain. Its treatment is most simply a gastrojejunostomy. It has been a striking observation in our experience that duodenal and biliary obstruction occur almost exclusively in patients with the large-duct form of chronic pancreatitis and not in the small duct form [1]. Among 58 consecutive patients whom I have operated on and reported in 1985, 38 had a dilated pancreatic duct suitable for pancreatojejunostomy, and 20 had a small pancreatic duct which had to be treated by pancreatic resection. Among these 58 patients there were 21 functionally significant biliary strictures and four duodenal obstructions. All of the biliary obstructions and all of the duodenal obstructions occurred in the group with large pancreatic duct. All of the duodenal obstruction patients occurred in those who also had biliary obstruction. There would appear to be a strong tendency from these manifestations to cluster in the large-duct form, suggesting that the large-duct form is different from the small-duct form. It is also known that the large-duct form is not an outgrowth or later stage of the small-duct form but characterizes a separate population of patients. The reason for this is not known. Pseudocysts were equally distributed among the two forms of pancreatitis in this series. When obstruction of the bile duct and duodenum are found in patients with the dilated pancreatic duct, a triple drainage operation (pancreatojejunostomy, choledochoduodenostomy, gastrojejunostomy) is very effective and does not require sacrifice of pancreatic tissue. Of note, this observation would suggest that a biliary stricture in a patient with a small pancreatic duct on pancreatography should raise the suspicion of cancer rather than chronic pancreatitis.

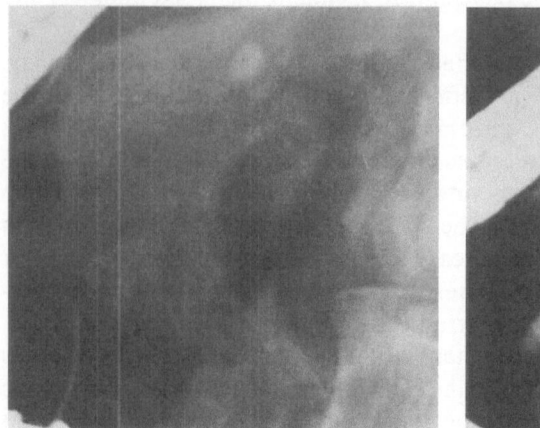 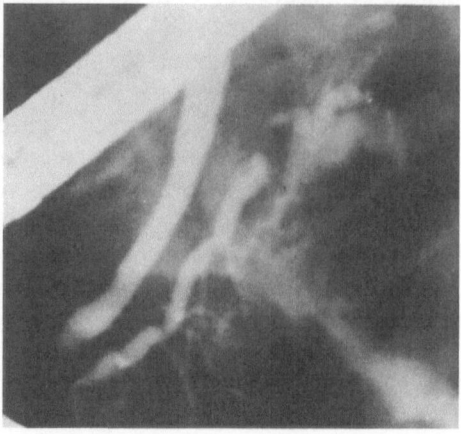

Fig. 1. *Left,* plain abdominal X-ray showing a stone in the pancreatic body. *Right,* pancreatogram showing obstruction of the pancreatic duct at the location of the stone

When pancreatojejunostomy fails to relieve pain, or when an initially successful operation fails later in the natural history of the patient, the cause of failure must be sought. In some cases, this may be a subsequent development such as biliary obstruction. In others in whom there is evidence of persistent or recurrent pancreatic duct obstruction, it may be possible to extend the pancreatojejunostomy to areas not adequately drained at the first operation. Most often in our experience, we have resorted to pancreatic resection at this stage in the natural history. If a Puestow-type drainage has been performed previously, resection of the pancreatic head by pancreatoduodenectomy is usually successful in achieving pain relief. We strongly prefer to avoid a total pancreatectomy in this patient population, which is often unreliable in insulin management because of drug or alcohol abuse.

It is not intended that this essay discuss in detail the results of pancreatic resection. Nonetheless, it should be commented that distal or left-sided resections tend to have poorer results than proximal or right-sided resections in current experience [6, 11, 12]. Exceptions occur when there is specific pathology in the tail of the gland to be resected. This is illustrated by Fig. 1 which shows a stone in the midportion of the pancreatic duct with distal obstruction. Resection of the obstructed tail in this patient successfully relieved his pain and recurrent pancreatitis.

Finally, the role of nonsurgical procedures which are now being introduced to compete with surgical treatment remains to be evaluated. The potential role for endoscopic manuevers such as stenting of the pancreatic duct, papillotomy or balloon dilatation of the papilla, and extracorporeal lithotripsy for pancreatic duct stones will be watched with great interest.

References

1. Warshaw AL (1985) Conservation of pancreatic tissue by combined gastric, biliary, and pancreatic duct drainage for pain from chronic pancreatitis. Am J Surg 149:563–569
2. Morrow CE, Cohen JI, Sutherland DER, et al. (1984) Chronic pancreatitis: long-term surgical results of pancreatic duct drainage, pancreatic resection, and near-total pancreatectomy and islet autotransplantation. Surgery 96:608–614
3. Ammann RW, Akovbiantz A, Largiader F, et al. (1984) Course and outcome of chronic pancreatitis. Longitudinal study of a mixed medical-surgical series of 245 patients. Gastroenterology 86:820–828
4. Nelson WH, Townsend CM Jr, Thompson JC (1988) Operative drainage of the pancreatic duct delays functional impairment in patients with chronic pancreatitis. Ann Surg 208:321–329
5. Warshaw AL, Jin G, Ottinger LW (1987) Recognition and clinical implications of mesenteric and portal vein obstruction in chronic pancreatitis. Arch Surg 122:410–415
6. Beger HG, Krautzberger W, Bittner R, et al. (1985) Duodenum-preserving resection of the head of the pancreas in patients with severe chronic pancreatitis. Surgery 97:467–473
7. Bradley EL III (1982) Pancreatic duct pressure in chronic pancreatitis. Am J Surg 144:313–316
8. Ebbehoj N, Borly L, Madsen P, et al. (1986) Pancreatic tissue pressure and pain in chronic pancreatitis. Pancreas 1:556–558
9. Bockman DE, Buchler M, Malfertheiner P, et al. (1988) Analysis of nerves in chronic pancreatitis. Gastroenterology 94:1459–1469
10. Warshaw AL, Schapiro RH, Ferrucci JT Jr, et al. (1976) Persistent obstructive jaundice, cholangitis, and biliary cirrhosis due to common bile duct stenosis in chronic pancreatitis. Gastroenterology 70:562–567
11. Rossi RL, Rothschild J, Braasch JW, et al. (1987) Pancreatoduodenectomy in the management of chronic pancreatitis. Arch Surg 122:416–419
12. Stone WM, Sarr MG, Nagorney DM, et al. (1988) Chronic pancreatitis. Results of Whipple's resection and total pancreatectomy. Arch Surg 123:815–819

Reducing the Risk of Pancreatic Surgery

M. Trede and G. Schwall[1]

Let us set the stage by making a few quotations. At the American Surgical Meeting 2 years ago, the Commissioner of Health for the State of New York stated: "The average general surgeon in New York State can expect to perform only two or three such operations [pancreatic resection] in 30 years of surgical experience with a likelihood of a 30% mortality rate at the current writing." And he went on, "These operations have been selected for discussion at an upcoming statewide New York Quality Insurance Meeting as models of *high*-risk, *high* morbidity and *low*-yield procedures" [2].

As regards "yield," a paper appeared last year which posed the question "Is resection appropriate for adenocarcinoma of the pancreas? A cost benefit analysis." The authors came to the conclusion that it was not [13]. Finally, in a Denver clinic a Saturday morning was spent debating whether or not "Congress should pass a law making it illegal to do a Whipple operation" [9]!

This is one side of the argument, the other clearly shows that practice improves performance. Recent statistics from surgical departments all over the world show that at least *operative mortality* for pancreatectomy can be brought well below 5% (Table 1). Even 21 years ago such results were possible, as shown by Howard's paper entitled "Forty-one consecutive Whipple resections without an operative mortality" [1]. Let us look at the risks of pancreatic surgery and see what can be done about them. As in

Table 1. Recent results of pancreatoduodenectomy

Carcinoma				Chron. Pancreatitis			
Author	Patients	Deaths	Mortality	Author	Patients	Deaths	Mortality
Braasch (1986)	87	2	2,3%	Beger (1987)	105	1	0.95%
Gall (1986)	30	2	6%	Cooper (1987)	83	4	4,3%
Christ (1987)	47	1	2,1%	Gall (1987)	289	3	1%
Grace (1987)	45	1	2.2%	Store (1988)	15	0	0
Bittner (1988)	69	3	4.3%				

[1] Department of Surgery, Klinikum Mannheim, Heidelberg University, Theodor-Kutzer-Ufer, 6800 Mannheim 1, FRG

Chronic Pancreatitis
Ed. by Beger, Büchler, Ditschuneit, and Malfertheiner
© Springer-Verlag Berlin Heidelberg 1990

all operative medicine, the risk comes from three directions: from the *patient* himself, from his *disease*, and from his *surgeon*.

Risks from the Patient

Among the 362 patients who had pancreatoduodenectomy performed in our clinic over the past 16 years, there were 260 with significant risk factors. Of these, 64 were over the age of 65; our oldest patient was 79 when she survived Whipple's operation for a pancreatic carcinoma. In our group, 169 patients – mainly those with complicated chronic pancreatitis – had had previous abdominal operations, which posed an additional technical risk. A further 27 had serious concomitant disease, predominantly hepatic cirrhosis.

One man was on chronic renal dialysis because of bilateral cystic disease when he became jaundiced due to a papillary carcinoma. He had adapted so well to creatinine levels above 8 mg% that he became the first dialysis patient to survive more than 5 years following Whipple's operation.

Risks Due to the Disease

In all published series, the risk (morbidity and mortality) seems to be higher when pancreatic resection is done for malignancy, which was the case in two-thirds of our patients (Table 2).

Table 2. Risk due to disease in 362 pancreatectomies

	Patients
1. Malignancy	241
2. Infiltration beyond pancreas	31
Vascular resections	24
Right hemicolectomy	4
Hepatic segmentectomy	2
Total gastrectomy	1
3. Obstructive jaundice	201

Part of the explanation lies in the fact that malignant infiltration involving adjacent organs may require additional and risky resections as was necessary in 31 cases. The patient requiring total gastrectomy died from ARDS.

Although the dangers of obstructive jaundice are known to all surgeons [3, 12, 17], we are taught that reduction of this risk by preoperative biliary drainage is superfluous and may indeed carry risks of its own. This teaching is based on three prospective, randomized studies, each of which failed to demonstrate any advantage in preliminary drainage (Table 3). Morbidity and mortality of pancreatic resection in patients with obstructive jaundice was not reduced by prior decompression of the biliary system. One might criticize these trials since bile was drained to the outside and was not drained for long enough to permit significant recovery of hepatic function.

Table 3. Preoperative biliary drainage

Author	Morbidity		Mortality	
	with PTD	without PTD	with PTD	without PTD
Hatfield (1982)	14%	15%	14%	15%
McPherson (1984)	33%	42%	32%	19%
Pitt (1985)	46%	53%	8%	5%

Our own experience and that of others [5] is different: The complete, albeit non randomized, documentation of 201 pancreatectomies in jaundiced patients is shown in Fig. 1. Comparison of those who had primary resection with those in whom resection followed biliary drainage reveals more favorable morbidity and mortality rates following drainage. This difference may be due to the method of endoscopic transpapillary drainage. Thus, bile drains into the gut, where it belongs.

A recent controlled trial reported from Amsterdam confirms this procedure. Nineteen patients with preliminary endoscopic drainage did far better on all counts – including bile and blood cultures – than did 19 patients who had resection without prior drainage [15].

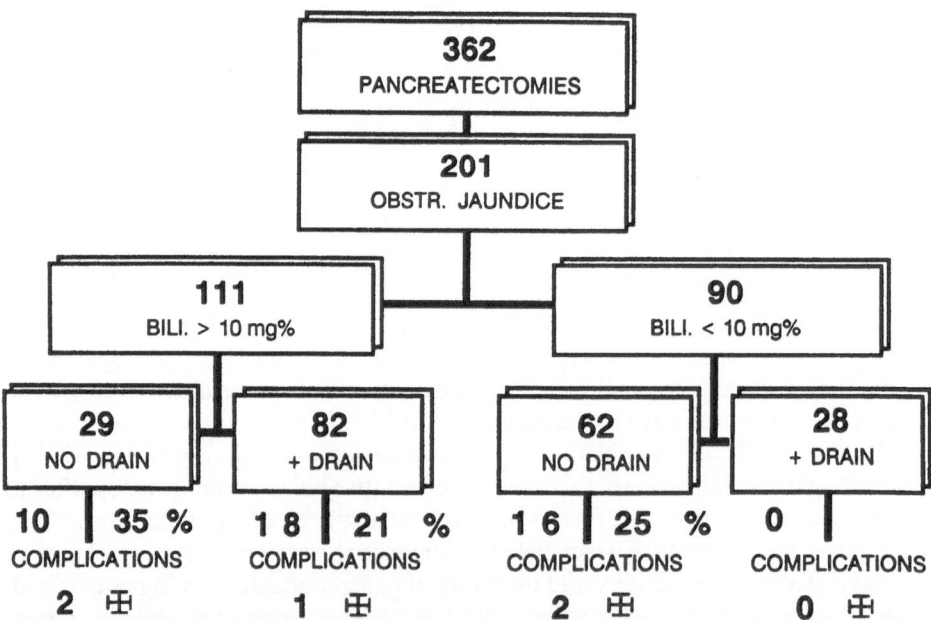

Fig. 1. The effect of preoperative biliary drainage on postoperative complications and mortality following pancreatoduodenectomy. BILI, bilirubin; †, deaths

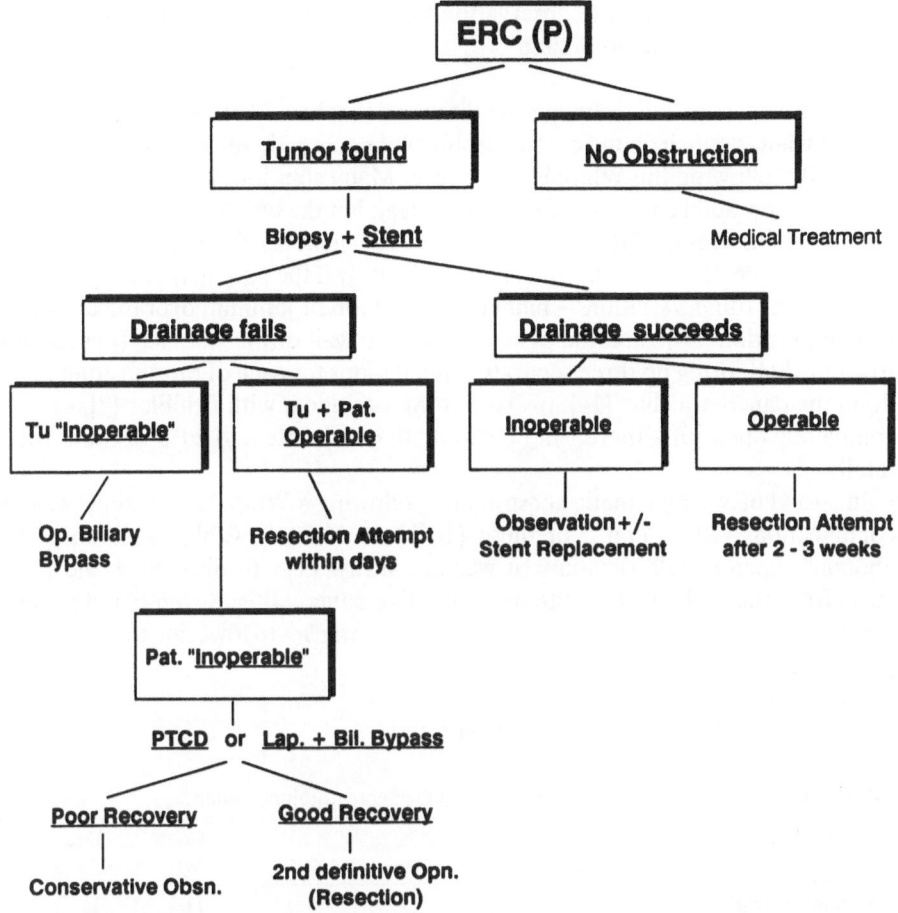

Fig. 2. Diagnostic and therapeutic algorithm for patients with malignant biliary obstruction. ERC(P), endoscopic retrograde cholangiopancreatography

To lower the risk of pancreatic surgery in the jaundiced patient it is our policy to let the endoscopist see the patient within 24 h of admission (Fig. 2). He can localize the obstruction and pass a transpapillary stent. If he fails, we operate anyway as soon as possible, doing a definitive resection if the local findings and the patient's general state of health permit. If endoscopic decompression is successful, we use the 2–3 weeks of drainage to assess operability – and then undertake pancreatic resection.

Risks from the Surgeon

Turning now to the surgeon, he can influence the course of events:
a) Preoperatively, by correct assessment and treatment of risk factors of the patient and his disease (see above)
b) During the operation, by correct tactics and meticulous technique

c) Postoperatively, by close observation of the patient to detect possible complications and combat them in time

Operative tactics and technique are discussed in other chapters in this volume. Here we just want to touch on the central problem of pancreatic surgery: *anastomotic leaks* especially following the Whipple procedure. Many solutions have been proposed to reduce the dreaded consequences of such a leak but the only really reliable method is *total* pancreatectomy. This is a real alternative whenever the pancreatic remnant is soft and friable, the duct is narrow, and particularly if the patient is already a diabetic.

As for the other variations – namely wrap a loop of jejunum over the anastomosis (jejunoplication [20], sink the pancreas into the wall of the stomach (pancreatogastrostomy [24], bring up three separate jejunal loops for each of the anastomoses [19], drain the pancreatic duct [14], oversew it [8], occlude it with Ethibloc [7], or leave it completely open [6] – there will be about 10% leak rate and 20% of these will end fatally.

In a total of 306 pancreatic anastomoses following a Whipple resection, we saw 30 complications (10%) and 5 of these (16%) were fatal (Table 4). Even with the abdomen open at relaparotomy, it was not always easy to distinguish the 11 overt leaks from the 12 bouts of acute postoperative pancreatitis. Seven bland pancreatic fistulae closed spontaneously. There are *two approaches* to lowering the risk from this particular complication:
a) prevention, if possible, and
b) early detection and treatment, if necessary.

Table 4. Complications occurring at or around 306 pancreatojejunostomies

Complication	Cases (n)	Deaths
Anastomotic leak	11	4
Acute pancreatitis	12	1
Pancreatic fistula	7	–
Total	30	5

Prevention involves surgical technique. We are convinced that it is not the type of anastomosis that matters so much as meticulous attention to detail in a standardized operation [21]. Thus, over the past 16 years, we have adhered to the technique of E-E telescope pancreatojejunostomy. Two-layered anastomoses – even using silk and cat gut! are admittedly rather old-fashioned but (as I hope to demonstrate) essentially effective.

We leave the pancreatic duct alone. If it is narrow, meaningful sutures or drains are impossible to place; if it is dilated, they are unnecessary [22]. However, we routinely drain the bile to the outside via a Völker drain, for the first postoperative week, in the hope that this will keep bile away from the pancreatic anastomosis.

Early detection is the key to successful treatment of pancreatic leaks should they occur. This involves close observation of the patient in the surgical intensive care unit.

Table 5. Diagnosis of postoperative pancreatic leaks

A. Laboratory tests	B. Imaging procedures
1. Leukocytes	1. Ultrasound (C.T.)
2. Creatinine	2. Fistulography
3. Amylase	
4. Prothrombin	
5. Transaminases	
6. Blood gas analysis	

C. Clinical Signs

1. Abdominal palpation/auscultation
2. The tongue!
3. Pulse rate
4. Respiration
5. Temperature
6. Urinary output
7. Psyche

The simple clinical signs are far more important than complicated imaging procedures (Table 5). Laboratory findings invariably lag behind the subtle clinical signs. The same applies to ultrasound imaging and a CAT scan, which are performed routinely 1 week postoperatively or earlier, if necessary.

We have all but abandoned routine contrast examination of the biliary and pancreatic anastomoses via the Völker drain, since this has caused spikes of temperature and pain in some patients (presumably iatrogenic ascending cholangitis). This examination is useful, however, for the detection and control of clinically benign pancreatic fistulae [23].

Table 6 summarizes our *treatment* of the 30 cases with pancreatic complications. Conservative observation was confined to 13 cases, 7 of whom had bland pancreatic fistulae which closed spontaneously after a maximum of 3 weeks.

Table 6. Treatment of 30 postoperative pancreatic complications

Complication	N	Treatment			Deaths (N)
		Conservative	Drainage	Total pancrea-tectomies	
Anastomotic leak	11	–	5 (2 deaths)	6 (2 deaths)	4
Acute pancreatitis	12	6 (1 death)	–	6	1
Pancreatic fistula	7	7	–	–	–
Total	30	13 (1 death)	5 (2 deaths)	12 (2 deaths)	5

The diagnosis of "acute pancreatitis" rested on raised postoperative amylase levels in six of the 12 cases. Misjudgement of the severity of the pancreatitis led to the death of the first patient early in the series. Thereafter, a policy of early intervention was followed, leading to two unnecessary but harmless relaparotomies.

Simple drainage is not really adequate treatment for most cases of pancreatic leak. Irrigation-suction drainage was, however, successful in two cases with minimal localized peritonitis. Here, the jejunum was oversewn, and the pancreatic duct was occluded with Ethibloc and then closed by suture. Renewed drainage was all that could be done for three further patients, two of whom died.

The most radical solution – total pancreatectomy – was attempted in 12 patients. Two of these died of severe retroperitoneal hemorrhage. But for 10 of 12 patients, removal of the remaining pancreas and spleen was a life-saving measure.

Prevention of complications by following a standardized technique, and practicing early detection and intervention should they occur, has reduced the risks of pancreatic resection as witness the *early results* of duodenopancreatectomy (Table 7).

Table 7. Early results of duodenopancreatectomy

Type of procedure	Patients (n)	Diagnosis		op. + hosp. mortality (n)
		neoplasm (n)	pancreatitis (n)	
Whipple's operation	306	202	104	6
Total pancreatectomy	56	39	17	3
Total	362	241 (7 †)	121 (2 †)	9 (2,5%)

Including 101 consecutive Whipple ops. without mortality

A total of 362 such operations were performed at the Surgical University Clinic in Mannheim over the past 16 years: 241 patients underwent surgery for carcinoma, and 121 for severe complicated chronic pancreatitis. There were 306 Whipple procedures and 56 total pancreatectomies. All but nine patients survived the operations and were discharged from hospital – an operative and hospital mortality of 2.5%. Furthermore, from November 1985 to date there have been 101 consecutive Whipple operations without mortality or serious morbidity.

In closing this section on risks from the surgeon, we ask ourselves, "Who should be doing this kind of pancreatic surgery?"

You may be familiar with the quotation about the resident who "wants to perform the Cadillac of abdominal operations – pancreatoduodenectomy . . . . Unfortunately, it frequently turns out for the resident, it is not really a Cadillac he is trying to drive, it is a Formula I racing car" [1].

John Braasch [4] asked: "Should we be training all general surgeons to do this procedure, and secondly, if we do train them, should they be allowed to do it, if they choose?"

At the Mannheim Surgical Clinic we have been training them. In 16 years, 14 different surgeons performed these 362 pancreatectomies – all of them adhering closely to the principles outlined above. In a way, pancreatic surgery is like mountaineering. It took 30 years and many costly expeditions to put two men on Everest.

Today a dozen will reach the summit on a fine day – including 60-year-olds. It is as if a spell has been broken. Similarly, with pancreatic resection no-one really knows why the risks have been so dramatically reduced in recent years. However, any surgeon with a mortality rate below 5% for this operation should be allowed to do it.

References

1. Baker RJ (1979) Discussion of AR Moossa. Arch Surg 114:502
2. Bernard HR (1987) Discussion of MM Connolly. Ann Surg 206:366–371
3. Blamey SL, Fearon KCH, Gilmour WH et al. (1983) Predictors of risk in biliary surgery. Br J Surg 70:535–539
4. Braasch J (1987) Discussion of DW Crist. Ann Surg 206:358–373
5. Carter DC (1989) Personal communication
6. Funovics J, Wenzl E (1985) Duodenopancreatectomie: Anastomosierung nicht notwendig. Langenbecks Arch Chir 366:613
7. Gebhardt C, Stolte M (1978) Pankreasgang-Okklusion durch Injektion einer schnellhärtenden Aminosäurenlösung. Langenbecks Arch Chir 346:149–166
8. Goldsmith HS, Ghosh BC, Huvos AG (1971) Ligation versus implantation of the pancreatic duct after pancreaticoduodenectomy. Surg Gynecol Obstet 132:87–92
9. Harken AH (1986) Presidential address: natural selection in university surgery. Surgery 100:129–133
10. Hatfield ARW, Terblanche J, Fataar S, Kernoff L (1982) Preoperative external biliary drainage in obstructive jaundice. Lancet 2:896–899
11. Howard JM (1968) Pancreatico-Duodenectomy: forty-one consecutive Whipple resections without an operative mortality. Ann Surg 168:629–640
12. Koyama K, Takagi Y, Ito K (1981) Experimental and clinical studies on the effect of biliary drainage in obstructive jaundice. Am J Surg 142:293–299
13. Lea MS, Stahlgren LH (1987) Is resection appropriate for adenocarcinoma of the pancreas? A cost-benefit analysis. Am J Surg 154:651–654
14. Longmire WP Jr (1966) The technique of pancreaticoduodenal resection. Surgery 59:344–352
15. Lygidakis NJ, van der Heyde MN, Lubbers MJ (1987) Evaluation of preoperative biliary drainage in the surgical management of pancreatic head carcinoma. Acta Chir Scand 153:665–668
16. McPherson GAD, Benjamin IS, Habib NA et al. (1982) Percutaneous transhepatic drainage in obstructive jaundice: advantages and problems. Br J Surg 69:261–264
17. O'Connor MJ (1985) Mechanical biliary obstruction. A review of the multisystemic consequences of obstructive jaundice and their impact on perioperative morbidity and mortality. Am Surg 51:245–251
18. Pitt HA, Gomes AS, Lois JF et al. (1985) Does preoperative percutaneous biliary drainage reduce operative risk or increase hospital cost? Ann Surg 201:545–553
19. Schreiber HW, Farthmann EH, Eichfuss HP, Kortmann KB (1977) Pankreasresektion, -exstirpation, Reparation durch isoperistaltische Segmentinterposition. Chirurg 48:607–612
20. Siedek M, Birtel F, Mitrenga I (1985) Pankreasganganastomose und Pankreatojejunoplicatio nach Rechtsresektion. Langenbecks Arch Chir 366:610
21. Trede M (1985) Technik der Duodenopankreatektomie nach Whipple. Chir Prax 34:611–633
22. Trede M (1986) Invited commentary to J. Schopohl et al. Chirurg 57:521
23. Trede M, Schwall G (1988) The complications of pancreatectomy. Ann Surg 207:39–47
24. Waugh JM, Clagett OT (1946) Resection of the duodenum and head of the pancreas for carcinoma – an analysis of thirty cases. Surgery 20:224–232

Surgical Treatment:
Denervation and Drainage

Denervation Procedures in the Management of Chronic Pancreatitis

C. W. Imrie[1]

The nerve supply of the pancreas largely follows blood vessels going to and from the gland. The main autonomic nerve fibres run through the greater splanchnic and lesser splanchnic nerves. Other branches run from the aortic plexus and in the fibres of the right vagus. In consideration of the main pancreatic pain pathways, there is agreement that the main ingoing fibres pass through the coeliac ganglia; it is therefore crucial to have an understanding of the anatomy of these ganglia.

The Anatomy of the Coeliac Ganglia

The coeliac ganglia are described as having a right and left grouping, with each bundle of ganglia typically lying on the anterolateral surface of the aorta between the close origins of the major vessels, the coeliac axis and the superior mesenteric artery. Very little is made of the variability of the anatomical disposition of the two major ganglia, but Ward et al. (1979) [1] found great variation in their 20-cadaver study, using CT scanning as the main monitoring modality but checking the findings at autopsy in all 20 patients. They found a *variation in diameter* between 0.5 cm and 4.5 cm in the individual ganglia and a *variation in number* from one to five. This paper is important in its emphasis on the range of findings in a relatively small group of patients. There was also a *variation in location* from the superior level at the T12–L1 disc interspace down to the L2 level of the body. Finally the authors made the comment that CT scans gave inconsistent results when they were used to locate optimum sites for nerve blocks.

When one considers the findings of the above study and then takes into the reckoning the effect of peripancreatic fibrosis, the surgical or percutaneous approaches to these ganglia represent a particular challenge in patients with chronic pancreatitis. Attempts have been made since 1943 to denervate the pancreas by interrupting the nerve pathways, with either total denervation or selective denervation being the target.

Total Denervation

The famous French surgeon, Mallet-Guy advocated combined splanchnicectomy and coeliac ganglion excision. He performed the operation in two stages: initial

---

[1] Consultant Surgeon, Department of Surgery, Royal Infirmary, Glasgow G4 0SF, UK

Chronic Pancreatitis
Ed. by Beger, Büchler, Ditschuneit, and Malfertheiner
© Springer-Verlag Berlin Heidelberg 1990

laparotomy and later, nerve section. This particular procedure denervates many organs in addition to the pancreas, but the results claimed for its efficacy are considerable [2, 3]. However, no controlled studies have been published from this approach to therapy.

Selective Denervation

In 1957 and 1958, Yoshioka and Wakabayashi described first class results of the selective denervation approach. They claimed to have cut two large nerve bundles going from the head and uncinate process of the pancreas to the coeliac ganglion [4, 5]. Excellent diagrams accompany these descriptions, but again the lack of controlled results makes analysis very difficult. An advantage over the earlier total denervation approach was the lack of effect on other organs, but the authors make light of the problem of peripancreatic fibrosis typically associated with chronic pancreatitis.

Total Denervation of Pancreas (Mark 2)

In 1986, Hiraoka et al. [6] from Japan described an alternative approach to that of Mallet-Guy to achieve complete denervation of the pancreas. The initial section of nerves was similar to the method described approximately 30 years earlier by the authors' countrymen Yoshioka and Wakabayashi, but that operation was considered insufficient by itself and a mobilisation of the body and tail of the pancreas with dissection away from the posterior abdominal wall was added. With this approach, nerve fibres around the major vessels were displayed and sectioned. The major problem with the credibility of this paper was that only two patients were reported and the follow-up varied from 10 to 24 months. Excellent results were claimed, but in such a very small study all that one can comment is that another idea has been advanced for denervation of the pancreas. The need to study more patients and the requirement for some sort of control data is obviously entirely lacking.

The Denervated Pancreatic Flap

An alternative approach was reported from Atlanta in the United States by Warren and colleagues in 1984 [7]. In their preliminary report on two patients, they described division of the neck of the pancreas, as performed in an early stage of Whipple's operation. They carefully preserved the gastro-epiploic vessels as well as the short gastric vessels to the upper pole of the spleen. Subsequently, the splenic artery and splenic vein were divided over the left anterolateral surface of the aorta, and the body plus tail of the pancreas were reflected off the posterior abdominal wall prior to anastomosis into the side or end of a Roux loop. In the head of the pancreas, a subtotal resection was performed, leaving only a rim of tissue close to the duodenal curve in a way analogous to subtotal pancreatectomy.

As with the Hiraoka paper, the paucity of patients makes this study of historical interest only. However, the radical nature of the resection belies the title of the operation, which suggests pancreatic preservation, while the truth is that this cannot be a simple operation or free from considerable hazard.

How Successful are These Operations?

Mallet-Guy reassessed 215 patients in his review of a lifetime's experience of as many operations [8]. The main follow-up comprised 177 patients and ranged from 5 years to 34 years after the initial procedure. An 85% success rate was claimed for what he described as "complete recoveries". The author's enthuasism for his operation is understandable but the 85% success rate, with little or no mention of patients who failed to reach this stage of follow-up through suicide or major ill health, is not really dealt with in any clear fashion.

Yoshioka and Wakabayashi [5] reported on 75 patients treated with selective denervation and claimed to have achieved excellent results. The real success of any operative procedure, however, depends on the disciples of the original protagonists obtaining satisfactory results in the course of time. In the case of the selective denervation approach [5], two Danish surgeons attempted to follow the Japanese lead. After five dissections in the autopsy room and a personal visit by one of the surgeons to Tokyo, six patients with severe pain due to chronic pancreatitis underwent selective denervation of the pancreas. The results were very disappointing indeed as Hoffman and Jensen [9] failed to find that this approach could provide any lasting pain relief.

I have been unable to find any critical repeat of the approach used by Mallet-Guy [8]. Likewise the newer methods described from Japan and Atlanta [6, 7] have not been critically assessed.

Personal Experience

My experience has been limited to direct anterior approach attempts to remove the ganglia in six patients with chronic pancreatitis. Three had additional surgical procedures carried out at the same operation. All but one of the six were improved at 6-month follow-up, but only two have enjoyed sustained benefit, one of whom is virtually free from requiring analgesics.

My conclusion at this stage is that there may well be some merit in interrupting the nerve pathways from the pancreas as a means of managing the pain suffered in chronic pancreatitis (and possibly in carcinoma as well). It is my belief that the whole subject requires re-examination and that studies should be set up to prospectively assess the place of neurectomy in modern surgery. Before embarking on a surgical procedure, a trial percutaneous nerve block may provide adequate indications of the likelihood of success, but the best modern paper known to us is not enthusiastic about the use of coeliac plexus blocking as a treatment for chronic pancreatitis [10]. Using 25 ml injections of alcohol on each side of the vertebral column, Leung et al. found effective pain relief in 11 out of 13 patients with pancreatic cancer, while in only 12 of 23 patients with chronic pancreatitis was pain relief achieved. In a further six patients, partial success was reported, with no effect being demonstrated in the remaining five patients. The minimal benefit was found in patients who had previously undergone pancreatic surgery, and repeat blocks were not found to be helpful. Postural hypotension of a transient nature occurred in the majority of patients, while two had nerve root pain after the treatment and one developed persistent weakness and anaesthesia of the left leg with bladder disturbance. Leung et al. concluded that the results warranted the continuing use of coeliac plexus blocking in cancer of the pancreas and (rarely) in patients with chronic pancreatitis.

References

1. Ward EM, Rorie DK, Nauss LA, Bahn RC (1979) The celiac ganglia in man: normal anatomic variations. Anesth Analg 58:461–465
2. Mallet-Guy P (1943) Resultats eloignés de la pancréatectomie gauche pour pancréatite chronique. Lyon Chir 38:339–350
3. Mallet-Guy P, Jeanjean R, Servettaz P (1945) Resultats eloignés de la splanchnicétomie unilatérale dans le traitement des pancréatites chroniques. Lyon Chir 40:293–314
4. Yoshioka H, Wakabayashi T (1957) Traitement de la douleur des pancréatites chroniques par le neurotomie de la tête du pancréas. Une technique nouvelle et ses resultats. Lyon Chir 53:836–845
5. Yoshioka H, Wakabayashi T (1958) Therapeutic neurotomy on head of pancreas for relief of pain due to chronic pancreatitis. A new technical procedure and its results. AMA Arch Surg 76:546–554
6. Hiraoka T, Watanabe E, Katoh T, Hayashida N, Mizutani J, Kanemitsu K, Miyauchi Y (1986) A new surgical approach for control of pain in chronic pancreatitis: Complete denervation of the pancreas. Am J Surg 152:549–551
7. Warren WD, Millikan WJ, Henderson JM, Hersh T (1984) A denervated pancreatic flap for control of chronic pain in pancreatitis. Surg Gynecol Obstet 259:581–583
8. Mallet-Guy P (1983) Late and very late results of resections of the nervous system in the treatment of chronic relapsing pancreatitis. Am J Surg 145:234–238
9. Hoffman J, Jensen HE (1986) Selective denervation of the pancreas for the pain of chronic pancreatitis. J R Coll Surg Edinb 31:37–39
10. Leung JWC, Bowen-Wright M, Aveling W, Shorvon PJ, Cotton PB (1983) Coeliac plexus block for pain in pancreatic cancer and chronic pancreatitis. Br J Surg 70:730–732

Why and When to Drain the Pancreatic Ductal System

C. F. FREY[1]

The underlying assumption behind pancreatic duct drainage procedures for the relief of pain in chronic pancreatitis is the belief that in many patients pain is caused by ductal hypertension. Therefore, decompression of the pancreatic ductal system would provide pain relief.

History of Pancreatic Duct Drainage Procedures

Obstruction of the major pancreatic duct may result from one or more multiple fibrotic strictures or calcium carbonate calculi frequently associated with chronic alcoholic pancreatitis or from an isolated, traumatically induced stricture of discontinuity of the major pancreatic duct resulting from necrosis and cyst formation due to biliary or other causes of necrotizing pancreatitis.

Treatment of an obstructed pancreatic duct was limited initially to those patients having calculi obstructing the major pancreatic duct. Caparelli in 1883, according to Haggard and Kirtley [1], described a baroness who ruptured a pancreatic abscess containing many calculi. Gould [2] in 1898 removed calculi from the duct of Wirsung, but the patient died 12 days after the last of two operations. Moynihan [3] in 1902 removed a pancreatic duct calculus; the patient survived. By 1939, Haggard and Kirtley [1] had collected 65 operative cases of pancreatic duct calculi that were removed, with a mortality of 18.4%. There was no long-term follow-up. They noted pancreatic calculi in 130 autopsy patients and 28 patients on the basis of radiologic studies.

The rationale stated by Moynihan in 1902 for the removal of the calculi which were noted to occur in both the duct of Santorini or Wirsung – by either the transpancreatic route described by Mayo-Robson [4] in 1904 or transductally through the papillae described by Moynihan – was to prevent "atrophy of the pancreas" and to relieve pain, nausea, and vomiting.

The concept of opening the main pancreatic duct to bypass obstruction by stricture or calculus rather than extracting calculi can be attributed to Coffey [5] in 1909 and Link [6] in 1911. In practice, duct decompressive procedures were initiated independently by Du Val [7] and by Zollinger et al. [8] in 1954. The tail of the pancreas was excised, and an end-to-side or end-to-end anastomosis was performed providing retrograde drainage of the major pancreatic duct. Retrograde drainage of the main

---

[1] University of California, Davis Medical Center, Department of Surgery, 4301 X Street, Sacramento, CA 95817, USA

Chronic Pancreatitis
Ed. by Beger, Büchler, Ditschuneit, and Malfertheiner
© Springer-Verlag Berlin Heidelberg 1990

pancreatic duct is effective if there is only one site of obstruction between the tail and the ampulla. However, in alcoholic pancreatitis, the most common cause of chronic pancreatitis, a single stricture is the exception rather than the rule. Puestow and Gillesby [9] in 1956, recognizing the need for an operation which would decompress multiple sites of obstruction in the main pancreatic duct "chain of lakes," described the longitudinal or side-to-side pancreaticojejunostomy performed in four patients.

Partington and Rochelle [10] in 1960 further modified the longitudinal pancreaticojejunostomy to its present form by not excising the tail of the pancreas. Splenectomy was no longer necessary.

Etiology of Pain in Chronic Pancreatitis

Evidence that ductal hypertension is a cause of pain is based on three lines of evidence: duct dilatation, measurements of duct pressure, and pain relief after decompression of the ducts.

Major Pancreatic Duct Dilatation

The normal pancreatic duct is 2–3 mm in diameter, increasing slightly with age [11]. The major pancreatic ductal system is dilated in most patients with chronic pancreatitis, even those with so-called small-duct disease. In the surgical literature, there has been imprecision about what is a large duct and what is a small duct. The definition of large and small duct, in fact, may be a surgical distinction based on what size duct the surgeon feels is technically big enough to perform a longitudinal pancreaticojejunostomy or as some believe, represent two different diseases characterized by large or small ducts? A survey of American Pancreas Club members indicated most felt the major pancreatic duct had to be 8 mm in diameter to make a longitudinal pancreaticojejunostomy technically feasible [12]. Some surgeons such as Keith et al. [13] require a duct 1 cm in diameter before performing a longitudinal pancreaticojejunostomy. We have used ducts as small as 5 mm in diameter and sewn the jejunum to the capsule of the pancreas rather than to the duct, as proposed by Jordan et al [14]. We do not feel it is necessary to perform a duct-to-mucosa anastomosis in the longitudinal pancreaticojejunostomy; conversely we feel it is essential in the end-to-side anastomosis.

Those surgeons willing to perform pancreaticojejunostomy on ducts as small as 0.5 cm in diameter carry out more longitudinal pancreaticojejunostomies than those who require ducts as large as 1 cm in order to perform an anastomosis. Even surgeons willing to perform longitudinal pancreaticojejunostomies on ducts as small as 0.5 cm in diameter must resect some patients whose ducts are in the 2–5 mm range. In my experience with 78 patients with chronic pancreatitis over the past 8 years, excluding the patients with pseudocysts and other miscellaneous procedures, it was possible to perform longitudinal pancreaticojejunostomy or the Frey procedure [15] on 40 patients while 13 (25%) required resection of either the distal or proximal pancreas.

Pressures in Major Pancreatic Duct

In most of the patients in whom drainage of the major pancreatic duct was performed, it was possible to obtain measurements of the intraductal pressure at the time of operation by puncture of the duct with manometric measurement. The average pressure was 33.4 cm, similar to the 35.4 cm reported by Bradley [16]. The pressure in the ducts less than 5 mm in diameter was virtually impossible to measure intraoperatively as it was not possible to locate the duct without dividing the pancreas. Therefore, we know little about the pressure in these 2- to 5-mm "small ducts." The validity of ERCP pressure measurements, plagued by technical and theoretical difficulties, limit their usefulness in resolving whether these small ducts are hypertensive in chronic pancreatitis. Measurements at the time of ERCP through the sphincter measures secretory pressure but not the pathophysiologic pressure reflecting impedance to outflow. Okazaki et al. [17] found pressures in the pancreatic duct to be higher in patients with chronic pancreatitis irrespective of the size of the main pancreatic duct. Ebbehoj et al. [18] using a small cannula connected to a transducer, showed in six patients a relationship between tissue pressures and intraductal pressure. The patients studied had either pseudocysts or obstructive pancreatitis by the 1988 Marseille-Rome classification [19], with the exception of one patient with a "nondilated" duct. The tissue pressures in the head and tail of the pancreas decreased in their patients after decompression of the pseudocysts or the main pancreatic duct. Pancreatic tissue pressures were not obtained in their patients with chronic pancreatitis who did not have cysts or a dilated duct. We have tried obtaining tissue pressures in patients with chronic pancreatitis in which the pancreas was very firm and fibrotic before and after duct decompression and were unable to obtain flows in these very fibrotic glands using pressures as high as 50 cm H_2O. The fact that duct decompression is not technically practical in the 25% of patients with ducts between 2–5 mm does not negate the possibility that ductal hypertension may exist in these ducts and in fact contribute to the pain which the patient experiences.

Pain Relief and Ductal Decompression

The results of decompression of the hypertensive pancreatic ductal system on pain relief also provide support for the belief that pain is associated with hypertension of the pancreatic ductal system. Most series report pain relief results in 80–90% of patients following longitudinal pancreaticojejunostomy, at least initially [20]. These results regarding pain relief do not differ significantly from those following resectional procedures, distal pancreatectomy and proximal pancreaticoduodenectomy, or total pancreatectomy (Table 1).

Table 1. Pain relief. (From [33])

	Good or fair	Poor or recurrence
Pancreaticojejunostomy	478/599 (79.8%)	121/599 (20.2%)
Distal pancreatectomy	242/328 (73.8%)	86/328 (26.2%)
Pancreatoduodenectomy	398/448 (88.8%)	50/448 (11.2%)
Total pancreatectomy	131/158 (82.9%)	27/154 (17.5%)

The failure of resectional procedures to provide significantly greater pain relief initially postoperatively than duct decompressions argues strongly for the significant role that ductal hypertension plays in the pain of chronic pancreatitis. Over time there is a significant failure rate in the pain relief provided by longitudinal pancratico-jejunostomy so that by 5 years, Taylor et al. [20] found only 54% of those surviving longitudinal pancreaticojejunostomy to be free of pain. Their follow-up of distal pancreatectomy at 5 years was dismal, showing only 25% to be free of pain. The poor results of distal pancreatectomy in these cases are most likely attributable to patient selection. When the disease focus is in the head of the pancreas, as it is most frequently in chronic pancreatitis, distal pancreatectomy will not help. Frey et al. [21], Eckhauser et al. [22], Morrow et al. [23] and Keith et al. [13] and other authors have shown that radical distal pancreatectomy (80%–95% distal pancreatectomy) provides excellent long-term relief in carefully selected patients.

The reasons for failure of longitudinal pancreaticojejunostomy are less related to patient selection than to (a) technical failure to carry the incision sufficiently close to the duodenum, a requirement of the operation, as described by Puestow and Gillesby [9] and Partington and Rochelle [10], or (b) the presence of a bulky head of the pancreas filled with multiple cysts and calculi in the ducts of Wirsung, Santorini, and that to the uncinate process and their associated tributary ducts. When the head of the pancreas is bulky, the main and tributary ducts in the head cannot be adequately decompressed by longitudinal pancreaticojejunostomy, even when the operation is properly performed, by opening the main duct to the duodenum.

The newer operations, the procedures of Beger et al. [24], Frey, and Smith [15] and Warren et al. [25], all address this problem of a large bulky head of pancreas in which there may be multiple cysts and impacted calculi not only in the ducts of Wirsung or Santorini or the duct to uncinate but in the tributary ducts as well. Prior to the development of these new operations, this problem could be dealt with only by pancreaticoduodenectomy or 95% distal pancreatectomy. The newer procedures make pancreaticoduodenectomy or 95% distal pancreatectomy unnecessary in many patients who might otherwise have been subjected to it in the past. However, long-term follow-up is not available on these new operations so that information regarding pain relief must still be considered preliminary. In our modest experience with 11 of these patients having a bulky head of the pancreas, four of whom had previously failed longitudinal pancreaticojejunostomy, our follow-up period ranges from 3 to 39 months, with an average of 2 years. Pain relief has been complete in eight patients, none of whom have required narcotics, and much improved in three, all of whom were addicted to narcotics prior to operation. Beger et al.'s [26] experience is much larger and follow-up longer as recently reported. Pain relief was achieved in 77% of 109 patients and pain reduced in 13 patients, or 12%.

While there is room for argument, these newer operations have achieved better results than longitudinal pancreaticojejunostomy primarily by improved drainage of the head rather than by the volume of diseased tissue resected. While there was pancreatic tissue removed in all three procedures, in the Beger and Warren procedures more tissue is resected than in the Frey procedure [15].

An additional advantage of these new operations is that it may be possible, as Beger pointed out, to decompress an obstructed common bile duct, one of the most frequent complications of chronic pancreatitis, by removing the restrictive fibrotic tissue constricting the common duct rather than performing a separate Roux-en-Y cholecy-stojejunostomy or choledochoduodenectomy.

Perineural Inflammation

In 1973 we [27] published photomicrographs demonstrating inflammation and fibrosis about some of the nerve endings in the pancreas in patients with "small" main pancreatic ducts. At that time, we assumed these ducts were not hypertensive because they were not dilated, an assumption which is probably incorrect. We theorized that the presence of this perineural inflammatory response might be a source of pain in patients with chronic pancreatitis whose ducts were not dilated. Recent work by Bockman et al. [28] using electronmicroscopy has confirmed the presence of damage to the nerve sheath in chronic pancreatitis. We have also noted neuromalike formations in some patients with chronic pancreatitis. Whether these perineural inflammatory and fibrotic reactions and neuromalike lesions initiate pain is neither proven nor disproven. It is certainly possible that there may be another, or more than one, source of pain in some patients with chronic pancreatitis aside from ductal hypertension. Numerous attempts have been made in the past to relieve the pain of chronic pancreatitis by interruption of the pain fibers to and from the pancreas, but good results have either not occurred or been short lived [29–31]. The most recent work reported by Stone [32] on 15 patients subjected to left transthoracic splanchnic nerve division (greater-lesser splanchnic) and bilateral vagotomy achieved pain relief. However, pain recurred in five which was relieved in four after right thoracic splanchnicectomy. He reported initially favorable results after an average follow-up of 15 months. There was one death.

There are other possible sources of pain in patients with chronic pancreatitis. We have noted periductal and intraductal inflammation and infection, perhaps similar to that which occurs in the biliary tract with cholangitis.

Factors Affecting the Selection of Operations

Operative Mortality

A major reason for considering a drainage procedure as opposed to pancreaticoduodenectomy in the management of patients with chronic pancreatitis is the lower operative mortality. Even in the most recent reports on the results of pancreaticoduodenectomy versus ductal decompression for chronic pancreatitis, the operative mortality of pancreaticoduodenectomy (5.9%) is significantly higher than that for longitudinal pancreaticojejunostomy (3.4%) or distal pancreatectomy (4.1%; Table 2 [33]. The newer procedures of Beger et al. [24], Frey and Smith [15], and Warren et al. [25] seem also to have a low operative mortality rate. (0.7%; Table 3) [33]. The number of late deaths following operation is dependent not on the operation performed but on the contributions of alcohol intake and progression of the pancreatitis (Table 4). Exocrine and endocrine insufficiency is also an important consideration in a patient population predominated by alcoholics, who are notoriously unreliable in their nutrition and insulin management.

Table 2. Operative mortality in chronic pancreatitis: collected series 1972–1988. (From [33])

	Number of patients	Deaths
Pancreaticojejunostomy	1194	41 (3.4%)
Distal pancreatectomy	1625	66 (4.1%)
Pancreaticoduodenectomy	1108	66 (5.9%)
Total pancreatectomy	324	31 (9.6%)

Table 3. Local resection of head of pancreas and denervated pancreatic flap and duodenal-preserving resection

Reference	n	Operative mortality	Late deaths	Average follow-up	Free	Pain Infrequent	Frequent
Beger et al. [26]	127	0.8%	4.7%	3.6	84/109 (77%)	12/109 (12%)	12/109 (11%)
Frey [15]	11	0	0	2.3	8/11 (73%)	3/11 (27%)	–
Warren et al. [25]	5	0	0	–	–	–	–

Table 4. Late deaths in chronic pancreatitis: collected series 1972–1988. (From [33])

	Number of patients	Deaths
Pancreaticojejunostomy	639	185 (28.9%)
Distal pancreatectomy	934	170 (18.2%)
Pancreaticoduodenectomy	805	171 (21.2%)
Total pancreatectomy	250	62 (24.8%)

Exocrine and Endocrine Function

One reason for favoring a drainage procedure in operating to relieve the pain of chronic pancreatitis is to avoid creating either exocrine or endocrine insufficiency. In our experience and that of others, approximately 30% of patients are diabetic preoperatively. In patients undergoing 80%–95% distal resection, the incidence of diabetes postoperatively is 72%, and four-fifths of these diabetic patients will be insulin dependent diabetics [24]. In patients undergoing a 40%–80% resection of the distal pancreas, 32% become diabetic postoperatively, and 60% of these patients are insulin dependent. After longitudinal pancreaticojejunostomy about 20%–40% of patients can be expected to become insulin-dependent diabetics during follow-up over several years (Table 5) [33]. The incidence of diabetes immediately after pancreaticoduodenectomy is similar to that following 40%–80% distal resection of the pancreas. While irreversible brain damage and death from hypoglycemic attacks are reported in every large series, there is no significant difference in the incidence of late

Table 5. Endocrine function pre- and postoperation – cases with insulin therapy. (From [33])

Reference	Follow-up time	n	PJ Pre	Post	n	DP Pre	Post	n	PD Pre	Post
Frey (1976)	8.2 years	–	–	–	53	3.8%	19%	19	15%	26%
Frey (1976)[a]	–	–	–	–	77	9.1	58%	–	–	–
Grodsinsky (1980)	12 months	–	–	–	30	26%	50%	–	–	–
Taylor (1981)	5 years	19	–	21%	38	–	37%	26	–	42%
Prinz (1981)	7.9 years	87	11%	28%	–	–	–	–	–	–
Gall (1982)	12 months –10 years	–	–	–	–	–	–	116	18%	44%
Eckhausen (1984)[a]	10 years	–	–	–	87	11.5%	62%	–	–	–
Kiviluoto (1984)	3.2 years	13	8%	67%	24	8%	39%	4	–	75%–
Morrow (1984)	5 years	46	24%	59%	29	7%	55%	–	–	–
Morrow (1984)[a]	9 years	–	–	–	8	0%	100%	–	–	–
Escallon (1986)	2 years	19	16%	32%	–	–	–	–	–	–
Hanyu (1987)	5 years	37	27%	48%	36	14%	39%	62	24%	27%
Williamson (1987)	4.5 years	–	–	–	16	50%	56%	6	50%	67%
Morrel (1987)	5–9 years	15	–	10%	57	–	57%	17	–	47%
Cooper (1987)	3 months –10 years	–	–	–	–	–	–	83	23%	36%
Kerremans (1987)	1–3 years	–	–	–	–	–	–	12	8%	50%
Frick (1987)	6.5 years	–	–	–	100	7%	36%	72	2%	29%
Rossi (1987)	4.9 years	–	–	–	–	–	–	73	25%	45%
Keith (1988)	4–9 years	–	–	–	32	9.3%	45%	5	–	25%

PJ, Pancreaticojejunostomy; DP, distal pancreatectomy; PD, pancreaticoduodenectomy
[a] Report in which 80%–95% pancreas was resected

deaths following either 80%–95% distal pancreatectomy, pancreaticoduodenectomy, or longitudinal pancreaticojejunostomy. In summary, endocrine deficiency is most common after 80%–95% distal resection of the pancreas but seems to have little influence on survival. This may be in part due to continued progressive destruction of the pancreas from chronic pancreatitis in patients whose pancreas has been drained but not resected. Over time the incidence of endocrine insufficiency requiring insulin replacement approaches that seen immediately postoperatively in patients undergoing proximal or distal resection of the pancreas.

Clinically apparent steatorrhea develops in 38% of patients after 80%–95% distal resection. The incidence of clinically apparent steatorrhea after longitudinal pancreaticojejunostomy and 40%–80% distal pancreatectomy is similar at 30% (Table 6). Fecal fat loss after pancreaticoduodenectomy is 22%–76% of ingested fat. This loss is reduced if the pylorus and antrum are preserved, as advocated by Traverso and Longmire [34].

Table 6. Exocrine function pre- and postoperation – incidence of steatorrhea. (From [33])

Reference	Follow-up time	PJ			DP			PD		
		n	Pre	Post	n	Pre	Post	n	Pre	Post
Frey (1976)	8.2 years	–	–	–	53	3.7%	19%	19	5.2%	55%
Frey (1976)[a]	8.2 years	–	–	–	77	9%	37.6%	–	–	–
Prinz (1981)	7.9 years	87	20%	33%	–	–	–	–	–	–
Morrow (1984)	5 years	46	9%	24%	21	23%	47%	–	–	–
Morrow (1984)[a]	5 years	–	–	–	8	50%	100%	–	–	–
Kiviluoto (1984)	3.2 years	–	–	–	24	13%	28%	–	–	–
Escallon (1986)	2 years	19	–	16%	–	–	–	–	–	–
Rossi (1987)	5 years	–	–	–	–	–	–	73	26%	75%
Williamson (1987)	4.5 years	–	–	–	16	19%	31%	6	33%	50%
Keith	4–9 years	–	–	–	32	25%	90%	5	25%	100%
Stone (1988)	6 years	–	–	–	–	–	–	15	27%	53%

PJ, Pancreaticojejunostomy; DP, distal pancreatectomy; PD, pancreaticoduodenectomy
[a] Report in which 80%–95% of pancreas was resected

Preservation of Exocrine and Endocrine Function

A yet unsubstantiated but potentially important and compelling indication for longitudinal pancreaticojejunostomy has been advanced by Nealon et al. [35]. They reported that pancreaticojejunostomy in patients with large ducts in whom severe morphologic changes and exocrine and endocrine insufficiency had not already occurred slowed further progression of exocrine and endocrine insufficiency regardless of whether the patients abstained from alcohol.

Should Nealon et al.'s [35] thesis be confirmed by others, it could have a profound impact on the present indications and timing of longitudinal pancreaticojejunostomy. Any patient with chronic pancreatitis with or without pain whose duct was sufficiently large to technically perform longitudinal pancreaticojejunostomy would be a candidate for longitudinal pancreaticojejunostomy as early as possible in the course of the disease in hopes of slowing the progression of exocrine and endocrine insufficiency. In contrast, the indication for longitudinal pancreaticojejunostomy and the Beger and Frey procedures at present are persistent or frequently recurring pain sufficiently severe to require narcotics for pain relief.

Complications of Chronic Pancreatitis in Patients with Pain

Other than for pain, duct decompression can be very useful in dealing with some of the complications of chronic pancreatitis such as pseudocysts. Depending on the location of these pseudocysts, they can often be drained with the same Roux-en-Y limb used to drain the main pancreatic duct or, if the pseudocyst is in continuity with the main pancreatic duct, by draining the main pancreatic duct.

Common Bile Duct Obstruction in Chronic Pancreatitis. The Beger and Frey procedures [15, 24] can be used not only to drain the ducts of Wirsung, Santorini, and that to the uncinate process, but to relieve the cicatrix engulfing the intrapancreatic portion of the common duct, thus negating the need for either a separate Roux-en-Y choledochojejunostomy or choledochojejunostomy.

Duodenal Obstruction in Chronic Pancreatitis. Longitudinal pancreaticojejunostomy in conjunction with the Frey and Beger procedures might in some cases reduce the fibrotic inflammatory reaction stricturing the duodenum.

Pancreatic Duct Fistulas. Pancreatic ascites and pleural or pericardial pancreaticothoracic fistulas are best managed initially by nothing by mouth and total parenteral nutrition (TPN). If the fistulas persist after 2–3 weeks, decompression of the main pancreatic duct with a Roux-en-Y limb of jejunum is required [36]. Once the main pancreatic duct is decompressed, the fistulas will close.

Contraindications to Ductal Decompression in Chronic Pancreatitis. Ductal decompression procedures in the absence of some other additional procedures are not definitive in the management of either left-sided portal hypertension from splenic vein thrombosis, or that of pseudoaneurysms of the splenic and other peripancreatic vessels usually associated with pseudocysts.

Suspicion of Cancer

In approximately 5%–12% of patients with noncalculus obstruction of the common bile duct it may not be possible on the basis of preoperative evaluation to establish whether one is dealing with chronic pancreatitis or cancer. The surgeon's level of suspicion regarding cancer must remain high as pancreatic carcinoma can masquerade as a pseudocyst or chronic obstructive pancreatitis. Every large series of longitudinal pancreaticojejunostomies contains some patients who are found later to have pancreatic cancer not chronic pancreatitis. In the past year, we have managed three patients with large pseudocysts, one patient with common duct obstruction and two with a markedly dilated pancreatic duct, all of whom were treated operatively for chronic pancreatitis at other hospitals, but whose primary problem was a carcinoma of the head of the pancreas or distal common bile duct.

While this article does not address the diagnosis, preoperative assessment, verification of the diagnosis of chronic pancreatitis, the role of CT scan, ERCP, and angiography, the team approach, the selection and commitment of the surgeon, and patient selection including the role of alcohol and drug addiction on outcome, it is important to note that these factors are very important in the management, and that they influence the operative results in patients with chronic pancreatitis.

Summary

We can summarize our observations regarding duct decompression in chronic pancrceatitis in the following points:
1. The major pancreatic duct is usually enlarged. A "small" duct of 2–5 mm is small only for the surgeon.

2. Intraoperative duct pressure measurements are invariably elevated, on the average three to four times normal in ducts 5 mm or larger.
3. Decompression of the pancreatic ductal system provides excellent clinical pain relief.
4. Recurrence of pain after duct decompression is due to incomplete decompression of the main and tributary ducts due to failure to perform longitudinal pancreaticojejunostomy as recommended or to a bulky thick head of pancreas.
5. A bulky thick head of pancreas 2–5 cm or more is best managed by the Beger or Frey procedure.
6. Complications of chronic pancreatitis which may be amenable to correction by longitudinal pancreaticojejunostomy or the Beger or Frey procedure are pseudocysts, common bile duct obstruction, duodenal obstruction, pancreatic ascites, intrapleural intrathoracic or intrapericardial fistulas.
7. Complications of chronic pancreatitis which are not amenable to correction by longitudinal pancreaticojejunostomy or the Beger or Frey procedures include left-sided portal hypertension secondary to splenic vein thrombosis, pseudoaneurysms of splenic and peripancreatic vessels, and main pancreatic ducts 2–5 mm in size.
8. Longitudinal pancreaticojejunostomy or the Beger or Frey procedure have a lower mortality than pancreaticoduodenectomy and are less likely to induce endocrine and exocrine insufficiency.
9. With regard to longitudinal pancreaticojejunostomy, pancreaticoduodenectomy or distal pancreatectomy, the incidence of late deaths is a reflection not of the operation performed but the effects of continued alcoholism and pancreatitis.

References

1. Haggard WD, Kirtley JA (1939) Pancreatic calculi: a review of 65 operative and 139 non-operative cases. Ann Surg 109:809–826
2. Gould AP (1898) Pancreatic calculi: transactions of the Clinical Society of London. Lancet 2:1532
3. Moynihan SB (1902) Pancreatic calculus. Lancet 2:335
4. Mayo-Robson AW (1904) The pathology and surgery of certain diseases of the pancreas. Lancet 1:733
5. Coffey R (1909) Pancreaticoenterostomy and pancreatectomy. Ann Surg 50:1238–1264
6. Link G (1911) Treatment of chronic pancreatitis by pancreatostomy. Ann Surg 53:768–782
7. DuVal MK (1954) Caudal pancreaticojejunostomy for chronic relapsing pancreatitis. Ann Surg 140:775–785
8. Zollinger RM, Keith LM Jr, Ellison EH (1954) Pancreatitis. N Engl J Med 251:497–502
9. Puestow CB, Gillesby WJ (1956) Retrograde surgical drainage of pancreas for chronic relapsing pancreatitis. Arch Surg 76:898–907
10. Partington PF, Rochelle REL (1960) Modified procedure for retrograde drainage of the pancreatic duct. Ann Surg 152:1037–1043
11. Skandalakis JE, Gray SW, Rowe JS, et al. (1979) Anatomical complications of pancreatic surgery. Contemporary Surg 15:17
12. Prellor T, Frey CF, Zaiss C (1981) Toxicity of ascitic fluids from pigs with hemorrhegic pancreatitis. J Surg Res 33: 136–137
13. Keith RG, Saibil FG, Sheppard RH (1989) Treatment of chronic pancreatitis by pancreatic resection. Am J Surg 157:156–162
14. Jordan GL, Strug BS, Crowder WE (1977) Current status of pancreaticojejunostomy in the management of chronic pancreatitis. Am J Surg 133:46–51

15. Frey CF, Smith GJ (1987) Description and rationale of a new operation for chronic pancreatitis. Pancreas 2:701–707
16. Bradley EL (1982) Pancreatic duct pressure in chronic pancreatitis. Am J Surg 144:313–316
17. Okazaki K, Yamamoto Y, Kagiyama S, et al. (1986) Pressure of papillary sphincter zone and pancreatic main ductal pressure in patients with chronic pancreatitis. Gastroenterology 91:409–418
18. Ebbehoj N, Borly L, Madsen P, et al. (1986) Pancreatic tissue pressure and pain in chronic pancreatitis. Pancreas 1:556–558
19. Singer MV, Gyr KE, Sarles H (1985) Revised classification of pancreatitis. Report of the Second International Symposium on the Classification of Pancreatitis in Marseille, France, March 20–30, 1984. Gastroenterology 89:683–690 and: Sarles JC, Adler G, Dani R et al. (1988) Pancreatitis. Definition and Classification. The revision of the Marseille Classification. International Congress of Gastroenterology and Digestive Endoscopy, Rome
20. Taylor RH, Bagley FH, Braasch JW, Warren KW (1981) Ductal drainage or resection for chronic pancreatitis. Am J Surg 141:28–33
21. Frey CF, Child CG, Fry WF (1976) Pancreatectomy for chronic pancreatitis. Ann Surg 184:403–414
22. Eckhauser FE, Strodel WE, Knol JA, et al. (1984) Near total pancreatectomy for chronic pancreatitis. Surg 96:599–607
23. Morrow CE, Cohen JL, Sutherland ER, et al. (1984) Chronic pancreatitis: long-term surgical results of pancreatic duct drainage, pancreatic resection, and near-total pancreatectomy and islet authotransplantation. Surgery 96:608–616
24. Beger HG, Krautzberger W, Bittner R, et al. (1985) Duodenum-preserving resection of the head of the pancreas in patients with severe chronic pancreatitis. Surgery 97:467–473
25. Warren WD, Millikan WJ Jr, Henderson JM, et al. (1984) A denervated pancreatic flap for control of chronic pain in pancreatitis. Surg Gynecol Obstet 159:581–583
26. Beger HG, Büchler M, Bittner RR, et al. (1989) Duodenum-preserving resection of the head of the pancreas in severe chronic pancreatitis. Ann Surg 209:273–278
27. Frey CF (1973) 95% pancreatectomy. In: The pancreas. Mosby, St Louis, pp 96–123
28. Bockman DE, Büchler M, Malfertheiner P, Beger HG (1988) Analysis of nerves in chronic pancreatitis. Gastroenterology 94:1459–1469
29. Howard J, Jordon GL (1960) Surgical disease of the pancreas. Lippincott, Philadelphia
30. Ribet M, Prost M, Quandale P, et al. (1975) Traitement chirurgical des pancréatites autonomies. J Chir (Paris) 110:25–38
31. Sarles JC, Trink DG (1976) Surgical treatment of chronic pancreatitis. Biol Gastroenterol (Paris) 9:76
32. Stone H (1988) Pancreatic denervation for pain relief in chronic alcohol associated pancreatitis. Pancreas Club Meeting, May 6, New Orleans
33. Frey CF, Suzuki M, Isaji S, Zhu Y (1989) Pancreatic resection for chronic pancreatitis. Surg Clin North Am 69:499–528
34. Traverso LW, Longmire WP (1978) Preservation of the pylorus during pancreaticoduodenectomy. Surg Gynecol Obstet 146:959–962
35. Nealon WH, Townsend CM Jr, Thompson JC (1987) Operative drainage of the pancreatic duct delays functional impairment in patients with chronic pancreatitis: a prospective analysis. American Society of the Alimentary Tract, San Francisco
36. Pottmeyer EW III, Frey CF, Matsuno S (1987) Pancreaticopleural fistulas. Arch Surg 122:648–654

Pseudocyst Drainage in Chronic Pancreatitis

R. A. Prinz[1]

Since pancreatic pseudocysts and chronic pancreatitis are both problems caused by alcohol abuse, it is not surprising that they can occur simultaneously in the same patient. The question arises as to whether pseudocyst disease is the same insofar as presentation, natural history, and results of treatment when it occurs in patients with chronic pancreatitis. To evaluate this, we have reviewed our experience and that of other investigators to determine the incidence of pseudocyst in patients with chronic pancreatitis, the likelihood of pseudocyst regression in these patients, the incidence of cyst recurrence and persistent abdominal pain after simple internal drainage, and the efficacy of combined pseudocyst and pancreatic duct drainage for their management.

Pancreatic pseudocysts occur in 2%–10% of patients with acute pancreatitis [1]. A higher incidence of pancreatic pseudocyst has been noted in patients with chronic pancreatitis. Grodsinsky [2] reported that 37% of his patients undergoing operation for chronic pancreatitis had a history of pancreatic pseudocyst or one found at operation. Potts and Moody [3] also found that 35% of their patients operated on for chronic pancreatitis had pseudocyst disease. In our own experience with 87 consecutive patients undergoing lateral pancreaticojejunostomy for intractable pain of chronic pancreatitis, 39% had pseudocyst disease [4]. This included 26 patients whose pseudocysts were indentified preoperatively (21 patients) or intraoperatively (5 patients) and 8 patients who had previously undergone surgery for pseudocyst drainage. In this study, pancreatic pseudocysts were defined as encapsulated fluid collections 3 cm or greater in diameter, the presence of which was confirmed by surgical exploration in each case.

Crass and Way [5] have pointed out that the main differene in the presentation of an acute pancreatic pseudocyst and a pseudocyst in a patient with chronic pancreatitis is that the acute cyst is associated with a definite recent attack of acute pancreatitis. Patients with chronic pancreatitis and a pancreatic pseudocyst usually have a prolonged history of abdominal pain and recurrent attacks of abdominal distress and pancreatitis. Aside from this one aspect of the history, there is little difference in the manifestations of an acute pancreatic pseudocyst and those in the setting of chronic pancreatitis. In our own series of patients with chronic pancreatitis undergoing lateral pancreaticojejunostomy, there was no difference in the clinical characteristics of the patients with chronic pancreatitis alone and those with chronic pancreatitis and a pseudocyst in terms of abdominal pain, diabetes, steatorrhea, weight loss, nausea and

[1] Department of Surgery, Loyola University Medical Center, 2160 S. First Avenue, Maywood, Il 60153, USA

Chronic Pancreatitis
Ed. by Beger, Büchler, Ditschuneit, and Malfertheiner
© Springer-Verlag Berlin Heidelberg 1990

Table 1. Clinical characteristics of 87 consecutive patients undergoing lateral pancreaticojejuno-stomy for intractable abdominal pain secondary to chronic pancreatitis (percentages)

	Total	Chronic pancreatitis and pseudocyst	Chronic pancreatitis alone
Age (mean years)	47	45	48
Abdominal pain	100	100	100
Diabetes	24	31	21
Steatorrhea	26	31	25
Weight loss > 4.5 kg	33	35	33
Nausea and vomiting	20	19	20
Abdominal tenderness	35	38	34
Amylase level > 250 U/l	26	31	25
White blood cell count > 10000/mm^3	21	23	20

vomiting, abdominal tenderness, elevation of serum amylase, and elevated white blood cell count [4] (Table 1). Thus, pseudocyst diasese in chronic pancreatitis presents primarily with the symptoms of chronic pancreatitis.

Even though it is difficult if not impossible to differentiate a bland fluid collection from a pseudocyst initially, it is well accepted that 15%–30% of acute pancreatic pseudocysts resolve spontaneously [6]. However, this does not hold true for patients with chronic pancreatitis. Crass and Way [5] emphasized the difference between an acute pancreatic pseudocyst and those associated with chronic pancreatitis. They recommended prompt operative therapy of pseudocysts in patients with chronic pancreatitis, since spontaneous regression is so unlikely to occur in this group. In our own experience with 105 patients with pancreatic pseudocyst, 28% or 29 patients had spontaneous regression of their pseudocyst [6]. However, none of the eight patients with chronic pancreatitis, as evidenced radiographically by pancreatic calcifications, had spontaneous resolution of their pseudocyst. In the series reported by McConnell and coworkers [7], pseudocysts resolved spontaneously in 9 of 44 patients with a pseudocyst occurring in the setting of acute pancreatitis, while only one patient had spontaneous pseudocyst regression among the 30 patients with chronic pancreatitis.

Patients with chronic pancreatitis who undergo pseudocyst drainage alone have a higher incidence of cyst recurrence and persistent abdominal pain. Traverso and coworkers [8] demonstrated a high incidence of reoperation in patients with chronic pancreatitis undergoing pseudocyst drainage. In this series and that of pseudocyst patients reported by Frey [9], cyst recurrence and persistent abdominal pain were the most frequent causes for reoperation. Of 120 patients at the University of Michigan undergoing operation for pseudocysts, Frey reported that 40 patients required a second operation and 5 patients a third operation. Of these 40 patients, 26 had a second operation for persistent or recurrent pseudocysts and 11 were operated on for persistent or recurrent abdominal pain.

Pseudocyst recurrence in the setting of chronic pancreatitis has been noted after both resection and internal drainage. Kiviluoto and colleagues [10] noted recurrent pseudocyst development in 4 (13%) of 32 patients with chronic pancreatitis who were treated primarily with pseudocyst resection by distal pancreatectomy. In addition, four other patients needed subsequent extensive pancreatic resection because of progression of chronic pancreatitis. Of the seven patients with chronic pancreatitis reported by Grodsinsky [2] undergoing internal drainage of a pancreatic pseudocyst, one had a recurrent cyst and three had persistent or recurrent abdominal pain. In our own experience, 4 of 12 patients who had undergone prior pseudocyst drainage had a recurrent or persistent cyst noted at the time of lateral pancreaticojejunostomy [4]. In addition to pseudocyst recurrence, reoperation because of unrelenting abdominal and back pain has also been a problem in our patients. Among 81 patients whom we have thus treated surgically for pancreatic pseudocyst, 15 have required reoperation [11]. In seven of these, the cause of pain was continued intractable abdominal pain. Lateral pancreaticojejunostomy was effective in relieving this pain in each patient. Way and coworkers [12] also noted that 7 of 16 patients with chronic pancreatitis undergoing pseudocyst drainage continued to suffer from chronic abdominal pain.

These findings convince us that pseudocyst disease in the setting of chronic pancreatitis is different than acute pseudocyst disease. This difference is important because of the implications that it has for therapy. We believe that optimum treatment for pancreatic pseudocysts in patients with chronic pancreatitis should include therapy for both problems. Since our preferred method of treating chronic pancreatitis in patients with a dilated pancreatic duct is to obtain complete ductal drainage with a lateral pancreaticojejunostomy [13], we have favored combined drainage of the pancreatic duct and pseudocyst as definitive therapy for this complex of problems. In our experience, patients with a pancreatic pseudocyst and chronic pancreatitis have a dilated pancreatic duct, and in at least one-third to one-half of patients the pseudocyst communicates with the main pancreatic duct.

It thus becomes important to recognize the presence of chronic pancreatitis in patients with pseudocyst. Chronic pancreatitis should be suspected in the patient with excessive alcohol consumption and a history of recurrent abdominal pain. Coexisting diabetes, steatorrhea, and weight loss suggest pancreatic endocrine and exocrine insufficiency, which supports a diagnosis of chronic pancreatitis. Detection of pancreatic calcifications on a plain abdominal radiograph of a CT scan would also indicate chronic pancreatitis. For patients with a pancreatic pseudocyst in whom chronic pancreatitis is suspected, we believe that ERCP is indicated. This procedure can delineate pancreatic ductal obstruction and dilation. If the pancreatic duct is enlarged, we believe it should be decompressed at the time of pseudocyst drainage. We do not believe it is necessary to obtain ERCP routinely in the diagnostic evaluation of pancreatic pseudocysts, but we think the therapeutic ramifications of a pseudocyst in the setting of chronic pancreatitis is so important that ERCP should be done whenever this is a serious consideration. We would omit the ERCP if pancreatic duct dilatation is identified on CT scan in the patient with chronic pancreatitis.

Kiviluoto and associates [10] have emphasized the frequency of silent or asymptomatic pseudocysts in patients with chronic pancreatitis. Three of their 32 patients with chronic pancreatitis treated with distal pancreatectomy for pseudocyst disease had a silent cyst revealed on follow-up radiographic studies. This, coupled with the above-noted finding that the symptoms in patients with chronic pancreatitis and a pseudocyst are the same as those in chronic pancreatitis alone, emphasizes that pseudocysts can be missed if not specifically looked for in the patient with chronic pancreatitis.

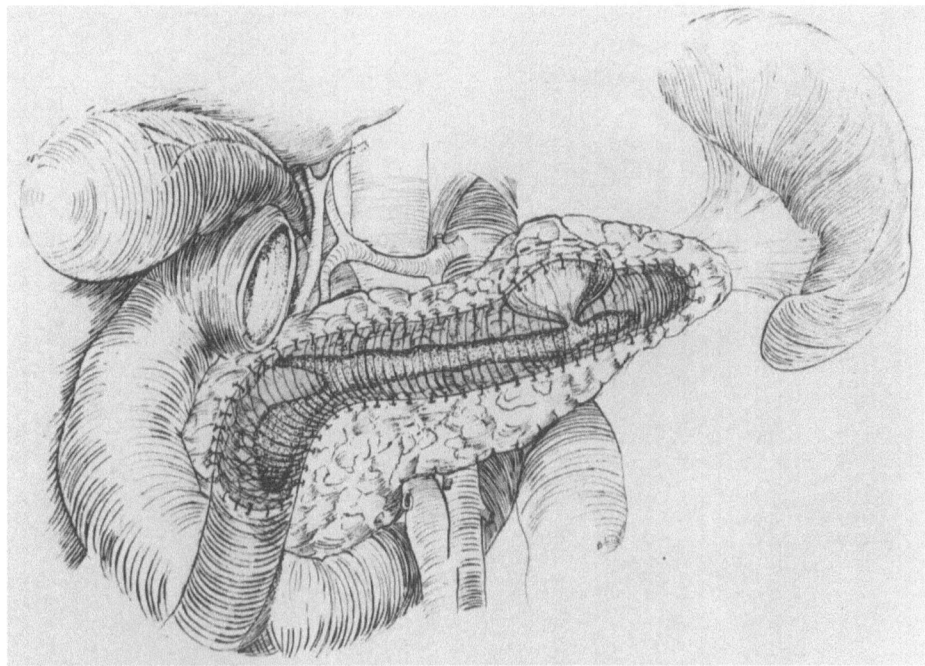

Fig. 1. Intrapancreatic pseudocysts are drained by extending the pancreatic ductal incision into the pseudocyst and incorporating the opening into the overlying jejunal limb. (From [4])

Since both pseudocyst disease and chronic pancreatitis require treatment, we believe this is best accomplished with lateral pancreaticojejunostomy. Most pseudocysts are suitably located for incorporation into the Roux-en-Y loop used for lateral pancreaticojejunostomy. Intrapancreatic pseudocysts and those linked to the main pancreatic duct can be drained by extending the pancreatic ductal incision to include the cyst or widening the communication of the cyst with the pancreatic duct (Fig. 1). Since the pseudocyst is frequently in continuity with the ductal system, it can be used as a window to find the main pancreatic duct. Once this is accomplished, the entire ductal system, including both the ducts of Wirsung and Santorini, are opened from as close as possible to the duodenum to the tail. The opening of the pseudocyst is then incorporated into the overlying Roux-en-Y loop used for the pancreaticojejunostomy. A single layer of interrupted sutures is used for this side-to-side anastomosis. The jejunum is sewn to the capsule of the pancreas and the wall of the pseudocyst; we do not attempt a duct-to-mucosa anastomosis. The jejunojejunostomy is performed in a routine matter. External drainage of the pancreatic bed is usually not necessary after pancreaticojejunostomy for chronic pancreatitis. Larger or extrapancreatic cysts that are not in continuity with the main pancreatic duct can be drained by opening a dependent portion of the pseudocyst and extending the end or side of the Roux-en-Y loop over for a similar one layer anastomosis (Fig. 2).

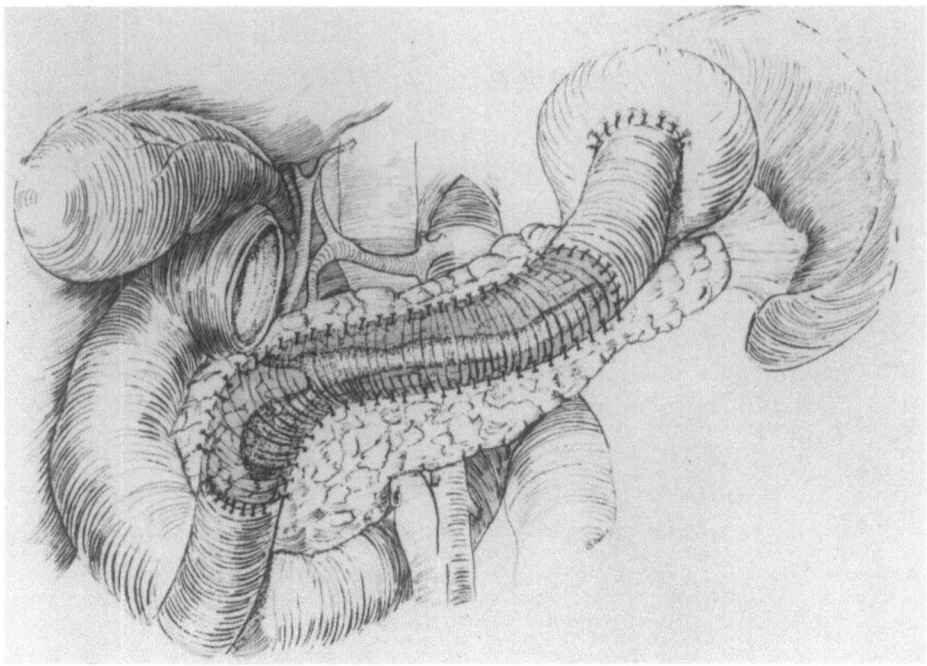

Fig. 2. Extrapancreatic pseudocysts are drained by anastomosing the free end of the Roux-en-Y loop of jejunum to the dependent portion of the cyst. (From [4])

This approach has been used in 87 consecutive patients undergoing lateral pancreaticojejunostomy. Among these patients, 26 had a coexistent pseudocyst and underwent combined drainage of the cyst and pancreatic duct. The remaining 61 patients had lateral pancreaticojejunostomy alone. Follow-up ranged from 3 months to 10 years (mean follow-up, 2.5 years). Fifty-seven percent of patients undergoing combined drainage and 48% of patients undergoing lateral pancreaticojejunostomy alone were pain free at the time of follow-up. Patients were judged to be improved if their abdominal pain was lessened, and if they had regained weight, sought employment, and no longer required frequent hospitalizations for exacerbations of their symptoms. Twenty-three percent of patients with combined drainge and 36% patients with pancreatic duct drainage alone were pain free after operation. Overall 81% of patients with combined drainage of 84% of patients with ductal drainage alone benefited from operation. Patients who had no pain relief, who went on to require additional surgical procedures for pain of chronic pancreatitis, or who suffered operative mortality were classified as poor results. Nineteen percent of patients with combined drainage and 16% of pancreaticojejunostomy alone patients fell into this class. Five patients, including one with combined drainage, have required additional surgical procedures related to pancreatitis. These included near-total pancreatectomy (one patient), splanchnic ganglionectomy (one patient), and revision of lateral pancreaticojejunostomy (three patients). No recurrent pseudocysts have been detected in the follow-up period to date in either group.

An objection to pseudocyst drainage in combination with lateral pancreaticojejunostomy would be the possibility of increasing the risk of operation. The evidence from our series does not support this contention. The morbidity and the mortality in patients undergoing simultaneous pseudocyst and pancreatic duct drainage were the same as in patients with pancreatic duct drainage alone. Complications occurred in five patients with simultaneous drainage (19%). These complications included one episode each of pneumonia, wound infection, urinary tract infection, anastomotic bleeding, and pancreatic fistula. This compares favorably to 11 complications (18%) in patients undergoing lateral pancreaticojejunostomy alone. These included four cases of pneumonia and intra-abdominal abcesses, two episodes of bleeding requiring reoperation and one case of wound infection. There were two deaths in patients with simultaneous drainage (8%). The first death occurred in a patient who developed an anastomotic leak, and who died of overwhelming staphylococcal sepsis. The second death was the result of complications of severe peptic ulcer disease in a patient who also had external drainage of an infected pseudocyst. There was one death among the patients having pancreatic duct drainage alone (2%); this resulted from mesenteric infarction in a patient with chronic renal failure. There was no significant difference in the morbidity and the mortality rates between these two groups of patients. Simultaneous lateral pancreaticojejunostomy does not appear to increase the risk of internal pseudocyst drainage. The 19% morbidity and 8% mortality found in our 26 patients undergoing simultaneous lateral pancreaticojejunostomy and pseudocyst drainage compares favorably with the results of morbidity and mortality in our patients undergoing pseudocyst drainage alone and those reported by other investigators.

This review concludes that appropriate treatment of pseudocyst disease in the patient with chronic pancreatitis must deal with both problems. Simultaneous pseudocyst and pancreatic duct drainage with lateral pancreaticojejunostomy is an effective, efficacious method of treatment which does not increase morbidity and mortality. Long-term results with this approach are favorable in decreasing the rate of cyst recurrence and intractable abdominal pain.

Acknowledgement. We appreciate the help of Frances M. Rinaldo in preparing this manuscript.

References

1. Bradley EL II, Clements JL, Gonzalez AC (1979) The natural history of pancreatic pseudocysts: a unified concept of management. Am J Surg 137:135–141
2. Grodsinsky C (1980) Surgical treatment of chronic pancreatitis. Arch Surg 115:545–551
3. Potts JR, Moody FG (1981) Surgical therapy for chronic pancreatitis: selecting the appropriate approach. Am J Surg 12:654–659
4. Munn JS, Aranha GV, Greenlee HB, Prinz RA (1987) Simultaneous treatment of chronic pancreatitis and pancreatic pseudocyst. Arch Surg 122:662–667
5. Crass RA, Way LW (1981) Acute and chronic pancreatic pseudocysts are different. Am J Surg 142:660–663

6. Aranha GV, Prinz RA, Esguerra AC, Greenlee HB (1983) The nature and course of cystic pancreatic lesions diagnosed by ultrasound. Arch Surg 118:486–488
7. McConnell DB, Gregory JR, Sasaki TM (1982) Pancreatic pseudocyst. Am J Surg 143:588–601
8. Traverso W, Tompkins RK, Urrea PT, Longmire WP Jr (1979) Surgical treatment of chronic pancreatitis. Ann Surg 190:312–319
9. Frey CF (1977) Pancreatic pseudocyst-operative strategy. Ann Surg 188:652–662
10. Kiviluoto T, Kivisaari L, Kivilaakso E, Lempinen M (1989) Pseudocysts in chronic pancreatitis. Arch Surg 124:240–243
11. Aranha GV, Prinz RA, Freeark RJ, Kruss DM, Greenlee HB (1982) Evaluation of therapeutic options for pancreatic pseudocysts. Arch Surg 117:717–721
12. Way LW, Gadacz T, Goldman L (1974) Surgical treatment of chronic pancreatitis. Am J Surg 127:202–209
13. Prinz RA, Greenlee HB (1981) Pancreatic duct drainage in 100 patients with chronic pancreatitis. Ann Surg 194:313–320

Operative Therapy of Pancreatic Pseudocysts

R. Häring and P. Dollinger[1]

The treatment of pancreatic cysts is no longer purely operative since there are now CT- and sonography-directed as well as endoscopic puncture and drainage procedures which permit emptying of the cyst. This raises the question of whether an operation may still be appropriate, or whether it has become superfluous. As a matter of principle, however, the indications for one approach or another must be carefully considered. In addition to a discussion of operative procedures and their results, the decision whether or not to operate will be an important topic of this chapter.

Incidence and Causes

One must distinguish between true cysts, pseudocysts, and cystic neoplasias. Of central interest are the pseudocysts, defined as fluid-filled cavities with walls made up of granulation tissue and adjacent tissue structures. They do not have an epithelial lining. Pseudocysts have a reported incidence of 1%–4.5% among all occurrences of chronic or acute pancreatitis. In our patients they constitute about 12% of all interventions in the pancreas. Warren et al. [19] have compiled the etiology of pancreatic cysts from their own patients (Fig. 1). This etiological distinction is important for the prognosis and for choosing the operative procedure.

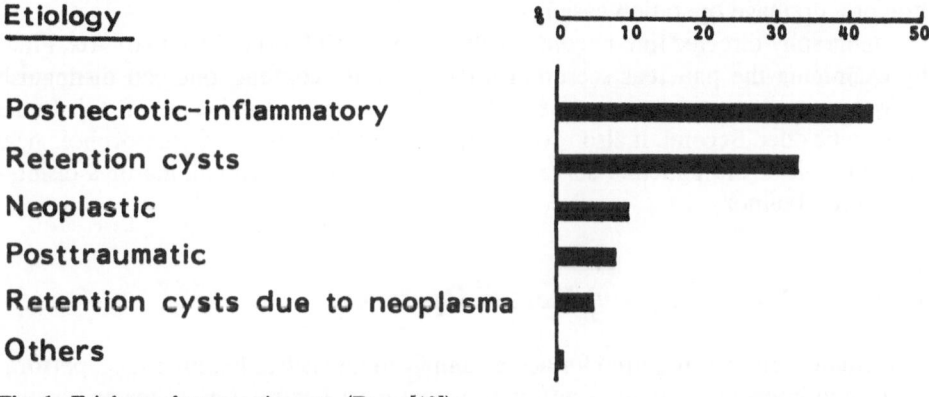

Fig. 1. Etiology of pancreatic cysts. (From [19])

---

[1] Department of Surgery, Steglitz Medical Center, Free University of Berlin, Hindenburgdamm 30, D-1000 Berlin (West), Germany

Chronic Pancreatitis
Ed. by Beger, Büchler, Ditschuneit, and Malfertheiner
© Springer-Verlag Berlin Heidelberg 1990

Complications

The clinical course and complications are dependent upon size, and localization of cysts. Postnecrotic pseudocysts, which are the vestige of an acute pancreatitis, recede spontaneously in 10%–40% of all cases within 6–8 weeks. If this does not occur, they develop a hard callous wall, as clinical experience and experimental studies have shown [17]. This is important because it is only at this stage that a surgical suture for the anastomosing becomes possible. For cysts developing from a chronic relapsing pancreatitis, on the other hand, a regression can hardly be expected.

Complications occur in up to 55% of all cases [4, 18, 21]. Particularly noteworthy are the following:

- Hemorrhages, particularly from the splenic artery
- Erosion of the duodenum, stomach or colon
- Infections with abscess formation
- Rupture with ascites and pleural effusion
- Compression of the common bile duct, the duodenum, and the colon with corresponding signs of stenosis, most frequently icterus

The incidence of such complications, according to Wade [18], ranges from 30% to 55%. These include: rupture, 6.6%; bleeding, 6.5%; abscess, 14.4%; fistula, 1.3%; obstruction, 1.4%; and ascites, 10.0%.

A few brief comments should be made in regard to diagnostics. CT and sonography show the number, localization, and size of the pseudocysts and permit assessment of wall thickness, which is important for scheduling the time of operation. While it is advantageous to visualize the pancreatic duct system, which can reveal stenoses, dilations, and fistulae, the disadvantage is the risk of infection associated with the instillation of contrast medium. We favor ERCP for cysts developing in connection with a chronic relapsing pancreatitis, since this makes the decision between a resection or a drainage operation easier.

Sonography-directed fine-needle puncture provides information of two sorts. First, by examining the pancreas secretion for its amylase content, one can distinguish between true cysts and pseudocysts. A high amylase content indicates a fistula to the pancreatic duct. Second, it also reveals the status of the process. Cytomorphological examination of the punctate serves to exclude a cystadenocarcinoma or a disintegrated solid tumor.

Indication for Surgery and Time of Operation

Immediate surgery is required for acute complications such as hemorrhages, perforations, and infections. Opinion differs as to the most favorable time for an elective operation [6]. Can a wait-and-see attitude be assumed or should surgery be performed as early as possible? The former position is supported by the fact that approximately half of the postacute cysts recede spontaneously within 6 weeks; if this is not the case, the cyst wall stabilizes in this interval so as to make it more suitable for a suture. In addition, mortality is higher in the early stage. Arguments for the latter, on the other hand, include the high complication rate of up to 40% and the associated higher surgical mortality rate, as well as the possibility of overlooking or neglecting a cystadenocarcinoma.

Surgical Procedures

The choice between draining and resecting surgical procedures should take into consideration the following aspects: (a) complications of pseudocysts; (b) correct timing with respect towards wall stability; and (c) size and, above all, cause of the cyst. The draining methods include: (a) external drainage and marsupialization; and (b) internal drainage – cystogastrostomy, cystoduodenostomy, and cystojejunostomy. Suitable resecting procedures are left pancreas resection and partial duodenopancreatectomy with and without preservation of the duodenum.

A number of points should be made about choosing from the various methods of operation. First, drainage to the outside is only necessary, in our opinion, for "fresh cysts" which are infected. Second, marsupialization is now obsolete due to complications such as pancreatic fistulae and maceration of the skin, as well as to the usually very protracted clinical course. And, third, if an internal drainage procedure is not to be considered, we place a drain in the cyst that is directed outward. If a pancreatic fistula develops later, it should be examined if drainage of the pancreatic duct via the papilla is unobstructed. If this is the case, the fistula usually closes spontaneously; otherwise surgery must be performed, but not immediately.

Preference should always be given to internal drainage for anastomosable cyst walls (6-week waiting period and CT control). The method of choice is now cystojejunostomy with an Roux-en-Y loop [21] (Fig. 2). This technique is simple, and dangerous complications are rare. In the Federal Republic of Germany it has displaced gastrocystostomy, once a common method which is still routinely used in the United States. We still perform the latter in cases in which the cyst is situated directly behind the stomach so as to permit a simple transgastric access. Then, however, hemorrhages and infections are more frequent. Some surgeons [1] prefer cystoduodenostomy for head cysts and duodenal wall cysts. The transduodenal access is simple and involves few complications.

Zirngibl et al. [21] have suggested that a resection be performed for all pseudocysts developing as a complication of chronic relapsing pancreatitis. They give the following reasons for this.

a) Internal cyst drainage is only a symptomatic therapy; many patients are not freed from symptoms, particularly pain.
b) It is unfavourable to wait for termination of chronic inflammation since new cysts can continue to develop.
c) Reoperations are technically more difficult and involve a higher risk for the patient.

It should be noted that, as a matter of principle, several biopsies should be taken from the cyst wall for each drainage operation in order definitely to exclude a cystadenocarcinoma.

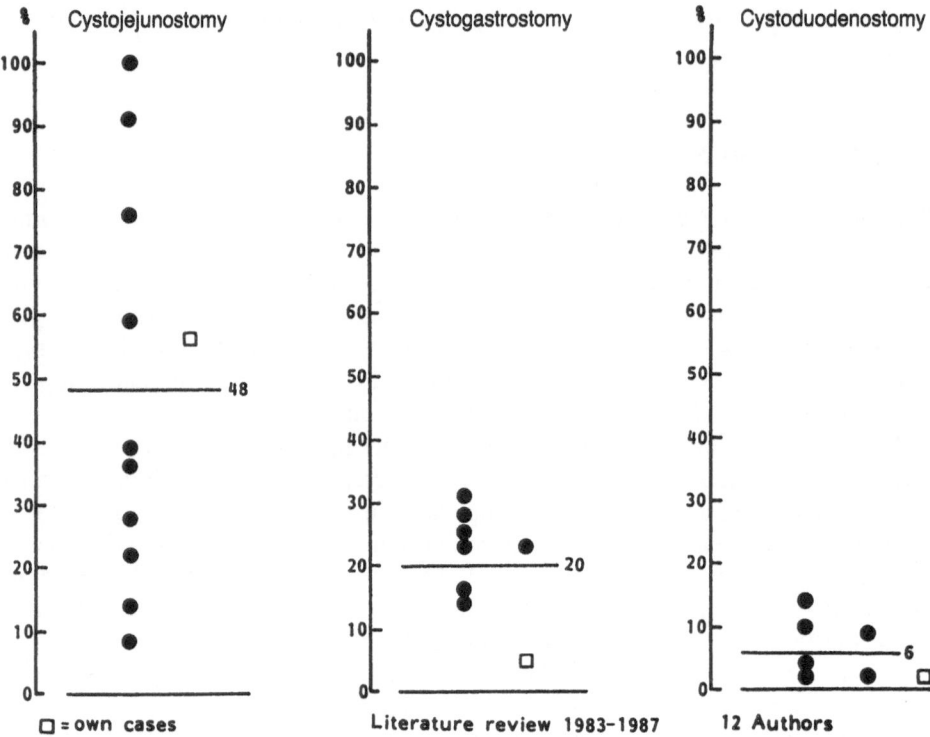

Fig. 2. Types of drainage procedures used in pancreatic cysts and reported frequencies in various studies [1–5, 7, 8, 10, 11, 18, 19, 21] (●) and in our own cases (□)

Interventional Puncture and Drainage Procedures

In recent years it has been possible with the aid of sonography, CT, and gastroscopy to develop various nonoperative puncture and drainage procedures for the emptying of pancreatic pseudocysts. These include: (a) Sonography-directed percutaneous fine-needle puncture, which is useful primarily in establishing the diagnosis and, at the same time, permits emptying of the cyst; (b) percutaneous insertion of a pigtail catheter as drainage to the outside [8]; and (c) percutaneous pancreaticogastric pseudocyst drainage [9–11, 13], a technically complex procedure of which, up to now, few reports have been presented.

Results

Regarding surgical results we must differentiate between early and late results. From 1975 to May 1989, our experience has involved operations on 122 patients with pancreatic pseudocysts. Eighty-nine were male and 33 female with a mean age of 44.7 years (range, 24–71). The operative modifications performed were: internal drainage in 79 (64.7%); external (pigtail) drainage in 4 (3.2%); and resection in 36 (29.5%) – including Whipple in 14, left resection in 21, and cyst excision in 11.

Of interest in considering the early results are postoperative complications and the postoperative mortality rate. The rate of specific early complications ranges between 4% and 40% in the literature and is 15% among our own cases [1–5, 7, 12, 14, 16, 20, 21]. These are essentially wound-healing impairments, pancreatic fistulae, subphrenic abscesses, interluminal and intra-abdominal hemorrhages, and peritonitis. A hospital mortality rate of between 0% and 8.1% is reported in the literature (1–5, 7, 12, 14, 15]; our own is 3.3%. This can be differentiated according to the type of operation and the cause of the pseudocysts. A literature review of various studies [1–5, 7, 12, 14, 15] shows an average rate of 4.0% for cystojejunostomy and one of 8.1% for cystogastrostomy. In particular, we know from the Erlangen Hospital study [21] that it is twice as high for chronic pancreatitis, at 8.4%, than for postacute cysts, at only 4.3%.

Regarding late results the following questions are of interest: (a) Is the patient asymptomatic? (b) How frequent are recurrences? (c) How many patients must undergo surgery a second time or even more often? (d) How high is the late mortality rate? Little information is available on freedom from symptoms achieved postoperatively. Reported rates vary between 23% and 47%, but no distinction has been made between postacute and chronic pseudocysts. The poorer results are due mainly to the fact that chronic pancreatitis continues to smolder. This also explains the poorer recurrence rate. The Erlangen Hospital study [21] reported a recurrence rate of 43.8% for chronic pancreatic pseudocysts as opposed to one of only 8.6% for postacute cysts; corresponding figures for late results were 39.1% and 11.1%. It is clear that alcoholism and diabetes also play an important role in this connection. The conclusion that must be drawn from these observations is that resection is preferable to a drainage operation for pseudocysts developing in connection with chronic pancreatitis.

In conclusion, we would like to recommend the following ten guidelines for pancreatic pseudocysts:

1. In cases of asymptomatic postnecrotic pancreatic pseudocysts, one can wait and observe the spontaneous development in the first 6 weeks. Clinical and sonographic control is, however, mandatory.
2. If the cyst does not regress, an operation is indicated.
3. Surgery is indicated for pseudocysts developing from chronic pancreatitis since regression cannot be expected.
4. Under controlled conditions, surgery can be dispensed with in the case of small pseudocysts (< 4 cm) if they are asymptomatic.
5. Percutaneous puncture and external catheter drainage can produce successful results in postacute cysts if the wall is still unstable, and the cyst can be collapsed.
6. Percutaneous decompression punctures, possibly with catheter drainage, are appropriate only for infected cysts or in patients whose general condition is very poor, particularly in cases in which an operative internal cyst drainage is not yet possible due to wall instability.
7. Punctures and external drainages are successful if the amylase values in the contents of the cyst are low, indicating that there is no fistula to the pancreatic duct.

8. It remains to be seen whether percutaneous pancreaticogastric drainage with a pigtail catheter will prove to be a successful approach.
9. A resection procedure is always better than internal cyst drainage for pancreatic cysts associated with chronic pancreatitis.
10. In our opinion, pancreatic cysts are still a surgical problem. We should, however, apply modern sonography as well as CT-directed puncture and external drainage procedures for appropriate indications and not leave them to other disciplines.

References

1. Altimari A, Aranha GV, Greenlee HB, Prinz RA (1986) Results of cystoduodenostomy for treatment of pancreatic pseudocysts. Am Surg 52:438
2. Andrén-Sandberg A, Evander A, Isaksson G, Ihse I (1983) Management of pancreatic pseudocysts. Acta Chir Scand 149:203
3. Belinkie SA, Russell JC, Deutsch J, Becker DR (1983) Pancreatic pseudocyst. Am Surg 49:586
4. Bradley EL (1984) Cystoduodenostomy. Ann Surg 200:698
5. Da Cunha JEM, Bacchella T, de Barros Mott C, Machado MCC (1985) Management of pancreatic pseudocysts in chronic alcoholic pancreatitis with duct dilatation. Int Surg 70:53
6. Ephgrave K (1986) Presentation of pancreatic pseudocysts: implications for timing of surgical intervention. Am J Surg 151:749
7. Fujita H, Konishi K, Miyazaki I (1985) Management of pancreatic pseudocysts in 42 patients with inflammatory or traumatic cysts. Jpn J Surg 15:266
8. Gerzof SG, Johnson WC, Robbins AH, Spechler SJ, Nabseth DC (1984) Percutaneous drainage of infected pancreatic pseudocysts. Arch Surg 119:888
9. Hancke S, Pedersen JF (1976) Percutaneous puncture of pancreatic cysts guided by ultrasound. Surg Gynecol Obstet 142:551
10. Henriksen FW, Hancke S (1987) Ultrasound-guided percutaneous pancreatic cystogastrostomy. Digestion 38:24
11. Heyder N, Domschke W (1987) Perkutane pankreatiko-gastrale Pseudozysten-Drainage. Dtsch Med Wochenschr 112:546
12. Köhler H, Schafmayer A, Lüdtke FE, Lepsien G, Peiper H-J (1987) Surgical treatment of pancreatic pseudocysts. Br J Surg 74:813
13. Mahlke R, Lübbers H, Lankisch PG (1988) Komplikation nach perkutaner pankreatiko-gastraler Pseudozystendrainage. Dtsch Med Wochenschr 113:78
14. Munn JS, Aranha GV, Greenlee HB, Prinz RA (1987) Simultaneous treatment of chronic pancreatitis and pancreatic pseudocyst. Arch Surg 122:662
15. O'Connor M, Kolars J, Ansel H, Silvis S, Vennes J (1986) Preoperative endoscopic retrograde cholangiopancreatography in the surgical management of pancreatic pseudocysts. Am J Surg 151:18
16. O'Malley VP, Cannon JP, Postier RG (1985) Pancreatic pseudocysts: cause, therapy, and results. Am J Surg 150:680
17. Salinas A, Triebling A, Toth L, Dreiling DA (1985) The pathogenesis of pancreatic pseudocysts – a canine experimental model. Am J Gastroenterol 80:126
18. Wade JW (1985) Twenty-five year experience with pancreatic pseudocysts. Am J Surg 149:705
19. Warren KW, Athanissiades S, Frederick P, Kune GA (1966) Surgical treatment of pancreatic cysts: review of 183 cases. Ann Surg 163:886
20. Warshaw AL, Rattner DW (1985) Timing of surgical drainage for pancreatic pseudocyst. Ann Surg 202:720
21. Zirngibl H, Gebhardt C, Faßbender D (1983) Drainagebehandlung von Pankreaspseudocysten. Langenbecks Arch Chir 360:29

What Type of Pseudocyst Should Undergo Surgery?

R. ROSCHER[1]

The history of surgical therapy of pancreatic pseudocysts is over 100 years old (Fig. 1) [1]. For more than 60 years, the preferred treatment has been internal drainage. Today, the development of endoscopic and radiologic techniques for interventional management of pseudocysts forces us to determine what type of cyst can be healed through interventional procedures, and which should be treated surgically. An analysis of our operated patients with pancreatic pseudocysts between the years 1982 and 1988 may contribute to the surgical decision-making as to whether an operation is necessary or not.

XII.

Zur operativen Behandlung der Pankreas-Cysten.

Von

Dr. Carl Gussenbauer,

Professor der Chirurgie in Prag.*)

---

*) Vorgetragen am 4. Sitzungstage des XII. Congresses der Deutschen Gesellschaft für Chirurgie zu Berlin, am 7. April 1883.

Fig. 1. Title of first paper on operative treatment of pancreatic pseudocysts

Pseudocysts were defined as encapsulated, amylase-rich, fluid collections, 20 mm or larger in diameter, that were verified by surgical exploration in each case. As postacute cysts we defined all those which evolved as sequelae of the first acute manifestation of pancreatitis. When multiple attacks of pancreatitis had been encountered before manifestation of pseudocysts, they were considered chronic cysts. For diagnosis of the pseudocysts we used sonography only as a screening method. The standard imaging methods were contrast-enhanced CT (our "gold standard," applic-

---

[1] Department of General Surgery, University of Ulm, Steinhövelstr. 9, D-7900 Ulm

Chronic Pancreatitis
Ed. by Beger, Büchler, Ditschuneit, and Malfertheiner
© Springer-Verlag Berlin Heidelberg 1990

able in all patients) and ERCP for the evaluation of pancreatic and bile ducts. An assessment of the endocrine and exocrine pancreatic function was part of the preoperative diagnosis in all patients with chronic pancreatitis.

A total of 125 patients with pancreatic pseudocysts – 92 with solitary and 33 with multiple cysts – were operated on. In only 3 patients (2.4%) did the pseudocysts have a traumatic cause, in 20 patients (16%) postacute forms were encountered, and in 102 patients (81.6%) chronic pancreatitis was the underlying disease. Altogether, we treated 183 pseudocysts with a median diameter of 66 mm, 40 intrapancreatic pseudocysts with one of 36 mm, 29 extrapancreatic cysts with one of 113 mm, and 114 cysts with one of 80 mm with both intra- and extrapancreatic extension (Table 1).

Table 1. Pseudocyst characteristics in 125 patients

Type of cysts	Number of cysts	Mean diameter
Intrapancreatic	40	36 mm
Extrapancreatic	29	113 mm
Intra- and extrapancreatic	114	80 mm
	183	66 mm (Av)

Cysts were solitary in 92 patients, multiple in 33.

The indications for operation were primarily pain and loss of weight as clinical symptoms, compression of the duodenum, bile duct and portal vein, and obstruction of the pancreatic duct as complications of the cysts (Table 2).

Table 2. Indication for surgery in 125 patients with pancreatic pseudocysts

Indication	n
Pain	121 (97%)
Loss of weight	77 (62%)
Compression of duodenum	50 (40%)
Compression of bile duct	45 (36%)
Obstruction of pancreatic duct	81 (36%)
Obstruction of mesenteric vein	22 (18%)
Mediastinal and intrasplenic extension	9 (7%)

The aim of surgical treatment in all cases was the elimination of pseudocysts and decompression of the pancreatic duct and the adjacent organs in combination with the greatest possible preservation of the gland parenchyma.

In consideration of this therapeutic goal, the following operations were performed: external drainage in 7 patients, internal drainage in 50, and partial pancreatic resection in 68.

In complicated forms of postacute cysts, external drainage sometimes is inevitable. Of 20 patients with postacute pseudocysts, five were found to have infection and three

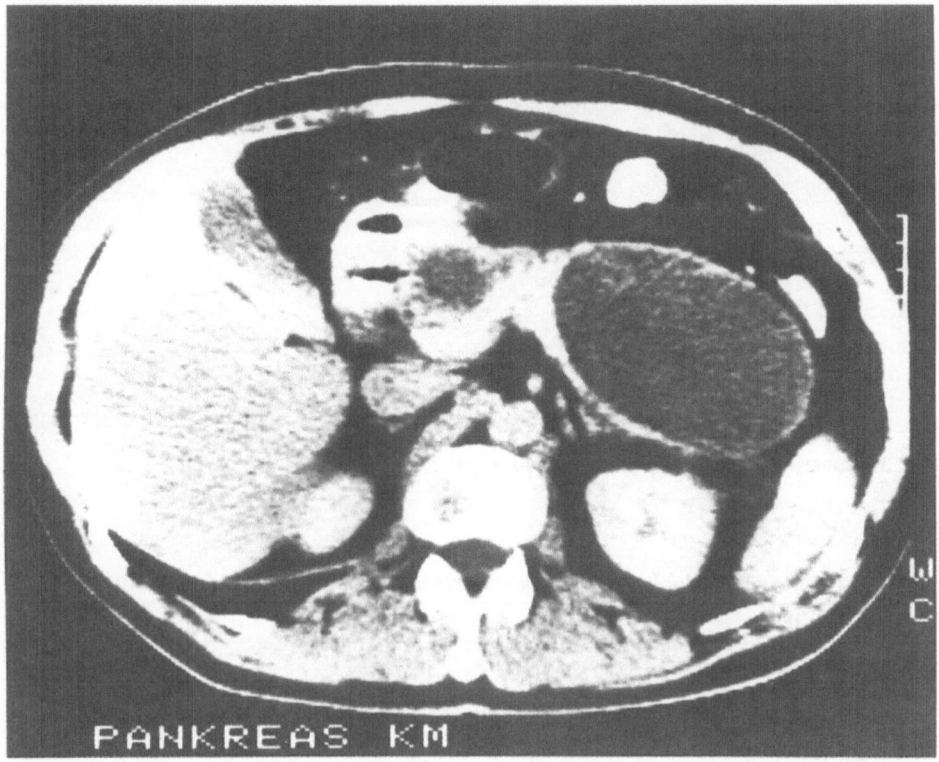

Fig. 2. Patient L. L., 61-year-old man. CT scan of postacute pseudocysts

cholestasis. All infected cysts were drained externally. The cases of postacute cysts treated with internal drainage were mainly results of a biliary pancreatitis in patients older than 60 years. In two-thirds of the cases, sequesters were found in the cyst fluid.

As a clinical example, a 61-year-old man was referred 3 months after an attack of biliary pancreatitis. The CT scan (Fig. 2) demonstrated a small, more extrapancreatic pseudocyst in the pancreatic head region and a large pseudocyst with a defined thick wall extending to the body and tail of the gland. Cholecystectomy was performed as well as excision of the cyst in the head. The larger cyst was drained internally through a cystojejunostomy. Extensive sequesters swimming in the cyst fluid were removed (Fig. 3).

In 102 of our operated patients (81%) with pseudocysts the underlying disease was chronic pancreatitis. In achieving our aforementioned therapeutic goal, internal drainage was sufficient in only one-third of the patients; the rest required a form of pancreatic resection (Table 3).

In the following, the different clinical situations encountered are demonstrated according to selected cases.

Internal drainage was performed in patients with cysts lying mainly extrapancreatically; further complications had to be excluded. A Roux-en-Y cystojejunostomy was

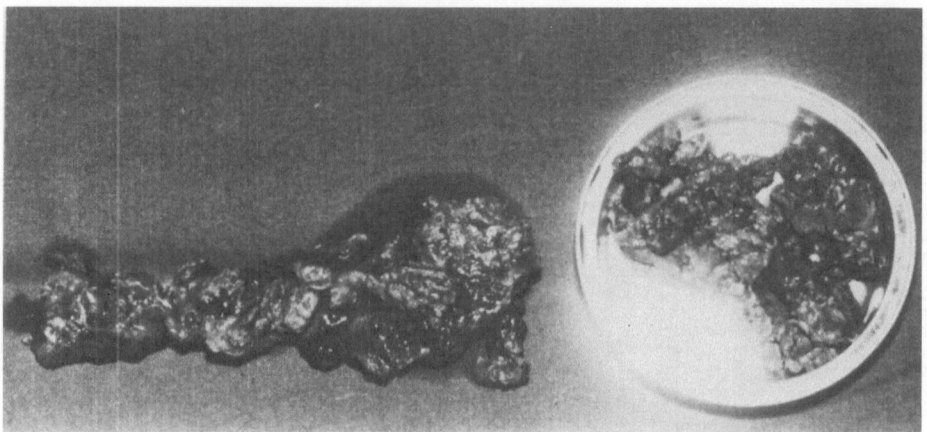

Fig. 3. Sequesters removed from the pseudocysts in Fig. 2

Table 3. Pancreatic pseudocysts: surgical procedures in 102 patients with chronic pancreatitis

Surgical procedure	n
Internal drainage	
Cystojejunostomy	30
Cystojejunostomy + cystoductojejunostomy	4
Pancreatic resection	
Duodenum-preserving pancreatic head resection	47
Distal pancreatectomy	20
Segmental pancreatic resection	1

carried out in all patients. In a case of such multiple cysts, Fig. 4 shows the CT scan of a 36-year-old man with alcohol-induced pancreatitis; Fig. 5 presents better illustration, with each cyst being anastomosed separately with the same Roux-en-Y loop. Such double cysts were encountered in six patients. A considerable group of 20 patients were treated with distal pancreatectomy. In our effort to preserve as much paren-chyma as possible, this indication was applied very restrictively. But pseudocysts in the pancreatic tail which are not apt for internal drainage still present a good indica-tion for distal resection. Of the 20 patients with distal resection, 11 were found to have multiple cysts (Table 4). We found an intrasplenic extension in six patients and a

Table 4. Pancreatic pseudocysts: features of 20 patients treated with distal cystopancreatectomy

Features	n
Multiple cysts	11[a]
Intrasplenic extension	6
Mediastinal extension	3
Combined operative procedures	9
Preservation of spleen	2

[a] Total number of pseudocysts treated: 33

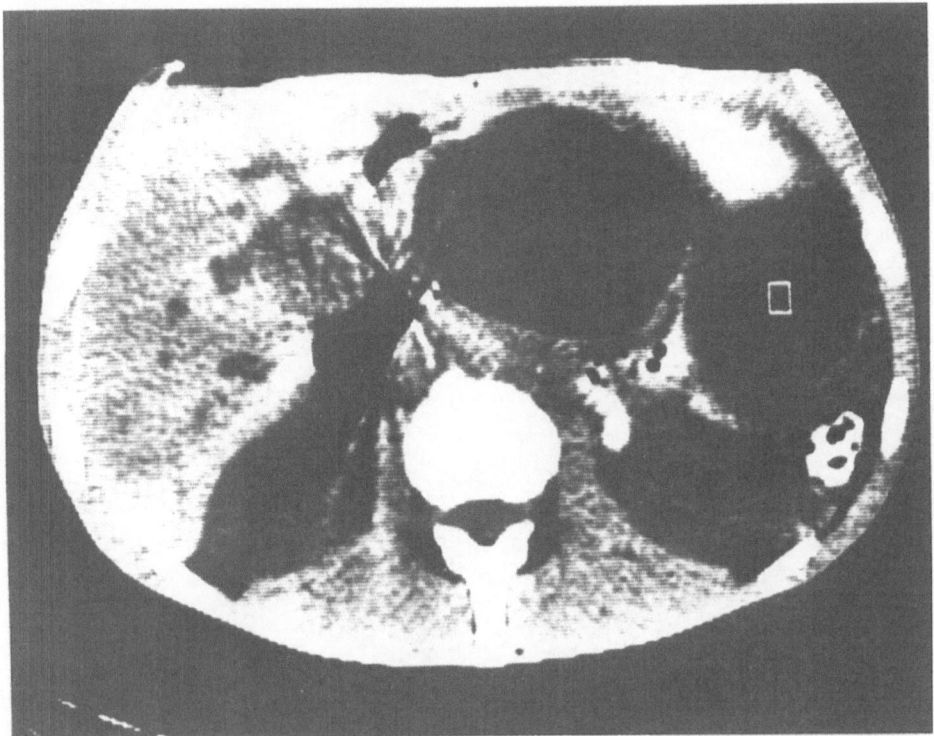

Fig. 4. Patient W.G., 36-year-old man. Chronic pancreatitis. CT demonstrates two large extra-pancreatic cysts

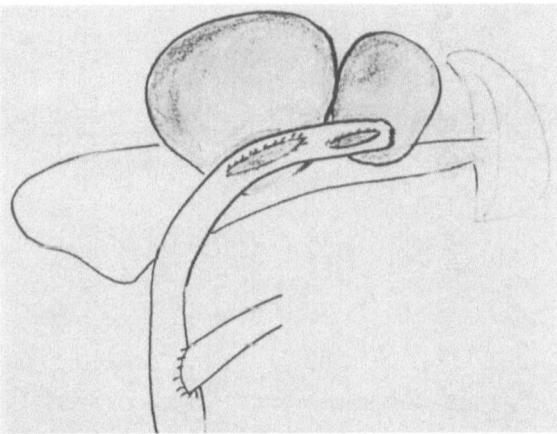

Fig. 5. Internal drainage procedure in multiple cysts: each cyst is anastomosed separately with the same Roux-en-Y jejunal loop

mediastinal in three. Simultaneous resection and drainage procedures were necessary in nine patients.

The following case examples serve to illustrate this kind of treatment.

A 45-year-old man with alcohol-induced chronic pancreatitis was hospitalized with dysphagia, loss of weight, and upper abdominal pain. Diagnostic measures revealed a

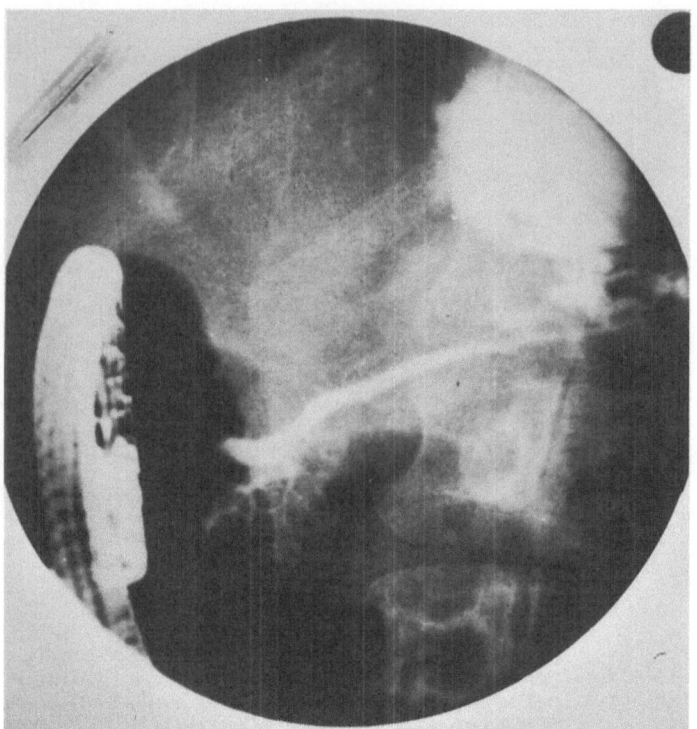

Fig. 6. Patient B. B., 45-year-old man. Chronic pancreatitis. ERCP fills up a mediastinal pseudocyst

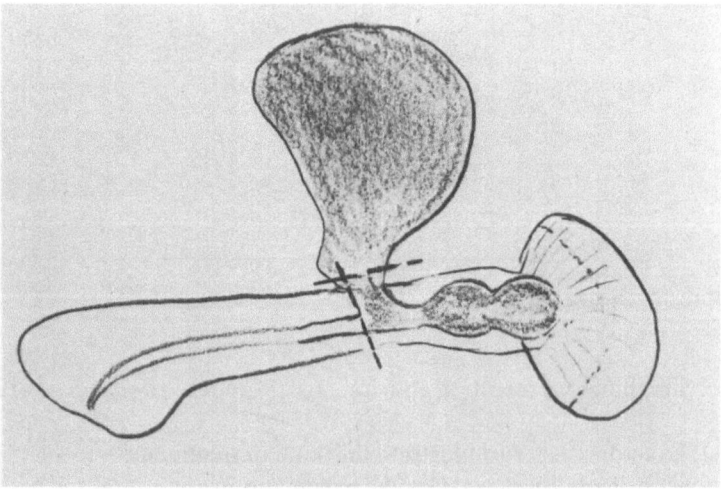

Fig. 7. Pathologic findings and resection lines at operation

pseudocyst with mediastinal extension, demonstrated through contrast-filling in ERCP (Fig. 6) and in CT. Two small intraparenchymatous cysts in the pancreatic tail were also seen. The latter two cysts were removed by means of distal pancreatectomy. Concomitantly, the communication of the main pancreatic duct to the mediastinal cyst was disconnected (Fig. 7). The mediastinal cyst was drained externally for several days. It then yielded to self-obliteration.

An example of an unsuccessful transcutaneous cyst puncture is offered by the case of a 62-year-old woman with a long history of pancreatitis of unknown etiology who developed cysts in the pancreatic head and tail region (Fig. 8). The cysts had been known for more than 1 year and several attempts of transcutaneous puncture had failed. The large cyst in the tail was removed with distal pancreatectomy (Fig. 9); internal drainage of the more extrapancreatic head cyst was performed with a Roux-en-Y loop (Fig. 10). Failure of the transcutaneous puncture was due to the rigid wall of the cyst.

Another example of a futile interventional cyst drainage is that of 28-year-old woman treated for recurrent pancreatitis for 2 years in a medical department. Pseudo-cysts had been known for over 1 year. The patient suffered from anorexia, loss of weight, and vomiting. Eight weeks before operation, the patient was admitted to a medical department with clinical sepsis. After 2 weeks of treatment a quantitative intraperitoneal hemorrhage was noted, and the patient was treated with blood transfusions. Tube drainages were placed transcutaneously in two cysts, but no progress was achieved, and the patient was transferred for surgery. We diagnosed two extra-

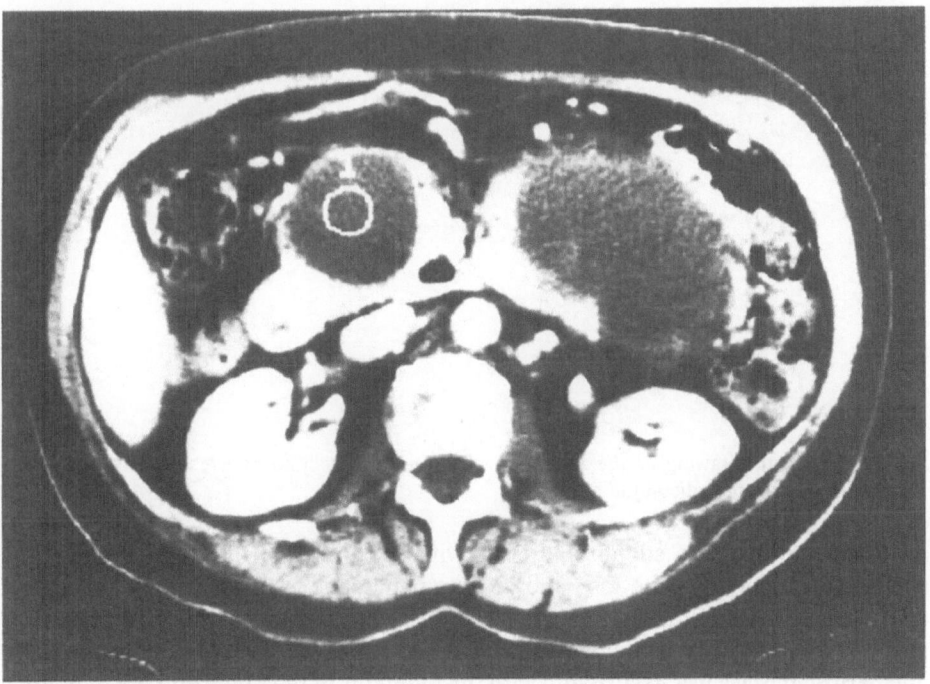

Fig. 8. Patient K.J., 62-year-old woman. Chronic pancreatitis. CT scan shows pseudocysts in the head and tail region of the pancreas

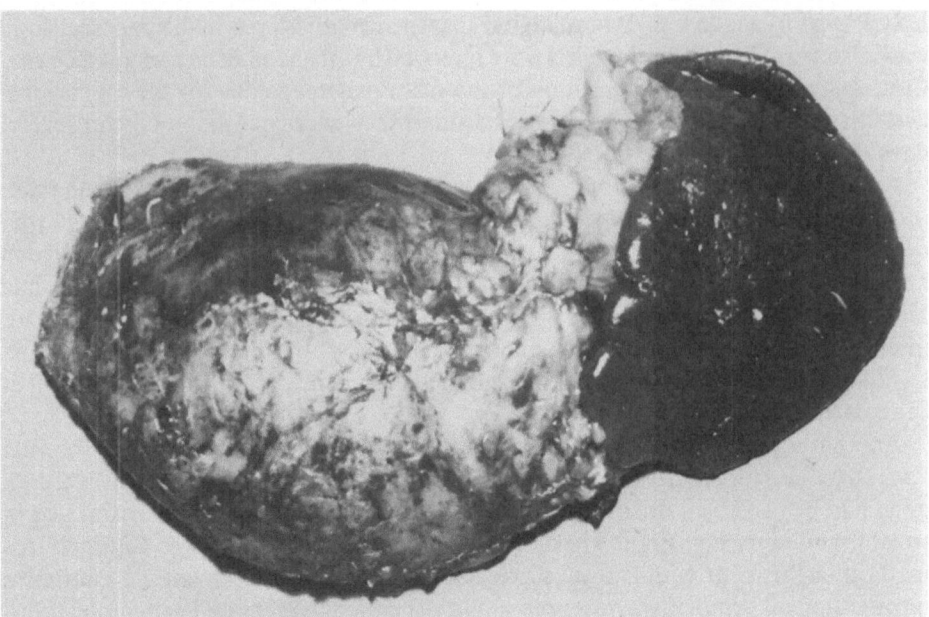

Fig. 9. Specimen removed at operation of the patient in Fig. 8

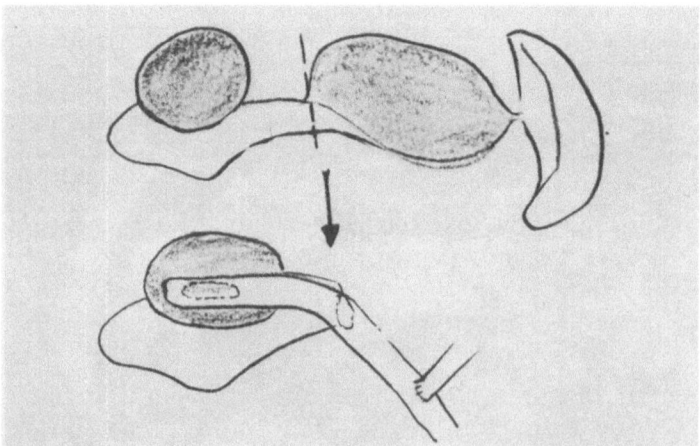

Fig. 10. Schematic drawing of the operation performed. Left cysto pancreatectomy plus cysto-jejunostomy and pancreaticojejunostomy

anatomic suprahepatic subphrenic cysts with the drainage tubes in situ, a more extrapancreatic cyst in the tail, and an intrapancreatic cyst with splenic extension (Figs. 11, 12). At operation, the catheters were removed and the suprahepatic cysts partially excised. They contained sterile pus. With a small distal resection, the intra- and perisplenic cyst was exstirpated with the remnants of the organ and the remaining juxtacaudal cyst partially excised (Fig. 13). A large, partially organized hematoma stemming from the splenic arrosion hemorrhage, was removed from the pelvis.

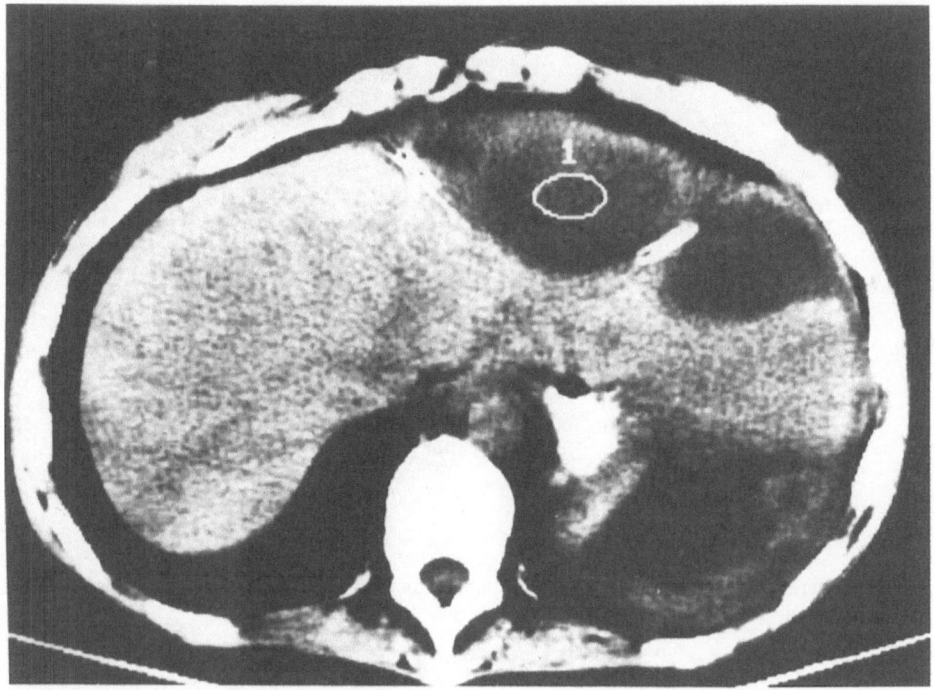

Fig. 11. Patient T.R., 28-year-old woman. Chronic pancreatitis. CT scan reveals two subphrenic, suprahepatic pseudocysts with transcutaneously inserted drainage tubes

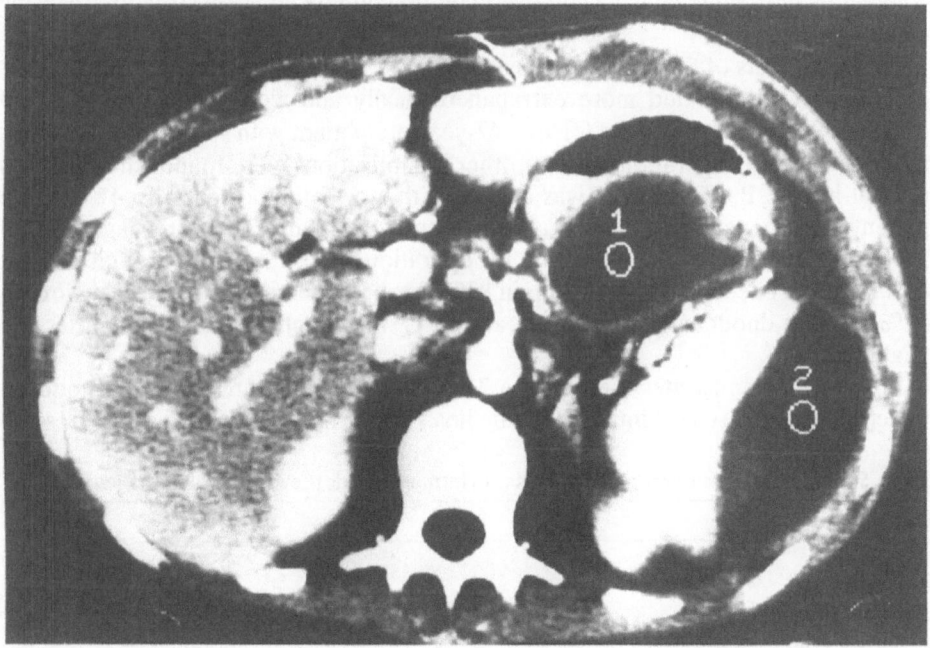

Fig. 12. A more caudal CT scan of the patient in Fig. 11 shows an extrapancreatic cyst at the tail and a pseudocyst with intra- and perisplenic extension

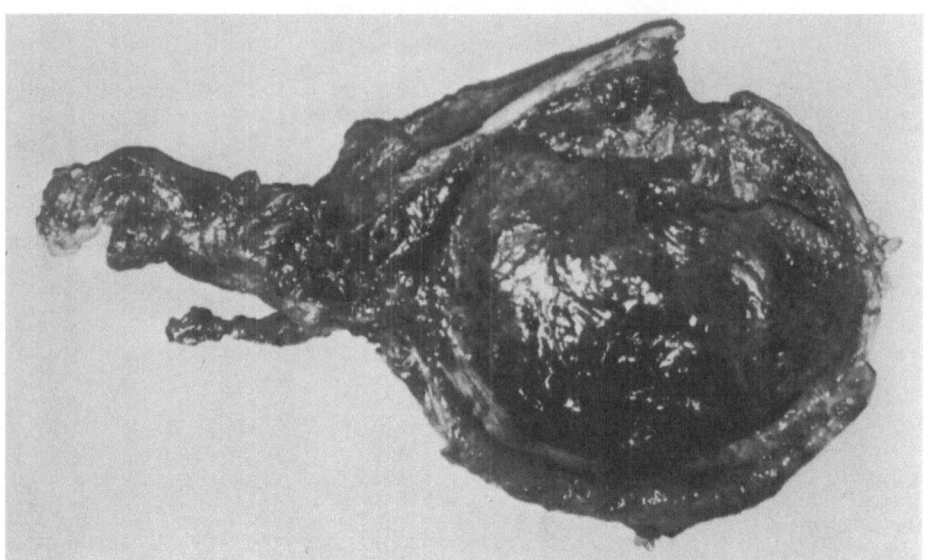

Fig. 13. Operative specimen after left distal pancreatectomy with the spleen encapsulated in the pseudocyst wall

Particular interest is dedicated to cysts in the pancreatic head. In most cases, they lie completely intrapancreatically and exert compression on adjacent structures causing complications.

We found cysts of the pancreatic head region in 55 of our patients. Of these cysts, only eight were situated more extrapancreatically and were treated via internal drainage. Figure 14 shows the CT of a 42-year-old patient with such a cyst. Pain was the indication for operation, and no other complications were found; the duct was normal in ERCP. The patient was treated with a cystojejunostomy. In 47 of these patients, intrapancreatic cysts with a diameter of more than 20 mm were diagnosed. In 98% of these patients, the indication for operation was established through pain, in 43% through bile duct compression, in 83% through pancreatic duct obstruction, in 57% through duodenal compression, and in 17% through portal vein compression (Table 5).

Figure 15 demonstrates the CT of a 31-year-old patient with an alcohol-induced pancreatitis and a typical intrapancreatic head cyst. This cyst induced a compression

Table 5. Indication for surgery in 47 patients with intrapancreatic pseudocysts of the pancreatic head

Indication	n
Pain	46 (98%)
Cholestasis	20 (43%)
Pancreatic duct obstruction	39 (83%)
Duodenal compression	27 (57%)
Portal vein compression	8 (17%)

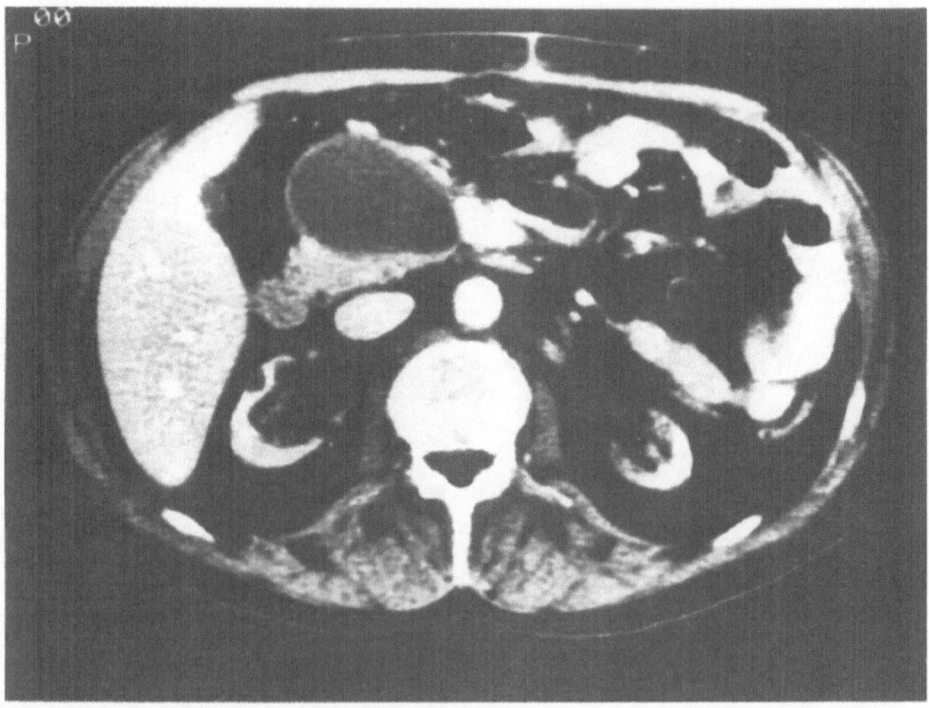

Fig. 14. Patient J.W., 42-year-old man. Chronic pancreatitis. CT scan demonstrates a more extrapancreatic pseudocyst at the head of the gland

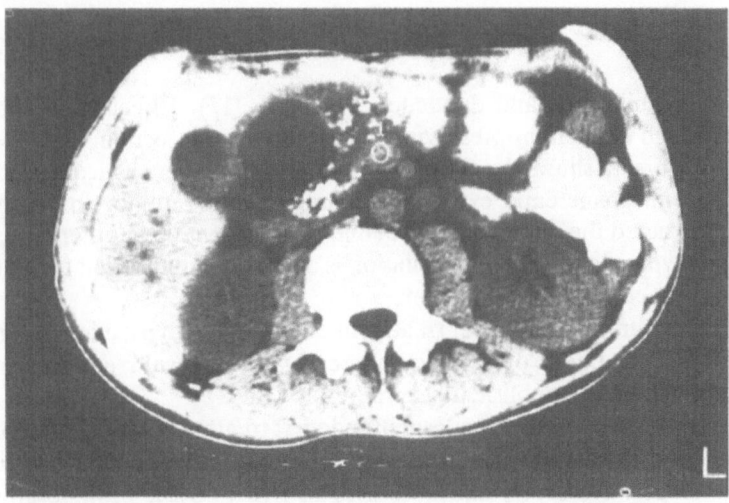

Fig. 15. Patient B.P., 31-year-old man. Chronic pancreatitis. CT scan shows an inflammatory head tumor of the pancreas with calcifications and a large intrapancreatic cyst

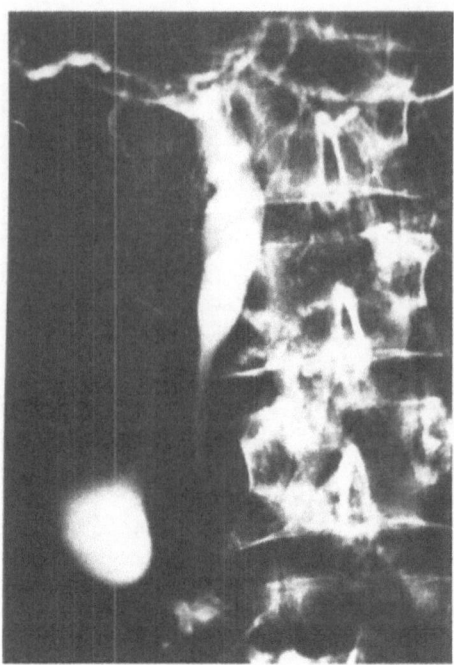

Fig. 16. Same patient as in Fig. 15, ERCP. Compression of distal bile duct

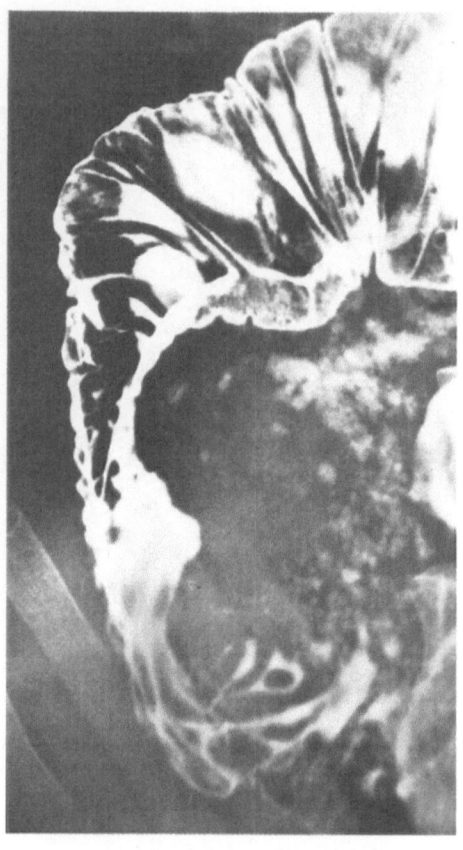

Fig. 17. Same patient as in Figs. 15 and 16, duodenography. Concomitant compression of the duodenum

of the bile duct and duodenum (Figs. 16, 17). Effective treatment was achieved through duodenum-preserving pancreatic head resection.

Figure 18 shows the CT of a 38-year-old patient with alcohol-induced pancreatitis. The intrapancreatic cyst and the inflammatory tumor in the head of the gland obstructed the pancreatic duct (Fig. 19), presenting another typical complication of this type of cyst. This constellation is also a good indication for a duodenum-preserving pancreatic head resection.

Long-term results after treatment of patients with pseudocysts are primarily results of the treatment of chronic pancreatitis. The results concerning our own patient population are published elsewhere [2].

The postoperative results of pseudocyst treatment of our entire patient group are as follows (Table 6). We encountered postoperative bleeding in three cases (2.4%), postoperative sepsis and abscesses in five (4.0%), postoperativel fistulas in two (1.6%), and miscellaneous other complications such as pleural effusion, pneumonia, urologic complications in 19 cases (15.2%). Seven patients had to be reoperated on

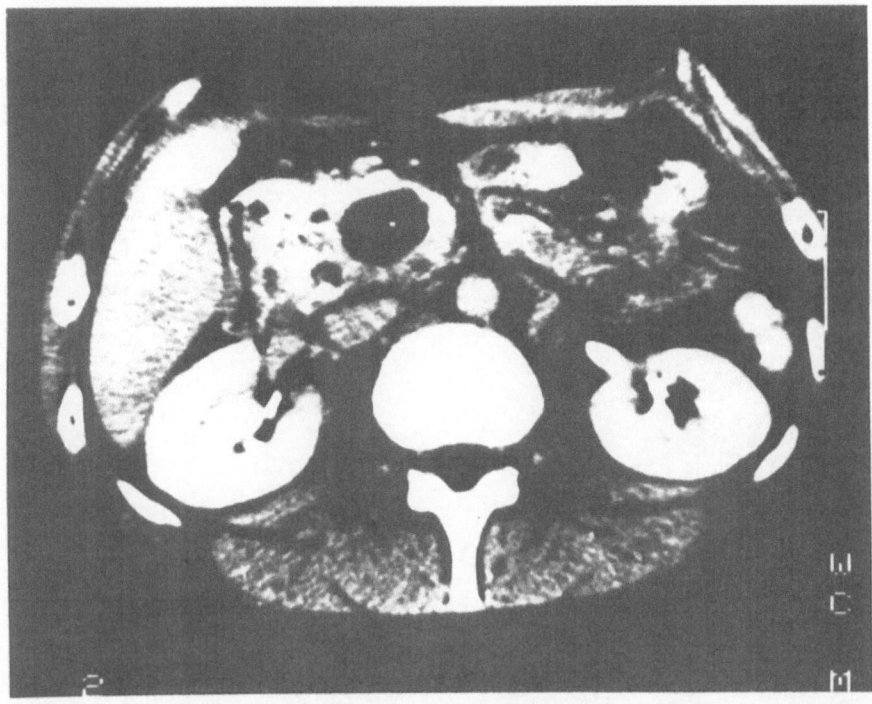

Fig. 18. Patient B. G., 38-year-old man. Chronic pancreatitis. CT scan reveals multiple, very small cysts and one large intrapancreatic cyst in the head of the gland

Table 6. Results after surgical treatment of 125 patients with pancreatic pseudocysts

Complication	n	
Postoperative hemorrhage	3	(2.4%)
Postoperative sepsis or abscess	5	(4.0%)
Postoperative fistula	2	(1.6%)
Miscellaneous	19	(15.2%)
Reoperations	7	(5.6%)
Postoperative deaths	1	(0.8%)

(5.6%). Only one patient died (mortality 0.8%). An overall morbidity rate of 23,2% and the low mortality compare favorably with data from recently published series concerning internal drainage of pancreatic pseudocysts (Table 7) [3]. Our results give evidence that today surgery for pseudocysts can be performed safely and present the surgical standards against which any interventional treatment ought to be measured.

To date, it has not yet been established which cases of pancreatic pseudocysts definitely require surgery, and in which cases interventional transgastric or trans-cutaneous treatment may present a valid alternative.

Summarizing our experience, we can point out that sequesters were often found in so-called postacute cysts. In 82% of the cases, the pseudocysts were complications of

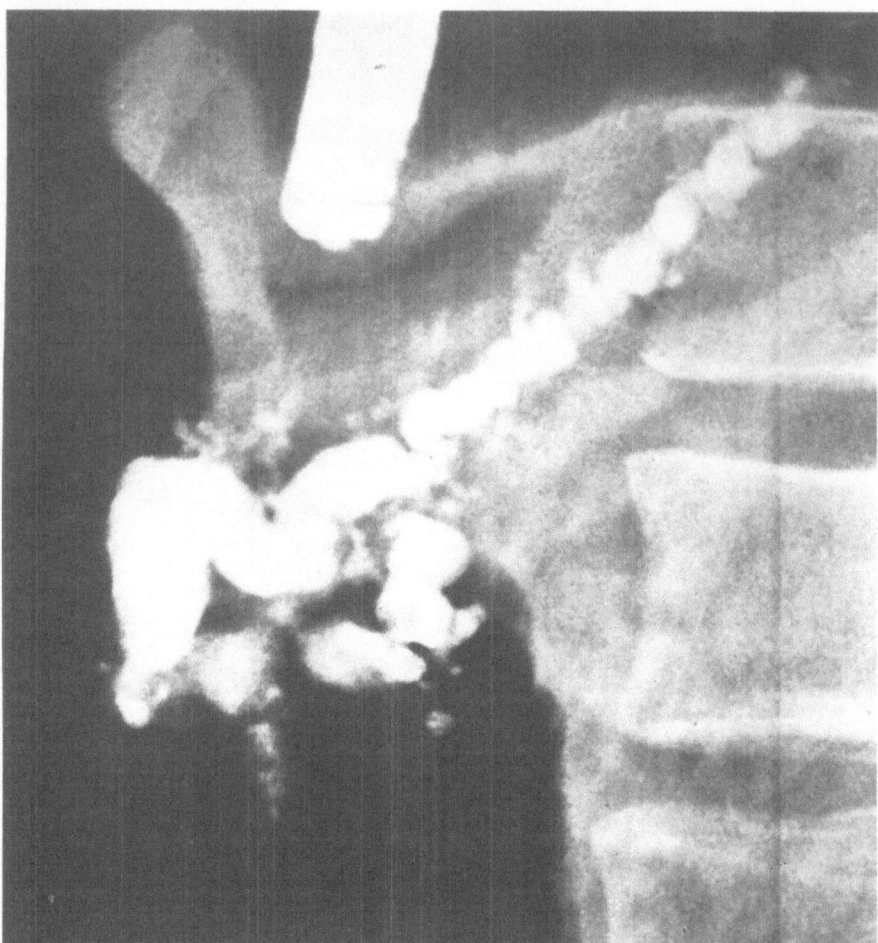

Fig. 19. Same patient as in Fig. 18. ERCP shows obstruction of the main duct

Table 7. Morbidity and mortality rates from seven recently published series concerning internal drainage of pancreatic pseudocysts. (From [3])

Source	Year	*n*	Morbidity	Mortality
Wade	1985	40	25 %	7.5%
Andren-Sandberg et al.	1983	20	25 %	0 %
Aranha et al.	1982	59	8.5%	6.7%
Bodurtha et al.	1980	18	44 %	6.0%
Boggs et al.	1982	16	31 %	0 %
Maruotti et al.	1982	22	27 %	4.5%
Schattenkerk et al.	1982	15	33 %	6.7%

an underlying chronic pancreatitis. In only one-third of these patients, internal drainage alone was sufficient. In two-thirds, resection was necessary for treatment of both the complications of the cysts and the underlying chronic pancreatitis.

In the face of our experience, we conclude that an interventional treatment for pancreatic pseudocyst is reasonable only if no other organ complications are present. Accordingly, surgical therapy of pancreatic pseudocyst is indicated in postacute cysts containing sequesters and in chronic cysts causing pancreatic duct obstruction, bile duct, duodenum or vein compression, or in cysts with intrasplenic and mediastinal extension.

References

1. Gussenbauer C (1883) Zur operativen Behandlung der Pankreas-Cysten. Arch Klin Chir 29:355–364
2. Beger HG, Büchler M, Bittner R, Oettinger W, Roscher R (1989) Duodenum-preserving resection of the head of the pancreas in severe chronic pancreatitis. Ann Surg 209:273–278
3. Munn JS, Aranha GV, Greenlee HB, Prinz RA (1987) Simultaneous treatment of chronic pancreatitis and pancreatic pseudocyst. Arch Surg 122:622–667

Pancreatojejunostomy in Combination with Transduodenal Pancreatic Sphincteroplasty

K. D. Rumpf[1] and H. Bunzendahl[2]

Long-standing chronic pancreatitis dramatically interferes with pancreatic function and the well-being of the patient. Digestion and metabolism are impaired, and resulting diabetes and malnutrition are often grave. Relapsing abdominal pain may be severe and long lasting, leading to impaired social function. Surgery has its place in treating disabling pain and possibly interfering with pancreatic self-destruction. The ideal operation for chronic pancreatitis is a low-risk procedure that releaves pain completely and predictably and preserves pancreatic function. Most surgeons have preferred pancreatic resections during the past 20 years. We now believe that complete drainage of the pancreas may come closer to those requirements. A complete decompression of the pancreas appears to be feasible in the treatment of severe pain without loss of organ function due to surgery.

Basic approach

Although drainage procedures have been used widely by some surgeons, their limitation is the lack of completeness of decompression, especially in the pancreatic head. We have tried to improve the standard drainage procedures by using a very long incision of the whole pancreas from the pancreatic head to the tail in order to open the duct of Wirsung (Fig. 1). Bleeding is controlled by oversewing; cautery is avoided as

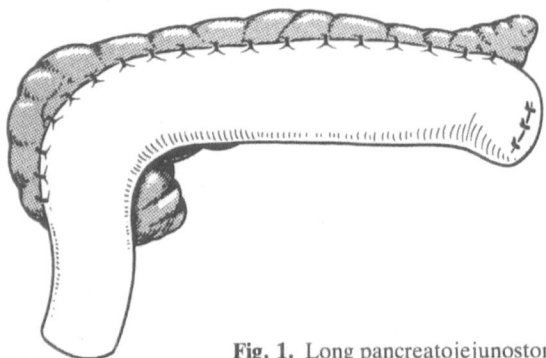

Fig. 1. Long pancreatojejunostomy side-to-side in CRP

[1] Klinik für Allgemein- und Abdominalchirurgie, Städtisches Klinikum, Pacelliallee 4, D-6400 Fulda, FRG
[2] Klinik für Abdominal- und Transplantationschirurgie, Medizinische Hochschule, Konstanty-Gutschow-Allee 9, D-3000 Hannover, FRG

Chronic Pancreatitis
Ed. by Beger, Büchler, Ditschuneit, and Malfertheiner
© Springer-Verlag Berlin Heidelberg 1990

much as possible. It is important to examine the inside of the duct carefully and to ensure complete removal of the segmental obstructions. Concrements are extracted, and scarring is excised if obstruction of major branches appears likely. The chance for normal passage of pancreatic secretion through the papilla of Vater is tested by passing a probe through the papilla. This maneuver also encourages to search for concrements in the duct of the unicante process.

We had to reoperate one case soon after complete drainage because of persistent pain. Left-sided small-duct disease inaccessable to drainage was the cause, in our opinion, and required resection of the pancreatic tail. This indicated the necessity of a *complete* drainage but also the potential limitation of drainage procedures.

To ensure completeness of drainage on the right side of the pancreas, we propose a simultaneous transduodenal papilloplasty with a generous opening of the duct of Wirsung. Quite frequently, previously undetected pancreatic stones can be detected and extracted. Hence this second step of the procedure is based on the frequent finding that significant duct obstruction may occur in the pancreatic head inaccessible from the left side (Fig. 2). This incompletely drained area obstructed by a diseased

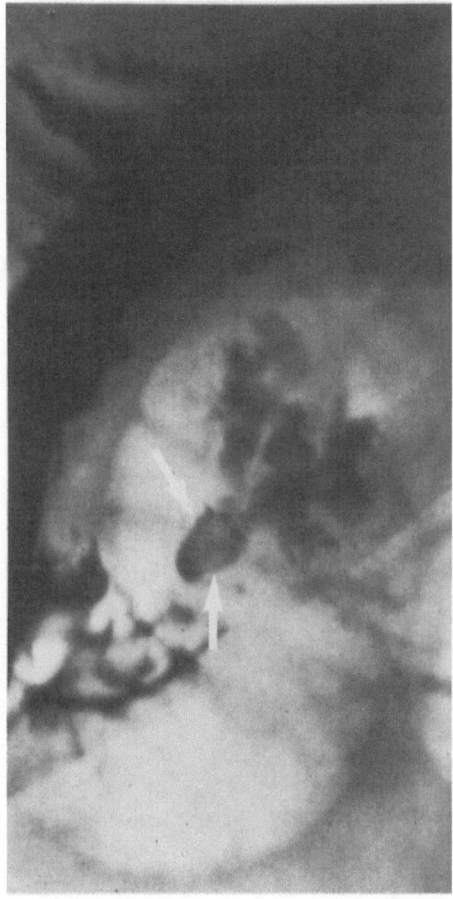

Fig. 2. Single stone incarceration in the prepapillary region

duct of Wirsung and possibly a scar to the papilla requires optimal drainage. This area is easily reached after a papillotomy of a sufficient size (Figs. 3, 4).

Technique of Transduodenal Pancreatic Papilloplasty

After a Kocher's maneuver and a long duodenotomy, the papilla of Vater is exposed. Two long incisions are performed in the papillary organ. The first one is a typical sphincterotomy into the common bile duct. It is helpful to releave the distal bile duct

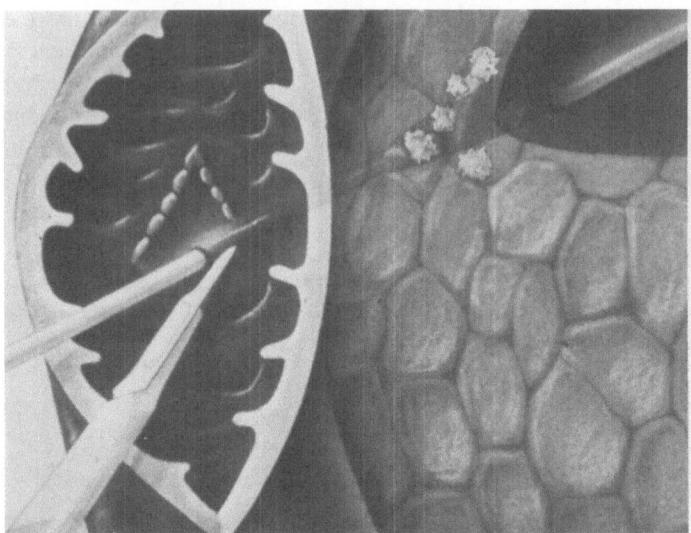

Fig. 3. Transduodenal-pancreatic papillotomy I

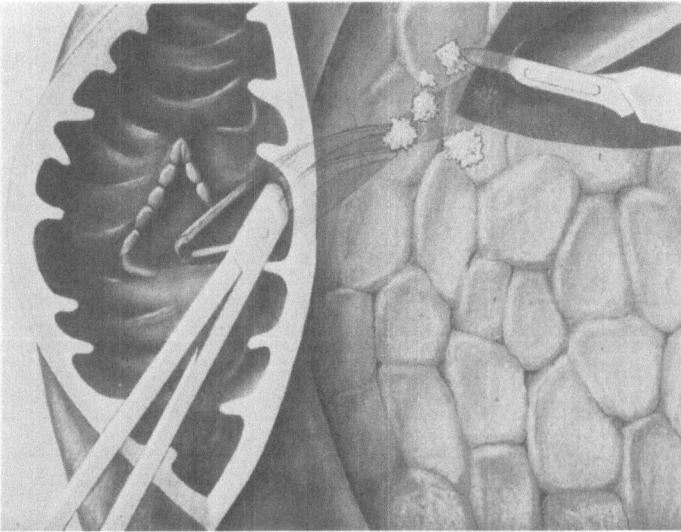

Fig. 4. Transduodenal-pancreatic papillotomy II

stenosis in some cases, and this prevents strictures after sphincteroplasty. It is always followed by a cholecystectomy. The second incision is a 2–3 cm papillotomy in the duct of Wirsung following a probe inserted from the left side of the pancreatic duct. Obstruction can easily be identified, and free flow of pancreatic juice can be restored. Duodenal mucosa is then sutured to the remnants of the papillary organ to avoid duodenal leaks. The procedure is used by itself very infrequently and in most instances it is combined with a long pancreatojejunostomy with a Roux-en-Y limb.

Results

After introduction of this concept 10 years ago, we abandoned pancreatic resections for most patients with severe chronic pancreatitis. A total of 34 patients were candidates for conventional drainage procedures who did not require a resection judged on conventional criteria. Between 1979 and 1985, however, 76 patients (66 men, 10 women; mean age 46 years) who clearly had been candidates for pancreatic resections before, were operated on with a long pancreatojejunostomy plus papilloplasty. This group has been subjected to a detailed follow-up and discussion. In more than 80% of cases alcoholism was at least in part an underlying cause. Hospital mortality was 5.3%. Causes of death were sepsis in three patients and pneumonia in one. Three of these deaths were related to the surgical technique at the very beginning of the series.

Long-lasting control of pancreatic pain was obtained in 66 patients (86.8%). Seven patients needed reoperations for pancreatic pain, usually resections. Three patients later required choledochojejunostomy because the transduodenal papilloplasty could not control cholestasis or cholangitis in the case of long stenosis of the distal bile duct. No death occured in this group of reoperations. Episodes of minor pains, distinctly different from pancreatic pains, were reported by 18 patients, but the frequency or intensity was sufficiently low that no therapy was necessary. Abdominal adhesions may be one reason for the complaints.

At the time of follow-up testing 32 of 76 patients (42%) were diabetic; 13 of these (40%) were treated with insulin, 15 (47%) with oral antidiabetic drugs, and four patients (13%) had not received any therapy for glucostasis. Repeated intravenous glucose tolerance testing revealed two important findings; even nondiabetics frequently showed an impaired glucose tolerance, as determined by a below-normal k value. Furthermore, postoperatively repeated k values do not show deterioration of glucose tolerance in nondiabetics (follow-up 24–56 months in eight patients).

Discussion

Since 1954 different drainage procedures for relief of pancreatic pain have been proposed to avoid resection of the pancreas for a benign lesion. Surgical risk has been only one aspect of this reconsideration. Loss of pancreatic tissue with detrimental endocrine and exocrine consequences is an important consideration as well.

Surgical drainage procedures compare favorably with resections in most series with respect to mortality and morbidity. Operation time and postoperative recovery of the patients are also very acceptable. In addition, patient acceptance is very good with nonresecting procedures. The sense of having "complete" organs should not be underestimated.

Impaired endocrine function of the diseased pancreas is, by definition, an essential feature of chronic pancreatitis. We could confirm this in our series even in nondiabetics. Parenchymal loss leads to overt diabetes in cases with boderline glucose tolerance and to further impairment in diabetics. Compliance is a problem in this group of patients. The presence or absence of glycemic control is likely to influence their survival. Even in diabetics residual endocrine function seems to be important for glucose hemostasis and longevity.

Although various drainage procedures have been used in the past, the procedures of DuVal [2], Leger et al. [3], Mercardier [4], and Puestow and Gillesby [7] have a major limitation in their relatively high risk of resulting in closure of their short anastomosis or incomplete drainage. A first step towards a more reliable drainage is that of Partington and Rochelle [5]. Although patient selection may have played a role in their series, the longer drainage area seems to offer long-term advantages. Many reports on nonresecting surgery for chronic pancreatitis lack a precise differentiation regarding how anastomoses were carried out. This may have obscured good results with proper drainage procedures in the past. White and Slavotinek [11] showed in 1979 that only long pancreatojejunostomies lead to freedom of pain in 87% after 3–20 years after operation. Warshaw et al. [10] and Prinz and Greenlee [6] have published data in agreement with these findings.

In order to carry the concept of completeness of drainage further, we propose the transduodenal pancreatic papilloplasty [8, 9], as described above. The procedure is not dangerous in experienced hands familiar with papillary surgery. Postoperative mortality was apparently not very low among our patients. It should be stressed, however, that mortality occurred early in this series. Increasing experience with this technique was followed by more than 60 operations without hospital mortality. Our results after a limited follow-up of 3–8 years seem similar to those reported by others [6, 10, 11]. Control of pancreatic pain with complete drainage procedure compares well with results after duodenopancreatectomy. The vast majority of our patients after internal drainage procedures live a pain-free life.

A possible limitation of the drainage procedures could be the presence of a small pancreatic duct. History of pancreatitis tends to be shorter in these cases. Uncertainty about success in controlling pain and sometimes the possibility of underlying malignancy cause us to decide in favor of pancreatic resection in a few cases.

The good chances to control pancreatic pain without resection in most of these relatively young patients without malignancy encourage us to propose the generous use of complete drainage procedures. The introduction of transduodenal papilloplasty together with a long pancreaticojejunostomy has expanded the use of drainage procedure to patients previously treatable only by major pancreatic resections. Early results are encouraging with respect to risk, pain control, and residual pancreatic function.

References

1. Cattel RB (1947) Anastomosis of the duct of Wirsung; its use in palliative operation for cancer of the head of the pancreas. Surg Clin North Am 27:636
2. Du Val MK (1954) Caudal pancreatico-jejunostomy for chronic pancreatitis. Ann Surg 140:775
3. Léger L, Détrie P, Chapuis Y (1961) Làvenir des wirsungojéjunostomies. A propos des 10 observations contrôlées. J Chir (Paris) 82:577
4. Mercardier M (1964) Affections du foire, des voies biliaires, de la rate et du pancréas. In: Traité de thérapeutique chirurgical, vol 4. Masson, Paris
5. Partington PF, Rochel REL (1060) Modified Puestow procedure for retrograde drainage of the pancreatic duct. Ann Surg 152:1037
6. Prinz RA, Greenlee HB (1981) Pancreatic duct drainage in 100 patients with chronic pancreatitis. Ann Surg 194:313
7. Puestow CB, Gillesby WJ (1958) Retrograde surgical drainage of pancreas for chronic relapsing pancreatitis. AMA Arch Surg 76:898
8. Rumpf KD (1984) Die chirurgische Therapie der chronischen Pankreatitis: Verfahrenstechniken und Indikationen. Aktuel Chir 6:19
9. Rumpf KD, Pichlmayr R (1983) Eine Methode zur chirurgischen Behandlung der chronischen Pankreatitis. Die transduodenale Pankreaticoplastik. Chirurg 54:722
10. Warshaw AL, Popp JW, Schapiro RH (1980) Long-term patency, pancreatic function, and pain relief after lateral pancreaticojejunostomy for chronic pancreatitis. Gastroenterology 79:289
11. White TT, Slavotinek AH (1975) Results of surgical treatment of chronic pancreatitis. Ann Surg 189:217

Surgical Treatment:
Resectional Procedures

Indication for and Results of Pancreatic Left Resection

CH. GEBHARDT[1]

Ten to twenty years ago pancreatic left resection was the standard procedure in the treatment of diffuse chronic pancreatitis with minimal dilatation of the ductal system. This is reflected in the relative frequency with which this procedure was used, both in our own patients and at other centers of pancreatic surgery. In Ann Arbor, Michigan, for example, 77 subtotal left pancreatic resections were performed in the 16 years between 1959 and 1975 while the same center reported only 10 such resections in the following 8 years [1]. In recent years various forms of resection of the pancreatic head have gained ground in the resectional treatment of chronic pancreatitis. Therefore, it seems appropriate to critically evaluate the importance which distal pancreatic resection has today, including the results which can be achieved by this method.

Basically, there are two forms of left resection which must be differentiated: partial left resection and subtotal pancreatectomy. In the latter the extent of resection comprises 80%–95% of the organ.

Operative mortality

Since 1969 more than 1000 cases of pancreatic left resection have been reported in the literature, and the average operative mortality is around 6% [1, 6–8] (collected series in [2]). It must be kept in mind, however, that in most hospitals with considerable experience in pancreatic surgery the results today are much better. In our own series of 18 patients who have undergone surgery during the past 4 years there has been no postoperative death.

Rate of Recurrence

As reported in the literature, pancreatic left resection leads to considerable improvement in or elimination of pancreatitis-associated symptoms in 66% of cases. In almost 30%, however, there is no improvement, or there is recurrence of pancreatitis [1, 7, 8] (collected series in [2]).

In analyzing our own series of patients we could determine that the late results depend mainly on the extent of pancreatitis, on the one hand, and on the extent of resection, on the other [4]. In diffuse pancreatitis, which was formally the classical indication for this procedure, we found poor results in 77% of the simple left

---

[1] Department of Surgery, City Hospital (Klinikum), Flurstrasse 17, D-8500 Nürnberg 90, FRG

Chronic Pancreatitis
Ed. by Beger, Büchler, Ditschuneit, and Malfertheiner
© Springer-Verlag Berlin Heidelberg 1990

resections and in 49% of the subtotal pancreatectomies – which of course are disappointing results. A different situation existed in patients with isolated segmental
pancreatitis of the tail region. Here, disappointing results were encountered, depending on the extent of resection, in only 33%, and 9% of cases respectively. The subtotal
pancreatectomy in these patients comprised an 80% resection of the organ with the
line of resection located above or just to the right of the portal vein (Tabelle 1).

Table 1. Late results after left resection for chronic pancreatitis. (From [4])

	n	No improvement or recurrence
Left-sided pancreatitis ($n = 58$)		
Partial resection	24	8 (33.3%)
Subtotal resection	34	3 (8.8%)
Diffuse pancreatitis ($n = 67$)		
Partial resection	24	16 (66.7%)
Subtotal resection	43	21 (48.8%)

Carbohydrate Metabolism

With regard to carbohydrate metabolism, pancreatic left resection leads to an average
postoperative increase in the rate of insulin-dependent diabetics of 50%. This is
considerably higher than after drainage procedures or even after partial duodenopancreatectomy. In our own 121 patients the rate of diabetics increased by 41%
during the late postoperative course (Table 2). It is of interest that in this series there
was no difference between partial and subtotal resection. This can be explained by the
fact that there were almost no true 95% subtotal resection in our patients; it also
signifies the importance of the cauda pancreatitis for carbohydrate metabolism.

Table 2. Carbohydrate metabolism after left resection for chronic pancreatits ($n = 121$). (From [4])

	Preoperative	Postoperative
Normal metabolism	53%	32%
Latent diabetes	32%	13%
Clinical diabetes	15%	56%

Different results have been reported by Morrow et al. [7]. In cases with 40%–80%
resection the results are similar to ours, with an increase in the incidence of diabetics
of 38%. The 95% resections, on the other hand, resulted in the occurrence of
postoperative insulin-dependent diabetes in all cases. Eckhauser et al. [1] found that
an 80%–95% left pancreatic resection increased the rate of diabetes among patients
by 50%. Of special importance is the fact that 82% of the 44 patients who developed
insulin-dependent diabetes in the postoperative period had a normal carbohydrate
metabolism preoperatively.

Based on these reports it can be expected that in general left pancreatic resection leads to an increase in the incidence of diabetes by about 40%, and that this rate increases to nearly 100% if the resection is very extensive.

Survival Rates

The cumulative, age-corrected, 5-year survival rate of our patients excluding the operative mortality was 78% ± 8%. These results are quite similar to those which can be achieved with a Whipple's procedure with ductal occlusion (75% ± 8%) or with drainage procedures (74% ± 11%) [5]. These results cast serious doubt on the frequently repeated view that late mortality is higher on principle in the more extensive resections such as the Whipple's procedure. In reality, survival does not seem to depend as much on the type of procedure performed as on the primary severity and extent of the disease and, on the other hand, on the postoperative behavior of the patients. Continued consumption of alcohol seems to be of paramount importance. Alcoholic patients with calcifying pancreatitis and preoperatively manifest diabetes mellitus had considerably lower 5-year survival rates than nonalcoholics without diabetes and without calcifications (Tabelle 3). The negative influence of continued alcohol consumption on survival after pancreatic left resection is especially evident in the series of patients reported by Eckhauser et al. [1]. Among our patients the cause of death was cirrhosis of the liver and hepatic coma related to continued alcohol abuse in 8 out of 40 patients (Table 4).

Table 3. Cumulative 5-year survival rate after left resection for chronic pancreatitis (operative mortality excluded). (From [5])

	n	5-year surival rate (± 2 SE)
Calcifying pancreatitis	47	71% ± 15%
No calcifying pancreatitis	113	81% ± 9%
Preoperative diabetes mellitus	64	73% ± 12%
No preoperative diabetes mellitus	96	82% ± 9%
Alcoholics	64	72% ± 13%
Nonalcoholics	96	83% ± 9%

Table 4. Late mortality and causes of death after left resection ($n = 40$; 23.9%). (From [5])

Hepatic coma	8
Hypoglycemia	4
Cardiac failure	4
Septic shock	4
Cachexia	3
Necrotizing pancreatitis	3
Gastrointestinal bleeding	3
Stroke	2
Trauma	2
Unknown	7

Conclusions

How should these data influence the indication for performing pancreatic left resection? An optimal indication with good late results in more than 90% of the cases seems to be the segmental pancreatitis with more or less isolated involvement of the tail of the pancreas. However, these good results can be expected only if an 80% resection is performed, i. e., dividing the organ in the region of the portal vein. We do not recommend more extensive resections because of the significant increase in metabolic problems in these patients. In addition to segmental pancreatitis of the tail region, we consider an indication to be given in persisting or bleeding pseudocysts and in chronic pancreatitis with splenic hypertension in splenic vein thrombosis.

Chronic pancreatitis of the diffuse type is not an indication for left resection because a low recurrence rate can be achieved only with a "near-total pancreatectomy," which in turn results in an extremely high rate of postoperative diabetes. Our method of choice in theses cases is a Whipple's procedure with occlusion of the ductal system of the remaining pancreas [7]. There are exceptions to this rule, however, for example, if a partial duodenopancreatectomy cannot be performed because of anatomical reasons such as arteriosclerotic occlusion of the common hepatic artery with collateral vessels which must be protected.

In conclusion, it can be stated that left pancreatic resection continues to have a place in the surgical treatment of chronic pancreatitis and can lead to favorable long-term results if it is performed for the right indications.

References

1. Eckhauser FE, Strodel WE, Knol JA, Harper M, Turcotte JG (1984) Near -total pancreatectomy for chronic pancreatitis. Surgery 96:599–607
2. Gebhardt C (1984) Chirurgie des exokrinen Pankreas. Thieme, Stuttgart
3. Gebhardt C(1987) Indications, techniques and results of surgical or endoscopic pancreatic duct occlusion in chronic pancreatitis. Tijdschr Gastroenterol 17:349–358
4. Gebhardt C, Zirngibl H, Gossler M (1981) Pankreaslinksresektion zur Behandlung der chronischen Pankreatitis. Langenbecks Arch Chir 354:209–220
5. Metzner K (1989) Spätsterblichkeit nach Eingriffen wegen chronischen Pankreatitis. Dissertation, University of Erlangen
6. Morel P, Rohner A (1987) Surgery for chronic pancreatitis. Surgery 101:130–135
7. Morrow CE, Cohen JI, Sutherland DER, Najarian JS (1984) Chronic pancreatitis: long term surgical results of pancreatic duct drainage, pancreatic resection, and near-total pancreatectomy and islet autotransplantation. Surgery 96:608–616
7. Ribet M, Quandalle P, Giard-Lefevre S, Pruvot FR, Watine O (1986) Traitement chirurgical de la pancréatite chronique. Étude rétrospective de 221 cas. J Chir (Paris) 123:559–562

Pancreaticoduodenectomy (Whipple Resection) in the Treatment of Chronic Pancreatitis: Indications, Techniques, and Results

J. M. Howard[1]

Introduction

Pancreaticoduodenectomy is excellent for the relief of pain in the patient whose lifestyle provides the probability of a stable, ongoing life. Furthermore, in the author's experience, if carcinoma of the head of the pancreas is suspected at operation, pancreaticoduodenectomy is the procedure of choice. The individual surgeon, however, must assess his own experience, for a low operation mortality risk is essential. A continuing alcoholic is not a good candidate for pancreaticoduodenectomy in this disease. The same limitation exists for the narcotic addict, but in the author's experience, narcotic addiction under these circumstances is largely a problem of bygone days. Most patients who do not stop drinking or who do not discontinue narcotics prior to operation are probably not acceptable candidates for pancreaticoduodenectomy.

As pancreatic centers evolve, it is increasingly possible to evaluate the role of radical approaches to the treatment of this benign disease; this is the case today, for example, at Ulm (FRG). Thus, resection in the case of a benign disease has become a practical option. The operative mortality now approaches zero. Recognizing that pancreaticoduodenectomy must be utilized carefully and selectively, the author presents his experience in this chapter.

Clinical Experiences

Thirty patients have undergone pancreatic duodenectomy for chronic pancreatitis by the author. These patients have been selected from several hundred patients treated for chronic pancreatitis. The majority of the patients had previously been operated upon, primarily by other surgeons, prior to referral. Eight of the patients were women, and 22 were men; ages ranged from 24 to 65 years. There was no peak in terms of distribution in any decade, but the median age was 40. Five of the patients were insulin dependent prior to operation, and four had experienced mild difficulties in maintaining their weight. Thirteen had pancreatic calcification. Five were ongoing alcoholics at the time of operation. None was a narcotic addict. Only one of the patients had cirrhosis, as recognized grossly at the time of laparotomy.

---

[1] Department of Surgery, Medical College of Ohio, Toledo OH 43699, USA

Chronic Pancreatitis
Ed. by Beger, Büchler, Ditschuneit, and Malfertheiner
© Springer-Verlag Berlin Heidelberg 1990

Other preoperative complications of the disease are shown in Table 1. Each of the patients had severe disease in the head of the pancreas. In 19 patients, severe pancreatic pain was present. At operation, the pancreatic mass was highly suggestive of malignancy in six and clinically compatible with cancer in eight others. A normal or small pancreatic duct was present in nine patients. One of the latter patients had a fibrotic section in the terminal common bile duct which was suspicious for malignancy. Five of the nine patients had stenosis of the duodenum and/or the common bile duct, and all nine had severe pancreatic pain. The inflammatory mass was dominant in the uncinate process in three patients.

Table 1. Preoperative status of patients ($n = 30$)

	n
Severe disease in head of pancreas	30
Severe pancreatic pain	19
Firm mass in head of pancreas	14
Mass in head of pancreas without severe pain	6
Pancreatic pseudocysts in head of pancreas	6
Predominance of disease in uncinate process	3
Failed longitudinal pancreaticojejunostomy	2
Duodenal stenosis	5
Common bile duct stenosis	9
Pancreatic calcification	13
Splenic vein thrombosis	3
Jaundice	6
Normal or small pancreatic ducts	9
Diabetes, insulin dependent	5
Malnutrition, mild	4
Cirrhosis of liver	1
Continuing alcoholism	5
Narcotic addiction	0[a]

[a] Questionable in one patient

Technique of Operation

Pancreaticoduodenectomy is generally easier technically in patients with chronic pancreatitis than in those with pancreatic cancer. Few patients reaching operation for chronic pancreatitis are obese, and few are in the geriatric age group. Long-standing disease complicated by repetitive prior operations can, very occasionally, make the pancreas technically unresectable because of loss of tissue planes, but this is extremely rare.

The author approaches pancreaticoduodenectomy by a long, bilateral subcostal incision. A liver biopsy is routinely obtained by wedge excision. The gallbladder is examined, and a complete exploratory laparotomy is performed. After mobilization of the hepatic flexure of the colon, a Kocher maneuver is performed, and the head of the pancreas is carefully palpated. The gastrocolic omentum is divided, and the entire panreas explored.

A decision as to biopsy of the pancreas is then made. In most patients, the prolonged preoperative course of the disease, the CAT scan, ERCP, and the operative findings make the diagnosis of chronic pancreatitis obvious, and biopsy may not be necessary. If the question is whether or not a mass in the head of the pancreas is benign or malignant, a needle biopsy, using the Tru-Cut needle technique, may be utilized, preferably transduodenally through the lateral and medial walls of the duodenum, avoiding the ampulla of Vater. If a wedge biopsy is elected, care is taken to avoid incision of the main pancreatic ducts. In the majority of patients, the anatomical outline of the common bile duct, the pancreatic duct, and the related gastroduodenal tract will have been obtained radiographically prior to operation. Early in the operation the pancreas is mobilized at the level of the superior mesenteric vessels by the identification of the superior mesenteric vein immediately inferior to its exit from behind the pancreas. Finger dissection is then performed anterior to the vein, resulting in the development of a plane behind the pancreas. Next, right-angle clamps are used to dissect a plane around the distal common bile duct, around which an umbilical tape is passed. The hepatic artery is similarly isolated, and another umbilical tape passed. Finally, an umbilical tape is passed around the portal vein, each dissection being carried out immediately craniad to the head of the pancreas.

At this stage, a decision is made to definitely proceed with resection. The lesser curvature and the greater curvature of the stomach are freed, and a stapler is used to transect the stomach proximal to the gastric antrum. Vagotomy is not performed. Next, stay sutures are inserted along the craniad and inferior border of the pancreas, immediately to the patient's left of the anticipated line of transection. These simple sutures are used to elevate the pancreas off the superior mesenteric vein so as to permit insertion of one's finger and transection of the pancreas by scalpel over the protecting finger. The size of the transected pancreatic duct is reassessed visually, and examination of the left half of the pancreas is further performed in order to decide whether the dissection is to be carried further to the left. In the majority of patients, further resection is not performed, although, in the past, patients with extensive calcareous deposits had the more radical resection of the body of the gland.

After transection of the neck of the pancreas, mobilization of the uncinate process then proceeds with the gland being dissected toward the right, away from the superior mesenteric and portal vessels. The inferior pancreaticojejunal arteries are divided at their origin. At this time the gastroduodenal artery and the right gastric arteries are ligated and hemostasis assured by transfixion sutures. The jejunum is then divided at a convenient distance, perhaps 15 cm, beyond the ligament of Treitz. The mesentery of the jejunum and the third and fourth portions of the duodenum are then divided so as to permit the passage of the jejunum and duodenum retrograde above the transverse mesocolon. If not previously divided, the common bile duct is then divided above the duodenum. If the blood supply to the cut edge of the bile duct appears adequate, the line of transection is kept low. If the blood supply is not rich, further resection of the common bile duct is carried towards the liver until an adequate supply to the common bile duct is assured.

Earlier, cholecystectomy was routinely performed. In many patients, it will have been performed at a prior operation. At present, it does not seem necessary to remove a healthy gallbladder. Care must be taken, however, to be certain that the cystic duct has not been transected at the time of transection of the common bile duct. If it has, it is probably safer to remove the gallbladder rather than to attempt any restorative anastomosis.

The antrum of the stomach, the duodenum, the head of the pancreas, and the first part of the jejunum are then removed.

Reconstruction

The end of the transected caudal pancreas is oversewn with 4.0 prolone sutures to prevent bleeding and to prevent the leakage of juice from small, secondary ducts (Fig. 1). Care is taken not to occlude the main pancreatic duct. The Roux-en-Y limb of the jejunum is then brought behind the transverse colon to lie comfortably along the pancreas and hilum of the liver. The pancreatic duct, per se, is then approximated to a small puncture wound in the side of the Roux-en-Y (jejunum), approximately 10 cm from the transected end of the jejunum (Fig. 2). Then, 5.0 prolene sutures are used to

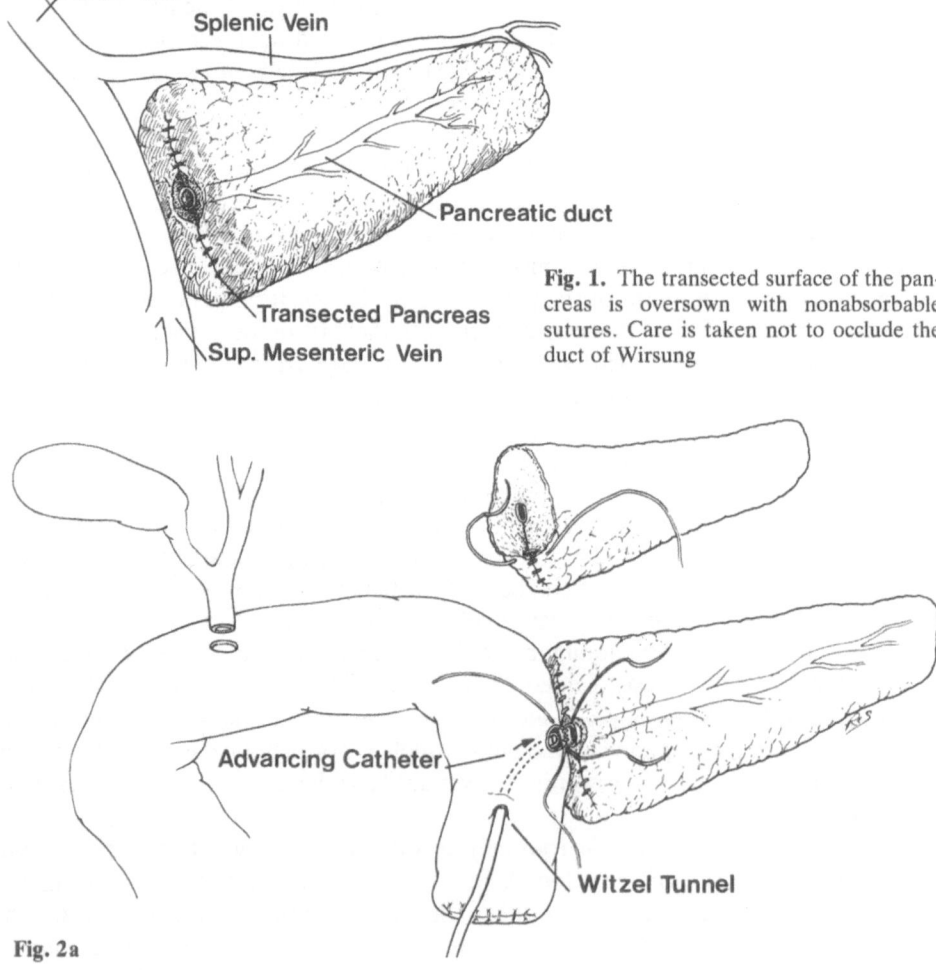

Portal Vein

Splenic Vein

Pancreatic duct

Transected Pancreas

Sup. Mesenteric Vein

Fig. 1. The transected surface of the pancreas is oversown with nonabsorbable sutures. Care is taken not to occlude the duct of Wirsung

Advancing Catheter

Witzel Tunnel

Fig. 2a

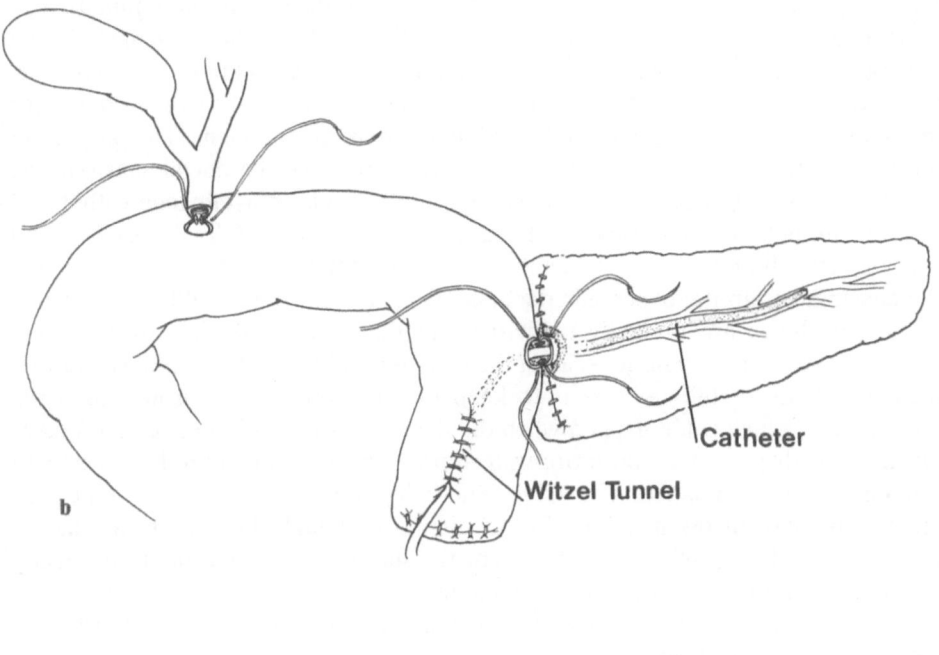

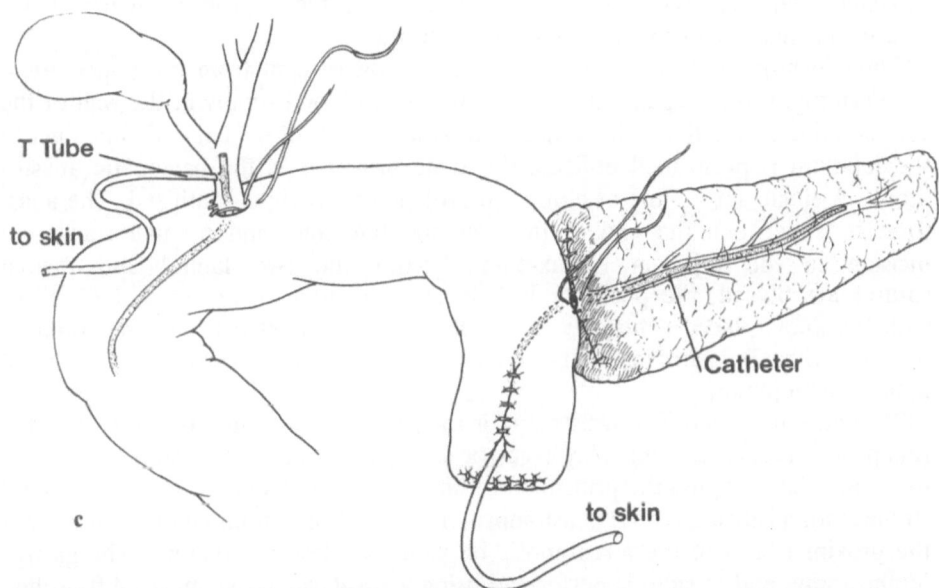

Fig. 2a–c. a Pancreaticojejunostomy. 5.0 prolene sutures are utilized to suture the posterior wall of the pancreatic duct to a small puncture wound of the jejunum. A small polyethylene catheter is positioned for cannulation of the anastomosis. **b** The catheter is then advanced through the incomplete anastomosis toward the tail of the pancreas. It is secured vie a Witzel tunnel. **c** The anterior wall of the pancreaticojejunostomy is sutured. Additional sutures (not shown) are utilized to abut the transected surface of the pancreas to the jejunal wall. Downstream, the common bile duct is anastomosed to the jejunum, utilizing a similar technique

create a precise anastomosis of the pancreatic duct to the side of the jejunum. The jejunal suture is through the full thickness with care being taken to include the mucosa. The sutures are placed on each lateral side of the pancreatic duct, and then its posterior wall is sutured to the jejunum. After this is secured, the oversewn ends of the transected pancreas are sutured to the jejunum as an abutment. The purpose in the latter step is fundamentally to take the tension off of the ductal anastomosis. Depending upon the size of the pancreatic duct, a small polyethylene catheter is inserted through the skin, "Whitzeled" through the blind limb of the Roux-en-Y, and carried inside the jejunum to the pancreaticojejunostomy. It is then passed through the anastomosis up the pancreatic duct almost as far as it will go. When the duct is small, side holes are probably inadvisable in the intrapancreatic portion of the catheter because they tend to weaken the catheter and cause it to kink. The fundamental purpose of the catheter is to keep the surgeon from suturing closed the anastomosis, which could happen when the duct is small even if great care is taken. Having already placed the posterior wall sutures, the anterior suture line of duct to jejunum is then completed. The suture line is usually quite secure in chronic pancreatitis because of the increased fibrous tissue. Although the author has characteristically used the principle of cannulating the anastomosis, it may not be necessary when the duct is 0.5 cm or greater in diameter.

When there is difficulty identifying the pancreatic duct in the transected surface of the pancreas, an intravenous injection of secretin, 1 μ/kg body weight, results in a flow of juice and permits identification of the small duct. Another technical point: when a small pancreatic duct is first transected, it is usually visible. A probe or small catheter inserted caudally can provide ongoing identification.

Choledochojejunostomy is then performed downstream from the pancreaticojejunostomy. Care is again taken to assure a good blood supply in the wall of the common duct at the line of its transection. Anastomosis of the common bile duct to the jejunum is performed utilizing the same principle as the pancreatic anastomosis. A single suture line of either 5.0 prolene or 5.0 vicro is utilized. The anastomosis is between the end of the common bile duct and a small transverse incision in the jejunum (Roux-en-Y). After the two lateral and medial sutures are placed, the posterior wall is approximated, again, as a single layer with the knots placed externally. A small T-tube is introduced into the common bile duct with a long arm inserted through the choledochojejunostomy into the distal limb of the jejunum.

The third anastomosis, downstream, is the gastrojejunostomy. Because of recurrent problems of a transient delay in gastric emptying during the convalescent period, the author has adopted the principle of utilizing the full diameter of the transected stomach for a Billroth type II anastomosis. The space limitations almost require that the proximal limb of the anastomosis be along the lesser curvature. The gastrojejunostomy, end-to-side, is performed using a two-layer anastomosis, 4.0 proline sutures on the serosa and 3.0 catgut as a continuous suture on the mucosa, the latter including the full thickness of the intestinal and gastric walls. Just beyond the greater curvature of the stomach, the jejunum must, almost of necessity, fold back on itself as it abuts the left side of the abdominal cavity. (This may be a disadvantage). Care is taken to fix the pancreaticojejunal catheter, as well as the T-tube, to the skin in a circular maneuver to add security to the fixation. Suction drains are brought to the skin, one placed adjacent to the choledochojejunostomy and one adjacent to the pancreaticojejunostomy, but neither touching the anastomosis.

Four patients in the current series had previously undergone gastrectomy with a Billroth II reconstruction. In order not to take down the gastrojejunostomy, an isolated jejunal limb was developed distal to the gastrojejunostomy and used as a conduit from the pancreas to the biliary tract. The afferent limb of the gastrojejunostomy was then divided and the gastrojejunal anastomosis left in situ. The new isolated jejunal limb was then anastomosed end-to-end to the afferent limb of the gastrojejunostomy. Distal to the area where the "Roux-en-Y" conduit was created, jejunal continuity was restored by end-to-end jejunojejunostomy.

In three patients, a previous Roux-en-Y had been constructed for internal drainage of a pancreatic pseudocyst or for longitudinal pancreatic jejunostomy. This preexisting Roux-en-Y limb was found to have foreshortened to such a degree that it could not be utilized. Resection of the preexisting Roux-en-Y was required and a new Roux-en-Y segment was created.

Results of Operation

There was no hospital mortality.

The complications occurring during the postoperative period of hospitalization are listed in Table 2. None of the complications proved life threatening. Convalescence was more rapid than in patients undergoing pancreaticoduodenectomy for cancer. A single, transient fistula from the choledochojejunostomy did not present a major problem.

Table 2. Postoperative hospital complications

	n
Choledochal fistula (transient)	1
Wound infection	2
Decubitus ulcers (heels)	1
"Insulin" diabetes (new)	2

The pancreaticojejunal stent was usually removed between 2 and 8 weeks postoperatively. Most of the patients had a common duct of normal diameter. The T-tube, having been inserted through the choledochal anastomosis was left in place for 4–6 months after operation in order to prevent the fibrous stricture which French surgeons have described.

The long-term postoperative complications after discharge from the hospital are shown in Table 3. One patient's reconstruction involved a cholecystojejunostomy with a long blind segment of common duct distal to the cystic duct. This stagnant column filled with sludge and soft stones. The patient became jaundiced with cholangitis. Reoperation required cholecystectomy and end-to-side choledochojejunostomy. She has remained well for the subsequent 5 years.

Table 3. Late postoperative complications

	n
Incomplete obstruction of Roux-en-Y	2
"Sump" syndrome with cholangitis	1
Breaking of pancreaticojejunal catheter (stent) within abdominal wall	1
Hematemesis requiring transfusion 2 months postoperatively	1
Delayed onset of diabetes (insulin dependent)	2
Delayed onset of nutritional insufficiency	1
Continued alcoholism	5
Choledochojejunal stenosis	0
Chronic marginal ulcer	0

Two other patients required rehospitalization for an unusual complication. The complication consisted of obstruction of the jejunal limb by kinking and adhesions between the pancreaticojejunostomy and the choledochojejunostomy. In each instance, operative correction 2 and 3 years, respectively, after pancreaticojejunostomy relieved the intermittent symptoms. No patient developed stricture of the choledochojejunostomy, nor has a stricture of the pancreaticojejunal anastomosis been recognized. Two patients developed delayed onset of insulin-dependent diabetes. Management of exocrine insufficiency following operation has not been a difficult problem. In fact, nutrition has been significantly better following operation than it was preoperatively. This improvement results from the fact that the patients felt better and took less pain medication following operation. In only one patient has there been an ongoing problem in maintaining an adequate nutritional status, although several of the patients are on pancreatic extracts.

Long-Term Results

No patient has required reoperation for control of the pain of chronic pancreatitis. As discussed above, three patients have required reoperation for other reasons. These three patients remain well. No patient has been lost to follow-up within the first 15 years after operation. During this time, there has been no fatality. Five patients are currently utilizing alcohol excessively, although four of them retain their ability to work fulltime. No patient currently complains of abdominal pain. No patient has been recognized as developing cirrhosis of the liver after operation, and no patient has developed evidence of a marginal ulcer, although one patient developed hematemesis requiring transfusion 2 months after operation. A source for the hematemesis was never determined as gastroscopy was negative; she has since remained well for 5 years. Follow-up data are shown in Table 4. It is to be emphasized that only one patient has required occasional narcotics following hospitalization, and this patient was one of the more emotionally labile in this series.

Table 4. Postresection follow-up in personal series ($n = 30$)

Duration of follow-up	Number of patients	Number living	Results good to excellent	Reoperation for chronic pancreatitis
Less than 5 years	12	12	10	0
5 years or longer	18	18	16	0[a]
10 years or longer	12[b]	12	12	0[a]
15 years or longer	5[b]	5	5	0

[a] Three patients required revisions of Roux-en-Y reconstruction but have remained well since
[b] Included also in the 5-year follow-up

Discussion

Operative Mortality

The operative mortality of pancreaticoduodenectomy for chronic pancreatitis compares acceptably to the mortality of other operations for this disease, (Table 5). During the period 1987–1989, the literature records reports of 467 patients undergoing this procedure for chronic pancreatitis. Among the eight reports included only three described fatalities. Five of the smaller series were without an operative mortality, and the overall mortality for the 467 patients was 1.7%. This operative mortality, reflecting to a large extent the experience of European surgeons, includes the experience of Gall [1], who occluded the pancreatic duct by the operative injection of prolamin. As always, it is important to stress that these low mortality rates reflect the experience of groups highly specialized in pancreatic surgery.

Table 5. Operative mortality of pancreaticoduodenectomy in chronic pancreatitis (1987–1989 reports)

Reference	Number of patients	Deaths
Gall [1]	289	3 (1%)
Köhler et al. [2]	24	3 (12%)
Morel et al. [3]	20	0 (0%)
Rossi et al. [4]	73	2 (3%)
Williamson et al. [5]	6	0 (0%)
Stone et al. [6]	15	0 (0%)
Mannell et al. [7]	10	0 (0%)
Current series 1989	30	0 (0%)
Total	467	8 (1.7%)

Postoperative Complications

The incidence of serious postoperative complications has also greatly diminished. Thus in the reports of the 1987–1989 series, of 433 patients in whom complications

Table 6. Acute postoperative complications (1987–1989 reports)

Reference	Number of patients	Anastomotic leakage	Other complications
Morel et al. [3]	20	–	4
Williamson et al. [5]	6	–	0
Rossi et al. [4]	73	5	8
Stone et al. [6]	15	1	3
Gall [1]	289	0	0
Current series (1989)	30	1	3
Total	433	7 (1.6%)	18

were delineated, a fistula from the pancreas or common duct was noted in only seven patients (1.6%) (Table 6). Again, this incidence is significantly influenced by the results of Gall [1]. Throughout the world, however, in pancreatic centers, the standard Whipple operation is resulting in a diminishing incidence of an anastomotic failure. Pancreaticojejunal fistula has almost disappeared. The incidence of other complications has been relatively nonspecific although intra-abdominal bleeding was significant in five of the reported patients after operation.

Follow-up Results

In the author's experience, the long-term (5–15 years) relief of pain has been good –quite good in those experiencing severe pain preoperatively. The recent literature (Table 7) reflects long-term pain relief in two-thirds of the patients. Standardization of follow-up reports, in terms of 5-, 10-, and 15-year periods, needs improvements. Such standardization does not compare favorably with the reports following operations for malignancy. Leger et al. [8] presented a classical report on the treatment of chronic pancreatitis which many should use as a model. They noted that of 15 patients followed for 8 years (mean) none required reoperation, whereas 43 required reoperation after pancreaticojejunostomy. We have not had to reoperate any patient for relief of pain for chronic pancreatitis, although three patients have required reopera-

Table 7. Long-term relief of pain of pancreaticoduodenectomy for chronic pancreatitis (1987–1989 reports)

Reference	Number of patients	Follow-up period (Years)	Percentages		
			Good	Fair	Failure
Rossi et al. [4]	33	5	61	18	21
Williamson et al. [5]	6	3.5	66.6	16.6	16.6
Gauthier-Benoit and Perissat [9]	237	3.8	65	–	–
Stone et al. [6]	15	6	53	27	20
Mannell et al. [7]	9	10	100	0	0
Köhler et al. [2]	24	–	61	–	–
Gall [1]	289	8	65	–	–
Current series (1989)	17[a]	5–15	94	–	6

[a] Limited to 17 patients with severe pain followed for longer than 5 years

Table 8. Reoperation rate after pancreaticoduodenectomy for control of pain in chronic pancreatitis (1987–1989 reports)

Reference	Number of patients	Number requiring reoperation
Gauthier-Benoit and Perissat [9]	237	3 (1.2%)
Morel et al. [3]	20	1 (5 %)
Rossi et al. [4]	71	8 (12 %)
Williamson et al. [5]	6	1 (17 %)
Mannell et al. [7]	10	0 (0 %)
Gall [1]	289	6 (2.1%)
Current Series (1989)	30	0 (0 %ᵃ)
Total	663	19 (2.9%)

ᵃ For control of pain. Three patients were reoperated on for other reasons

tion for late complications related to the reconstructive procedure. Table 8 reflects an incidence of reoperation for control of pain of 2.9% among 663 patients reported during the 1987–1989 period.

In our series, five patients required insulin prior to operation, and four additional patients currently require insulin. Gall et al. [10], noted that the incidence of clinical diabetes increased from 17% preoperatively to 44% postoperatively after pancreaticoduodenectomy with occlusion of the pancreatic duct. Rumpf et al. [11] found that of 48 patients, 31% were diabetic prior to operation and 40% (total) after operation. To reiterate, in the author's experience, the lack of pain after operation usually makes treatment of the diabetes easier to achieve after resection because of better standardization of diet and nutrition.

Exocrine insufficiency seldom presents a major problem in management after resection. In only one patient has the long-term follow-up presented a continuing nutritional problem, and this is more closely related to the problems of alcohol than to the problems of pancreatic insufficiency. One additional patient has an alcohol problem which limits his work schedule. Frey [12], in his 1981 review of the literature, noted the increased loss of fecal fat after pancreaticoduodenectomy but observed that the loss could be rather readily controlled by the addition of pancreatic supplements to the diet.

The life expectancy of the patient surviving pancreaticoduodenectomy for chronic pancreatitis has been reported to be perhaps shorter than that following other operations [13]. In their report, Leger et al. [8], described the 5-year survival after the Whipple resection to be approximately 50% compared to approximately 75% following pancreaticojejunostomy. These statistics included the operative mortalities. As the experience accumulates and with better selection of patients so as to avoid resection in the continuing alcoholic, the long-term survival rate is increasing. Table 9 indicates that currently the long-term survival rate after pancreaticoduodenectomy is about 80%–85% at 5 years, being lower in those series which included more alcoholic patients. In the author's experience with 18 patients, followed for longer than 5 years and a median of 10 years, there has been no late death.

Table 9. Late deaths in patients who underwent pancreaticoduodenectomy for chronic pancreatitis (1987–1989 reports)

Reference	Number of patients	Follow-up period (years, median)	Deaths
Williamson et al. [5]	6	4.5	1 (16%)
Rossi et al. [4]	73	5	17 (23%)
Mannell et al. [7]	10	8	1 (10%)
Stone et al. [6]	15	6	3 (20%)
Current Series	13	3	0 (0%)
Current Series	17	10	0 (0%)
Gall [1]	289	8	55 (19%)
Gauthier-Benoit and Perissat [9]	287	3.8	57 (24%)
Total	660	–	134 (20%)

None of the recent papers indicate a late development of pancreatic cancer in their series.

Indications of Pancreaticoduodenectomy

The author's experience, based on his clinical observations and *operative findings*, has convinced him that the suggestion made by several colleagues is probably correct: "chronic pancreatitis is driven from the right side of the pancreas."

If at the time of operation the surgeon believes the lesion to be chronic pancreatitis, *a benign inflammatory process*, he must carefully and thoughtfully consider all options. If he is experienced in the Whipple resection, and can approximate the currently reported operative mortality rate of 2%, he may well be justified in resection. Justifications for this procedure, however, for a known benign disease, carries a significant burden of responsibility.

A decision for any resection of the pancreas, including the Whipple resection, is made easier if the patient is already requiring insulin prior to resection. Chronic pancreatitis may result in a false-positive elevation of CA 19-9 serum titer, so that the elevation of this serum antigen requires further assessment before it can influence significantly the decision for resection.

An emotionally stable patient can almost always stop narcotics during the preoperative hospital evaluation. His refusal to do so points towards a bad postoperative prognosis. Currently, any patient who will not discontinue all alcohol while at home prior to operation is a bad candidate for any related operation, particularly pancreaticoduodenectomy.

A prerequisite to which the author has usually, but not always, adhered has been that the disease be manifested predominantly in the head of the pancreas. Pain has been present in most patients, but has not been the predominant factor in the decision in several instances.

Like most surgeons, the author continues to assess his experience, but our current indications for pancreatic duodenectomy in this disease include:

1. A chronic inflammatory mass involving the head of the pancreas. This indication is strengthened if the mass is hard and compatible with cancer, *in spite of a negative biopsy*. Additional weight is also given if the disease involves predominantly the uncinate process. The literature reflects numerous instances in which the diagnosis of carcinoma of the pancreas has been made a few months to a year following drainage procedures. Such experiences have been reported by mature pancreatic surgeons. Although the anatomical information is not always presented, the drainage procedures had been performed in at least several patients because a mass in the head of the pancreas had erroneously been considered to be inflammatory in nature.

2. Failure of longitudinal pancreaticojejunostomy is considered by the author to be an indication for pancreaticoduodenectomy. Numerous patients have been reported in whom a longitudinal pancreaticojejunostomy has been followed by recurrent pain, and who at the time of reoperation were found to have inadequate drainage of the uncinate process and the small ducts of the head of the pancreas. Currently, the author believes that resection, rather than secondary bypass drainage, may be a more effective operation.

3. Chronic pancreatitis with severe pain associated with small pancreatic ducts can usually best be treated by pancreaticoduodenectomy even though the disease is rather diffuse throughout the gland.

4. A chronic inflammatory mass in the head of the pancreas associated with stenosis of the duodenum and/or the common duct.

5. Multiple pseudocysts in the head of the pancreas and the uncinate process, particularly if complicated by stenosis of the duodenum or common bile duct.

Summary

Most operations performed on patients with chronic pancreatitis are designed to treat the complications of this disease. Since the anatomical complications vary widely, the availability of several operative approaches is essential. One of the essential approaches is pancreaticoduodenectomy. Its indications and its limitations are changing as experience evolves.

Resection of the head of the pancreas provides excellent relief of pain in most patients with advanced chronic pancreatitis. The need for subsequent reoperation for control of pain after pancreaticoduodenectomy is less than after drainage procedures. In the past 3 years, the reported postoperative mortality rate is less than 2%. It is evident that pancreatic resection of any type diminishes pancreatic function in the great majority of patients. These metabolic losses are partially compensated by the improved well-being of the patient following relief of pain and improved appetite.

It is essential, in performing pancreaticoduodenectomy in patients with a benign disease, that the anticipated mortality rate from the operation be low. This requires that the operation be performed by experienced surgeons. It would appear to be the operation of choice in patients with small pancreatic ducts requiring operation for relief of pain. In selected patients, pancreaticoduodenectomy appears to be a good procedure and possibly the operation of choice when the disease presents anatomically as a mass in the head of the pancreas.

Acknowledgement. The author gratefully acknowledges that this report is based on a review entitled "Pancreaticoduodenectomy (Whipple Resection) in the Treatment of Chronic Pancreatitis" prepared by the author in collaboration with Zhaoda Zhang, Ph. D. (Surgery) for publication in the *World Journal of Surgery*.

References

1. Gall FP (1988) Treatment of chronic pancreatitis. International Hepato-Biliary-Pancreatic Association, Nico
2. Köhler H, Schafmayer A, Peiper HH (1987) Follow-up results of surgical treatment of chronic pancreatitis. Dig Surg 4:67
3. Morel P, Rohner A (1987) Surgery for chronic pancreatitis. Surgery 101:130
4. Rossi RL, Rothschild G, Braasch JW, Munson JL, Remine SG (1987) Pancreatoduodenectomy in the management of chronic pancreatitis. Arch Surg 122:416
5. Williamson RCN, Cooper MJ (1987) Resection in chronic pancreatitis. Br J Surg 74:807
6. Stone WM, Sarr MG, Nagorney DM, McIbrath DC (1988) Chronic pancreatitis. Results of Whipple's resection and total pancreatectomy. Arch Surg 123:815
7. Mannell A, Adson MA, McIbrath DC, Ilstrup DM (1988) Surgical management of chronic pancreatitis: long-term results in 141 patients. Br J Surg 75:467
8. Leger L, Lenriot JP, Lemaigre G (1974) Five to twenty-five year follow-up after surgery for chronic pancreatitis in 148 patients. Ann Surg 180:185
9. Gauthier-Benoit C, Perissat J (1987) The treatment of chronic pancreatitis. In: 89ième Congrès de l'Association Francaise de Chirurgie, Masson, Paris
10. Gall FP, Gebhardt C, Zisngibl H (1982) Chronic pancreatitis-results in 116 consecutive, partial duodenopancreatectomies combined with pancreatic duct occlusion. Hepatogastroenterology 29:115
11. Rumpf KD, Antonschmidt J, Datan C, Lick R, Mitzkat HJ (1980) Long-term follow-up study of C cell function after partial duodenopancreatectomy. Langenbecks Arch Chir 351:285
12. Frey CF (1981) Clinical review: role of subtotal pancreatectomy and pancreaticojejunostomy in chronic pancreatitis. J Surg Res 31:361
13. Howard JM (1987) Surgical treatment of chronic pancreatitis. In: Howard JM, Jordan GL Jr, Reber HA (eds) Surgical Disease of the pancreas. Lea and Febiger, Philadelphia, p 504

Results of the Whipple Procedure in Combination with Pancreatic Duct Occlusion

H. Zirngibl and F. P. Gall[1]

Introduction

The results of operative treatment of chronic pancreatitis are disappointing, as shown in a literature survey by Gebhardt [7] (Table 1). The reason for the high number of recurrences – 30%–50% following pancreatic drainage procedures and 20%–30% following resection – lies in the continuing, independently progressing inflammation in the residual pancreas. In about 10–15 years this leads to complete atrophy and to a tissue alteration of the exocrine pancreas parenchyma. In 1984, Ammann et al. [1] were able to show that burning out of the glands in alcohol-induced chronic pancreatitis, in addition to an increasing calcification parallel with a reduction in the endocrine reserve capacity, leads ultimately to insulin-dependent diabetes mellitus. Surgical therapy can thus eliminate only the consequences and complications but not the cause of the pancreatitis.

A surgical approach for treatment of chronic pancreatitis must therefore aim not only to reduce early and late morbidity and mortality but also meet the challenge of continuous freedom from recurrence or pain. At the same time, the present residual endocrine function should be preserved. These goals could be only partially met using the standard operative treatments for chronic pancreatitis. The resective operative methods resulted in a lower recurrence rate than the draining procedures, but were associated with a higher operative mortality of 5%–6% (Table 1). Complete removal

Table 1. Results of various surgical procedures in operative treatment of chronic pancreatitis: collective literature review. (From [7])

Surgical procedure	n	Mortality rate		Recurrence rate	Follow-up period (years)
		Operative	Late		
Pancreatic duct drainage					
End-to-side (Du Val)	76	2.6%	31%	52%	8 –20
Side-to-side (Mercadier)	451	2.4%	26%	31%	5 –20
Resection					
Left resection	883	5.0%	17%	31%	9 –30
Whipple without duct occlusion	917	6.3%	19%	19%	6 –30
Total duodenopancreatectomy	259	16.0%	30%	0%	0.5–4

[1] Department of Surgery, Universitätsklinik, Friedrich-Alexander University of Erlangen–Nuremberg, Maximiliansplatz 1, D-8520 Erlangen, FRG

Chronic Pancreatitis
Ed. by Beger, Büchler, Ditschuneit, and Malfertheiner
© Springer-Verlag Berlin Heidelberg 1990

of the gland could prevent recurrence, however the high peri- and postoperative morbidity and mortality prohibited its use in so-called "benign" conditions such as chronic pancreatitis.

In order to make advances in operative treatment, development of a new method had to be attempted in which the advantages of pancreatectomy, namely freedom from recurrence, were retained, and the disadvantages in the form of high primary and secondary mortality and diabetes mellitus were eliminated.

Pancreas Duct Occlusion

For some time it has been known, based on animal experiments, that occlusion of the duct of Wirsung leads to an atrophy of the excretory parenchyma, with preservation of the islets of Langerhans (Table 2). The discovery of insulin by Banting and Best in 1922 [3] was facilitated by ligation of the pancreatic duct with consequent atrophy of the excretory pancreatic tissue. In 1946, Rienhoff (after [12]) became the first to perform a therapeutic pancreas ligation for treatment of chronic pancreatitis. Hoffmann and coworkers [9] reported an improved technique in 1977. This was, however, associated with a high number of pancreatic recurrences through recanalization in the suture site, incomplete duct occlusion, or a missed duct of Santurini. In 1977, Little et al. [10] reported on duct occlusion using injection of a cyanoacrylate glue. A complete occlusion was not possible due to the rapidly hardening acrylate glue, so the results of this methods were comparable to those of ligation. Dubernard and coworkers [6] used injection of neoprene, an artificial material which also hardened in the duct system, to suppress exocrine secretion as part of their transplantation experiments.

Table 2. History of pancreatic duct occlusion

Author(s)	Year	Type of occlusion	
Bernard [4]	1856	Ligature	Animal studies
Pawlow [13]	1878	Ligature	Animal studies
Banting and Best [3]	1922	Ligature	Animal studies
Rienhoff (after [12])	1946	Ligature	Therapeutic
Madding et al. [11]	1967	Ligature	Therapeutic
Hoffmann et al. [9]	1977	Ligature	Therapeutic
Little et al. [10]	1977	Acrylate glue	Therapeutic
Gebhardt and Stolte [8]	1978	Prolamin (Ethibloc)	Therapeutic
Dubernard et al. [6]	1978	Neoprene	Therapeutic

In 1978, Gebhardt and Stolte [8] were able to show in animal experiments that through the occlusion of the pancreas with a resorbable prolamin solution (Ethibloc), filling and obstruction of even the smallest branches of the pancreatic duct system were obtained. This led to an extensive atrophy and fibrosis of the excretory parenchyma with preservation of the islets of Langerhans.

Methods and Materials

Since 1978, the occlusion of the pancreatic remnant with Ethibloc during the Whipple operation has been established as a permanent concept at the Department of Surgery of the University of Erlangen. Using this, we attempt to prevent the usual course of simultaneous loss of exo- and endocrine parenchyma in chronic pancreatitis, in so far that only the inflamed exocrine portion is eliminated, freedom from pain and recurrence is ensured, and islet cells are preserved.

Technique. Ethibloc is highly viscous liquid which, following resection, is introduced under moderate pressure through a wide-bore cannula into the duct of Wirsung of the pancreatic remnant. Stones in the duct, which would prevent complete occlusion, must be removed in advance. After withdrawal of the cannula, the pancreatic duct is closed using a purse-string suture in order to prevent the occlusion material from leaking out. Initially, we anastomosed the pancreas resection surface to the small bowel. In recent years, we have foregone the pancreas anastomosis and close the pancreas resection surface blindly using single sutures.

Patients. Between January 1978 and February 1989, 321 patients with severe chronic cephalic pancreatitis were operated on using this technique. There were 297 men and 24 women (12.4-fold more men). Average age was 41.6 years. Patients had suffered pancreatitis symptoms on average for 44 months. The average follow-up of all patients was 5.8 years (range 0.25–10.5 years).

Previous Operations. A total of 123 patients, or 38% of the study group, had undergone previous operations (Table 3). The most common were operations on the pancreas itself ($n = 21$), or operations in the region, such as on the gallbladder or biliary ducts ($n = 48$) and resections of the stomach ($n = 25$).

Table 3. Previous surgery in 321 patients with severe chronic cephalic pancreatitis

Type of operation		
Biliary tract	48	(15%)
Gastric resection	25	(8%)
Pancreatic operation	21	(7%)
Necrosectomy	4	(1%)
Endoscopic duct occlusion	7	(2%)
Other	18	(6%)
Total	123	(38%)

Indication for Operation. The most frequent indication for operation was severe recurrent or intractable pain ($n = 190$, or 59%) which was often accompanied by other symptoms. As can be appreciated in Table 4, in patients in whom pain was the main indication, pseudocysts, calcifications, choledochus stenosis and duodenal stenosis were found in the resected specimens at the same rates as in the entire study group. From the remaining 131 patients, in 45 cases the indication was obstructive jaundice,

Table 4. Morphological findings in 321 resected specimens in severe chronic cephalic pancreatitis compared with the group of 190 specimens out of 321 in which the main operative indication was "intractable pain"

Morphological findings	All patients ($n = 321$)		Indication "pain" ($n = 190/321$)	
Pseudocysts	197	(61%)	126	(66%)
Pancreatic calcification	190	(59%)	125	(66%)
Choledochal stenosis	200	(62%)	121	(64%)
Duodenal stenosis	111	(35%)	66	(35%)
Duodenal wall cysts	109	(34%)	66	(35%)

duodenal stenosis in 32 cases, suspicion of malignant diseases in 44 cases, and pseudocystic complications in 10 cases. Of course, these patients also suffered from pain typical for pancreatitis. The morphological changes in the resection specimens – high degree of destruction of the head of the pancreas as an expression of a severe complicated chronic cephalic pancreatitis – underline the urgent need for surgical treatment in our study group.

Results

Mortality. Out of 321 patients who underwent Whipple's operation with duct occlusion, four patients died postoperatively as inpatients or after discharge within 60 days postoperatively. This represents a postoperative mortality of 1.3% (Table 5). During the follow-up period of on average 5.8 years, we found a relatively high late mortality of 21.8%. The high mortality, as shown in Table 5, was the result of continued alcohol and nicotine abuse with a correspondingly high percentage of liver damage and cardiac and circulatory diseases. The high percentage of carcinomas, all located in the upper respiratory and digestive tract, is remarkable.

Table 5. Early (0–60 days after operation) and late mortality (mean follow-up 5.8 years; range 2 months–10.5 years) following partial duodenopancreatectomy with pancreatic duct occlusion for severe chronic pancreatitis

Postoperative mortality: 4/321 (1.3%)	
1 Myocardial infarction	
2 Splenic artery hemorrhage	
1 *Candida* sepsis	
Late mortality: 69/317 (21.8%)	
Liver cirrhosis	34%
Heart diseases	16%
Carcinomas	14%
Diabetic coma and cachexia	12%
Lung diseases	8%
Sepsis, abscess	8%
Other	8%

Table 6. Nonlethal postoperative complications (0–60 days) and recurrences of pancreatitis (mean follow-up 5.8 years; range 2 months–10.5 years) after partial duodenopancreatectomy for severe chronic pancreatitis

	Total		Reoperation	
Nonlethal postoperative complications	41	(12.9%)	23	(7.3%)
Recurrences	7	(2.2%)	4	(1.3%)

Complications and Recurrences. We observed nonlethal postoperative complications at a rate of 12.9% (Table 6). The most common complication was hemorrhage ($n = 10$), which always required surgical revision. Three out of five anastomotic bile leaks needed surgical treatment. All except one out of eight pancreas fistulae healed spontaneously. During the follow-up period of 5.8 years, we observed only three pancreatitis recurrences with corresponding abnormal laboratory values and typical symptoms. We were able to treat these conservatively. Three patients required reoperation because of space-occupying pseudocysts, one other because of pancreas abscess with splenic vein thrombosis and gastric bleeding. The rate of pancreas-specific recurrences was 2.2%.

Clinical Late Results. Patients were followed-up at regular intervals, and late results were recorded. In all, 97% of surviving patients were followed-up. Presence of pain is one of the most important parameters in charting the course of chronic pancreatitis. Following operation, 53.6% of all patients became pain-free; 34.6% complained of occasional symptoms such as flatulence, pressure, or a feeling of fullness. These complaints were minor compared to the earlier pancreatitic pain; 10.8% of patients complained of frequently occurring symptoms of this kind. Only 1% of patients followed-up suffered from strong, pancreatitis-like pain (Table 7). Among all patients 80% considered the operative results as good, a further 16% as adequate, and 4%

Table 7. Patient evaluation of pain relief, operative success, and occupational rehabilitation after partial duodenopancreatectomy with duct occlusion (mean follow-up 5.8 years) for severe chronic pancreatitis

	Proportion of cases
Pain relief	
No pain	53.6%
Minor complaints	
Rare	34.6%
Frequent	10.8%
Severe pain	1.0%
Operative success	
Good	80%
Fair	16%
Poor	4%
Ability to work	
Back at work	50%
Temporary disablement	8%
Retired	42%

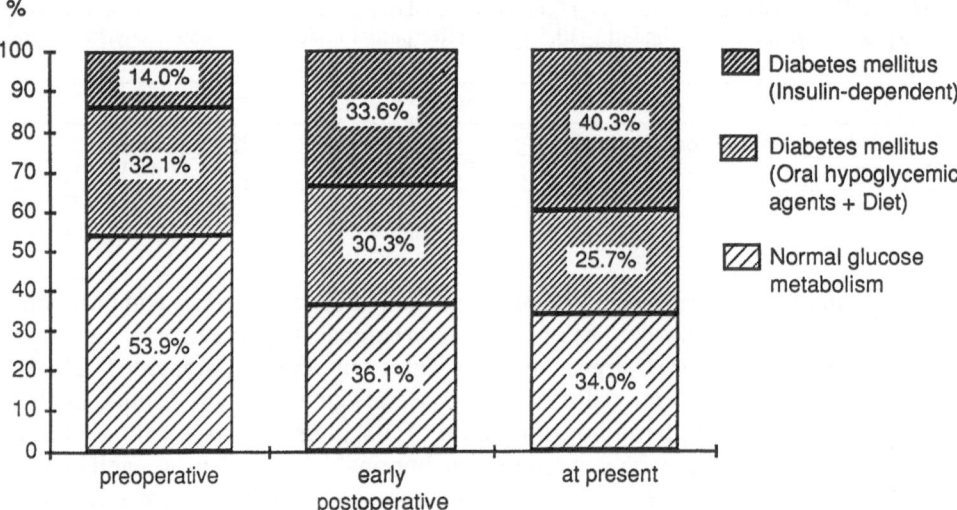

Fig. 1. Diabetic metabolic status in 321 patients with severe chronic pancreatitis – preoperative and immediately after Whipple operation and duct occlusion with Ethibloc (≤ 1 month) compared with at present (average follow-up time, 5.8 years)

were dissatisfied with the operation. One-half of patients are able to resume work, 42% retired from work, and 8% are temporarily on sick leave.

Metabolic Late Consequences. At the time of operation, 46.1% of our patients with chronic pancreatitis were diabetic (Fig. 1). This proportion rose, relative to the extent of resection of the head of the pancreas, of 63.9%. Follow-up shows that the endocrine situation has hardly changed; after 5.8 years, 66% of patients are diabetic. These numbers for the entire study group were supported by data obtained from a prospective study of a group of 23 patients which were consecutively operated from January 1983 to February 1984. Precise preoperative and postoperative examinations of exocrine and endocrine function as well as inflammatory activity, as done by Schneider and coworkers [14] from the Department of Internal Medicine, University of Erlangen, underline the fact that pancreas duct occlusion effectively eliminates the chronic inflammation. Preoperative pathologically elevated serum trypsin concentrations were clearly and permanently reduced following operation (Fig. 2).

Exocrine pancreas function, which preoperatively was 31% below the lower normal values, fell to a minimal remaining function of a median of 6.6% following partial duodenopancreatectomy with pancreas duct occlusion (Fig. 3). This emphasizes once again the complete atrophy of the exocrine pancreas following duct occlusion. Endocrine pancreas function, measured as increase of insulin and C peptide within the framework of maximal beta cell stimulation was preoperatively 65% below normal. Resection resulted in a further reduction of endocrine function of about 50%; postoperative follow-up to date has not shown any additional decline (Fig. 3).

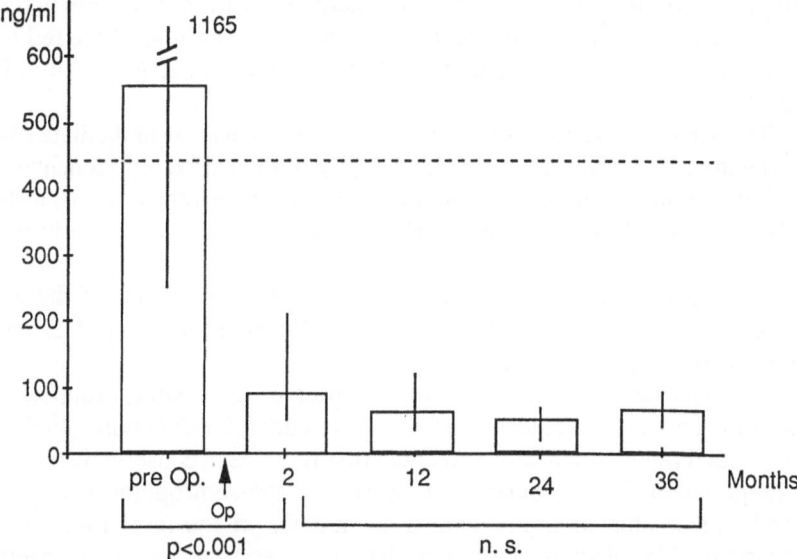

Fig. 2. Switching-off of inflammatory activity with Ethibloc duct occlusion of the remaining pancreas following partial duodenopancreatectomy for severe chronic pancreatitis: serum trypsin levels (ng/ml) pre- and postoperatively

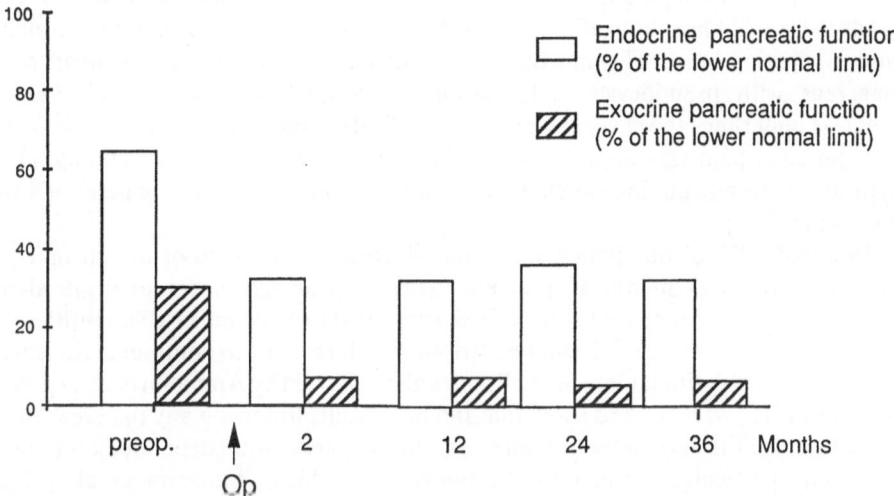

Fig. 3. Endo- and exocrine function before and after Whipple operation with duct occlusion for severe chronic pancreatitis ($n = 23$)

Discussion

Unsatisfactory early and late results following operation for treatment of chronic pancreatitis led us to introduce Ethibloc duct occlusion in our therapy concept. When complications arise in the course of chronic pancreatitis, these usually affect the area of the head of the pancreas. Adequate therapy consists of resection of the head of the pancreas. Through standardization of the operative technique, we reduced mortality in the Whipple procedure to under 2%, which fulfills the requirements of Ammann et al. [1].

The decisive advantage of pancreas duct occlusion is the immediate switching off of inflammatory activity by complete atrophy of the exocrine parenchyma and consequent creation of an effective protection against recurrence. In this fashion we were able to reduce the rate of pancreatitis recurrence to 2.2% in our study group. Because in our patients there was a considerable preexisting reduction in exocrine pancreas function preoperatively, and because the spontaneous course of the disease always leads to both exocrine and endocrine insufficiency, the loss of exocrine function postoperatively was negligible.

A special advantage of duct occlusion observed in our study group was the dissociation of the combined decline of exo- and endocrine function. While one expects continued reduction of exo- and endocrine reserves in conservatively treated disease [2, 5] as well as following classical drainage and resection operations [1], pancreas duct occlusion is able to freeze endocrine function at the level found at the time of operation. The blocking of the complete pancreatic duct system probably facilitates a rapid and gentle path to atrophy and therefore to preservation of the function of the islet cells, as compared with the course of scarring remodeling with calcification found in untreated disease.

A key problem in patients with chronic pancreatitis is intractable pain. This often leads to frequent hospitalization, to inability to work, and not uncommonly to alcohol and analgesic abuse. The morphological correlate of tumors of the head of the pancreas with pseudocysts, calcifications, choledochus stenosis, and duodenal stenosis underlines the severity and the complicated course of the disease. In 59% of our patients, pain was the main indication for operation; in these patients, all the typical severe morphological changes related to chronic cephalic pancreatitis were found (Table 4).

In about 90% of our patients, alcohol abuse was the cause of the chronic pancreatitis. Although nearly all patients swore convincingly never to drink alcohol again, one must assume that at least 50% continued to consume large quantities. The high late mortality of 21.8% can be attributed in large part to continued alcohol and nicotine abuse. A similar late mortality was also reported by Ammann et al. [1]. White and Keith [15] were able to show that the late results following any pancreas operation, but also the spontaneous course of chronic pancreatitis depended on patients' behavior, particularly regarding continued alcoholism. Ammann et al. [1] also observed a higher late mortality in alcohol-induced compared to non-alcohol-induced pancreatitis.

Summary

We feel that the Whipple procedure together with an intraoperative duct occlusion has proven to be the best treatment for severe chronic cephalic pancreatitis because perioperative morbidity and mortality can be clearly reduced, recurrences of pancreatitis seldom occur, and pancreatogenic pain can be reliably eliminated. Within the limitations imposed by a short follow-up time, it still seems possible to state that duct occlusion can stabilize the endocrine residual function in the long term. The effective suppression of inflammatory activity offers the patients the chance to be reintegrated into society with the possibility of leading a normal life. However, this requires willingness to cooperate and complete abstention from alcohol on the part of the patient.

References

1. Ammann RW, Akovbiantz A, Largadier F, Schueler G (1984) Course and outcome of chronic pancreatitis. Gastroenterology 86:820–828
2. Anderson BN, Krarup T, Pedersen NT, Faber OK, Hagen C, Worning H (1982) B-cell function in patients with chronic pancreatitis and its relation to exocrine pancreatic function. Diabetologia 23:86–89
3. Banting FG, Best CH (1922) Internal secretion of the pancreas. J Lab Clin Med 7:251–266
4. Bernard C (1856) Mémoire sur le pancréas et sur le rôle du suc pancréatique dans les phénomènes digestifs. C R Acad Sci [Suppl] (Paris) 1:379
5. Domschke S, Stock KP, Pichl J, Schneider MU, Domschke W (1985) Beta cell capacity in chronic pancreatitis. Hepatogastroenterology 32:27–30
6. Dubernard JM, Traeger J, Neyra P, Touraine JL, Tranchant D, Blanc-Brunat N (1978) A new method of preparation of segmental pancreatic grafts for transplantation: trials in dogs and in man. Surgery 84:633–639
7. Gebhardt C (1984) Chirurgische Therapie der chronischen Pankreatitis. In: Gebhardt C (ed) Chirurgie des exokrinen Pankreas. Thieme, Stuttgart, pp 139–191
8. Gebhardt C, Stolte M (1978) Pankreasgangokklusion durch Injektion einer schnell härtenden Aminosäurelösung. Langenbecks Arch Chir 346:149–166
9. Hoffmann E, Usmiani J, Gebhardt C (1977) Die Ausschaltung der exokrinen Funktion des Pankreas als Behandlungskonzept der chronischen Pankreatitis. Dtsch Med Wochenschr 102:392–395
10. Little JM, Lauer C, Hogg J (1977) Pancreatic duct obstruction with an acrylate glue: a new method for producing pancreatic exocrine atrophy. Surgery 81:243–249
11. Madding GF, Kennedy PA, McLaughlin B (1967) Obstruction of the pancreatic duct by ligature in the treatment of pancreatitis. Ann Surg 165:56–60
12. Martin L, Canseco JD (1947) Pancreatic calculosis. JAMA 135:1055–1060
13. Pawlow S (1878) Folgen der Unterbindung des Pankreasganges beim Kaninchen. Arch Gesamte Physiol 16:123–129
14. Schneider MU, Meister R, Domschke S, Zirngibl H, Strebl H, Heptner G, Gebhardt C, Gall FP, Domschke W (1987) Whipple's procedure plus intraoperative pancreatic duct occlusion for severe chronic pancreatitis: clinical, exocrine and endocrine consequences during a 3-year follow-up. Pancreas 2:715–726
15. White TT, Keith RG (1973) Long-term follow-up study of fifty patients with pancreaticojejunostomy. Surg Gynecol Obstet 136:353–358

Resection of the Head of the Pancreas in the Treatment of Chronic Pancreatitis

F. HANYU, M. SUZUKI, and T. IMAIZUMI[1]

In the past, chronic pancreatitis was regarded as a rare disease in Japan. However changing eating and drinking habits, especially concerning alcohol consumption and fatty foods, has led to an increased number of patients with severe chronic pancreatitis. About 20%–30% of patients with chronic pancreatitis have enlargement of the head of the pancreas due to inflammatory alteration of the gland [1, 2]. Surgical treatment of patients with this type of severe chronic pancreatitis needs resection of the most severely inflamed portion of the gland to relieve their debilitating pain [3, 4]. With the advance of preoperative diagnostic procedures such as ERCP, ultrasonography, and CAT scan structural abnormalities of the pancreas in patients with chronic pancreatitis can now be easily diagnosed. Surgical treatment of chronic pancreatitis can be more selective than in the past. We present here our experience with resection of the head of the pancreas in 90 patients with chronic pancreatitis.

Patients and Methods

Between 1968 and May 1989, surgical management was used in 216 patients with chronic pancreatitis in the Department of Gastroenterological Surgery, Tokyo Women's Medical College. Of the 216 patients, 90 (41.7%) underwent resection of the head of the pancreas. There were 82 men and 8 women; their mean age at the time of operation was 45.8 years, with a range of 15–83. The main cause of chronic pancreatitis was alcohol abuse in 59 patients; postacute pancreatitis was the cause in 16, pancreatic duct anomaly in 5, idiopathic pancreatitis in 8, and pancreatic trauma in 2. Preoperatively, 75% of patients had severe abdominal pain. Preoperative diabetes was present in 26 patients (28.9%), 11 of whom (12.2%) required insulin therapy preoperatively. Steatorrhea was present in 8 patients preoperatively. Of the 90 patients, 25 (27.8%) represented failure of previous operation. Structural abnormalities of the pancreas and peripancreatic region were evaluated preoperatively on the basis of diagnostic imaging procedures (Table 1). Inflammatory mass of the head of the pancreas was present in 44 patients (48.9%). Multiple pancreatic stones and multiple pseudocysts were seen in 51 and 32 patients, respectively. Complete obstruction of the common bile duct due to the mass in the head of the gland was found in five patients; these five required percutaneous transhepatic biliary drainage because of

---

[1] Department of Gastroenterological Surgery, Tokyo Women's Medical College, 8-1, Kawada-Cho, Shinjuku-ku, Tokyo 162, Japan

---

Chronic Pancreatitis
Ed. by Beger, Büchler, Ditschuneit, and Malfertheiner
© Springer-Verlag Berlin Heidelberg 1990

Table 1. Preoperative morbidity

Morbidity	Number of patients	
Inflammatory mass	44	(48.9%)
Multiple stones	51	(56.7%)
Multiple pseudocysts	32	(35.6%)
Stenosis of the choledochus		
Complete	5	(5.6%)
Incomplete	44	(48.9%)
Compression of the portal vein		
Severe	3	(3.3%)
Moderate	13	(14.4%)
Stenosis of the duodenum	2	(2.2%)

Table 2. Surgical procedures 1968–1989

Surgical procedures	1968–1983	1984–1989
Standard Whipple procedure	46	19
Pylorus-preserving procedure	0	25
Total	46	44

severe jaundice and acute cholangitis preoperatively. Severe stenosis of the portal vein or the superior mesentric vein was found in three patients. Of the 90 patients, 46 had a standard Whipple procedure between 1968 and 1983, 25 had a pylorus-preserving pancreatoduodenectomy, and 19 had the standard Whipple procedure between 1984 and 1989 (Table 2). After the pylorus-preserving procedure, 18 patients had end-to-end duodeno-duodenostomy, side-to-side pancreatico-jejunostomy, end-to-side choledocho-jejunostomy (Fig. 1). Four patients had the same gastrointestinal recon-

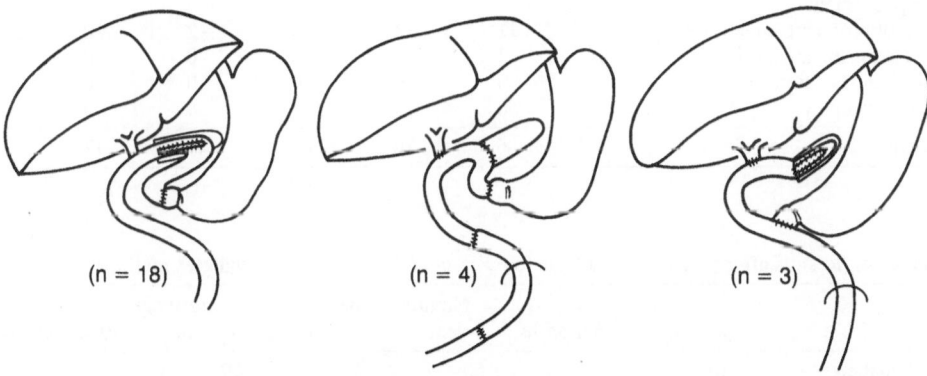

1) Duodeno-duodenostomy
2) Pancreatico-jejunostomy
3) Choledocho-jejunostomy

1) Duodeno-jejunostomy
2) Pancreatico-jejunostomy
3) Choledocho-jejunostomy with jejunal interposition

1) Pancreatico-jejunostomy
2) Choledocho-jejunostomy
3) Duodeno-jejunostomy

Fig. 1. Techniques of pancreatoduodenectomy for chronic pancreatitis using the pylorus-preserving procedure

struction with jejunal interposition segment between the second and forth portions of the duodenum. Three patients had gastrointestinal reconstruction similar to Traverso and Longmier's procedure.

Results

Two patients died on 9th and 25th postoperative days, respectively; the operative mortality rate was 2.2%. These two operative deaths occurred early in this series, with no further operative deaths occurring in the 55 patients operated on after 1982. Abdominal bleeding occurred in one patient and abdominal abscess in two. Following pancreatoduodenectomy, 86 patients were available for follow-up study longer than 6 months postoperatively. The mean follow-up time was 5.9 years, with a range of 6 months–22 years. Six months after the operation, 72 of 86 patients were completely free of pain (Table 3). Twelve patients had mild pain which did not require analgesics postoperatively. Two patients still needed analgesics postoperatively; these two patients had not stopped drinking alcohol. At 3-year follow-up data regarding relief of pain were not available in four patients. Complete relief of pain was obtained in 51 of 56 patients. At 5 and at 10 years, respectively, 95% of patients were free of pain. Insulin-dependent diabetes was present in 12.2% of patients preoperatively and developed in 17.7% at 6 months postoperatively (Table 4). At 1, 3, and 5 years, the proportion of patients who required insulin treatment was 17.9%, 29.5%, and 30%, respectively. Ten years after pancreatoduodenectomy, 28.6% of patients needed insulin treatment. Variations in body weight were recorded postoperatively. Post-

Table 3. Results after pancreatoduodenectomy: postoperative relief of pain

| Relief of pain | Number of patients postoperatively | | | | |
	6 months	1 year	3 years	5 years	10 years
Complete relief	72	61	51	35	12
Improvement					
Not requiring analgesics	11	12	5	2	0
Requiring analgesics	3	2	0	0	0
No improvement	0	0	0	0	0
No answer	0	3	4	4	0
Total	86	78	60	41	12

Table 4. Results after pancreatoduodenectomy: pre- and postoperative diabetes mellitus

| | Preoperatively | Number of patients postoperatively | | | | |
		6 months	1 year	3 years	5 years	10 years
No diabetes	63	60	50	29	19	5
Latent	14	5	5	2	2	0
Insulin dependent	11 (12.5%)	14 (17.7%)	12 (17.9%)	13 (29.5%)	9 (30.0%)	2 (28.6%)
No answer	0	7	11	16	11	5
Total	88	86	78	60	41	12

No diabetes, normal oral GTT; latent, diet therapy or oral medication

Table 5. Pre- and postoperative body weight

Change in body weight	Number of patients postoperatively				
	6 months	1 year	3 years	5 years	10 years
Increased (≥ 10%)	1	2	2	1	1
No change (± 10%)	41	37	27	19	6
Decreased (≥ 10%)	39 (48.1%)	25 (39.1%)	13 (30.9%)	9 (31.0%)	2 (22.2%)
No answer	5	14	18	12	3
Total	86	78	60	41	12

operative body weight was compared with preoperative weight. The proportion of patients who had less than 90% of preoperative weight was 39.0%, 30.9%, 31.0%, and 22.2% at 1 year, 3, 5, and 10 years, respectively (Table 5). Of the 86 patients followed-up for longer than 6 months, 17 died during the follow-up period for a late mortality rate of 19.8%. Three patients died of diabetic complications, three of malnutrition, and two of alcoholism. Eight of the 17 late deaths were thus related to complication of chronic pancreatitis (Table 6).

Table 6. Results after pancreatoduodenectomy: late mortality and morbidity ($n = 86^a$)

	Number of patients
Diabetic complication	3
Malnutrition	3
Alcoholism	2
Carcinoma	2
Myocardial disease	1
Others	2
Unknown	4
Late mortality	17 (19.8%)

[a] Two operative deaths were excluded

Discussion

Various surgical procedures have been chosen in patients with chronic pancreatitis. Previously, if the pancreatic duct was dilated, a ductal drainage procedure was the treatment of choice. It has been suggested that increased intraductal pressure is responsible for the pain in patients with dilatated pancreatitis duct. Current studies, however, indicate that ductal hypertension is only one of the causes of pain in patients with chronic pancreatitis [1, 5, 6]. Frey [7] reported that one-third of patients with pain and chronic pancreatitis do not have dilated duct. Frey and Bodai [1] also showed photomyographs demonstrating inflammation and fibrosis about some of the nerve endings in the pancreas in patients with a small duct and proposed that the pressure of this perineural inflammatory response might be a source of pain in patients with chronic pancreatitis whose ducts were not dilated. Recent work by Bockman et al. [8] has confirmed that the mean diameter of nerves in patients with chronic pancreatitis was significantly greater than in the normal control group, and the mean area of tissue served per nerve was significantly less than in controls. Keith et al. [6] described significant perineural inflammatory infiltrate in tissue removed from patients with chronic pancreatitis and demonstrated a significant correlation between the proportion of eosinophilic composition in the infiltrate and pain severity.

If a patient has debilitating pain and severe diseases, such as inflammatory mass, multiple pancreatic stones, pseudocysts, and abscess in the head of the pancreas, either with or without dilatation of the pancreatic duct, resection of the head of the pancreas is most effective and the preferred treatment for patients with debilitating pain.

Because of the technical difficulty of this procedure, many surgeons do not prefer pancreatoduodenectomy for the treatment in patients with chronic pancreatitis. Recent reports, however, have described a postoperative mortality rate of under 3% after pancreatoduodenectomy [9, 10]. This operation is no longer a very dangerous procedure.

Late mortality and morbidity after pancreatoduodenectomy depend on the duration of the follow-up period. Rossi et al. [10] reported a 5.6% late mortality rate in patients with a mean follow-up of 4.9 years. Moreaux [9] described a late mortality rate of 51% after pancreatoduodenectomy with a mean follow-up exceeding 10 years. The late postoperative mortality rate after pancreatoduodenectomy in our series was 22.7% and this is similar to that in other series [11]. Frey et al. [12] reported no major differences in the incidence of late deaths among patients with chronic pancreatitis receiving pancreatic resection and those receiving pancreatic duct drainage procedure. The survival rate following pancreatoduodenectomy and pancreatic ductal drainage did not differ at 10 and 15 years in our series.

New surgical procedures have been reported by several authors [3, 13, 14]. These new operations were used in the attempt to obtain relief of pain by resecting the head of the pancreas and to preserve pancreatic function. All patients in our series who underwent pancreatoduodenectomy had severe inflammatory changes in the head of the gland. In some patients, it was very difficult to dissect between the pancreatic gland and the portal vein. Three patients in our series required a segmental resection of the portal vein because of severe inflammation of the head of the pancreas. It is not clear whether these new procedure can be performed easily and safely in patients who have severe inflammatory changes between the chronically inflamed gland and the portal vein. It is also unclear whether all inflamed gland of the resection of the head of the pancreas can be resected by these new methods. The mortality rates after these new procedures are less than those with pancreatoduodenectomy, and the likelihood of endocrine and exocrine insufficiency developing following these operations is less because less tissue is removed compared with either pancreatoduodenectomy or distal resection. These new procedure can be indicated for some type of patients with chronic pancreatitis.

In our pylorus-preserving procedure, the extent of the duodenum is minimized. Usually, less than 10 cm of the duodenum is resected. The duodenum is divided at the third portion and is preserved as long as possible. The gastrointestinal tract is reconstructed by end-to-end duodeno-duodenostomy. In this type of gastrointestinal reconstruction, food and gastric juice can enter the third portion of the duodenum and upper jejunum. End-to-end duodeno-duodenostomy might prevent stomal ulceration postoperatively. The rate of postoperative ulceration after pylorus preserving procedure was less than 2% in our series. We routinely measure the acidity of the gastric juice preoperatively for every patient who is a candidate for pylorus-preserving pancreatoduodenectomy. If a patient has high acidity of the gastric juice preoperatively, or if a patient has a history of peptic ulcer, the standard Whipple resection is the choice of the procedure in our institution.

The gastrointestinal tract is reconstructed in the most physiological fashion by end-to-end duodenostomy. This type of gastrointestinal reconstruction has no blind loop of the jejunum. Some patients experienced late postoperative cholangitis after pancreatoduodenectomy due to the stasis of bile in the blind loop of the jejunum. This type of reconstruction may prevent late postoperative cholangitis.

References

1. Frey CF, Bodai BI (1984) Surgery in chronic pancreatitis. Clin Gastroenterol 13:913
2. Grodsinsky C (1980) Surgical treatment of chronic pancreatitis – a review after a ten year experience. Arch Surg 115:545
3. Beger HG, Krautzberger W, Bittner R, et al. (1985) Duodenum-preserving resection of the head of the pancreas in patients with severe chronic pancreatitis. Surgery 97:467–473
4. Hanyu F, Nakamura M, Suzuki M (1985) Surgical treatment of chronic pancreatitis with special reference to pancreatectomy. In: Toshio Sato Pancreatitis: its pathophysiology and clinical aspect. Tokyo University Press, Tokyo, p 424
5. Beger HG, Büchler M, Bittner RR, et al. (1989) Duodenum-preserving resection of the head of the pancreas in severe chronic pancreatitis. Early and late results. Ann Surg 209:273–278
6. Keith RG, Saibil FG, Sheppard RH (1989) Treatment of chronic alcoholic pancreatitis by pancreatic resection. Am J Surg 157:156–162
7. Frey CF (1981) Clinical review: role of subtotal pancreatectomy and pancreaticojejunostomy in chronic pancreatitis. J Surg Res 31:361
8. Bockman DE, Buchler M, Malfertheiner P, et al. (1988) Analysis of nerves in chronic pancreatitis. Gastroenterology 94:1459–1469
9. Moreaux J (1984) Long-term follow-up study of 50 patients with pancreaticoduodenectomy for chronic pancreatitis. World J Surg 8:346–353
10. Rossi RI, Rothschild J, Braasch JW, et al. (1987) Pancreatoduodenectomy in the management of chronic pancreatitis. Arch Surg 122:416–420
11. Gebhardt C (1984) Chirurgische Therapie der chronischen Pancreatitis. In: Gebhardt C, et al. (eds) Chirurgie des exocrinen Pancreas. Thieme, Stuttgart, pp 139–191
12. Frey CF, Suzuki M, Isaji S, et al. (1989) Pancreatic reection for chronic pancreatitis. Surg Clin North Am 69:499–528
13. Frey CF, Smith GJ (1987) Description and rationale of a new operation for chronic pancreatitis. Pancreas 2:701
14. Warren WD, Millikan WJ, Henderson JM, et al. (1984) A denerved pancreatic flap for control of chronic pain in pancreatitis. Surg Gynecol Obstet 159:581

Recent Findings Following Pancreas Head Resection for Chronic Pancreatitis

H. Wolff and H. Lippert

Chronic pancreatitis is a progressive disease with a pathomechanism that is not well understood. The fact that the progress of the disease differs from case to case makes it difficult to come to conclusions about treatment. The objective of surgery is to determine whether the condition in question is benign or malignant and to remove symptoms such as pain and stenoses. Of the two forms of surgical treatment – drainage and resection – neither is favoured more than the other; which method is adopted is still something to be decided in each individual case and is determined by pathomorphological changes (Horn 1987).

The results of the form of surgical treatment adopted in each case must be measured against the extent to which early or late sequelae, in addition to the basic disease, are caused. Operation mortality is said to be lower following drainage than following resection. The reverse, on the other hand, seems to be the case with delayed mortality. In the latter case, drainage, with a 30% later mortality, produces clearly worse results than resection, with 20% (Gebhardt 1984). The most significant later disorders arising from chronic pancreatitis are diabetes and digestive malfunctioning. Surgical treatment, above all resection, is scarcely able to halt these developments. The goal of our study was to establish what the late sequelae are following pancreas resection carried out in patients with chronic pancreatitis. At the same time, in our study we gave special attention to the changes in glucose metabolism.

Patients and Methods

From 1979 to 1988 we carried out operations on 227 patients with chronic pancreatitis. Among the various forms of surgery adopted, 98 cephalic pancreatoduodenectomies were carried out (Table 1). The average age of patients undergoing cephalic pancreatoduodenectomy was 47 years. The proportion of men to women was 5:1. The most common cause of the chronic pancreatitis was alcohol abuse of many years' standing. Typical for the progress of chronic pancreatitis with our patients were, in 49% of the cases, preliminary operations in the region of the bile duct and the upper alimentary canal (Table 2).

We concluded that cephalic pancreatoduodenectomy should be carried out when we either diagnosed severe inflammation of the pancreas head with duodenal stenosis

Chirurgische Klinik der Charite, Humboldt University, Schumannstrasse 20/21, 1040 Berlin (East), Germany

Chronic Pancreatitis
Ed. by Beger, Büchler, Ditschuneit, and Malfertheiner
© Springer-Verlag Berlin Heidelberg 1990

Table 1. Surgical therapy in patients with chronic pancreatitis

Surgical therapy	Number
Cephalic pancreatoduodenectomy (with ductal occlusion 56)	98
Total pancreatoduodenectomy	17
Pancreatectomy (95%)	7
Distal pancreas resection	10
Pseudocyst-jejunostomy	65
Pancreatico-jejunostomy	14
Bile duct drainage, papillotomy	16
Total	227

Table 2. Preliminary operation in patients with chronic pancreatitis

Preliminary Operation	Number
Cholecystectomy	19
Pancreatitis and abscess drainage	13
Cholecystectomy, choledochojejunostomy	5
Pseudocyst-jejunostomy	8
Stomach resection	10
Cholecyst-jejunostomy	2

and/or cholestasis, or strongly suspected the presence of a malign disorder of the distal choledochus, the papillae, the duodenum and the head of the pancreas. Attacks of pain were observed in cases of recurring pancreatitis that could not be controlled conservatively. We carried out resection along with gastrectomy of the distal two-thirds of the stomach, the duodenum, the distal ductus choledochus, the gall bladder and the first 15 cm of the proximal jejunum. Pancreaticojejunostomy and choledochojejunostomy were performed on the loop leading to the remaining part of the stomach. In 56 of the 98 patients we occluded the remainder of the pancreas with Ethibloc. A hepatic biopsy was performed in every case.

Since there remains the question of late changes, only those patients were included in this study whose operation had taken place at least 5 years earlier, which meant that 77 patients were considered. The object of the investigation was to establish the general condition of the patients and above all to gather information about changes in glucose metabolism. In our comparative study, we considered patients who had developed no insulin-dependent diabetes prior to the operation.

To establish carbohydrate tolerance, a glucose tolerance test was carried out with glucagon stimulation. In addition, regular follow-up examinations were carried out, including sonography, computed tomography and endoscopy.

Results

Of the 77 patients in this study who underwent cephalic pancreatoduodenectomy, eight (10%) died during the course of the 1st year following the operation. The main causes of death were infection (pneumonia, peritonitis) and failure of the liver and remaining pancreatitis. Among early complications, there were four cases of fistulae of the pancreas, two cases of peripancreatic fluid accumulation, which were punctured under CT control, and a subphrenic abscess. There were four cases of gastric haemorrhage which it was possible to check conservatively. Further complications included four cases of pneumonia, two cases of pleural effusion, two cases of diffuse thrombopathy and two cases of delirium tremens.

Among late complications which were first observed 12 months after the operation, we registered four cases of pancreatitis regression, two cases in which a fistula of the pancreas had existed for more than 6 months and one case of regressive bronchopneumonia. Of 69 patients, 51 required enzyme substitution in order to keep the daily excretion of stool fats below 20 g.

Within 5 years, and with changing degrees of severity, patients experienced pain, loss of weight, diarrhoea, meteorism, motility disturbance and cholangitis, mostly linked with a markedly adverse effect on well-being, inability to work or a stay in hospital. Four patients of the 69 developed hepatitis. In a further three cases, virus pneumonia and a herpes infection made a hospital stay necessary. With two patients we were compelled to perform a further resection because of a jejunal peptic ulcer. Of 51 patients in this study, 90% were disabled 5 years following the operation. The other 6 had limited disability, were dependent on exocrine ferment substitution and did light work. There were grounds for believing that only one-third of the patients abstained from alcohol.

Observation of the glucose metabolism was of interest. With some patients who came for an operation while suffering from pronounced jaundice, we observed a stabilization of metabolism within 6 months following the operation.

The precise examination of glucose tolerance from the 1st to the 6th year following cephalic pancreatoduodenectomy clearly revealed, however, that deterioration took place. In 46% of the patients operated on insulin substitution was necessary. Within 3 years, a significant deterioration of glucose tolerance was observed (Fig. 1), and this deterioration became more marked after a further 3 years. Insulin measurements revealed a similar progression. Six years after cephalic pancreatoduodenectomy, 28 patients had only a very low insulin level, which it was possible to raise (Fig. 2) by means of glucose stimulation. We were able to demonstrate a similar progression in our measurement of C peptide levels.

Over the whole of the period in question, we were not able to make a significant distinction with regard to glucose metabolism between patients on whom occlusion of the pancreas remainder had been performed and those on whom it had not been carried out. The two groups had a similar need of exocrine substitution. Endoscopic control examinations of the choledocho- and pancreatojejunostomies showed that while a slight diminution of biliodigestive anastomosis occurred, there was in no case a functionally effective stenosis. The endoscopic picture of the pancreatojejunostomy showed an area, largely covered by the intestinal epithelium, on which a pancreatic secretion was demonstrable in 14 from 31 patients examined.

All the patients examined reported varying pain symptoms, which were particularly marked post-prandially, often combined with diarrhoea. A recurrence of pancreatitis with marked increase in calcification of the pancreas remainder was demonstrable in only 10% of the cases. The determination of progressive steatosis of the liver follow-

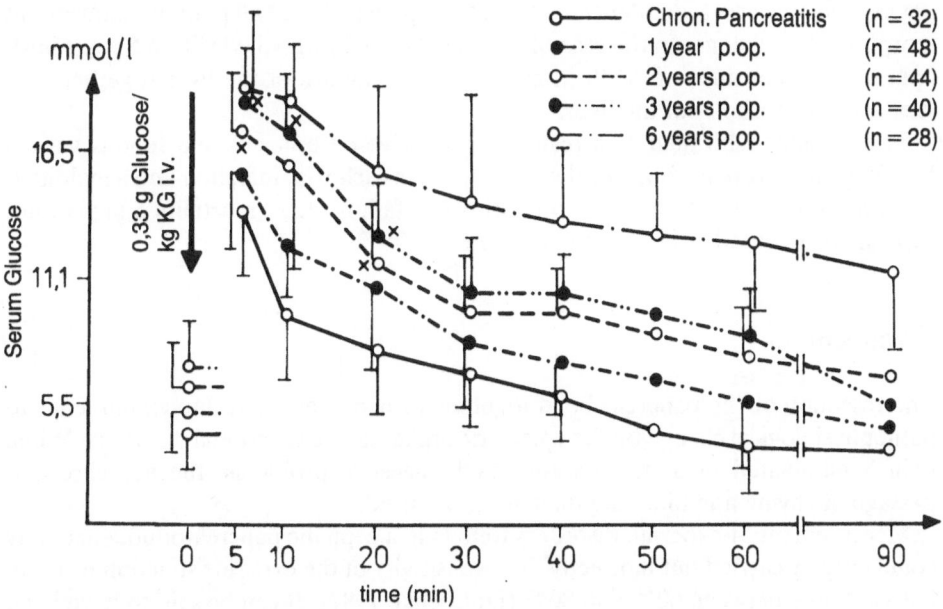

Fig. 1. Intravenous glucose tolerance test in patients with chronic pancreatitis and 1–6 years following cephalic pancreatoduodenectomy

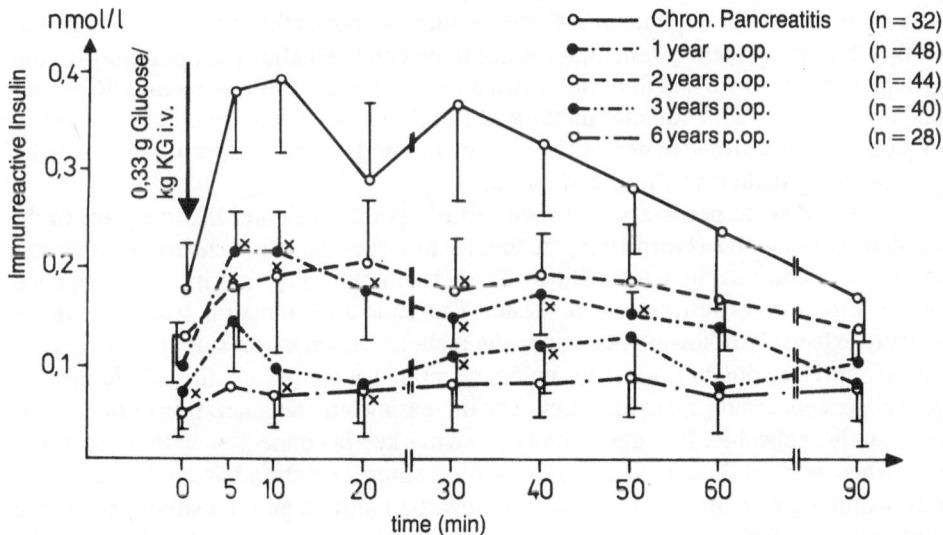

Fig. 2. Insulin level in the blood of patients with chronic pancreatitis and 1–6 years following cephalic pancreatoduodenectomy (iv. GTT)

ing cephalic pancreatoduodenectomy seems serious; 60% of all patients showed this morphological change. In the case of 18 patients (25%) who died within 5 years post-operatively, the cause of death in nine cases was failure of the liver together with steatosis and cirrhosis of the liver.

Two patients who died as a result of regressive oesophagus and fundus varices bleeding had severe cirrhosis of the liver. Serious cachexia, infection and a maldigestion syndrome led in four cases to multi-organ failure. Late mortality 5 years after cephalic pancreatoduodenectomy amounted to 25%.

Discussion

The resection of the pancreas head together with stomach and duodenum leads to pathophysiological changes in the epigastric organs and to functional disorders. While pain is eliminated or a stenosis corrected, digestive problems, the asynchronous passage of chyme and bile, and diabetes are caused.

Measurement of exocrine disorders following a cephalic pancreatoduodenectomy could only by carried out indirectly. The sensitivity of the exocrine function test is in any case only between 60% and 80% (Domschke 1987). It can be said to have been confirmed, however, that in 55% of the cases following Whipple's operation and in 100% of the cases following total pancreatoduodenectomy, steatorrhea is to be expected (Frey 1976). We found steatorrhea in 74% of our patients. After 5 years, this digestive disorder was difficult to compensate in 25% of cases, despite ferment substitution. Chronic pancreatitis is accompanied by alteration in carbohydrate metabolism as well as other endocrine functions of the pancreas (Kalk 1979; Staszenwicz 1980). If the endocrine pancreas part, as well as the existing damage, is reduced by resection, a deterioration in post-operative carbohydrate tolerance is generally to be expected (Keitz 1989; Lippert 1984; Moreaux 1984).

Within 3–5 years following Whipple's operation because of chronic pancreatitis, we registered insulin-dependent diabetes mellitus in 46% of the cases. A regeneration of B cells in the pancreas remainder is not to be expected after the operation. In the group of patients who had undergone drainage, we found after 6 years only 16% who had insulin-dependent diabetes mellitus. After the same period, a comparative group of patients with chronic pancreatitis who had not undergone an operation revealed a proportion of diabetes sufferers of 20%.

It does not seem necessary that methods of operation should take account of an incidence of diabetes (Horn 1985). It should, however, be made clear that resection induces or manifests diabetes mellitus. Diabetes mellitus is primarily a consequence of the progressive destruction of tissue. The endocrine function reserve is more quickly exhausted following resection; the diabetes which as a result appears earlier and is more serious has a not insignificant influence on the quality of life and on prognoses concerning life expectancy. The increasing fatty degeneration of the liver is not clearly explicable. It is significantly more marked in connection with resection of the pancreas head than in comparative groups where resection has not been carried out. Continuing alcohol abuse cannot be regarded only as an intensifying noxa. We also found similar changes in 75% of the patients who were operated on because of a pancreas head carcinoma.

Altogether, the later consequences of pancreas resection in cases of chronic pancreatitis are the cause of a higher late mortality rate. Siewert (1988) indicates a 5-year mortality rate of 30.5% following pancreaticoduodenectomy; following a left resection, this proportion rises, in fact, to 45%. The comprehensive statistics gathered by Gebhardt [3] show a late mortality of 18.6% following cephalic pancreatoduodenectomy. In our study, we registered a late mortality of 25% after 5 years.

Our investigations lead us to the conclusion that accurate diagnosis is imperative when pancreas head resection comes into consideration. The patient's fate is influenced by this life-style, in particular his indulgence in alcohol. The functionally healthier pancreas tissue that can be saved when an operation is carried out, the less the endocrine function will be adversely affected.

References

1. Domschke W, Domschke H (1981) Funktionsdiagnostik des exocrinen Pankreas. Diagnostischer und differentialdiagnostischer Stellenwert. In: Grabner W, Männl HFK (eds) Klinik der chronischen Pankreatitis. Perimed, Erlangen
2. Frey CF, Child CG, Fry W (1976) Pancreatectomy for chronic pancreatitis. Am Surg 186
3. Gebhardt C (1984) Chirurgie des exocrinen Pankreas. Thieme, Stuttgart
4. Horn J (1985) Therapie der chronischen Pankreatitis. Springer, Berlin Heidelberg New York Tokyo
5. Horn J, Hohenberger P (1987) Chronische Pankreatitis – Drainage und Resektionsverfahren. Standortbestimmung. Chirurg 58:14–24
6. Kalk WJ, Vinik AJ, Jackson WPU, Bank S (1979) Insulin secretion and pancreatic exocrine function in patients with chronic pancreatitis. Diabetologia 16:355–358
7. Keith RG, Saibil FG, Sheppard RH (1989) Treatment of chronic alcoholic pancreatitis by pancreatic resection. Am J Surg 157:156–162
8. Lippert H, Wolff H, Lorenz D, Wojczik H, Kühn F (1984) Erfahrungen mit der Pankreasokklusion nach kephaler Duodenopankreatektomie. Zentbl Chir 109:1112–1121
9. Moreaux J (1984) Long-term follow-up study of 50 patients with pancreatoduodenectomy for chronic pancreatitis. World J Surg 8:346–353
10. Siewert JR (1988) Stellung der Duodenopankreatektomie in der chirurgischen Behandlung der chronischen Pankreatitis. In: Grabner W, Männl HFK (eds) Klinik der chronischen Pankreatitis. Perimed, Erlangen, pp 126–132
11. Stasienwicz J, Adler M, Decourt A (1980) Pancreatic and gastrointestinal hormones in chronic pancreatitis. Hepato-Gastroenterol 27:152–160

Surgical Treatment: New Horizons

Preservation of the Pylorus During Pancreaticoduodenectomy for Chronic Pancreatitis

L. W. Traverso[1]

Introduction

This chapter analyzes the indications for removal of the head of the pancreas in patients with symptomatic, chronic pancreatitis. Several methods can be utilized to remove the pancreatic head, including pancreaticoduodenectomy with hemigastrectomy [1], pancreaticoduodenectomy with preservation of the pylorus [2], and excision of the pancreatic head with duodenal preservation [3]. An additional goal of this report is to examine the most current results of the author's preferred method to excise the pancreatic head in patients with chronic pain of chronic pancreatitis, i. e., pancreaticoduodenectomy with pylorus preservation (PDPP).

The surgeon treating chronic pancreatitis can obtain superlative pain results with the support of the rapidly progressing technologies of therapeutic endoscopy, interventional radiology, and anesthesiology. Therefore, only the past 3 years of experience with PDPP for chronic pancreatitis is reviewed in the personal series of the author. Utilizing modern diagnostic and therapeutic techniques combined with proper patient selection, the procedure of PDPP should result in almost every patient obtaining pain relief with little gastrointestinal sequelae. The mortality rate of PDPP approaches zero.

Materials and Methods

Technique of Pylorus Preservation

Instead of antrectomy or hemigastrectomy during pancreaticoduodenectomy (Whipple's procedure), the pylorus is widely dissected free of the hepatoduodenal ligament (Fig. 1). The right gastric artery (if present) is divided at its origin, and the neurovascular supply to the pylorus is protected. Dissection of the duodenal bulb is continued until the pancreas and duodenum merge. Many shared blood vessels are observed at this point. About 5 cm of duodenum will have been freed, and the GIA stapling device is used to divide the duodenum. Wide dissection of the pylorus and duodenum adjacent to the head of the pancreas makes PDPP less than ideal for pancreatic cancer, but uniquely suited for chronic pancreatitis. The stomach and stapled-over first part of the duodenum is placed in the left upper quadrant until antecolic end-duodeno-to side-jejunostomy is constructed.

---

[1] Virginia Mason Medical Center, 1100 Ninth Avenue, Seattle, Wa 98111, USA

Chronic Pancreatitis
Ed. by Beger, Büchler, Ditschuneit, and Malfertheiner
© Springer-Verlag Berlin Heidelberg 1990

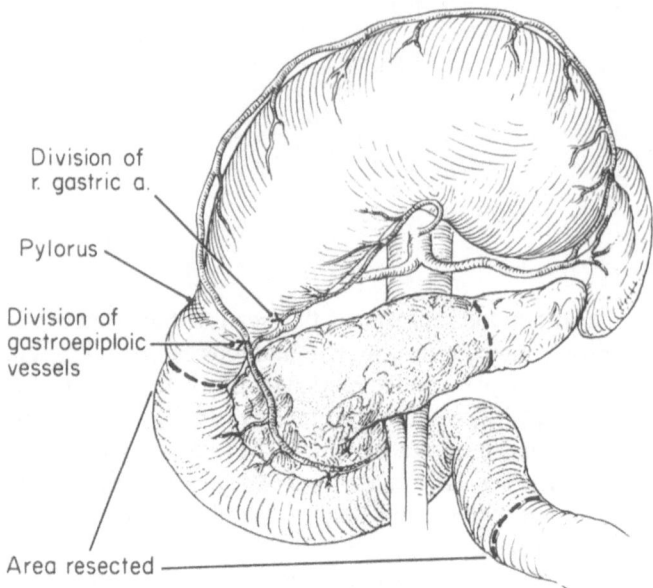

Division of
r. gastric a.

Pylorus

Division of
gastroepiploic
vessels

Area resected

Fig. 1. Area of the pancreas and duodenum resected. Ligation of the right gastric and gastropyloric vessels preserve the vascular arcade on the lesser and greater curvature of the stomach. An intact neurovascular supply to the pylorus and first portion of the duodenum is mandatory for a functioning pylorus. A vagotomy or history of vagotomy precludes pylorus preservation. (From [2])

The entire vagus nerve supply to the stomach is mandatory to preserve a functioning pylorus. A vagotomy or history of vagotomy does not allow for pyloric preservation. After excision of the pancreatic head, remaining duodenum, and distal common bile duct, the anastomoses are positioned to isolate potential leakage of the bile or pancreatic duct connections from the duodenojejunostomy. This maneuver may help to prevent gastric outlet dysfunction. The proximal jejunum is directed toward the pancreatic and bile duct remnants by a retrocolic route, and the stomach with preserved pylorus and duodenum are brought antecolic to the left transverse colon, allowing for a remote duodenojejunostomy. If the chain of lakes type dilatation is present in the pancreatic tail, the pancreatic anastomosis is constructed with a side-to-side technique (Fig. 2).

Patient Data

Between January 1986 and April 1989, seven patients with chronic pancreatitis have required excision of the head of the pancreas. One of these patients (L. C.) had undergone a previous vagotomy and antrectomy and therefore underwent standard pancreaticoduodenectomy. The remaining six patients underwent PDPP. Preoperative data are presented in Table 1. An overview of indications for excision of the pancreatic head in these patients is listed in Table 2.

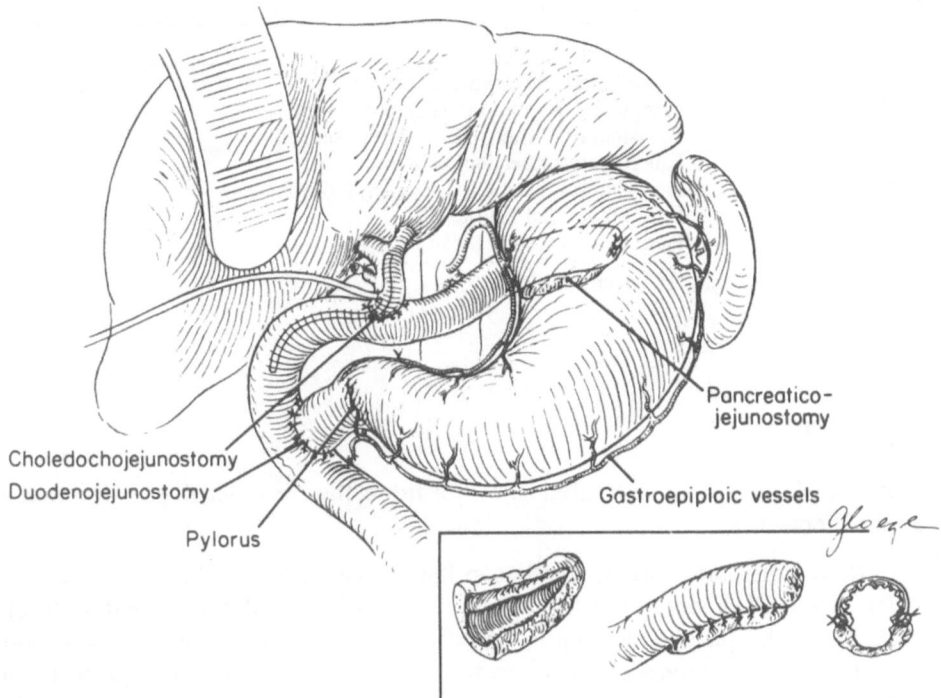

Fig. 2. Reconstruction with retrocolic anastomoses to the pancreatic duct and then bile duct. The pancreatic duct connection should be made with a side-to-side technique if a "chain of lakes" type of ductal dilatation is present *(inset)*. The end-duodenal to side-jejunal anastomosis is made antecolic (usually left transverse colon) to isolate the pancreatic from the duodenal anastomosis and prevent gastric outlet obstruction. (From [2])

Table 1. Preoperative patient data

Patient	Age	Male	ETOH	ABD pain	Panc. calcif.	Preop. Dia-betes	Pseudo-cyst (head)	PD fistula	Bil. obst.	Prior op.
RR	46	+	+	+	0	0	+	+	+[b]	0
LC	59	+	+	+	+	0	+	0	+[b]	0
TD	39	+	+	0	0	+	0	+	+[b]	+
DJ	48	+	+	+	0	0	+[a]	0	+[b]	+
KL	41	0	+	+	+	0	0	0	+	+
GH	44	0	0	+	+	0	0	0	0	0
KB	35	+	+	+	+	0	0	0	0	0
Ave. or %	44	71%	86%	86%	57%	14%	43%	29%	71%	43%

ETOH, Alcohol; ABD, abdomen; Panc. Calcif., pancreatic calcifications; PD Fistula, pancreatic duct fistula to skin or bile duct; Bil. Obst., biliary obstruction (chemical or clinical), all had bile duct stenosis by ERCP; Prior Op., prior operation on pancreas. Ave. or %, the average or percentage of all patients
[a] Percutaneously drained
[b] Clinical jaundice

Table 2. Patients' indications for operation

Patient	Indications for operation
R.R.	Sepsis, CBD-PD cloaca, CBD obstruction
L.C.	Pain, jaundice, pseudocyst on portal vein
T.D.	Persistent PD fistula, CBD obstruction
D.J.	Failed central resection, pain, pseudocyst
K.L.	Pain, duodenal and CBD stenosis, failed Puestow
G.H.	Pain, obliterated PD (head)
K.B.	Pain, obliterated PD (head)

CBD, Common bile duct; PD, pancreatic duct

Case Histories

More specific details are presented below regarding the events leading to resection in each patient.

1. *R.R.* This hard-working gentleman had a long history of heavy alcohol use. After a 4-month history of right upper quadrant abdominal pain, radiating to the back, he was hospitalized for sepsis, jaundice, and abdominal bloating. An arteriogram showed a hypervascular mass in the head of the pancreas thought to be an endocrine tumor. Endoscopy showed a large duodenal ulcer just proximal to the ampulla of Vater. An endoscopic retrograde cholangiopancreatogram (ERCP) showed a communication between the pancreatic duct and common bile duct through a 3-cm cavity in the pancreatic head [4]. Both alkaline phosphatase and transaminase levels were over ten times elevated. During his pancreatic resection, a cloaca-like cavity was found just above the junction of the common bile duct and the pancreatic duct that communicated freely with both structures (Fig. 3). The cavity had enlarged

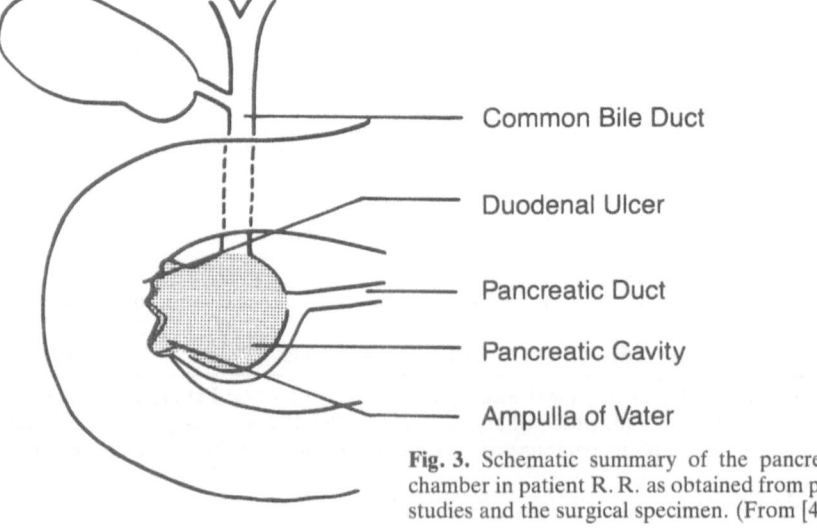

Common Bile Duct

Duodenal Ulcer

Pancreatic Duct

Pancreatic Cavity

Ampulla of Vater

Fig. 3. Schematic summary of the pancreaticobiliary chamber in patient R.R. as obtained from preoperative studies and the surgical specimen. (From [4])

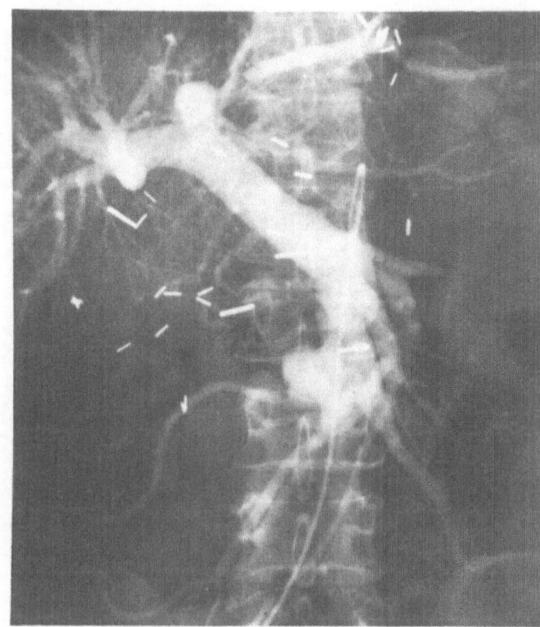

Fig. 4. An arteriovenous fistula is demonstrated in patient L.C. immediately after injection into the superior mesenteric artery. The A-V mesenteric to portal vein fistula was located in the wall of a pseudocyst contiguous with the right side of the portal vein and within the head of the pancreas

to cause local necrosis of the duodenum (as seen by the duodenal ulcer). Bile was present in the pancreatic duct when the pancreas was divided over the portal vein. Histologic examination of the resected specimen showed the intense inflammation to be benign.

2. *L. C.* This patient had a long history of alcohol-related pancreatitis and recent abdominal pain with biliary obstruction. During a prior admission for abdominal pain, he had undergone embolization of a superior mesenteric artery to portal vein fistula within the wall of a pseudocyst (Fig. 4). The 3-cm necrotic cyst was located within the head of the pancreas to the right of the portal vein. Resolution of abdominal pain led to discharge, but 6 months later he was readmitted for increasing abdominal pain, jaundice, nausea, and vomiting. A percutaneous transhepatic biliary stent was placed. An arteriogram showed absence of mesenteric portal fistula. CT scan showed persistent pseudocyst. The abdominal pain had to be managed with a chronic epidural catheter. After total parenteral nutrition for 10 days, the patient underwent standard pancreaticoduodenectomy (past history of antrectomy). The medial wall of the pseudocyst was the portal vein.

3. *T. D.* Alcohol abuse and associated gallstones resulted in necrotizing pancreatitis for this American Indian. Six months prior to PDPP, a pancreatic phlegmon penetrated the transverse colon requiring colon resection, ileostomy, and débridement of the pancreas. A chronic but controlled pancreatic fistula developed from the main pancreatic duct just adjacent to the pancreatic duct sphincter (Fig. 5). The fistula volume of 120 ml per day could be decreased 50% but not stopped with subcutaneous somatostatin. Insulin-dependent diabetes developed. Exploration was required for persistent pancreatic fistula, bile duct obstruction requiring endoscopic stent, and

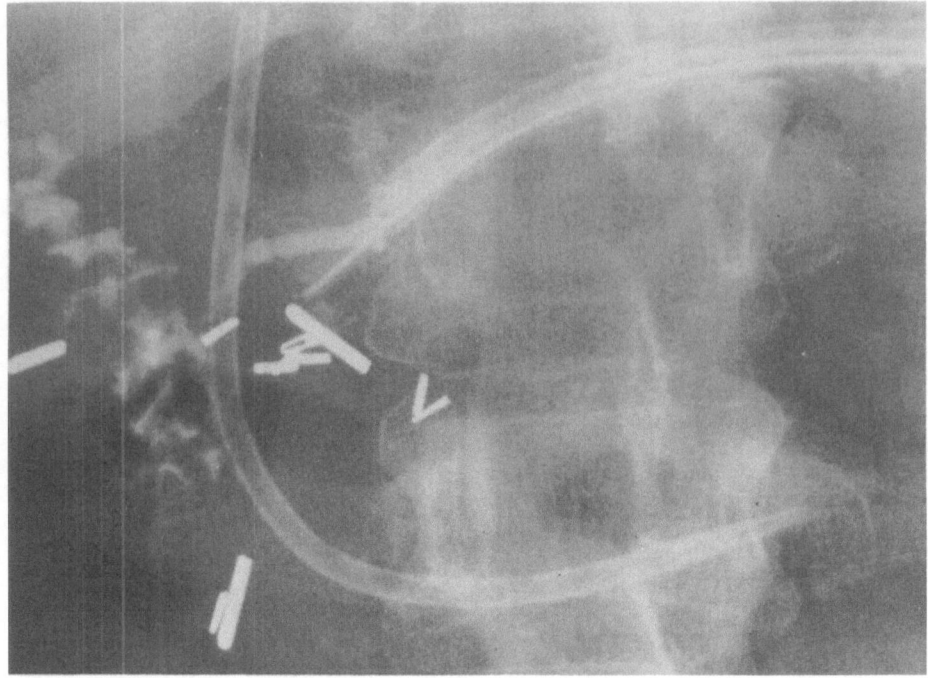

Fig. 5. In patient T.D., an endoscopically placed bile duct stent is in place while a surgically placed drain lies on the anterior surface of the pancreatic head to exit the skin in the left upper quadrant (off this figure). The end of the pancreatic drain is adjacent to the patient's remaining pancreatic duct after necrotizing pancreatitis and débridement. Contrast introduced into the pancreatic drain outlines the short pancreatic duct and rapidly enters the duodenum

take-down of the ileostomy. Almost all of the pancreas was found to be atrophic, with a small rim of chronically scarred pancreas in the duodenal curve. This was the site of the pancreatic fistula, and the remaining head was excised by PDPP.

4. *D.J.* Because of long-term alcohol abuse, this man developed chronic calcific pancreatitis. Abdominal pain was associated with a 6-cm pseudocyst connected to the main pancreatic duct as it passed over the portal vein. Endoscopic transampullary pancreatic stent decompression into the cyst was accomplished through the pancreatic duct. The pseudocyst resolved over several weeks, but recurred with stent removal. A central pancreatic resection was performed to eliminate the pseudocyst/pancreatic duct connection, and the tail of the pancreas was drained with a pancreaticojejuno-stomy. Within 6 months, abdominal pain and jaundice occurred. Another pseudocyst anterior and cephalad to the pancreatic head was found (Fig. 6). An endoscopic biliary stent decompressed the biliary tree. Percutaneous drainage of the new 6-cm cyst allowed temporary decompression, but abdominal pain persisted. At explora-tion, the patient required PDPP.

5. *K.L.* Heavy alcohol use was associated with a 10-year history of chronic calcific pancreatitis in this woman. A Puestow procedure for a chain of lakes pancreatic duct

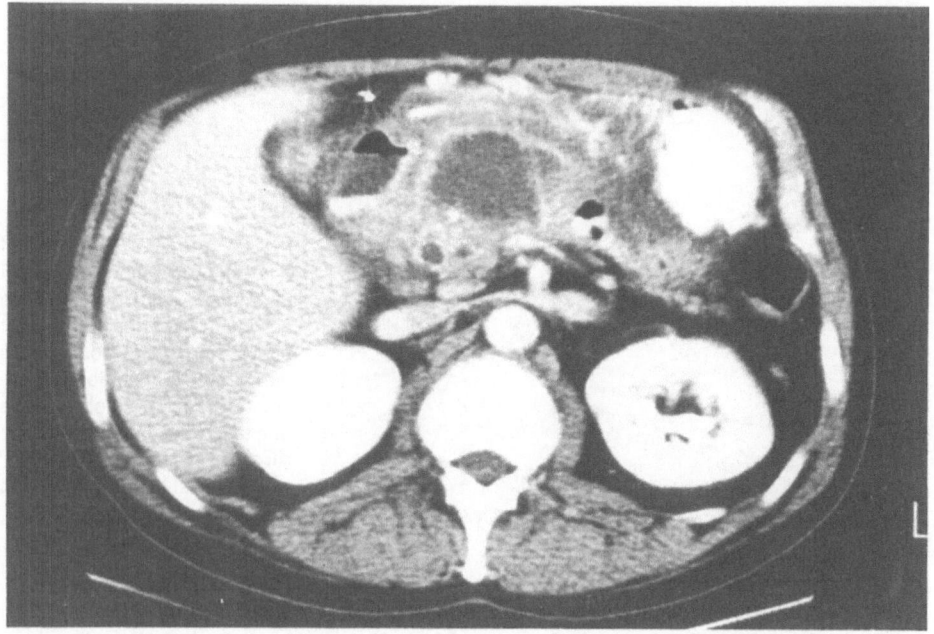

Fig. 6. In patient D. J., another pseudocyst is observed 6 months after central pancreatic resection. This 6-cm cyst was associated with bile duct stenosis requiring endoscopic stent. The new cyst was drained percutaneously, but pain persisted and resection of the head was required

had not been successful in relieving her abdominal pain. The smoldering inflammatory process in the pancreatic head resulted in duodenal obstruction just below the ampulla. She had been managed at home on total parenteral nutrition until she could not handle her own gastric secretions, resulting in nausea, vomiting, and more abdominal pain. Resection was indicated for increasing duodenal stenosis, common bile duct stenosis, and persistent abdominal pain. Four months after the Puestow procedure, PDPP was required. The Puestow pancreaticojejunostomy was left in place with the end of the jejunal limb fashioned to cover the fresh stump of the remaining pancreas.

6. *G. H.* Pancreatitis of unknown etiology resulted in complete pancreatic ductal obstruction due to stenosis and stones throughout the head of the pancreas. The common bile duct was also stenotic by ERCP. Pancreatic stenting was not possible. Intractable abdominal pain induced by eating required total parenteral nutrition preoperatively. A CT scan showed a diffusely enlarged pancreatic head. After PDPP, histologic examination of the head of the pancreas showed severe inflammation and a benign process.

7. *K. B.* A 5-year history of abdominal pain was associated with heavy alcohol use in this man. ERCP showed multiple pancreatic duct calcifications and a totally obstructed pancreatic duct at the midportion of the head of the pancreas (Fig. 7). CT scan showed a dilated pancreatic duct in the body and tail. There was a small

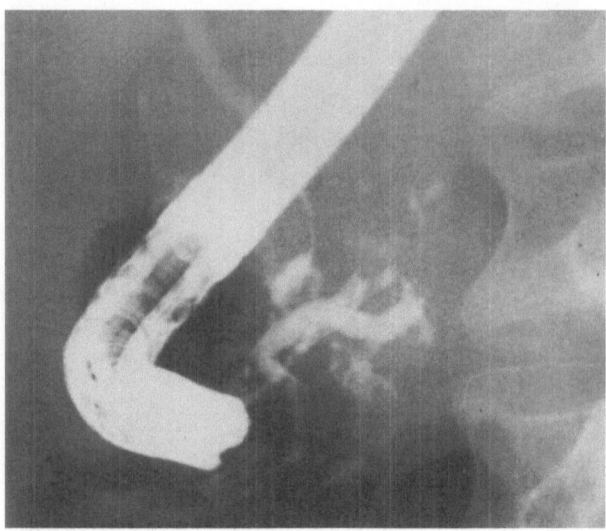

Fig. 7. An ERCP in patient K. B. showed a short segment of main pancreatic duct and an abrupt termination. Miniscope pancreatoscopy from both duodenum and midbody pancreatotomy showed obstruction due to stones and scarring. The surgical specimen after PDPP was involved histologically with marked chronic pancreatitis

pseudocyst on the tail of the pancreas. Distal common bile duct stenosis was present. Because of the dilated pancreatic duct in a chain of lakes pattern in the tail and body, a Puestow procedure and transduodenal septoplasty were planned. Intraoperative miniscope pancreatoscopy through the duodenum and the opened pancreatic duct in the body showed the majority of the duct in the pancreatic head to be totally obstructed with stenosis and stones associated with an intense inflammatory mass. Excision of the pancreatic head was performed by PDPP and lateral pancreatico-jejunostomy.

Results

Short Term

Short-term operative results are presented (Table 3) in regards to the length of operation, estimated blood loss, intraoperative or subsequent need for blood transfusion, use of a chronic epidural catheter during the operation and postoperatively, and the 30-day hospital mortality rate. Morbidity in the postoperative period was seen in four of seven patients. The most common complication resulting in delay of hospital discharge was gastric outlet obstruction seen in three of seven patients. This included

Table 3. Short-term operative results

Duration of operation	10.7 h (7–14)
Estimated blood loss	1374 ml (120–2800)
Blood transfusion	71%
Chronic epidural catheter	71%
Mortality	None
Morbidity	57%

the sole patient with previous gastrectomy. One patient (R. R.) developed adult respiratory distress syndrome and ventilator dependence for 10 postoperative days. The etiology was probably preoperative sepsis plus the volumes of fluid required during his 14-h operation. There were no instances of wound infections or bleeding complications. No instances of new diabetes were observed.

Long Term

Long-term operative results were obtained with a 100% follow-up on an average of 14.6 months after operation (range 2–41 months). All patients were alive, and during a personal interview all of them indicated that their preoperative symptoms were gone. No patient was taking pain medications for abdominal pain, but two required oral analgesics for chronic low-back pain. No patient had returned to alcohol abuse. Only one patient had not returned to work but planned to do so in the near future.

In regards to the long-term gastrointestinal sequelae, all patients indicated they were eating "everything" or had "no problem" with eating. Every patient's weight was stable, except for two who complained of being overweight. No patient complained of persistent diarrhea, but two indicated diarrhea would occur when not taking pancreatic enzyme supplements. Two patients indicated they had had temporary postprandial diarrhea for 6 months and 1 year postoperatively. One patient (G. H.) described dumping symptoms prevented by avoiding a high-carbohydrate meal, particularly of milkshakes or chocolate. Insulin-dependent diabetes was present in three patients (T. D., D. J., K. L.), as compared to one patient (T. D.) preoperatively.

The sequelae of preserving the pylorus during pancreaticoduodenectomy were assessed by examining potential symptom complexes from either excision of the duodenum and distal common bile duct, or the preserved pylorus.

In regards to the excision of the duodenum and the distal common bile duct, there had been no episodes of cholangitis, biliary fistula, persistent dumping, or permanent diarrhea in patients receiving PDPP.

In regards to sequelae of pyloric preservation, no patient has developed a marginal ulcer with the lack of gastrectomy. Gastric outlet obstruction developed in two of six PDPP patients (G. H., K. B.) in the postoperative period, and they were able to resume a regular diet 21 days postoperatively. Those patients not developing gastric outlet obstruction resumed a diet on an average of the 11th postoperative day. In both patients with gastric outlet obstruction, a CT scan showed a retrogastric or peripancreaticojejunostomy fluid collection, which was percutaneously drained. One fluid collection (K. B.) was associated with an elevated amylase (7800 IU/ml). Both patients began eating within a week of percutaneous drainage. The remaining gastric outlet obstruction patient (L. C.) had had prior antrectomy and a similar CT finding of peripancreatic fluid collection. Effective drainage resulted after repositioning a nearby drain on the 22nd postoperative day, however, he did not resume a diet until the 36th postoperative day.

Discussion

Excision of the head of the pancreas was required in these patients for one of two situations: progressive disease in the pancreatic head after prior pancreatic operation, or significant fibrosis in the pancreatic head on initial presentation. Examples of progressive disease in the head of the pancreas despite prior treatment is the abdominal pain due to continued smoldering inflammation or pseudocyst that also caused duodenal or biliary stenosis following a Puestow procedure or central pancreatic resection. Examples of significant disease initially presenting in the pancreatic head that required resection are stenosis of the common bile duct or the duodenum combined with obliteration of the pancreatic duct in the head (particularly without distal ductal dilatation that would allow a Puestow procedure). Other examples are persistent pseudocyst with arteriovenous fistula, later to be associated with jaundice, or intrapancreatic cavity with perforation into the common bile duct resulting in sepsis.

These cases emphasize that the head of the pancreas was the pacemaker of chronic pancreatitis. A continuous smoldering inflammatory process within the head of the gland results in persistent symptoms even after ductal decompression procedures. The latter procedure is incapable of draining the multiple major ductal connections within the head of the gland and therefore cannot interrupt the process. The current report indicates that excision of the head of the gland relieved symptoms in all patients, was associated with zero mortality, and little permanent gastrointestinal dysfunction.

Pain relief was immediate. In addition, PDPP solved distressing clinical problems of sepsis, jaundice, or dependence on parenteral nutrition. No patient reported attacks of recurrent pancreatitis or reoperations. Previous experience with pain relief following a Whipple procedure has been superior if patients abstained from alcohol [5]. These latter patients also had statistically superior results (as compared to pseudocyst drainage) with fewer readmissions and recurrent pancreatitis. However, follow-up in the latter study was 3.2 years and only 14 months in the current series. Beger and colleagues [3] reported a 14% recurrent pancreatitis rate after a median follow-up of 24 months following duodenal preservation and pancreatic head excision. Chronic pain relief was complete or near complete in 93%. The advantages of this operation should be considered in future studies.

Marginal ulceration was not seen, although follow-up averaged only 14.6 months. Five years may be necessary to follow patients to reliably assess the incidence of marginal ulceration [6]. No higher incidence has been observed after PDPP when compared to standard pancreaticoduodenectomy [7, 8].

There is a significant morbidity, however, as with any series of pancreaticoduodenectomy. In contrast to excision of the head for periampullary tumors, the patient with chronic pancreatitis has a marked inflammatory or fibrotic process. An obligate intraoperative blood loss results. Blood transfusions were therefore the rule in treating these chronic pancreatitis patients with excisional procedures. The operative difficulty with this inflammatory process is also significant, as explained by the increased operating time. However, the major cause of morbidity was not related directly to chronic pancreatitis associated inflammation.

The major cause of morbidity was gastric outlet obstruction. Investigation with CT scanning found peripancreatic fluid collections in all patients with obstruction. Once the fluid was drained, the gastric outlet obstruction resolved. PDPP has been reported to have a high incidence of delayed gastric function [9], but the only patient in the current series with pancreaticoduodenectomy *without* pylorus preservation also had this problem. The common factor appears to be an inflammatory process (temporary or subclinical leak from the pancreatic anastomosis) locally irritating the new gastric connection. The pancreatic anastomosis techniques associated with gastric outlet obstruction was reviewed. One lateral pancreaticojejunostomy (K.B.) and two end pancreaticojejunostomy (G.H., L.C.) procedures were utilized. The latter two were performed with silicone rubber stents, a technique that I have found in the dog pancreas to be associated with a 40% leak rate as compared to no leaks using a multiple perforated polyvinyl chloride (Teflon) stent (unpublished data) manufactured by Wilson-Cook (Winston-Salem NC, USA).

Advances in anesthesia through the use of epidural catheters have significantly decreased the need for large concentrations of inhalation anesthetics. The epidural catheter is utilized for excellent pain control in the postoperative period, although it may prolong postoperative ileus. Improved postoperative pain control with regional administration of narcotics undoubtedly improves the patients' respiratory function in these chronically debilitated and usually tobacco-smoking (six of seven) individuals. No episodes of persistent atelectasis or pneumonia were seen in these patients. The one pulmonary complication (ARDS) was related to sepsis.

The advances of interventional radiology and therapeutic endoscopy are evident in the case histories of these patients. Preoperatively, one patient underwent percutaneous drainage of a new pseudocyst while one underwent embolization of an arteriovenous fistula contained within a pseudocyst. Six of seven patients had clinical or chemical biliary obstruction, and three of these individuals underwent preoperative biliary stent placements, either endoscopically or transhepatically. One patient underwent endoscopic transduodenal decompression of a large pseudocyst, utilizing a pancreatic stent placed from the duodenum through the pancreatic duct into a pseudocyst [10]. The cyst had developed from a rupture of the main pancreatic duct in the body of the gland and the stent allowed for resolution of the pseudocyst and ultimate operative management. Three patients required postoperative percutaneous drainage of fluid collections around the pancreatic anastomosis.

Because of significant inflammation, fibrosis, and ductal obliteration in the head of the gland, the pathology in these patients resulted in stenosis of the duodenum and/or common bile duct. Disruption of the bile duct occurred in one case. Therefore, a procedure that preserved the duodenum and distal common bile duct was felt not indicated, and PDPP was performed without mortality. In this small series, no significant or permanent sequelae from removal of the duodenum and preserving the pylorus were seen, while all patients experienced relief of symptoms.

The concept of conserving portions of the gastrointestinal tract traditionally removed during the standard Whipple procedure deserves attention by pancreatic surgeons. Future studies are required to compare the results of PDPP to the duodenal preserving resection of the head of the pancreas.

References

1. Child CG, Frey CF (1966) Pancreaticoduodenectomy. Surg Clin North Am 46:1201–1213
2. Traverso LW, Longmire WP (1978) Preservation of the pylorus during pancreaticoduodenectomy. Surg Gynecol Obstet 146:959–962
3. Beger HG, Krautzberger W, Bittner R, Büchler M, Limmer J (1985) Duodenum-preserving
   resection of the head of the pancreas in patients with severe chronic pancreatitis. Surgery
   97:467–473
4. Miller BM, Traverso LW (1988) Intrapancreatic communication of bile and pancreatic ducts
   secondary to pancreatic necrosis. Arch Surg 123:1000–1003
5. Traverso LW, Tompkins RK, Urrea PT, Longmire WP (1979) Surgical treatment of chronic
   pancreatitis. Twenty-two years experience. Ann Surg 190:312–319
6. Grant CS, van Heerden JA (1979) Anastomotic ulceration following subtotal and total pancreatectomy. Ann Surg 190:1–5
7. Itani KM, Coleman RE, Akwari OE, Meyers WC (1986) Pylorus-preserving pancreaticoduodenectomy. Ann Surg 204:655–665
8. Traverso LW, Longmire WP (1980) Preservation of the pylorus in pancreaticoduodenectomy.
   A follow-up evaluation. Ann Surg 192:306–310
9. Warshaw AL, Torchiana DL (1985) Delayed gastric emptying after pylorus-preserving pancreaticoduodenectomy. Surg Gynecol Obstet 160:1–4
10. Kozarek RA, Patterson DJ, Ball TJ, Traverso LW (1989) Endoscopic placement of pancreatic
    stents and drains in the management of pancreatitis. Ann Surg 209:261–266

Endocrine Function after Duodenum-Preserving Resection of the Head of the Pancreas With or Without Segmental Pancreatic Autotransplantation: An Experimental Study in Dogs*

H. G. Gooszen, O. R. Guicherit, M. P. M. van der Burg, J. B. M. J. Jansen, M. Frölich, and C. B. H. W. Lamers[1]

Introduction

Effective treatment for the relief of pain remains the major challenge in surgical management of chronic pancreatitis. The exact mechanism of how chronic pancreatitis leads to the well-known severe pancreatic pain has yet to be elucidated and for this reason a causal surgical approach to patients suffering from chronic pancreatitis is currently not available. Different types of operations have been devised in the past decennia but a well-outlined strategy about what type of operation should be conducted under different circumstances has not emerged and selection of the type of operation is a matter of personal preference and experience. We have learned from a retrospective survey of our own patient material [1] that minor resection (less than 50%) is usually ineffective and that major resection is effective but carries high morbidity in terms of loss of exo- and endocrine function.

Two alternatives that meet the criteria of combining effectiveness with maintenance of at least part of the pancreatic function deserve closer attention: segmental pancreatic autotransplantation with preservation of the duodenum and the so-called duodenum-preserving resection of the head of the pancreas. Clinical experience with segmental pancreatic autotransplantation is limited and the largest series has been described by Rossi et al. [2]. They describe a 100% success rate in terms of pain relief, with some patients in their series being free of pain after a second operation for completion pancreatectomy, i. e., resection of the small remnant of the pancreatic head with the duodenum. Our experience is limited, but the four patients we treated along these lines are all completely free of pain. Our technique is different from the technique described by Rossi et al. [2] since we place the graft intraperitoneally with a Roux-en-Y pancreaticojejunostomy for exocrine drainage and in Rossi's patients the pancreatic duct was injected to induce exocrine atrophy (ductobliteration). Two of our four patients do not need exocrine substitution, and all are insulin independent. The major drawback of the procedure is that it is a large and technically demanding operation. The other alternative, the duodenum-preserving resection of the pancrea-

* This study was supported by grants from the Dutch Kidney Foundation and from Immuno Chemie France.
[1] From the Departments of Surgery, Gastroenterology and Endocrinology, University Hospital, PO Box 9600, 2300-Leiden, The Netherlands.

tic head, as described by Beger, is as promising and not as demanding as segmental pancreatic autotransplantation.

The indication for both procedures is slightly different and we follow Beger and coworkers in proposing the duodenum-preserving resection of the head of the pancreas as the option of first choice if the inflammatory mass is localized in the head of the pancreas.

Segmental pancreatic autotransplantation should be considered if a previous Puestow operation or Beger procedure has failed, or if there is diffuse chronic inflammation without ductal dilatation or a localized inflammatory mass.

We have studied endocrine function after segmental pancreatic autotransplantation and after duodenum-preserving resection of the head of the pancreas in two different groups of dogs (beagles weighing 9–17 kg). Body and tail of the pancreas were injected to induce exocrine atrophy. Neoprene-Latex or Tissucol were used for ductobliteration.

In the group of dogs that underwent segmental autotransplantation, the effect of operation on endocrine function was tested with pre- and postoperative intravenous glucose tolerance tests (IVGTTs) with insulin response curves.

In the dogs that were subjected to duodenum-preserving resection of the pancreatic head, a more detailed analysis of endocrine function was carried out and not only IVGTTs were performed, but a standard test meal was also administered (TMA). At the different test intervals hormone profiles for insulin, glucagon, pancreatic polypeptide (PP), and cholecystokinin (CCK) were analyzed. Peripheral serum levels of insulin and glucagon were determined throughout the test period of 5 h. Plasma PP and CCK levels were analyzed on a limited scale for logistical reasons.

For the IVGTT, 0.5 g/kg glucose was injected intravenously. Before and up to 60 min after glucose injection, blood glucose and plasma insulin levels were determined. The glucose response was expressed in K-values (%/min) and the insulin response in incremental area under the plasma concentration-time curve (integrated insulin response; $\triangle$ AUC). The test meal consisted of 45% carbohydrate, 30% protein, and 24% fat (energy %) as a semiliquid mixture. Before and up to 5 h after completion of the meal, venous blood samples were taken for the determination of glucose, insulin, glucagon, pancreatic polypeptide (PP), and cholecystokinin (CCK). Results of glucose, insulin, and glucagon responses were calculated as basal levels and as incremental $\triangle$ AUC (integrated postprandial response). The responses of CCK and PP to the test meal were expressed as basal and incremental levels (t_{60}–t_0). Pilot studies have shown that peak levels for CCK and PP were reached at about 60 min after completion of the test meal.

The radioimmunological determination of plasma insulin was performed according to Berson and Yalow [3]. Plasma glucagon was radioimmunoassayed using a specific antiserum to synthetic pancreatic glucagon, not crossreacting to enteroglucagon. Plasma PP was measured by a sensitive and specific radioimmunoassay as described previously [4]. Plasma CCK was measured by a sensitive and specific radioimmunoassay using antibody T_{204}, which binds to biologically active carboxy-terminal CCK peptides containing the sulfated tyrosine region [5]. Results were calculated as means ± SEM. One-way analysis of variance and Student's t test were used for statistical analysis of the results. Differences were considered nonsignificant (NS) at $P > 0.05$.

Glucose Homeostasis After Segmental Autotransplantation

For the evaluation of postoperative glucose metabolism, segmental pancreatic auto-transplantation in humans can stand comparison with experimentally performed segmental pancreatic autotransplantation, a technique usually performed in combination with removal of the remaining part of the pancreas. Much experience has accumulated from the work performed in Minneapolis by Baumgartner et al. [6], by Cutfield et al. [7], by Jonung et al. [8], by Calhoun et al. [9], and by Gooszen et al. [10, 11]. Several factors, however, compromise the comparison between the experimental data and those obtained in patients with chronic pancreatitis. In patients, usually 5% of the pancreas has been left in situ and it is impossible, other than by invasive sampling techniques, to decide whether the insulin sampled from peripheral blood is secreted by the autograft or by the small brim of pancreas along the duodenum. It is remarkable that "only" 80% of patients become insulin dependent after 95% distal pancreatectomy, and it must be concluded that the remaining 5% of pancreas has a higher insulin-secreting potential than expected in 20% of patients who remain insulin independent after a major resection. The other pathophysiological mechanism interfering with the interpretation of the effect of segmental autotransplantation on glucose tolerance is the slowly progressive spontaneous deterioration of endocrine function as a consequence of the natural history of chronic pancreatitis.

Especially if ductobliteration is performed, the ensuing histological changes will frustrate even more the interpretation of the effect of segmental autotransplantation on endocrine function. In the detailed description of Rossi et al. [2], there is no distinct pattern of a change in K-values after operation. Some patients have been followed up for 2 years or more and no decrease in K-value with time was observed. These patients, however, were nonalcoholics and it may be that in these patients there is not such an easily recognizable progressive deterioration in endocrine function with time. At any rate, the ductobliteration performed in these patients did not lead to a demonstrable progressive loss in endocrine function.

The peripheral insulin levels, obtained during intravenous glucose tolerance test in some of the patients studied by Rossi, show an interesting pattern. The early insulin peak occurring as a result of the so-called first phase insulin release seems to have been abolished whereas there is a distinct rise after 30 min. Unfortunately no preoperative insulin data are available for comparison.

In our experiments to investigate the applicability of ductobliteration in clinical pancreas allotransplantation we have analyzed the long-term results of ductobliteration on endocrine function in different experimental conditions in dogs. After in situ ductobliteration of the left lobe of the pancreas in combination with removal of the right lobe in dogs, we found that K-values ($\pm$ SD) of intravenous glucose tolerance test were severely reduced from 2.8 $\pm$ 0.6 to 1.5 $\pm$ 0.6 at 1 month after operation. No further decrease with time was observed up to 1 year after operation [11]. On histological examination, the exocrine tissue had completely disappeared and the architecture of the islets of Langerhans was disrupted. At 1 year after ductobliteration the homone-producing cells were rearranged into clusters, without showing the original islet configuration.

After ductobliterated segmental pancreatic autotransplantation in combination with removal of the right pancreatic lobe, K-values ($\pm$ SD) were significantly but only moderately reduced from 3.2 ± 0.5 to 2.2 ± 0.8. These postoperative K-values still fell in the lower limits of normal and are significantly higher than those observed after in situ ductobliteration. We have explained these apparently contradictory findings from the data which were obtained from the peripheral insulin response curves registered during intravenous glucose tolerance tests. After in situ ductobliteration the integrated insulin output ($\pm$ SD) amounted to 650 ($\pm$ 299) and was significantly lower than in unmodified animals (2036 $\pm$ 822). After segmental ductobliterated pancreatic autotransplantation the integrated insulin response ($\pm$ SD), amounting to 1875 ($\pm$ 893), fell in the same range as before operation. It was concluded that liver bypass caused by caval venous drainage of the ductobliterated autograft was responsible for the quantitatively normal integrated insulin response after operation. Apparently the insulin made available to the peripheral circulation was appropriated to glucose withdrawal from the peripheral blood as manifested from the near-normal K-values after autotransplantation. Although these K-values thus obtained fell in the lower limits of the normal range, we feel that such K-values should not be interpreted as reflecting normal or near-normal glucose metabolism. If the peripheral insulin response curves after ductobliterated autotransplantation were looked at in a qualitative fashion, it was found that the initial insulin peak was not as high as before operation and that the return of the peripheral insulin levels to normal was delayed as compared to the pattern observed in unmodified dogs.

These findings are in keeping with those described by Rossi et al. after ductobliterated autotransplantation in patients wich chronic pancreatitis and support our hypothesis that ductobliteration leads to quantitative and qualitative changes in endocrine function mainly as a result of the histological changes in the endocrine compartment [11].

Endocrine Function After Duodenum-Preserving Resection of the Pancreatic Head

The results of basal glucose and hormone levels are presented in Table 1. Basal blood glucose levels and plasma CCK levels did not change during the course of the experiment. Basal plasma glucagon and PP levels, however, showed a significant decrease at 6 weeks without a further decrease at 12 weeks postoperatively ($p < .05$ and $p < .001$ respectively). The fall in basal plasma insulin levels was significant only at 12 weeks after operation ($p < .05$).

The results of IVGTT and TMA are presented in Table 2 with IVGTT, a decrease in K-value at 6 and 12 weeks ($p < .001$) was observed. Integrated insulin response showed a drop at 6 weeks and 12 weeks after operation ($p < .001$).

At test meal stimulation, a decrease in glucose tolerance was observed also with an increase in integrated glucose response at 6 and 12 weeks ($p < .001$). Meal-stimulated incremental PP levels showed a drop to an almost absence of stimulation at 6 and 12 weeks respectively ($p < .001$). No significant changes in integrated insulin and glucagon responses or on incremental CCK levels were observed (n. s.).

Table 1. Effect of removal of the right lobe of the pancreas with ductobliteration of the left lobe on basal plasma glucose, insulin, glucagon, pancreatic polypeptide (PP), and cholecystokinin (CCK) levels. Results are presented as mean ± SEM

	Before operation	Postoperative	
		6 weeks	12 weeks
Glucose (mM)	5.8 ± 0.1	6.0 ± 0.1	5.9 ± 0.1
Insulin (uU/ml)[a]	14 ± 3	11 ± 2	8 ± 1
Glucagon (pg/ml)[b]	86 ± 23	60 ± 13	44 ± 10
PP (pM)[c]	75 ± 11	29 ± 8	24 ± 3
CCK (pM)	4 ± 1	4 ± 2	3 ± 1

[a] Only at 12 weeks postoperatively are basal insulin levels significantly lower than before operation ($p < .05$)

[b] Basal plasma glucagon levels are significantly lower at 6 and 12 weeks after operation than those observed in unmodified dogs ($p < .05$)

[c] Basal plasma PP levels showed a progressive decline and plasma levels at 6 and 12 weeks are significantly lower than before operation ($p < .05$ and $p < .02$ respectively)

Table 2. Effect of removal of the right lobe of the pancreas with ductobliteration of the left lobe on i.v. glucose and test meal stimulated plasma glucose and hormone levels ($n = 9$). Results are presented as mean ± SEM

	Preoperation	Postoperation	
		6 weeks	12 weeks
IVGTT			
K value (%/min)[a]	3.4 ± 0.3	1.5 ± 0.2	1.6 ± 0.1
$\triangle AUC_{Ins}$ (uU)[a]	1488 ± 235	701 ± 108	470 ± 90
Test meal			
$\triangle AUC_{Glucose}$ (mM)[b]	0.7 ± 0.2	4.9 ± 1.1	6.2 ± 1.3
$\triangle AUC_{Insulin}$ (uU)[c]	132 ± 37	209 ± 39	188 ± 46
$\triangle AUC_{Glucagon}$ (pg)[c]	310 ± 54	225 ± 19	307 ± 52
PP (pM)[d]	363 ± 39	6 ± 3	10 ± 4
CCK (pM)[c]	9 ± 2	10 ± 2	11 ± 1

[a] K values and integrated insulin response ($\triangle$ AUC, min uU/ml over 60 min) are significantly lower at 6 and 12 weeks than preoperative levels ($p < .001$)

[b] Integrated glucose levels ($\triangle$ AUC, h mM over 5 h) are significantly higher at 6 and 12 weeks than before operation ($p < .001$)

[c] Integrated insulin ($\triangle$ AUC, h uU/ml over 5 h), integrated glucagon ($\triangle$ AUC, h pg/ml over 5 h) response and incremental CCK levels (CCK, pM) do not show significant changes over the observation period (n.s.)

[d] Incremental PP response (PP, pM) is almostly completely abolished at 6 and 12 weeks after operation ($p < .001$)

Discussion

It has been shown from our own results [1] and from those of others that for effective pain relief in chronic pancreatitis major operations cannot be avoided in a distinct proportion of patients.

Total pancreatectomy is effective but has unacceptable morbidity. Whipple's operation may be less effective and morbidity is not as high as reported after total pancreatectomy. Late complications like peptic ulceration, reflux gastritis, and the dumping syndrome are not avoidable and hard to treat effectively. Segmental pancreatic autotransplantation and duodenum-preserving resection of the pancreatic head share the advantage that the pylorus, the duodenum, and the gallbladder are left intact. The clinical impression that the nutritional status of these patients is better may be tentatively explained from the fact that both alternatives interfere less with upper gastrointestinal physiology than total pancreatectomy and Whipple's operation.

Our experiments were performed to investigate some aspects of the enteropancreatic axis to further substantiate our clinical impression suggesting the superiority of both surgical alternatives that were tested. After segmental pancreatic autotransplantation quantitatively normal peripheral insulin levels were observed and K-values after operation fell in the normal range. So initially we felt that caval drainage of the insulin secreted by the autografted segment was of benefit to glucose tolerance and could thus be explained as an argument in favor of autotransplantation.

More recently we conducted a study with autotransplantation after previous partial pancreatic resection and we found no such advantage in caval drainage over portal drainage of the insulin secreted [12].

After duodenum-preserving resection of the pancreatic head, a decrease in basal plasma insulin, glucagon, and PP is observed, while basal plasma CCK levels are unaffected. This observation can be explained by a combination of removal of the right lobe of the pancreas and ductobliteration-induced histological changes of the left lobe. High tissue concentrations of especially PP are observed in the right lobe, whereas insulin concentrations are highest in the left lobe. Tissue concentrations of glucagon show a significant gradient between the left lobe and right lobe of the pancreas with highest concentrations in the left lobe also [13, 14]. Ductobliteration leads to severe qualitative histological changes [15] and although destruction and reduction of number of hormone-producing cells has not been documented, insulin secretion studies support the occurrence of such a phenomenon [16], and a reduction in hormone-producing cells by the combination of removal of the right lobe and ductobliteration of the left lobe may therefore serve as an explanation for the decrease in basal plasma glucagon and insulin levels. In the decrease in basal plasma PP levels, removal of the right lobe is undoubtedly the most important factor. It is not surprising that basal plasma CCK levels are unchanged since CCK is secreted mainly in the duodenum and the upper gastrointestinal tract is left intact by duodenum-preserving resection of the pancreatic head in man and in dogs.

The second finding of this study is that both at i. v. glucose bolus injection and at TMA a decrease in glucose tolerance is observed. At IVGTT, this decrease is accompanied by a severely reduced insulin response, whereas after test-meal stimulation the insulin and glucagon response are left quantitatively intact. The presence of the duodenum with an unaffected postprandial secretion of CCK and probably other incretins may explain the quantitatively unchanged insulin response. Although the data on the incretin effect of CCK are still controversial, some authors have reported a modulating role of CCK in the release of insulin after administration of a test meal in man [17, 18] as well as in dogs [19, 20]. The importance of leaving the duodenum in situ for optimal CCK release is supported by the study of Inoue et al. [21]. They found a decrease in integrated CCK response to a test meal after Whipple's operation. If the continuity of the gastrointestinal tract was restored by a B_I-type anastomosis between the gastric remnant and proximal duodenum this decrease was less pronounced than after B_{II}-type reconstruction. In duodenum-preserving resection of the pancreatic head as performed in our study no effect of operation on meal-stimulated CCK release has been observed.

The meal-stimulated insulin release may be quantitatively unaffected in this experiment, possibly as a result of intact postprandial CCK release, the insulin secreted being insufficient to provide for normal glucose tolerance as reflected by an increase in integrated glucose response after test meal administration. Glucose insensitivity or ineffective insulin delivery may be responsible for this finding. Pulsatile insulin delivery seems an important mechanism for optimal glucose uptake by the peripheral tissue and there are data to stress that an intrinsic pancreatic neural network plays an important role in the regulation of pulsatile insulin delivery [22, 23]. Destruction of islet architecture by ductobliteration with subsequent intrinsic denervation may be the mechanism responsible for interference with pulsatile insulin delivery and decrease in glucose tolerance in combination with a quantitatively normal insulin response. Although the meal-stimulated insulin and glucagon response are left unaffected, an almost complete abolishment of the PP response is observed. The explanation for this finding may be threefold. With the operation performed, the PP-rich right lobe of the pancreas is removed and vagal denervation of the left lobe is a consequence of removal of the right lobe since the majority of the parasympathetic nerves enter the pancreas through a plexus localized in the duodenal flexure [24]. All these fibers are transected when the right lobe is taken out and, since vagal stimulation is the main drive for PP secretion, a significant decrease in PP response is the understandable consequence of the operation. Additionally, we have previously observed that, after removal of the right pancreatic lobe, high PP concentrations can still be measured in the splenic vein [25]. This indicates that the left lobe is containing and still secreting PP but that these cells are relatively insensitive to stimulation. Intact humoral stimulation mechanisms and an intact CCK response may explain the presence of a minimal PP response at 6 and 12 weeks. Our study indicates that preservation of the duodenum in the case of resection of the pancreatic head (with or without autotransplantation) interferes less with CCK and pancreatic hormone release than cephalic pancreaticoduodenectomy with either B_I- or B_{II}-type reconstruction. Whether this pays in terms of decreased postoperative morbidity remains to be established in detailed clinical studies.

Acknowledgments. The technical assistance of Mrs. K. H. van der Nat-van der Mey, Ms. G. M. van Brakel, Mr. H. F. Dudart, I. van Starkenburg, and Mr. J. P. Gilliams is gratefully acknowledged. The authors thank Ms J. F. N. Visser for typing the manuscript.

524   H. G. Gooszen et al.

References

1. Gooszen HG, Schmidt JH, van Heurn LWE, Terpstra JL, Jansen JBMJ, Lamers CBHW (1989) The effectiveness of operative treatment for pain relief in chronic pancreatitis. Scand J Gastroenterol (in press)
2. Rossi RL, Soeldner JS, Braasch JW, et al. (1986) Segmental pancreatic autotransplantation with pancreatic ductal occlusion after near total or total pancreatic resection for chronic pancreatitis. Ann Surg 203:626–636
3. Berson SA, Yalow RS (1959) Quantitative aspects of the reaction between insulin and insulin-binding antibody. J Clin Invest 38:1996–2000
4. Lamers CBHW, Diemel JM, van Leer E, van Lensen R, Peetoom J (1982) Mechanisms of elevated serum. Pancreatic polypeptide concentrations in chronic renal failure. J Clin Endocrinol Metab 55:922–926
5. Jansen JBMJ, Lamers CBHW (1983) Molecular forms of cholecystokinin in human plasma during infusion of bobesin. Life Sci 33:2197–205
6. Baumgartner D, Sutherland DER, Najarian JS (1980) Studies on segmental pancreatic autotransplants in dogs. Transplant Proc [Suppl 2] 12:163–171
7. Cutfield RG, Kyriakides GK, Olsou L, Condie RM, Mintz DH, Miller J (1984) Late observations of canine segmental pancreatic autografts. Transplant Proc 16:762–763
8. Jonung M, Berlatzky Y, Chen MH, et al. (1984) Appraisal of endocrine function of segmental autotransplanted pancreas in dogs. Acta Endocrinol (Copenh) 105:72–77
9. Calhoun P, Brown KS, Krusch DA, et al. (1986) Evaluation of insulin secretion after pancreas autotransplantation by oral or inravenous glucose challenge. Ann Surg 204:585–593
10. Gooszen HG, van Schilfgaarde R, Frölich M, Cramer-Knijnenburg GF, van der Burg MPM (1984) Long-term function of in situ autografted, ductobliterated canine left pancreatic segments. Transplant Proc 16:766–768
11. Gooszen HG, van Schilfgaarde R, Frölich M, van der Burg MPM (1985) The effects of ductobliteration and of autotransplantation on the endocrine function of canine pancreatic segments. Diabetes 34:1008–1013
12. Gooszen HG, van der Burg MPM, Guicherit OR, Jansen JBMJ, van Schilfgaarde R, Lamers CBHW, Frölich M (1989) A crossover study on the effects of ductobliteration, coeliac denervation, and autotransplantation on glucose and meal stimulated insulin, glucagon and pancreatic polypeptide levels. Diabetes [Suppl] 38:114–116
13. Gersell DJ, Gingerich RL, Greider MH (1979) Regional distribution and concentration of pancreatic polypeptide in the human and canine pancreas. Diabetes 28:11–15
14. Frölich M, van der Burg MPM, Gooszen HG, Jansen JBMJ, Lamers CBHW (1989) Distribution of insulin, glucagon, pancreatic polypeptide and somatostatin in the canine pancreas. Diabetes [Suppl 1] 38:257
15. Gooszen HG, Bosman FT, van Schilfgaarde R (1984) The effect of ductobliteration on the histology and endocrine function of the canine pancreas. Transplantation 38:13–17
16. Gooszen HG, van Schilfgaarde R, van der Burg MPM, Lawick van Pabst WP, Frölich M, Bosman FT (1988) Quantitative assessment of changes in insulin secretion after canine ductobliterated pancreas transplantation in relation to their histological background. Transplantation 46:793–799
17. Rushakoff RJ, Goldfine ID, Carter JD, Liddle RA (1987) Physiological concentrations of cholecystokinin stimulate amino acid-induced insulin release in humans. J Clin Endocrinol Metab 65:395–401
18. Schusdziarra U, Lenx N, Schick R, Maier U (1986) Modulatory effect of glucose, amino acids, and secretin on CCK-8-induced somatostatin and pancreatic polypeptide release in dogs. Diabetes 35:523–529
19. Frame CM, Davidson MB, Sturdevant RAL (1975) Effects of the octapeptide of cholecystokinin on insulin and glucagon secretion in the dog. Endocrinology 97:549–553
20. Meyer FD, Gyr K, Häcki WH, Beglinger C, Jeker L, Varga L, Kayasseh L, Gillessen D, Stalder GA (1981) The release of pancreatic polypeptide by CCK-octapeptide and some analogues in the dog. Gastroenterology 80:742–747

21. Inoue K, Tobe T, Suzuki T, Hosotani R, Kogire M, Fuchigami A, Miyashita T, Tsuda K, Seino Y (1987) Plasma cholecystokinin and pancreatic polypeptide response after radical pancreatoduodenectomy with Billroth I and Billroth II type of reconstruction. Ann Surg 206:148–154
22. Weigle DS (1987) Pulsatile secretion of fuel-regulatory hormones. Diabetes 36:764–775
23. Opara EC, Atwater I, Go VLW (1988) Characterization and control of pulsatile secretion of insulin and glucagon. Pancreas 3:484–487
24. Tiscornia OM, Martinez JL, Sarles H (1976) Some aspects of human and canine macroscopic pancreas innervation. Am J Gastroenterol 66:353–361
25. Gooszen HG, Jansen JBMJ, van Suylichem PTR, van Haastert FA, Guicherit OR, van der Burg MPM, van Schilfgaarde R, Lamers CBHW (1986) Are intra-insular pancreatic polypeptide producing cells not reactive to bombesin stimulation (Abstr)? Digestion 35:25

Duodenum-Preserving Resection of the Head of the Pancreas: A 20-Year Experience

R. Bittner, M. Büchler, and H. G. Beger[1]

Opinions are divided on the surgical therapy of chronic pancreatitis. It is feared, on the one hand, that resective procedures cannot prevent chronic destruction of the gland, and moreover that they lead to an acute deterioration of endocrine and exocrine capacity. On the other hand, there is no doubt that surgical therapy is the only remedy for a considerable number of patients.

Some 20% of patients with chronic pancreatitis develop an inflammatory mass at the head of the pancreas [1]. In more than 80% of these patients (predominantly males under 45 years of age) it is caused by ethyl toxicity. Almost all these patients suffer from severe, medically intractable pain. Stenosis of the common bile duct with concomitant elevation of cholestatic parameters, and in some cases even jaundice, occurs frequently. Compression of the duodenum or the portal vein and thrombosis with portal hypertension are also observed quite often. Obstruction or stenosis of the Wirsung's duct is encountered in over 90% of these patients.

In general, surgical management is indicated in cases where the patient suffers from medically intractable pain, or when one or more of the above mentioned complications caused by the inflammatory mass are observed. Partial duodenopancreatectomy, i. e. Whipple's operation, is the standard surgical procedure even today, except when patients present with a significant enlargement of the pancreatic duct (> 7–8 mm).

Whipple's operation, however, includes not only resection of the pancreatic head but also resection of two-thirds of the stomach, the duodenum, and the common bile duct. Mortality and morbidity rates following this operation cannot be disregarded, although some improvement has been reported more recently. To avoid the disadvantages implicit in Whipple's operation – in particular removal of the duodenum, which plays a major role in the intake of food and its utilisation – a duodenum-preserving resection of the head of the pancreas was introduced into clinical practice in 1972 [2].

Duodenum-preserving resection of the head of the pancreas (DPRHP) seeks to relieve patients of their pain by removing the inflammatory tumour in the pancreatic head, provide decompression of the common bile duct; restore pancreatico-intestinal secretory flow; and last but not least protect endocrine capacity. This new surgical procedure is characterized by its very low morbidity and mortality.

The present study – partly retrospective and partly prospective – was designed to investigate to what extent these goals have actually been achieved. A separate, experimental investigation focused on possible alterations of the endocrine capacity resulting from DPRHP.

[1] Department of General Surgery, University of Ulm, Steinhövelstrasse 9, 7900 Ulm, W-Germany

Chronic Pancreatitis
Ed. by Beger, Büchler, Ditschuneit, and Malfertheiner
© Springer-Verlag Berlin Heidelberg 1990

Surgical Techniques of Duodenum-Preserving Resection

The surgical procedure includes two major steps [3]. The first is transection of the pancreas at the border between the head and the body and subtotal resection of the head of the pancreas. The remaining small disk-like head of the pancreas (5–8 mm) between the common bile duct and the duodenal wall maintains the blood supply to the duodenum. The fibrotic, tumorous-type tissue in the central sections of the pancreatic head is completely removed so that the anterior part of the common bile duct is freely accessible. The second important operative step is restoration of the pancreatic secretory flow from the left pancreas into the upper intestinum by interposition of a jejunal loop, preserving the gastroduodenal unit and its food passage (Fig. 1).

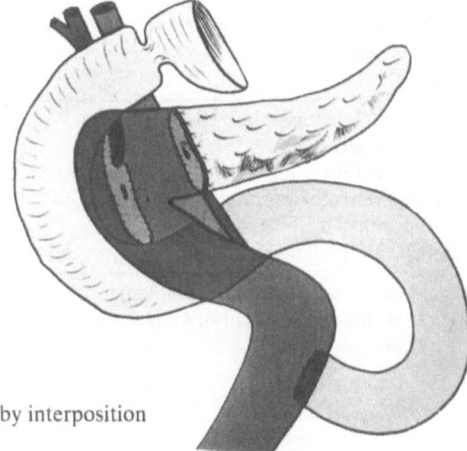

Fig. 1. Restoration of pancreatic secretory flow by interposition of a jejunal loop

Patient Population and Preoperative Morbidity

Since 1972, DPRHP has been performed in 141 of 148 patients with an inflammatory mass in the pancreatic head. Whipple's operation was necessary in only seven patients. Chronic pancreatitis was associated with alcohol consumption in 82% of the patients and was due to a biliary disease in only 11%. The median time interval from onset of symptoms to surgery was 3.6 years (2 months to 15 years). A total of 80% of patients experienced daily, sometimes severe pain. Cholestasis was demonstrated in 60% of the patients, obstruction of the duodenum in 11.4%, and some degree of portal hypertension in 13% (Table 1).

Insulin-dependent diabetes mellitus was present in 21% of the patients at the time of operation.

Special Modification of the Standard Operative Procedure

Where decompression of the stenosed intrapancreatic segment of the common bile duct is not possible because of severe intramural fibrotic development, the incision is

Table 1. Morbidity in 141 patients with chronic pancreatitis and an inflammatory mass in the head of the pancreas. Preoperative and intraoperative observations

	Patients (n)	Frequency (%)
Stenosis of the common bile duct[a]	84/141	59.6
cholestasis	37/ 84	
jaundice	47/ 84	
Stenosis of the duodenum[b]	48/132	11.4
slight/moderate	33/ 48	
severe	15/ 48	
Portal hypertension[c]	25/141	12.8
PV[d] compression	16/ 25	
PV thrombosis	2/ 25	
liver cirrhosis	7/ 25	
Stenosis of the pancreatic duct[e]	141/141	37.6
single, head	53/141	
multiple	88/141	

[a] ERCP/cholangiography; cholestasis. alk. phosphatase $> 2 \times$ the norm; jaundice, bilirubin > 1.2 µmol/dl
[b] hypotonic duodenography in 132 patients
[c] intraoperatively observed 11/25 patients
[d] portal vein
[e] ERCP, 132 patients; intraoperatively evaluated 9 patients

ERCP, endoscopic retrograde cholangiopancreatography
Data from the Department of General Surgery, University of Ulm, Federal Republic of Germany, June 1988

extended to the dilatated area. Subsequently, the upper circumference of the opened duct is included in the end-to-side anastomosis of the pancreatic head and interposed jejunal loop. Fourteen of 84 patients required such a modification of the DPRHP.

When the pancreatic duct exhibits multiple stenoses or stones in the body and tail area, it is longitudinally incised and reconstruction is performed by a Puestow modification, i. e. placement of longitudinal pancreaticojejunostomy instead of end-to-end anastomosis to the pancreatic body (Fig. 2).

Early Postoperative Complications

The most frequently observed early postoperative complication was an episode of pancreatitis which occurred in 14 of 141 patients. In 8% of the patients, there was an intestinal haemorrhage from the cut surface of the pancreas. Three patients developed leakage of the pancreatic anastomosis with fistulization; in 1 patient a duodenal fistula occurred. Nine of 141 patients had to be reoperated. The median hospitalization time was 15 days. One of the 141 patients died on the 9th postoperative day because of a fulminant pulmonary embolism.

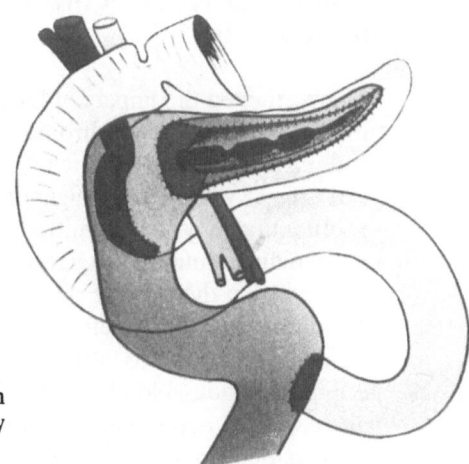

Fig. 2. When the pancreatic duct shows multiple stenoses in the body and tail area, restoration of pancreatic secretory flow is performed via a Puestow modification

Late Results after Duodenum-Preserving Resection

After a median follow-up period of 3.6 years (range 3 months to 16 years), 77% of the patients were free of abdominal pain and 12% complained occasionally of abdominal pain, while 11% continued to suffer frequently from attacks of pain (Table 2). In only 11% of 109 patients was further hospitalization necessary due to an acute attack of the underlying pancreatitis. Regarding glucose metabolism, 84% of the patients demonstrated stable glucose metabolism. In 11%, glucose metabolism deteriorated, and in 5% it showed improvement. An increase in weight was exhibited by 80% of patients (median 8.7 kg). About 18% had the same body weight as preoperatively, and only 2% of 109 patients showed weight loss. Occupational integration was appraised for 101 patients; 67% of the patients had complete professional rehabilitation, 20% were in a state of limited or full retirement, and 13% were unemployed (Table 2). Late postoperative mortality was 5%.

Table 2. Late results after duodenum-preserving resection of the head of the pancreas

	Patients (n)	(%)
Abdominal pain		
free	84/109	77
seldom	13/109	12
frequent	12/109	11
Professional rehabilitation[a]		
complete	68/101	67
unemployed	13/101	13
full/limited retirement	20/101	20

[a] Date: Dec. 31, 1987; 109 patients followed-up (96%)
patients ≥ 6 mo postoperatively:
       6 mo–1 year, 20%
       1– 2 year, 15%
       2– 3 year, 15%
       3–16 year, 50%

Clinical Experimental Investigation on the Endocrine Function after DPRHP

We investigated the impact of DPRHP on glucose tolerance and endocrine pancreas function in patients with chronic pancreatitis and inflammatory mass in the pancreas head. Fifteen patients (14 males, 1 female) entered the study; the mean age was 47.5 years (36–65 years), and weight 61.5 kg (42.6–79 kg). The patients were examined in the order that they were admitted to hospital for the DPRHP procedure. Patients with known diabetes mellitus or a fasting blood sugar of over 120 mg/dl on admission were excluded from the study. Endocrine function was studied using oral and intravenous glucose tolerance tests before the operation, on the 10th or 11th postoperative day, and at least 3 months after the operation. In addition to glucose levels in the peripheral venous blood, levels of insulin, C-peptide, glucagon, somatostatin, and pancreatic polypeptide were determined.

One patient (6.6%) developed diabetes mellitus immediately postoperatively and was excluded from further tests.

As indicated by the k-value, glucose tolerance improved in 11 patients (73.3%), two patients (13.3%) showed no postoperative change, and one (6.6%) was worse. The pre- and postoperative levels of insulin and C-peptide showed no significant differences. The fasting levels of glucagon and somatostatin were significantly lower postoperatively than before the operation ($p < 0.01$). The stimulation of pancreatic polypeptide after oral glucose was significantly lower postoperatively ($p < 0.01$). According to these results, improved glucose tolerance is not due to increased insulin secretion but rather to a normalization of the preoperative concentrations of the antiinsulin hormones glucagon and somatostatin [4].

Discussion

Chronic pancreatitis is characterized by a painful progressive destruction of the gland with increasing loss of exocrine and endocrine function. Surgery is only indicated by local complications in the pancreatic head area, such as compression of the common bile duct or the duodenum, or in case of medically intractable pain. In contrast to Whipple's operation, the major advantage of DPRHP is the limited resection, the objective of which is the removal of only the inflammatory tumour in the pancreatic head. In this way, preservation of the duodenum in the food passage and, consequently, the synergism of the upper abdominal organs are secured. In light of these facts, the duodenum-preserving resection of the pancreatic head presents an organ-saving alternative to Whipple's operation. Our large patient population indicates that both early and late postoperative morbidity and mortality are relatively low.

Diabetes mellitus is a major problem following resective surgical procedures, and its incidence after Whipple's operation is reported to range between 20% and 40% [5, 6]. By contrast, development of diabetes mellitus was seen in only 10% of all of our patients with DPRHP. It is particularly remarkable that of the patients investigated in the prospective study, 70% experienced an improvement in glucose tolerance, suggesting that preservation of the duodenum and thus the enteroinsular axis might be responsible. At least 50% of total insulin secretion in response to a defined glucose stimulus is caused by intestinal stimulation of the beta cells [7].

Although the loss of pancreatic parenchyma in DPRHP is similar to that in Whipple's operation, the nutritional functions of the duodenum are preserved, as are consequently the complex neurohumoral regulatory mechanisms of food consumption and metabolism.

References

1. Beger HG, Krautzberger W, Bittner R, Büchler M, Limmer J (1985) Duodenum-preserving resection of the head of the pancreas in patients with severe chronic pancreatitis. Surgery 97:467
2. Beger HG, Witte C, Krautzberger W, Bittner R (1980) Erfahrung mit einer das Duodenum erhaltenden Pankreaskopfresektion bei chronischer Pankreatitis. Chirurg 51:303
3. Beger HG (1987) Die duodenumerhaltende Pankreaskopfresektion bei chronischer Pankreatitis. Langenbecks Arch Chir 372:357
4. Bittner R, Butters M, Büchler M, Nägele S, Roscher R, Beger HG (1988) Glucose homeostasis and endocrine pancreatic secretion in patients with chronic pancreatitis before and after surgical therapy. Biomed Res 9:28
5. Frey C, Child CG, Frey W (1976) Pancreatectomy for chronic pancreatitis. Ann Surg 184:403
6. Lankisch PG, Fuchs K, Peiper HF, Creutzfeld W (1981) Pancreatic function after drainage or resection for chronic pancreatitis. In: Mitchel CJ, Kallcher L (eds) Pancreatic disease in clinical practice. Pitman, London, pp 362–369
7. Bittner R, Butters M, Ebert R, Beger HG (1988) Entero-insular axis and surgical trauma. Scand J Gastroenterol 23:633

Duodenum-Preserving Resection of the Head of the Pancreas in Treatment of Chronic Pancreatitis: The Munich Experience

D. K. Wilker, L. Schweiberer, W.-T. Knoefel, J. R. Izbicki, K. Geissler, and B. Eibl-Eibesfeldt[1]

Introduction

The surgical approach to chronic pancreatitis is by either drainage operation or resection [4, 7]. If the entire pancreas is affected by the chronic inflammation, only drainage procedures such as the Puestow-Mercadier procedure [9], possibly combined with biliary-enteric anastomosis are indicated. By contrast, in localized chronic pancreatitis resection procedures should be favored. Distal resection is indicated if the chronic inflammatory process is confined to the tail of the pancreas. Patients with predominant involvement of the head of the pancreas should undergo proximal resection. The most commonly performed proximal resection is a partial pancreatoduodenectomy [14]. The sacrifice of adjacent structures, i.e., distal stomach, distal common duct, duodenum, and first jejunal loop, which are not diseased, is the major disadvantage of this procedure.

In order to minimize this sacrifice stomach-preserving resections of the head of the pancreas were developed [11]. The subtotal resection of the pancreas, where only a small part of the pancreas is left in the duodenal knee [5], is aimed at the same goal. A new step towards structure-preserving surgery of the pancreas was the duodenum-preserving resection of the head of the pancreas [2, 3, 6]. We report on our experience with this procedure in treatment of chronic pancreatitis of the head of the pancreas.

Patients and Methods

Between 1984 and 1988, 24 patients with chronic pancreatitis located predominantly in the head of the pancreas were treated by duodenum-preserving resection of the head of the pancreas. Of these 24 patients 20 were men and 4 were women. Ages ranged from 28 to 58 years with an average of 41. The time interval between onset of symptoms of pancreatitis and surgery varied from 12 months to 8 years with an average of 3.9. Twenty-two patients had a history of heavy alcohol ingestion. In two patients an alcoholic or biliary etiology could be ruled out, and the pancreatitis was considered to be of idiopathic origin.

[1] Department of Surgery, University of Munich, Nussbaumstrasse 20, 8000 Munich 2, FRG

Chronic Pancreatitis
Ed. by Beger, Büchler, Ditschuneit, and Malfertheiner
© Springer-Verlag Berlin Heidelberg 1990

Preoperative Assessment

Preoperative assessment in all patients included abdominal ultrasound and computed tomography of the abdomen. Endoscopic retrograde cholangiopancreatography was performed in 17 patients, upper GI series in 9, and digital subtraction angiography (DSA) in 6. All patients presented with severe abdominal pain due to chronic pancreatitis and tumorous enlargement of the pancreatic head. All required frequent treatment with analgetics, and some had severe analgetic abuse. At the time of operation 8 patients presented with obstructive jaundice, 17 had pancreatic calcification, and 3 suffered from duodenal obstruction. In three patients DSA revealed compression of the portal vein with segmental portal hypertension.

Operative Procedure

The technique of the stomach- and duodenum-preserving resection of the pancreatic head has been extensively described by Beger et al. [2, 3]. Our modification is an initial choledochotomy and insertion of a metal bile duct probe for identification of the intrapancreatic common bile duct. In our experience this facilitates an effective decompression of the common bile duct.

Postoperative Assessment and Follow-Up

The postoperative course of all 24 patients was evaluated for mortality, postoperative complications, and hospitalization period. Every patient was reassessed in our out-patient clinic. Follow-up ranged from 9 months to 5 years postoperatively, with an average of 31 months. Patient responses to operation were evaluated by direct examination and communication with referring physicians. Relief of obstructive jaundice was evaluated by ultrasonographic assessment of the width of the common bile duct and postoperative course of alkaline phosphatase. Occupational rehabilitation, development of diabetes mellitus, and weight gain were other parameters.

Results

There was no surgical mortality in the 24 patients who underwent duodenum-preserving pancreatic head resection.

In the immediate 30-day postoperative period one patient developed pneumonia which was treated successfully by antibiotics. One patient developed a perforation of the duodenum which required reoperation. Two patients exhibited bleeding from the resection site, which was treated conservatively. In one patient a cholangitis developed as well as a pancreatic fistula. Both were successfully treated by conservative means.

In the late postoperative period one patient developed a stenosis of the common bile duct which was treated by percutaneous dilatation. Three patients suffered from another attack of pancreatitis in the tail.

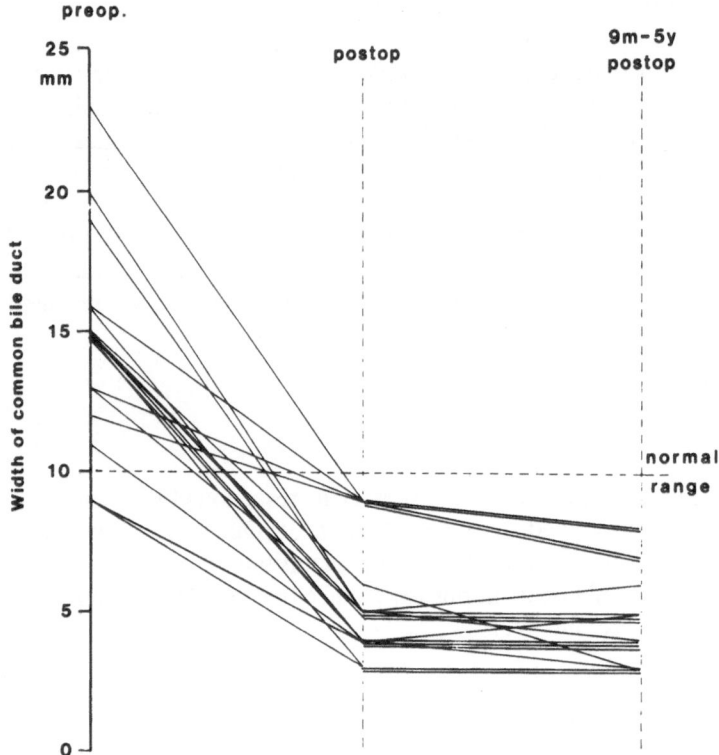

Fig. 1. Ultrasonographic assessment of the width of the common bile duct. Only patients with stenosis of the common bile duct are included

The overall mortality rate in this follow-up period was three of 24 patients. One patient died in a hypoglycemic shock 4 years postoperatively. He was an insulin-dependent diabetic and alcohol intoxicated when he became hypoglycemic. One committed suicide 5 years postoperatively but had had no recurrence of pancreatitis. The third patient died 5 years postoperatively of metastatic bronchial carcinoma.

Figure 1 shows the ultrasonographic assessment of the width of the common bile duct. In all but two patients the common bile duct had a width of more than 10 mm preoperatively. The operation led to an effective and permanent decompression of the common duct in all patients. This is also reflected by the postoperative decrease of serum alkaline phosphatase, which is shown in Fig. 2.

In two of eight diabetic patients a change in the diabetic state was observed. One patient exhibited a marked improvement, whereas the diabetic state in one patient deteriorated (Fig. 3).

In the follow-up period 22 patients have become asymptomatic. In these patients pain had been eliminated after the operation, except for four patients who experienced pain when not keeping to their diet (e.g., heavy alcohol ingestion, major amounts of fat). This was considered a good response. Two patients complained of mild attacks of pain, which were occurred less often than once a week. This was judged to be a fair response to the operation.

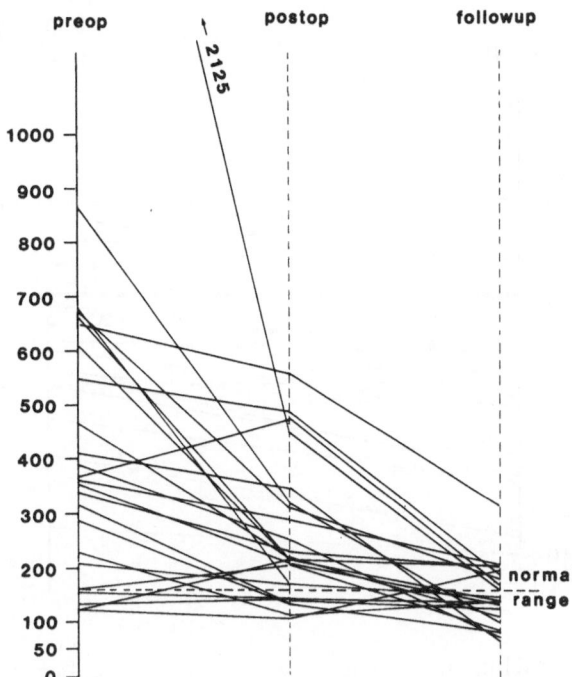

Fig. 2. Pre- and postoperative alkaline phosphatase

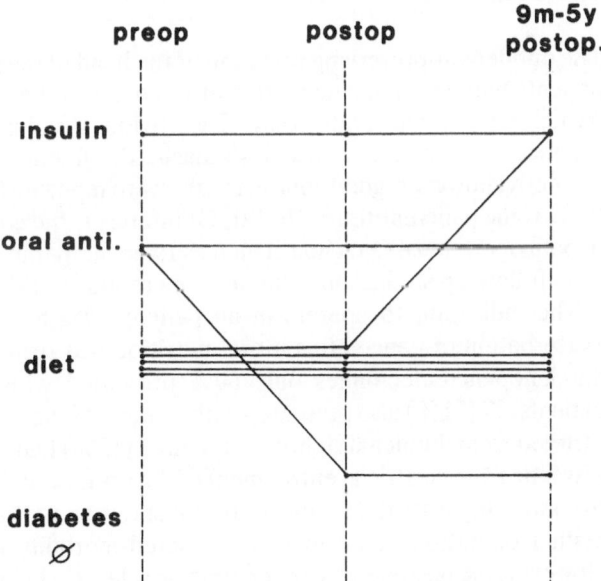

Fig. 3. Glucose metabolism in diabetic patients. Patients with normal glucose metabolism pre- and postoperative are not included. (*Oral anti.*, patient on oral antidiabetics)

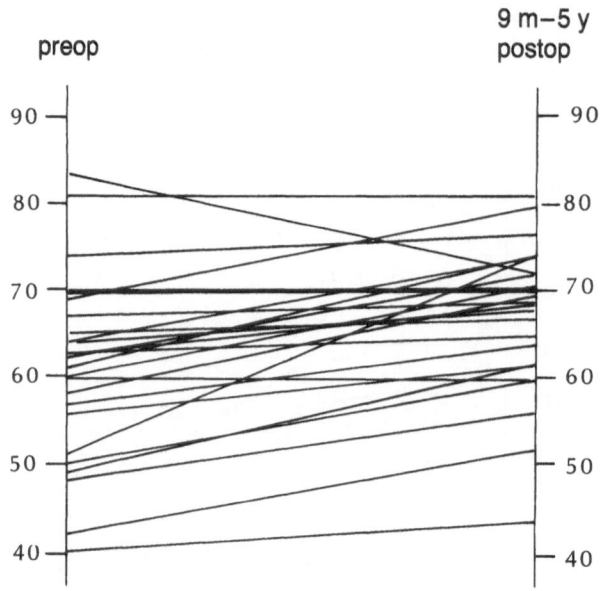

Fig. 4. Patients' weight gain after duodenum-preserving resection of the head of the pancreas for chronic pancreatitis

All but one patient gained in body weight after the operation; this increase in body weight averaged 12% of the preoperatively measured body weight (Fig. 4). Assessment of occupational rehabilitation showed that 20 patients have a full-time job after the operation; it must be mentioned that 2 of these 20 patients were on social welfare before the operation. Four patients retired after the operation; one of these has a part-time job.

Discussion

The duodenum-preserving resection of the head of the pancreas is one alternative for patients with chronic pancreatitis of the head of the pancreas. Another option is a partial duodenopancreatectomy. The obvious disadvantage of this procedure is the sacrifice of duodenum, distal stomach, distal bile duct, and first jejunal loop. Recently, however, good clinical results were reported following Whipple's operation for chronic pancreatitis [8, 10, 12]. Of interest is the comparison of long-term results of both operations. Our clinical material was comparable to that of retrospective long-term follow-up studies on Whipple's operation [8, 12].

The indication to operate in all patients was heavy persistent pain with acute exacerbation of pancreatitis if oral nutrition was restarted. In comparable series of duodenopancreatectomies only 60% presented with persistent pain [8]. Of our patients, 17 (71%) also presented with stenosis of the common bile duct. Three (13%) suffered from duodenal stenosis, and three (13%) had segmental portal hypertension resulting from cicatricial entrapment of the portal vein [13]. Early and late postoperative mortality was comparable to recent series on partial duodenopancreatectomy as neither operation- nor pancreatitis-related mortality was seen in the past 5 years. However, the postoperative complication rate was slightly higher following Whipple's operation. Major nonsurgical complications such as bronchopneumonia were seen after partial duodenopancreatectomy in 9%, among our patients in only 4% (one patient). Surgical complications after partial duodenopancreatectomy occurred in 24%, two-thirds of whom required relaparotomy. Following duodenum-preserving resection of the head of the pancreas four patients (16%) developed surgical complications, and only one patient (4%) required relaparotomy for an early postoperative complication. This patient on admission had a duodenal stenosis and developed ischemic problems of the duodenum intraoperatively; finally, duodenal insufficiency urged us to relaparotomy.

Recurrence of pancreatitis is a well-known risk in all operative procedures for chronic pancreatitis but in total pancreatectomy. Our rate of pancreatitis of the tail was 13%. However, only one patient underwent surgery, and all of these patients were asymptomatic at the latest follow-up. Pancreatitis of the tail was reported at comparable rates after duodenopancreatectomy [8, 12]. Especially in view of the chronicity of alcohol abuse of most patients recurrence of pancreatitis is not surprising [1].

The only other late postoperative complication was a symptomatic common bile duct stenosis. It was treated by percutaneous transhepatic bile duct dilation. In this case the common bile duct was severely obstructed by the inflammatory tumor. Thus a resection of the intrapancreatic common duct was performed as recommended in the original description of this procedure [2]. In order to avoid this and to preserve the intrapancreatic common bile duct we modified the operation. We perform a choledochotomy and insert a metal bile duct probe before we start to resect the head of the pancreas. This enables us to identify the intrapancreatic common bile duct in order to prevent an injury. Thus, decompression of the common duct is facilitated. To avoid postoperative cholestasis due to edema of the common bile duct, a T-tube was inserted in all cases. Although two patients had nearly complete obstruction of the common bile duct no biliary-enteric anastomosis was necessary. Our follow-up showed normal values for the width of the common bile duct in all patients. Even the patient after percutaneous transhepatic dilation is now asymptomatic for 4 years. In view of the risks of a biliodigestive anastomosis the insertion of a bile duct probe seems to be an important modification for long-term survivors. Although the mentioned retrospective studies on partial duodenopancreatectomy found late postoperative complications neither from choledocho-jejunostomy nor from gastro-jejunostomy, these complications are known from other operations involving these procedures.

The most important parameter for the patient is whether he is free of symptoms or not. Among our 24 patients only two (8%) complained of having minor symptoms less often than once a week. The others were completely asymptomatic except for four patients having mild symptoms when not keeping to their diet. Following partial duodenopancreatectomy 11% continued to have significant symptoms that were less heavy than before the operation, however, rather frequently [8].

After duodenopancreatectomy the glucose tolerance usually deteriorates [8]. This is not seen after duodenum-preserving resection of the head of the pancreas. Among our patients one became insulin dependent after surgery. One was on oral antidiabetics before the operation and being without a diet postoperatively has no glucosuria. In all other patients the glucose metabolism did not change.

Another important parameter in long-term results is the social function that patients achieve after treatment. After duodenopancreatectomy not more than 50% of patients can be expected to work again [8]. Our experience with the duodenum-preserving resection is that 83% of patients have a full-time job after the operation, and 75% have the same or an equivalent job as before the first manifestation of pancreatitis. This strongly advocates the duodenum-preserving resection of the head of the pancreas.

Comparison of duodenum-preserving resection of the head of the pancreas and partial duodenopancreatectomy for severe chronic pancreatitis of the head of the pancreas shows that both operations can alleviate the majority of symptoms. Complication rates are grossly comparable. The following guidelines for comparing the two procedures should be considered in surgery of the pancreas:
1. To have a low rate of recurrence of pancreatitis
2. To preserve as much pancreatic tissue as possible for endocrine and exocrine function
3. To preserve neighboring structures
4. To provide the highest possible quality of life.

In terms of these criteria the duodenum-preserving procedure seems to be superior to partial duodenopancreatectomy.

References

1. Ammann RW, Akovbiantz A, Lardiader F, et al. (1984) Course and outcome of chronic pancreatitis: longitudinal study of a mixed medical-surgical series of 245 patients. Gastroenterology 86:820–828
2. Beger HG, Witte J, Kraas E, Bittner R (1980) Erfahrung mit einer das Duodenum erhaltenden Pankreaskopfresektion bei chronischer Pankreatitis. Chirurg 51:303
3. Beger HG, Krautzberger W, Bittner R et al. (1985) Duodenum-preserving resection of the head of the pancreas in patients with severe chronic pancreatitis. Surgery 97:467–473
4. Bradley EL III (1987) Long-term results of pancreatojejunostomy in patients with chronic pancreatitis. Am J Surg 153:207–213
5. Child CG, Frey CF, Fry W (1969) A reappraisal of removal of 95% of the distal portion of the pancreas. Surg Gynecol Obstet 129:49–56
6. Frey CF, Smith GJ (1987) Description and rationale of a new operation for chronic pancreatitis. Pancreas 6:701–707
7. Frey CF, Child CG III, Fry W (1976) Pancreatectomy for chronic pancreatitis. Ann Surg 184:403–414
8. Gall FP (1987) Chirurgische Therapie durch Resektionsverfahren (Kongreßbericht). Langenbecks Arch Chir 372:363–368
9. Puestow CB, Gillesby WJ (1958) Retrograde surgical drainage of pancreas for chronic relapsing pancreatitis. Report of 142 cases. Arch Surg 76:898–906
10. Rossi RL, Rothschild J, Braasch JW, et al. (1987) Pancreatoduodenectomy in the management of chronic pancreatitis. Arch Surg 122:416–420
11. Traverso LW, Longmire WP (1978) Preservation of the pylorus during pancreaticoduodenectomy. Surg Gynecol Obstet 146:959–862
12. Trede M, Schwall G (1988) The complications of pancreatectomy. Ann Surg 207:39–47
13. Warshaw AL, Jin G, Ottinger LW (1987) Recognition and clinical implications of mesenteric and portal vein obstruction in chronic pancreatitis. Arch Surg 122:410–415
14. Whipple AO, Pearson WB, Muullius CR (1935) Treatment of carcinoma of the ampulla of Vater. Ann Surg 102:763–779

Preservation of the Duodenum in Total Pancreatectomy for Chronic Pancreatitis

R. C. G. RUSSELL[1]

Introduction

To date the role of surgery in the management of chronic pancreatitis is debatable [1]. Undoubtedly, a conservative treatment is preferable for the primary management, and surgery should be reserved for the complications of chronic pancreatitis. Unfortunately, the clinical problem is that of a patient with severe pain, often on an increasing dose of analgesics and whose life quality is destroyed by the effects of both pain and analgesics. There is a group of patients who fail to respond or who relapse after non-surgical procedures, such as, nerve blocks or endoscopic sphincterotomies; among these there are some whose clinical features are not helped by subtotal pancreatectomy or a drainage procedure. In the patient with pancreatic pain which has not responded to other surgical measures, including resection, the question of total pancreatectomy arises. In fact, for the failures of partial pancreatectomy, there is little more to offer the patient than ablation of the pancreas.

In the management of a benign disease, it is appropriate, when considering major ablative resection, to minimise the consequences which follow such an operation. For instance, when Whipple [2] in 1946 introduced resection of the head of the pancreas, he resected the pylorus and left the antrum and stomach largely intact. However, Warren [3] showed that this original procedure had a 17% incidence of anastomotic ulceration, and that by incorporating a more radical gastrectomy, with or without vagotomy, the duodenal ulcer rate was reduced to 7.5%. Unfortunately, partial gastrectomy is associated with significant morbidity in terms of dyspepsia, diarrhoea and the dumping syndrome. On account of dissatisfaction with the quality of life achieved by a pancreatoduodenectomy, Traverso and Longmire [4, 5] introduced the pylorus-preserving pancreatoduodenectomy. However, pylorus preservation involves duodenal resection with loss of the alkaline duodenal secretions which may prevent duodenal ulceration. Both Traverso et al. [6] and Newman et al. [7] have reported patients suffering acute upper gastrointestinal bleeding following the pylorus-preserving procedure.

In order to overcome the disadvantage of removal of the duodenum a subtotal resection of the head of the pancreas with duodenal preservation was introduced by Beger et al. [8]. It was apparent that the rim of pancreatic tissue maintained around the inner border of the C loop of the duodenum maintained the viability of the duodenum due to the preservation of the arcade of vessels which runs within the

---

[1] Middlesex Hospital, London W1N 8AA, UK

Chronic Pancreatitis
Ed. by Beger, Büchler, Ditschuneit, and Malfertheiner
© Springer-Verlag Berlin Heidelberg 1990

pancreatic substance. Unfortunately, 14% of these patients have gone on to have further attacks of pancreatitis, and thus it cannot be counted as a true total pancreatectomy.

It was Whipple, in one of his original articles, who said that is was necessary to resect the duodenum because "complete removal of the head of the pancreas so compromises the blood supply to the duodenum as to favour necrosis and fistula formation." [9] Nevertheless, work with children who have nesidioblastosis has shown that a 98% pancreatectomy could be performed with preservation of the duodenum.

Eloy et al., while undertaking experimental work on pancreatic transplantation, simplified the total pancreatectomy animal model and described excising the pancreas by meticulous dissection of the pancreas off the duodenum, leaving the duodenum intact. [9 a] This simplified the animal model as it avoided the usual duodenal resection and major reconstruction involved. Biochemical study of the animals showed no detectable insulin or insulin activity, thereby indicating that the pancreatectomy was complete. Further, the duodenum remained vascularised and appeared to function normally.

Harken et al. in 1971 [10] described a total pancreatectomy performed in infants with idiopathic hypoglycaemia in whom a 50% pancreatectomy had failed to control the symptoms. All the identifiable pancreatic tissue within the C loop of the duodenum was removed. The spleen was preserved, relying on the blood supply via the short gastric vessels. It was apparent that the duodenum would survive after sacrifice of both the superior and inferior pancreatoduodenal arteries. Subsequent descriptions of this procedure by Gough [11] confirmed that this operation was safe in infants, and that it was in fact the only procedure which would satisfactorily relieve the symptoms of infantile hyperinsulinism. My own experience with this procedure in nine infants [12] confirmed that the duodenum could be well separated from the pancreas in the infantile state, and that a plane of cleavage could be developed along the pancreatic border of the duodenum by careful dissection. In the infant, the colour of the duodenum was completely normal at the end of the operation. Further, the growth of these children has remained normal over a 4-year observation period, indicating that there are no major long-term sequelae from this procedure.

Injection studies in the human suggest that there is an arcade of vessels within the mucosa of the duodenum similar to those vessels in the stomach [13]. These injection studies suggested that contrast injected at the superior pancreatoduodenal artery would perfuse through this submucosal plexus down to the fourth part of the duodenum [14]. On the basis of these experimental results on the blood supply of the duodenum, it was felt appropriate to proceed in the young adult with a duodenal-preserving total pancreatectomy in order to reduce the consequences of the loss of the duodenum and pylorus.

At the outset, it was decided that the patients for this operation should be carefully selected and that the ideal subject was the person with a long history of severe pancreatitis with much fibrosis and minimal inflammatory change around the head of the pancreas. With the patient who has a fibrosing reaction to their pancreatic disorder the pancreas occasionally contracts away from the duodenum, giving the surgeon a tissue plane for dissection. The typical patient who has chronic pancreatitis from excess alcohol and has a large inflammatory mass in the head of the pancreas is unsuitable for this procedure; in this instance the vessels cannot be identified, and an accurate dissection is not possible. There are also patients who have minimal-change pancreatitis presenting with severe pain. Such patients, if they cannot be managed by conservative therapy, are suitable candidates for this preservation procedure.

Operative Technique

The pancreas is approached through a long transverse upper abdominal incision, and a full laparotomy is undertaken to assess the extent of disease and its complications. If this assessment suggests that disease is localised to the pancreas with no evidence of complication, and that the operation of duodenal preservation is technically satisfactory, then the pancreas is exposed further by dividing the gastrocolic omentum within the epiploic arch and so opening the lesser sac. If a distal pancreatectomy has not previously been performed, the body and tail of the pancreas are mobilised in the usual way. Having assessed and mobilised the distal pancreas, attention is turned to the head of the pancreas and an assessment made as to whether the vessels to the pancreas can be clearly identified and separated from the duodenum. The superior mesenteric vein and the portal vein should be clearly identified at this stage. The middle colic and left colic vessels should be defined and separated from the inferior border of the pancreas and uncinate process so that they do not become damaged or compromised during the procedure.

The omentum is cleared from the head of the pancreas by dividing the right gastroepiploic artery. The hepatic flexure of the colon and its mesocolon is dissected easily inferiorly, well away from the operating field. The front of the pancreas and the whole of the duodenum should now be clearly exposed and dissection commenced. Before commencing dissection it is essential not to mobilise the head of the duodenum by dividing the peritoneum on the lateral surface of the C loop. Further assessment is made of the pancreas to ensure that a preservation procedure is technically possible, and that there is no inflammatory mass preventing dissection between the duodenum and the pancreas itself.

In order to ease the dissection, if the body and the tail are still present, it is useful to divide the neck of the pancreas with a GIA stapler so that the portal vein is clearly exposed. The portal vein and superior mesenteric vein are dissected free of their branches to the pancreas, so further exposing the vessels and defining their relationship to the pancreatic tissue. The uncinate process of the pancreas at the junction of the duodenum with the mesenteric vessels is inspected and all adhesions from this area divided. A clamp is placed on the apex of the pancreas which is then lifted forwards. With mosquito forceps, each vessel between the pancreas and the duodenum or the pancreas and the mesenteric vessels is dissected out and tied as near to the pancreas as possible. Ties are preferable to ligaclips as they are less prone to slip during handling. The dissection is continued posteriorly to ensure that the duodenum is free from the pancreatic tissue, but this posterior dissection should not be sufficiently deep as to destroy the vessels running on the surface of the posterior aspect of the pancreas and conveying blood from the superior mesenteric artery to the duodenum. The tip of the uncinate process can be brought further fowards and a finger inserted onto the posterior surface of the uncinate process. With the finger lifting the pancreas forward and tensing the vessels it is more easy to dissect out the small vessels passing from the pancreas directly to the superior mesenteric and portal veins. This dissection is continued until the upper border of the pancreas is reached. The dissection is now continued along the fourth part of the duodenum continuing with the left hand to lift forward the pancreas and individual vessels divided up to the point of the entry of the ampulla of Vater. Dissection is difficult near the ampulla of Vater, for the tissue planes at this point between the pancreas and the duodenum are obliterated. When near the ampulla, it is wise to lift the pancreas forward and inspect the posterior part of the pancreas, for occasionally the bile duct lies superficial. Otherwise, in the angle between the first part of the duodenum and the portal vein a dissection is made until the bile duct is found. It is dissected away from both structures. The bile duct is traced down to the ampulla of Vater gently teasing the pancreas off the bile duct and entering the tunnel around the biliary tree. Once the ampulla is reached, it is easy to define the pancreatic duct and continue working the pancreas off the duodenum. Attention is now turned to the attachment of the pancreas to the first and second part of the duodenum. By careful dissection, avoiding the bile duct and the main pancreato-duodenal artery, which is tied as far from the duodenum as possible, the dissection is continued down to the second part of the duodenum at which point the accessory duct may be present. This is dissected out, tied and oversewn. All that remains attaching the pancreas to the duodenum is the segment of tissue between the accessory and main pancreatic ducts. Careful removal by sharp dissection enables a clear dissection of the structures to be achieved.

The duodenum is now carefully inspected to ensure that there are no perforations present. If there is bleeding from the medial wall of the duodenum, it is wise to oversew rather than to use diathermy. The bile duct is inspected to ensure that there are no perforations present; if there are, accurate suture with 6-0 prolene is advised. Packs are now placed on the duodenum and the colour assessed after 5 min in which no handling takes place. There is usually a normal colour of the fourth and second parts of the duodenum, but the third part has a dusky hue. With time this colour resolves, and the duodenum remains viable. Once meticulous haemostasis has been achieved, a drain is placed within the C loop.

The procedure takes between 2.5 and 4.5 h to complete. Intraoperative blood loss varies between 200 and 900 ml (median 550 ml). In two patients, the bile duct has been opened during dissection, and in one the duodenum was opened. The bile duct was repaired with 6-0 polydioxanone and the duodenum with two layers of 3-0 polydiox-anone. In the post-operative period patients are monitored carefully and the arterial PO_2 maintained at a high level to ensure adequate tissue oxygenation. A period of gastric stasis may be encountered post-operatively, and for this gastric aspiration is advised with intravenous infusion. The median time before a return of gastric empty-ing occurs is 14 days and has been as long as 34. The post-operative appearances of the duodenum on barium examination suggests ischaemia, but this appearance returns to normal after a variable period of 2–4 weeks. In one patient, a cannula placed in the gallbladder to monitor the appearance of the bile duct showed gross oedema around the ampulla of Vater with narrowing of the terminal portion of the bile duct, yet returning to a normal appearance within a 6-week period.

Results of Duodenal-Preserving Procedures

Since 1976, 241 patients have had a pancreatic resection for chronic pancreatitis. Of these, 99 have had a proximal pancreatectomy, 133 have had a distal pancreatectomy, and 9 have had a total pancreatectomy primarily. Of the 99 patients who had a proximal resection as their primary treatment 13 have proceeded to a distal pancreatectomy so ablating their pancreas, whilst of the 133 distal pancreatectomies 30 patients have proceeded to a proximal pancreatectomy so ablating their pancreas. Thus, 52 patients have had a total pancreatectomy; of these, 28 patients have had a duodenal-preserving procedure and 24 have had a total pancreatectomy with excision of the duodenum. However, in all 30 duodenal-preserving procedures have been performed, 5 having had a total excision of the pancreas as a one-stage procedure, 20 patients having had a proximal completion pancreatectomy with duodenal preservation and 5 a primary duodenum-preserving proximal pancreatectomy; of these 3 have gone on to develop subsequent symptoms necessitating removal of the distal part of the pancreas.

In the presentation of the results, the outcome of the standard resections is given alongside that of the duodenal-preserving procedures in order to compare the merits of the operations. Table 1 shows that the mean age of the duodenal preservation patients was 33, compared to 38 in the standard total resection. Length of history was similar in both groups, and the aetiologies were comparable. Many of the patients with unknown aetiology had a minimal-change pancreatitis with previous

Table 1. Basic data: comparisons between the two groups

	Duodenal preserving	Standard total
Number of patients	28	24
Age (years)		
Median	32.5	40
(range)	(19–51)	(22–51)
Mean	33	38
Sex		
Male	13	17
Female	15	7
Aetiology		
Acute: idiopathic trauma	–	3
Chronic		
Alcohol	9	13
Unknown	7	2
Divisum	4	5
Gallstone	2	1
Trauma	2	–
Hereditary	2	–
Viral	1	–
Other	1	–
Length of history (years)		
Median	6.5	6
(range)	(2–22)	(0.1–15)
Mean	8	6

documented evidence of raised amylase levels, following which pancreatic pain started with great severity. The large number of patients with pancreas divisum portrays the interest of this condition in our unit. Most of the patients whose pancreatitis was of an alcohol aetiology had been weaned off alcohol by the time that they had their total pancreteactomy performed; indeed, this was a prerequisite in our selection of such patients.

Table 2. Pre-operative non-operative procedures

	Duodenal preserving ($n = 28$)	Standard total ($n = 24$)
Nil	3	6
Total parenteral nutrition	20	13
Percutaneous nerve blocks	11	5
Endoscopic pancreatic therapy	2	5
Endoscopic biliary therapy	4	2
Percutaneous drainage pseudocyst/phlegmon	2	1
Percutaneous biliary drainage	1	0
Percutaneous, other	0	1
Number of procedures per patient		
0	3	6
1	13	12
2	9	3
3	3	2
4	0	1

Table 3. Prior surgical procedures

	Duodenal preserving ($n = 28$)	Standard total ($n = 23$)
Nil	1	1
Cholecystectomy	9	14
Drainage cyst/abscess	3	6
Pancreatic sphincteroplasty	8	3
Diagnostic laparotomy	2	3
Pancreato-jejunostomy	4	1
Biliary procedure	6	1
Appendicectomy	6	4
Pancreatic, other	1	0
Laparotomy, other	6	9
Distal pancreatectomy	22	10
Proximal pancreatectomy	–	10
Number of operative interventions per patient		
0	1	1
1	7	6
2	12	10
3	4	5
4	2	2
5	1	0
6	1	0

Many of the patients had had previous procedures, both operative and non-operative (Tables 2, 3). Eleven of our patients who had a duodenal-preserving pancreatectomy were diabetic pre-operatively, and 12 of the standard total pancreatectomy patients were already diabetic. Thus, more than half the patients were not diabetic preoperatively, and these patients were willing to accept the disadvantages of diabetes in a quest to alleviate their severe pain. Steatorrhoea was present in 18 of the 28 patients receiving the duodenal-preserving procedure and in 15 of the 24 receiving standard total pancreatectomy; all such patients were taking enzyme supplements preoperatively.

Perioperative Complications

The mortality for the 28 patients who had a duodenal-preserving total pancreatectomy was nil, while three patients who had a total pancreatectomy died, two as a consequence of the severe complications of an acute attack of pancreatitis in patients who already had chronic pancreatitis. Two patients died of the adult respiratory distress syndrome while the third died of severe sepsis within 36 h of a salvage procedure for a massive pancreatic abscess involving the whole pancreas following a transduodenal sphincteroplasty. The complications of both procedures are outlined in Table 4, sepsis being the commonest complication. In the nine patients who had sepsis

Table 4. Post-operative morbidity

	Duodenal preserving ($n = 28$)	Standard total ($n = 21$)
Nil	12	13
Sepsis	9	13
Chest	3	5
Wound	1	3
Central venous catheter	2	2
Urinary tract infection	1	2
Septicaemia	1	1
Pyrexia of unknown origin	1	0
Delayed gastric emptying	4	1
Haemorrhage		
Major	0	0
Minor	1	1
Leak		
Biliary	1	0
Enteric	3	0
Hepatic abscess	1	0
Other	1	1
Morbidity: number of complications per patient		
0	12	13
1	12	4
2	4	1
3	0	1
> 3	0	1
Unknown	0	1

following a duodenal-preserving procedure three had chest infections necessitating treatment with antibiotics, two had infection of their central venous feeding line which resolved following removal of the line, and one had a urinary tract infection. A duodenal leak occurred in three patients, but in none was this serious, and in each it settled with conservative management without re-operation. The delayed gastric emptying was a problem and accounts for the prolonged in-patient stay in the case of some patients. In time it invariably resolves. The length of stay was similar in the two groups of patients, with means of 22 and 21 days. Apart from the delayed gastric emptying, the reason for the prolonged post-operative hospital stay was the policy not to discharge patients until their diabetes was under control, their steatorrhoea treated with enzyme tablets, and their analgesic requirements reduced to nil or minimal quantity. It has been found that if patients are discharged on pethidine or other similar major analgesics, then they tend to remain on narcotics for a long period of time.

Long-term Assessment

An appropriate yardstick by which to assess the success of a procedure is to determine the number of times such patients are readmitted to hospital (Table 5). Few patients avoided such readmissions, and in some many hospital admissions were not necessarily in order to solve their problems. The vast majority of these patients were admitted on account of narcotic abuse and nutritional difficulties, with poor diabetic control being a frequent reason. There have been four late deaths; three of these occurred in the standard total pancreatectomy group whilst one occurred in the duodenal preserving patients. In one patient, a carcinoma of the oesophagus developed, requiring an oesophagogastrectomy at his local hospital, from which he died. One patient died at 9 months of sepsis; a further patient died of alcohol intoxication at 24 months while a final patient died some 74 months after the original operation of a perforated gastric ulcer.

Table 5. Number of post-operative readmissions

	Duodenal preserving ($n = 28$)	Standard total ($n = 21$)
Nil	5	7
1	2	2
2	3	1
3	4	2
4	1	1
> 4	13	5
(range)	(5–15)	(5–12)
unknown	0	3

Bile Duct Stricture

The major later surgical complication associated with duodenal-preserving procedures has been the development of a bile duct stricture which has occurred in six patients. In two patients an endoscopic sphincterotomy, at 1 month and 29 months, has been sufficient to control the problem. In a further patient insertion of stents has been found to be suitable, and these remained patent on a long-term basis. Three patients have required a choledochojejunostomy. These operations have been performed at 6, 16 and 30 months after the original procedure. A predisposing factor to bile duct stricture was damage at the time of the original operation. The other strictures were undoubtedly related to ischaemia, and it is these that have required bypass procedures. Subsequent follow-up of these six patients has been good.

Long-Term Follow-up

It is our standard practice to see all patients following duodenal-preserving pancreatectomy in a special pancreatic clinic. At this clinic standard questions are asked regarding such factors as pain, analgesic requirements, bowel function, pancreatic enzyme supplements and requirement and level of activity.

The results of the questionnaire are stored in the computer and kept for subsequent analysis. Pain is divided into nil or minimal, moderate and severe, while the analgesics required for their pain are subdivided into minor (panadol, codeine), intermediate (pentazocine or buprenorphine) and major, which is a continual requirement for a narcotic.

Taking the 1-, 3- and 5-year results (Table 6), it is noted that after duodenal-preserving pancreatectomy 9 of 23 patients were completely pain free, with a further 5 requiring only moderate analgesics. This good response continued throughout the 3- and 5-year follow-up periods. A similar proportion had pain relief following a standard total pancreatectomy. Nevertheless, nine patients had severe pain, with six of these requiring major analgesics. From the point of view of pain relief, there was no significant difference between those patients who had had a duodenal-preserving procedure and those who had had a standard total pancreatectomy.

Table 6. Long-term results of duodenal-preserving and total pancreatectomy

	Duodenal preserving			Standard total		
	1 year ($n = 23$)	3 years ($n = 17$)	5 years ($n = 3$)	1 year ($n = 15$)	3 years ($n = 9$)	5 years ($n = 6$)
Pain						
Nil/minimal	9	6	2	5	4	4
Moderate	5	5	1	4	1	1
Severe	9	6	0	6	4	1
Analgesics						
Minor	9	5	3	6	2	3
Moderate	8	7	0	3	4	2
Major	6	5	0	5	3	1

Diabetic Status

The patients are all managed by "normal", that is, twice-daily, injection of a combination of rapidly absorbed and intermediate insulins with the exception of two patients
who are controlled using an insulin pump. One of these patients was an anorexic, and
one is a young fit man. Patients routinely monitor their blood glucose with a reagent
strip and also test their urine, thus assessing possible calorie loss.

   One patient who has been insulin dependent since 1977 and had a total pancreatectomy performed in 1983 had peripheral neuropathy; this was represented only by loss
of the ankle jerks. A further patient who had been diabetic only since a total
pancreatectomy in 1984 has possible peripheral neuropathy, the diagnosis being
complicated by the carpal tunnel syndrome. Neither of these patients has any history
of alcohol abuse.

   There were no other long-term complications of diabetes, but the follow-up period
was too short to draw conclusions. The frequency of hypoglycaemic episodes tends to
occur more frequently in those who have had a standard total pancreatectomy than in
the duodenal-preserving group. Although mild hypoglycaemic episodes are not
routinely recorded by the patients, many of these mild episodes of hypoglycaemia are
associated with diarrhoea and malabsorption.

   In patients who have had a duodenal-preserving procedure, good control was
achieved in 11 patients while 15 had fair control, whereas after a standard total
pancreatectomy 8 of 15 patients had good control and the remaining 7 poor control.

   It is of interest that the overall requirement of insulin was 42 units in the duodenal-
preserving group and 30 units in the standard total pancreatectomy group.

Pancreatic Enzyme Replacement Therapy

In the management of patients after a total pancreatectomy, the control of steatorrhoea appears important, and many patients have a less than optimal outcome
because they do not master sensible control of their pancreatic enzyme supplements.
The amount of enzyme replacement varies markedly between individuals, as illustrated by the range of capsules in the duodenal-preserving pancreatectomy group
from 8 to 130, with a mean of 60 capsules/day. However, for those who have had a
standard total pancreatectomy the median requirement is only 30 capsules/day, with a
range of 0–150 capsules/day. It is interesting to speculate whether the higher insulin
requirement in the duodenal-preserving group and the higher enzyme requirements
indicate that there is better tolerance of food with better absorption of the food
requiring more insulin.

   In order to test this hypothesis the weight of the patients was compared with that at
their original operation. It can be seen from Table 7, there is a far higher weight gain in
the patients who had a duodenal-preserving procedure than in those who had the
standard excisional procedure. It is apparent that the patients who had a standard
total pancreatectomy were thinner compared to their height than those who were
selected for a duodenal preservation. Therefore, the weight difference may merely
indicate that a more severe form of pancreatitis was chosen for those who had the
larger surgical procedure. This fact is indisputable, but the continued weight gain of

Table 7. Long-term changes in body weight after duodenal-preserving and after total pancreatectomy

| | Percentage of ideal body weight | | Post-operative weight gain/loss (kg) | |
	Duodenal preserving	Standard total	Duodenal preserving	Standard total
At operation				
n	21	14		
median	99.5	83		
range	75–138	64–129		
At 1 year				
n	21	14	21	14
median	105	89	+ 1.5	+ 3.2
range	72–143	70–112	− 8.2– +9.2	−18.5– + 12.1
At 3 years				
n	17	8	17	8
median	108	88	+ 3.8	+ 3.5
range	74–142	63–117	− 3.2– + 14.1	−13.5– + 15.0
At 5 years				
n	3	6	3	6
median	116	82	+ 4.4	− 1.6
range	106–121	67–103	+ 2.3– + 9.0	−15– + 2.5

the duodenal-preserving group suggests that this operation is compatible with a more normal life-style and is achieving the desired outcome, namely a normal diet, good insulin control and normal weight.

In the maintainence of these patients the importance of overcoming pancreatic enzyme insufficiency cannot be over emphasised. Our current practice is to use only three enzyme replacement products, standard enteric coated tablet preparation (Pancrex V Forte, Paines and Byrne), an enteric coated granular preparation (Creon, Duphar Laboratories), and an enteric coated microsphere preparation (Pancrease, Johnson and Johnson). Patients are usually started on the standard preparation as it is cheaper, and the dose is increased until diarrhoea is controlled. If control is not possible with reasonable doses, the enteric coated preparation is substituted at the same dose. If this fails to control the diarrhoea, then the enteric coated microsphere preparation is used. A reasonable dose is determined by the patient after guidance in clinics.

Conclusions

Duodenal-preserving pancreatectomy can be performed safely in the correctly selected patients. Selection is important, and the procedure should be performed only in those patients in whom technical risks of doing the operation are reasonable. Whether this rather tedious dissection is appropriate and preferable to a standard total pancreatectomy is at present difficult to determine. Certainly, there are no more immediate complications, and the only specific complication related to duodenal-preserving pancreatectomy is an incidence of biliary stricture, seen in 6 of our 28 patients. Undoubtedly this complication could be reduced by a more careful dissection of the bile duct and after a difficult dissection with perhaps perforation of the biliary tree, performing an elective choledochoduodenostomy at the time of the original procedure.

The advantages of this procedure are fewer long-term complications with improved gastrointestinal function and diabetic control. The work of Linehan et al. [15] has shown that patients with duodenal-preserving total pancreatectomy have a more normal weight than those after a standard total pancreatectomy and a better control of their diabetes. Further, Linehan et al. [16] have shown that no dumping occurs with this operation. These are all factors which suggest that gastrointestinal function is more normal after this procedure, but assessment is so difficult in these patients, and only prolonged studies with large numbers of patients will determine the merit of the procedure. Nevertheless, the argument is strong that the duodenal alkaline tide and pacemaker function may well provide a more physiological setting for long-term management. Finally, this study has shown no contra-indication to perform the procedure, and it is felt that as this operation may have advantage over the standard duodenal resection, it should be tried in appropriately selective patients as a way of offering a better quality of life in the long term.

References

1. Sato T, Miyashita E, Matsuno S, Yamauchi H (1986) The role of surgical treatment for chronic pancreatitis. Ann Surg 203:266–271
2. Whipple AO (1946) Radical surgery for certain cases of pancreatic fibrosis associated with calcareous deposits. Ann Surg 124:991–1006
3. Warren KW (1969) Surgical management of chronic relapsing pancreatitis. Am J Surg 117:24–32
4. Traverso LW, Longmire WP (1979) Preservation of the pylorus in pancreatico-duodenectomy. Surg Gynaecol Obstet 146:959–962
5. Traverso LW, Longmire WP (1980) Preservation of the pylorus in pancreatico-duodenectomy. A follow-up evaluation. Ann Surg 190:312–316
6. Traverso LW, Tompkins RK, Urrea PT, Longmire WP (1979) Surgical treatment of chronic pancreatitis. Ann Surg 190:312–316
7. Newman KD, Braasch JW, Rossi RL, Campo-Gonzales S (1983) Pyloric and gastric preservation with pancreatoduodenectomy. Am J Surg 145:152–156
8. Beger HG, Krautzberger W, Bittner R, Büchler M, Limmer J (1985) Duodenum-preserving resection of the head of the pancreas in patients with severe pancreatitis. Surgery 97:467–473
9. Whipple AO (1946) Observations on radical surgery for lesions of the pancreas. Surg Gynecol Obstet 82:623–631
9a Eloy R, Bouchet R, Clendinnen G, Daniel J (1980) New technique of total pancreatectomy without duodenectomy in the dog. Am J Surg 140:409–412
10. Harken AH, Filler RM, Auruskin TW, Crigler JF (1971) The role of total pancreatectomy in the treatment of unremitting hypoglycaemia of infancy. J Pediatr Surg 6:284–289
11. Gough MH (1984) The surgical treatment of hyperinsulinism in infancy and childhood. Br J Surg 71:75–78
12. Murphy JP, Russell RCG (1988) Operative treatment of nesidioblastosis. Br J Surg 75:930
13. Thomas LM, Langford RM, Russell RCG, Le Quesne LP (1978) The anatomical basis for gastric mobilisation in total oesophagectomy. Br J Surg 65:356–360
14. Lambert MA, Linehan IP, Russell RCG (1987) Duodenum preserving total pancreatectomy for end stage chronic pancreatitis. Br J Surg 74:35–39
15. Linehan IP, Lambert MA, Brown DC, Kurtz AB, Cotton PB, Russell RCG (1988) Total pancreatectomy for chronic pancreatitis. Gut 29:358–365
16. Linehan IP, Russell RCG, Hobsley M (1988) The dumping syndrome after pancreatoduoden-ectomy. Surg Gynaecol Obstet 167:114–118

Pancreatic Resection and Segmental Pancreatic Autotransplantation for Chronic Pancreatitis

R. L. Rossi[1]

Introduction

All patients who undergo total pancreatectomy and 80% of patients who undergo a 90%–95% resection for chronic pancreatitis become diabetic [1]. Twenty-four of 26 patients treated at the Lahey Clinic who underwent total pancreatectomy for chronic pancreatitis required multiple hospital admissions primarily because of poorly controlled diabetes. Half of the patients had died at a mean follow-up of 5 years [2].

Since 1981, in an attempt to prevent or delay the onset of diabetes we have performed segmental autotransplantation of the body and tail of the pancreas as a vascularized and denervated graft in patients who are thought to be candidates for extensive distal resections of the gland.

Method

The body and tail of the pancreas were autotransplanted to the left thigh, anastomosing the splenic vessels to the common femoral vessels. The pancreatic duct was suture ligated and injected with neoprene [3]. Patency of the graft was assessed by angiography and Doppler studies. Function of the graft was studied by percutaneous selective venous assays of insulin from both iliac veins, oral and intravenous glucose tolerance tests, glucagon stimulation studies, and late graft biopsies.

Results and Discussion

Segmental pancreatic autotransplantation was performed in 13 patients, three of whom had alcoholic pancreatitis and ten of whom had idiopathic pancreatitis [4]. The median follow-up was 62 months, with nine patients being followed until death or for 5 or more years. All patients were disabled and used narcotics. All had pancreatic ducts of small diameter, and nine patients had undergone 16 previous pancreatobiliary operations. Five patients required oral pancreatic enzymes.

The transplant was technically successful in 11 patients (84%) and failed in two patients (16%), presumably because of graft thrombosis.

---

[1] Department of General Surgery, Lahey Clinic Medical Center, 41 Mall Road, Burlington, MA 01805, USA

Chronic Pancreatitis
Ed. by Beger, Büchler, Ditschuneit, and Malfertheiner
© Springer-Verlag Berlin Heidelberg 1990

Early complications included eight pancreatic graft fistulas that were transient (lasted less than 6 weeks) in five patients but lasted 3, 7, and 39 months, respectively, in three patients. Two patients had bleeding from the pancreatic graft. There were no operative deaths.

In the two patients whose grafts failed, the patient who underwent a 60% resection does not require insulin; however, the patient who underwent a 90% resection requires 10 U neutral protamine Hagedorn (NPH) insulin.

Of 11 patients with technically successful grafts, six do not require insulin (insulin independent). Three of these patients underwent a 90% resection and were followed for 27, 71, and 56 months, respectively; three patients underwent an initial or staged total pancreatectomy and were followed for 94, 39, and 33 months, respectively.

Five patients with successful grafts require insulin (insulin dependent). Two of the five patients underwent a 90% resection and began requiring 20 and 8 U NPH insulin at 23 and 40 months, respectively, with a total follow-up of 51 and 43 months each. Three patients underwent an initial or staged total pancreatectomy. One of these patients began requiring 10 U NPH insulin immediately, one patient began requiring 12 U NPH insulin at 27 months, and one patient began requiring 0–15 U regular insulin per day at 56 months, with a follow-up of 21, 64, and 64 months, respectively.

The k value, the glucose clearance rate after an intravenous glucose load expressed in percent per minute (normal, greater than 1.2% per minute), was used as an indicator of islet cell function. Of the six patients who underwent initial or staged total pancreatectomy, one patient with a very low preoperative k value of 0.71% per minute became diabetic after total pancreatectomy and autotransplantation, requiring 10 U supplemental NPH insulin per day. One patient with a normal postoperative k value continued to be insulin independent at 94 months. Two patients with a mildly decreased k value (approximately 1% per minute) who were followed for a limited time of 33 and 39 months, respectively, did not require insulin; however, two other patients with similar mildly decreased postoperative k values but followed for a longer period of time (64 months each) became diabetic late in the course of follow-up.

The procedure failed to control pain in the two patients who had a 60% distal resection. Both patients subsequently had pancreatoduodenectomy with pain improvement.

All nine patients who had a 90% resection and autotransplantation had transient improvement of pain. However, pain recurred in five of the nine patients at 7, 20, 24, 26, and 54 months, respectively. Three of these five patients underwent pancreatoduodenectomy with pain improvement. The two patients who had total pancreatectomy initially had improvement of pain.

All 13 patients were using narcotics before operation and were not actively working. At the time of the last follow-up, only six patients required narcotics at a decreased dose, and six patients had returned to active employment.

Of the six patients who had initial or staged total pancreatectomy, all patients had improvement of pain. Three patients remained insulin independent at 94, 39, and 33 months, respectively; three patients are insulin dependent, requiring insulin at 0, 27, and 56 months in doses of 10, 12, and 10 U insulin daily, respectively.

Late complications occurred in the groin and included late abscess in one patient, delayed fluid collection in one, and mild thigh and leg discomfort in three patients.

Ten of the 13 patients underwent late reoperations. Pancreatoduodenectomy for pain relief was the most common procedure, and groin procedures were the next most common.

There were three late deaths in patients who had undergone 90% resection and had had improvement of pain. The first patient committed suicide 27 months after operation. The second patient had fulminating pneumococcal pneumonia at 56 months despite pneumococcal vaccine. The third patient died of acquired immunodeficiency syndrome at 51 months.

In our experience with 73 patients who underwent pancreatoduodenectomy for the management of chronic pancreatitis, 80% of the patients had improvement of pain at 5 years, and the incidence of newly developed diabetes, which was easy to control, was 44% at 5 years [5]. Resection of the head of the pancreas has become, in our experience, the operation that is associated with the best long-term results of pain relief.

We concluded that segmental pancreatic transplantation can prevent or delay the onset of diabetes and that when insulin is required, the diabetes is stable. However, recurrent pain is frequent after subtotal distal resection, and, therefore, in selected patients we currently favor the increased use of pancreatoduodenectomy or a procedure that removes the head of the pancreas as the initial operation. Total or near total pancreatectomy should be used very selectively and only as a last resort procedure. The addition of segmental transplantation offers definitive, although sometimes transient, benefits in glucose homeostasis.

References

1. Rossi RL, Heiss FW, Braasch JW (1985) Surgical management of chronic pancreatitis. Surg Clin North Am 65:79–101
2. Braasch JW, Vito L, Nugent FW (1978) Total pancreatectomy of end-stage chronic pancreatitis. Ann Surg 188:317–322
3. Rossi RL, Soeldner JS, Braasch JW, Heiss FW, Shea JA, Nugent FW, Watkins E Jr, Silverman ML, Bolton J (1986) Segmental pancreatic autotransplantation with pancreatic ductal occlusion after near total or total pancreatic resection for chronic pancreatitis. Results at 5- to 54-month follow-up evaluation. Ann Surg 203:626–636
4. Rossi RL, Soeldner JS, Braasch JW, Heiss FW, Shea JA, Watkins E Jr, Silverman ML (1990) Long-term results of pancreatic resection and segmental pancreatic autotransplantation for chronic pancreatitis. Am J Surg 159:51–58
5. Rossi RL, Rothschild J, Braasch JW, Munson JL, ReMine SG (1987) Pancreatoduodenectomy in the management of chronic pancreatitis. Arch Surg 122:416–420

A New Alternative for Chronic Pancreatitis

N. J. Lygidakis and M. N. van der Heyde[1]

Introduction

Chronic pancreatitis is a challenging clinical problem, and the results after surgical management are controversial [1–6]. It is distressing and disappointing for both the surgeon and the patient to learn soon after a time-consuming operation that the complaints and symptoms are coming back, and that a new operation or a new modality of management is warranted. How can we possibly avoid such a situation? On the basis of our experience in the Hepato-biliary-pancreatic unit of the Academic Medical Centre, we developed a new surgical technique that is applicable in a number of patients suffering of chronic pancreatitis.

The present contribution is directed to the basic technical steps of this procedure.

Surgical Technique

The pancreas is reached and freed along its inferior and superior borders to the left of the superior mesenteric vessels. We continue with mobilization of the posterior surface of the pancreas from the underlying splenic artery and splenic vein (Fig. 1). We then transect the pancreas (Fig. 2), and split it into two parts. If advanced changes of chronic pancreatitis are confined centrally, pancreatic resection can be pursued either distally or proximally, or both distally and proximally. The central pancreatic transection can be combined with resection of the pancreas centrally, in a simple technical way. A Roux-en-Y loop is now transferred in the upper abdomen and is interposed between the two pancreatic segments (Fig. 3). A double seromyotomy is carried out in the lateral surface of the jejunal loop exactly opposite to the rough surface of the pancreatic remnants (Fig. 3). Both pancreatic segments are drained via an end-to-side pancreaticojejunostomy (Fig. 4). We start with interrupted absorbable sutures interposed between the posterior surface of one pancreatic segment and the seromuscular layer of the corresponding seromyotomy (Fig. 4). For the other pancreatic segment we do exactly the same (Fig. 5).

Now an opening is made in the jejunal mucosa exactly opposite the pancreatic duct of the one pancreatic segment. The anastomosis between the pancreatic duct and the jejunal mucosa opening is carried out with interrupted absorbable sutures (Fig. 5).

[1] Department of Surgery, Academic Medical Centre, University of Amsterdam, Meibergdreef 9, 1105 AZ Amsterdam, The Netherlands

Chronic Pancreatitis
Ed. by Beger, Büchler, Ditschuneit, and Malfertheiner
© Springer-Verlag Berlin Heidelberg 1990

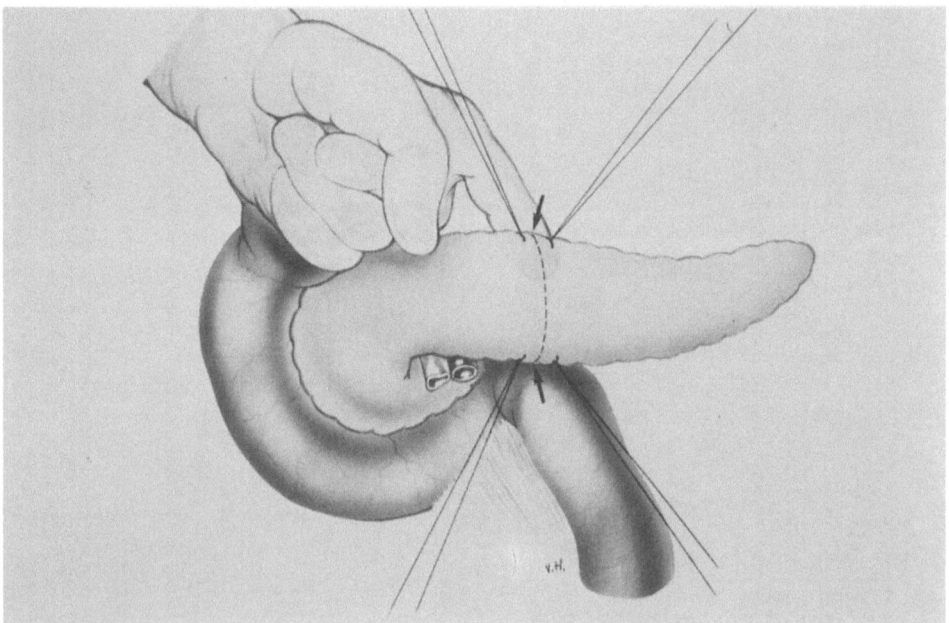

Fig. 1. Mobilization of the posterior surface of the pancreas from the underlying splenic artery and splenic vein

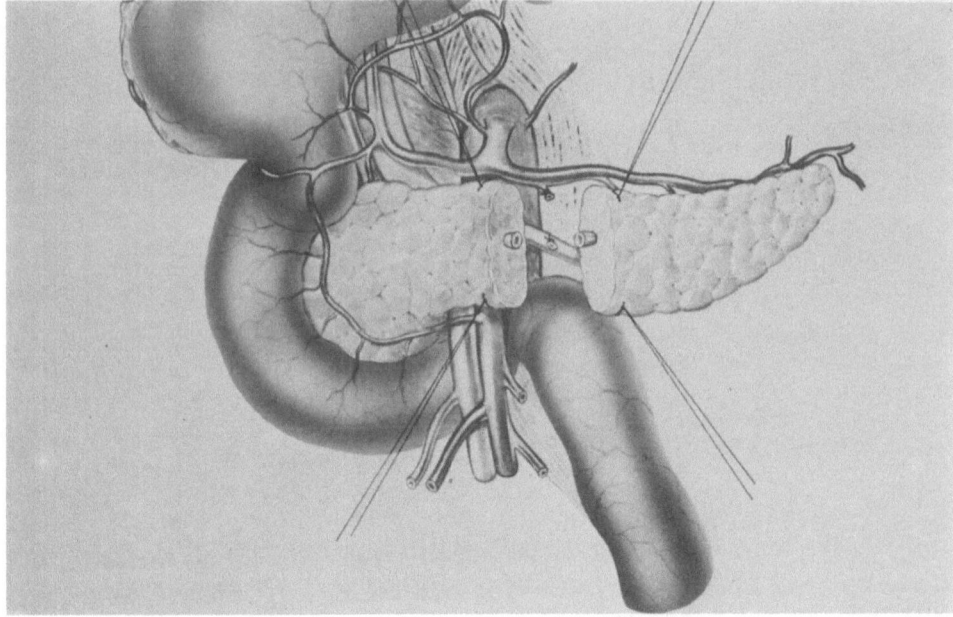

Fig. 2. Transection of the pancreas

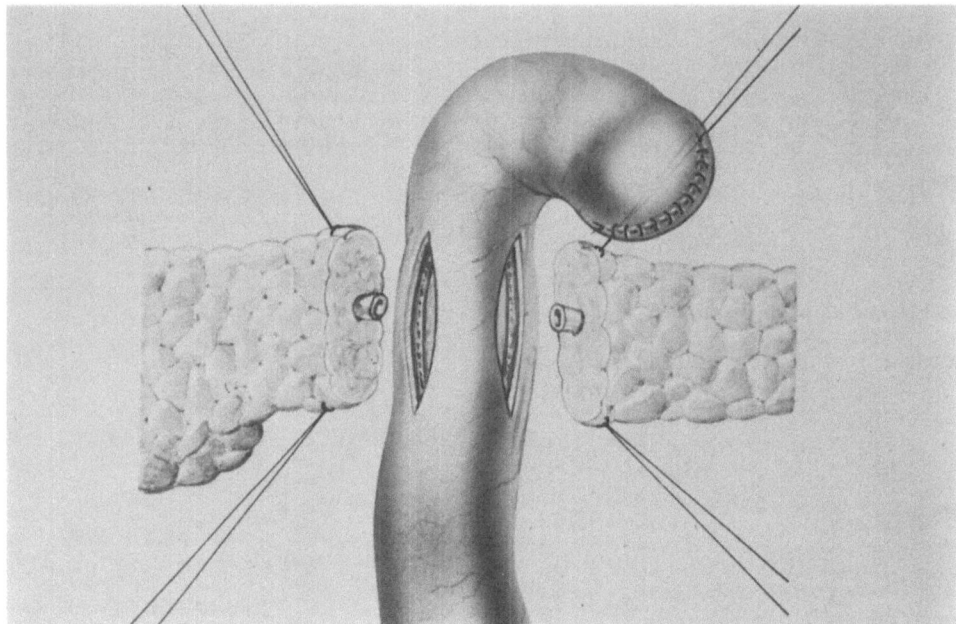

Fig. 3. Interposition of Roux-en-Y loop between the two pancreatic segments

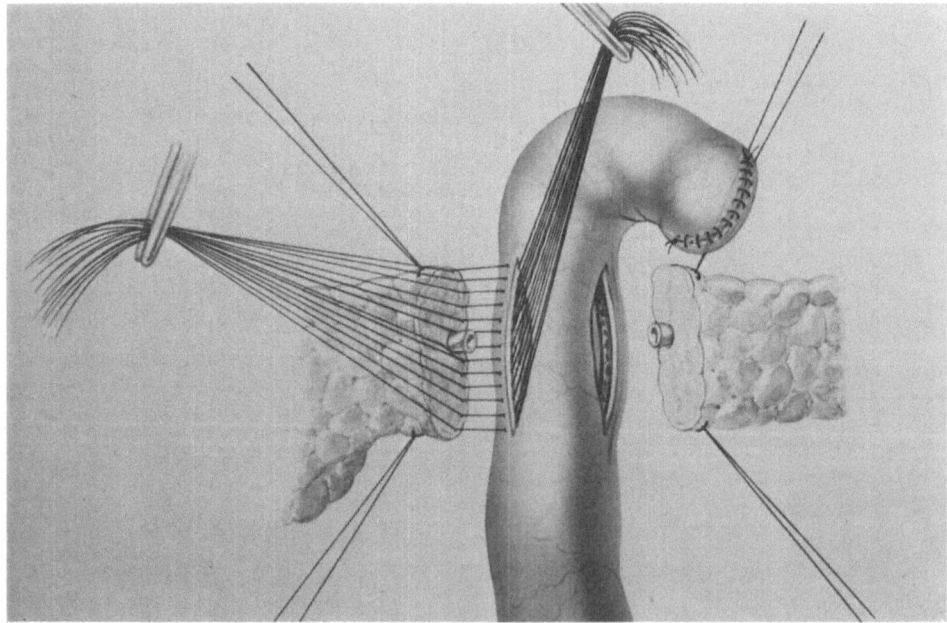

Fig. 4. Draining of both pancreatic segments via end-to-end pancreaticojejunostomy

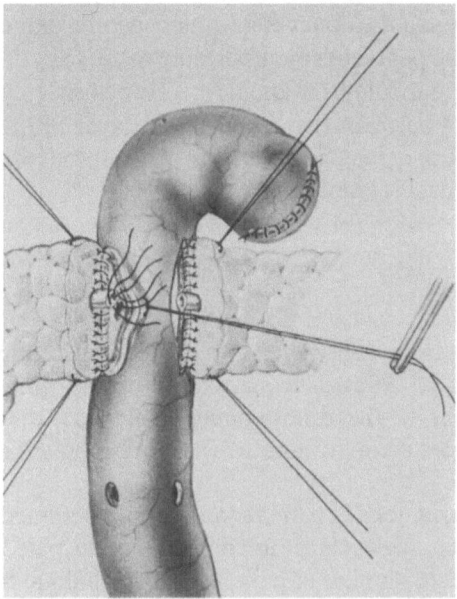

Fig. 5. Interposition of absorbable sutures between posterior surface of one pancreatic segment and the seromuscular layer of the corresponding seromyotomy

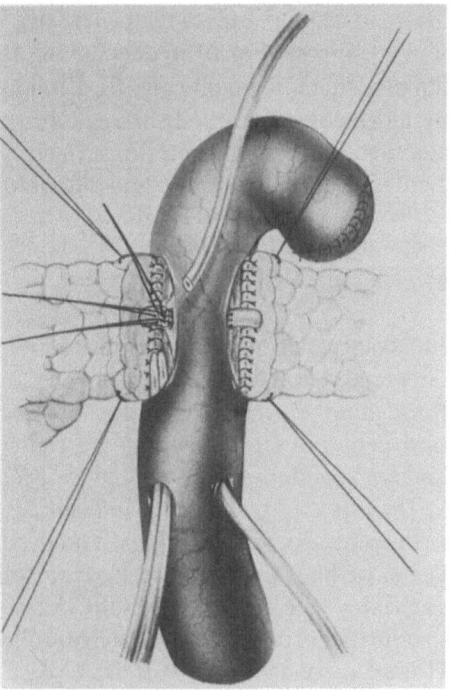

Fig. 6. Same procedure as in Fig. 5, for the other pancreatic segment

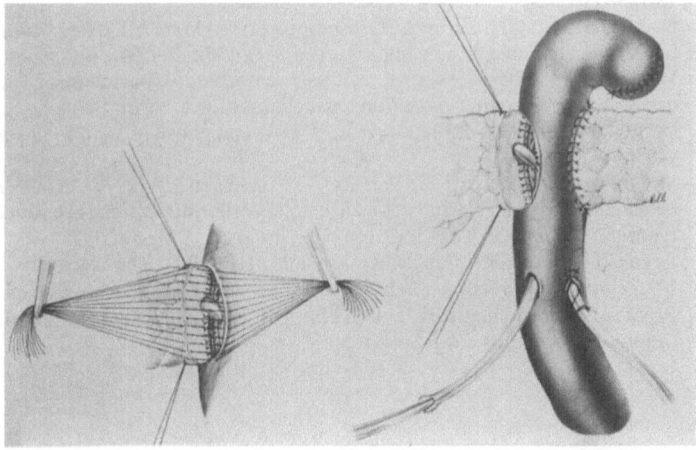

Fig. 7. Interposition of sutures between the seromuscular layer of the seromyotomy and the anterior surface of the pancreas

The anastomosis is stented and completed by using interrupted sutures interposed between the upper tip of the pancreatic duct and the upper edge of the opening of the jejunal mucosa (Fig. 6). We repeat this for the pancreaticojejunostomy of the remaining pancreatic segment (Fig. 6). Both pancreaticojejunostomies are now completed by means of interrupted sutures interposed between the seromuscular layer of the seromyotomy and the anterior surface of the pancreas (Fig. 7). Both anastomoses are stented using silicon tubes and a double Witzel jejunostomy.

Discussion

In advanced chronic pancreatitis, either a narrow constricted or a dilated pancreatic duct tends to be identical for a given patient [4]. Fibrosis seems to develop uniformly throughout the gland. Fibrotic obstructions of the distal common bile duct and obstruction of the duodenum are well-known complications of chronic pancreatitis and are sometimes both present [5–8].

The reported technique is indicated for a number of patients with lesions confined to the central pancreas and in whom the pancreatic ducts are not dilated. For the past 3 years, we have used this technique in a limited number of patients. The technique is associated with good early results with regard to mortality and morbidity. We believe that further experience and a longer follow-up is essential for an objective evaluation. However, we assume that it has a place in the surgical armamentarium of technical options and alternatives for the treatment of chronic pancreatitis.

References

1. Moossa AR (1987) Surgical treatment of chronic pancreatitis: an overview. Br J Surg 74:661–662
2. Gall FP, Mühe E, Gebhardt C (1987) Chronic pancreatitis. Results in 116 consecutive partial duodenopancreatectomies combined with pancreatic head occlusion. Hepatogastroenterology 29:115–119
3. Napnick S, Hadas N, Purow E, Grosberg SJ (1979) Mass in the head of the pancreas in cholestatic jaundice, carcinoma or pancreatitis. Ann Surg 190:587–591
4. Warshaw AL (1985) Conservation of pancreatic tissue by combined gastric biliary and pancreatic duct drainage for pain from chronic pancreatitis. Am J Surg 149:563–569
5. Lygidakis NJ (1983) Biliary strictures as a complication of chronic pancreatitis. Am J Surg 146:254–256
6. Warshaw AL, Shapiro RH, Ferrucci JT, Galdabini JJ (1976) Persistent obstructive jaundice, cholangitis and biliary cirrhosis due to common bile duct stenosis in chronic pancreatitis. Gastroenterology 70:562–567
7. Aranha GV, Prinz RA, Fileart RJ, Greenlee HB (1984) The spectrum of biliary tract obstruction from chronic pancreatitis. Arch Surg 119:595–600
8. Bradley E, III, Clements JR Jr (1981) Idiopathic duodenal obstruction. An unappreciated complication of pancreatitis. Ann Surg 193:638–643

Subject Index